4th *edition*

Periodontology
for the Dental Hygienist

DOROTHY A. PERRY, RDH, MS, PhD
Professor and Associate Dean for Education
  and Student Affairs
School of Dentistry
University of California, San Francisco
San Francisco, California

PHYLLIS L. BEEMSTERBOER, RDH, MS, EdD
Professor and Associate Dean
School of Dentistry
Oregon Health & Science University
Portland, Oregon

GWEN ESSEX, RDH, MS, EdD
HS Clinical Professor
Preventive and Restorative Dental Sciences
Director of Educational Technology
School of Dentistry
University of California, San Francisco
San Francisco, California

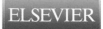

ELSEVIER

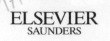

7/13
76.95
MATT

3251 Riverport Lane
St. Louis, Missouri 63043

PERIODONTOLOGY FOR THE DENTAL HYGIENIST, FOURTH EDITION   978-1-4557-0369-2

Notices

Library of Congress Cataloging-in-Publication Data

Perry, Dorothy A.
    Periodontology for the dental hygienist / Dorothy A. Perry, Phyllis L. Beemsterboer, Gwen Essex.—4th ed.
      p. ; cm.
    Includes bibliographical references and index.
    ISBN 978-1-4557-0369-2 (pbk. : alk. paper)
    I. Beemsterboer, Phyllis.   II. Essex, Gwen.   III. Title.
    [DNLM: 1. Periodontal Diseases.   2. Periodontics—methods.   WU 240]
    617.6′32—dc23
                                                                                    2012039137

Vice President and Publisher: Linda Duncan
Executive Content Strategist: Kathy Falk
Content Manager: Kristin Hebberd
Content Development Specialist: Joslyn Dumas
Publishing Services Manager: Jeff Patterson
Senior Project Manager: Tracey Schriefer
Design Direction: Jessica Williams

Printed in China

Last digit is the print number: 9 8 7 6 5 4 3 2 1

The fourth edition of *Periodontology for the Dental Hygienist* is dedicated to Fermin A. Carranza for his enormous contributions to the discipline of periodontics and his mentorship of many dental and dental hygiene educators. We strive to carry on his commitment to excellence in the preparation of the next generations of health care professionals.

PREFACE

OVERVIEW

Periodontology is an integral part of the practice of dental hygiene, and the fourth edition of *Periodontology for the Dental Hygienist* provides the dental hygiene student with the contemporary knowledge necessary to achieve the essential goal of preserving teeth in comfort and function. The concepts provided in this textbook reflect current thinking and a collection of updated content, detailed clinical images, and electronic ancillary products provide the basis for the understanding and application of modern periodontal therapy. It is our hope that faculty and students will find the supplemental materials available on the Evolve website to be welcome tools as they work through this newest edition and prepare for clinical practice.

FEATURES

This book is grounded in evidence-based practice as it relates to the treatment of gingival and periodontal diseases and conditions. Evidence-based medicine is defined as "the integration of the best research evidence with clinical expertise and patient values."* Evidence-based thinking summarizes issues into answerable questions, which are then addressed by identifying the best evidence, integrating it into our knowledge base, and evaluating our effectiveness as clinicians. Each chapter in this book represents the answer to one of these questions, asked in logical sequence, from Chapter 1 (How did dental hygiene develop as a profession?) to Chapter 18 (What is the prognosis for patients who have periodontal treatment provided by the dental hygienist?). The chapters progress in sections from essential background information, the foundations of therapy, assessment of diseases and conditions, treatment of diseases and conditions, to the results of therapy. Throughout this sequence, the authors have collected and evaluated the best available evidence to support the information presented in each chapter.

The terminology used in this edition reflects the contemporary understanding of dental plaque as a biofilm; the significance of this understanding has profound implications for treatment, including the reemergence of the importance of mechanical plaque control. The terms *plaque biofilm* or *dental plaque biofilm* have been used throughout the book, although where appropriate the simpler term *plaque* has been used. The use of these terms emphasizes the significance of the contemporary wording while still using the older terminology.

NEW TO THIS EDITION

The fourth edition is a revised, concise, and complete review of current literature and thinking in periodontology. The chapters emphasize clinical relevance throughout and include case scenarios specific to the topics in each chapter. The material is clearly written for easy assimilation. End of chapter questions reflect the new national board approaches that emphasize higher order learning. The format for the fourth edition is attractive and displays complex material in a manner that supports study and comprehension.

ABOUT EVOLVE

The Evolve website provides a variety of resources for both instructors and students. For instructors, included is an image collection, case scenarios, answers to the study questions and case scenarios found in the textbook, PowerPoint lecture slides, and a much larger test bank. Also included are plaque control challenge images that emphasize the variety of approaches for dental hygienists. Learning strategies are presented to emphasize the unique attributes of adult learning to assist both faculty and students. Students will find clinical case studies (previously on the companion CD-ROM), flashcards, image identification exercises, and weblinks.

The reader is provided with an integrated presentation of facts, analysis of contemporary data, and practical ways to assess and treat patients requiring dental hygiene care. The end point of using the book is for the dental hygienist to be confident in applying a comprehensive understanding of diseases and treatment in daily clinical practice. Dental hygiene care is extremely valuable to patients in maintaining dental health and improving the quality of life.

The half-life of scientific data is thought to be 5 years or less. With a strong educational background, and practice and experience in the profession, students will be prepared to incorporate evidence-based information into the practice of dental hygiene.

Dorothy A. Perry, RDH, MS, PhD
Phyllis L. Beemsterboer, RDH, MS, EdD
Gwen Essex, RDH, MS, EdD

---

*Sackett DL, Straus SE, Richardson WS, et al. *Evidence-Based Medicine*. 2nd ed. St Louis: Churchill Livingstone; 2000:1.

ACKNOWLEDGMENTS

The authors would like to acknowledge our friends and family who supported us in the preparation of the fourth edition. We also had excellent contributors and colleagues who assisted with this edition. They are Dr. Gary Armitage (Chapter 9), Dr. Cheryl Cameron (Chapter 8), Ms. Gina Evans (Chapter 8), Dr. Fritz Finzen (Chapter 15), Dr. Peter Loomer (Chapter 4), and Dr. Mark Ryder (photographic images).

In particular the authors want to recognize significant persons in our lives who gave up time with us to make this edition possible:

DR. PERRY—MR. JIM OWENS
DR. BEEMSTERBOER—DR. JOE JEDRYCHOWSKI
DR. ESSEX—MR. MASON LANCASTER

ABOUT THE AUTHORS

Dorothy A. Perry, RDH, MS, PhD is a graduate of the USC Dental Hygiene Program. She has a master's degree and Doctorate in Education, also from USC. Dr. Perry has been teaching in dental hygiene and dental education for over 30 years and, although now retired from active practice, practiced dental hygiene from 1970 until 2002. Dr. Perry is a professor at UCSF School of Dentistry. In this capacity she has engaged in clinical and translational research primarily relating to dental hygiene practice, taught many clinics and courses, and chaired the UCSF Dental Hygiene Program for 10 years. She currently serves as Associate Dean for Education and Student Affairs at the UCSF School of Dentistry, responsible for the educational activities in the school, student services, and continuing education.

Phyllis L. Beemsterboer, RDH, MS, EdD holds a bachelor's and master's degree from the University of Michigan and a Doctorate in Education from Pepperdine University, with a specialty in bioethics education. Dr. Beemsterboer has been actively teaching dental hygiene and periodontics for over 30 years. She is past president of the National Dental Hygiene Directors and former chairman of the Council on Allied Dental Directors, and has served on the Commission on Dental Accreditation representing dental hygiene. Dr. Beemsterboer's academic activities include journal publications in ethics, occlusion, and temporomandibular disorders and service on numerous dental hygiene editorial review boards and educational associations. Currently, Dr. Beemsterboer is a Professor and Associate Dean for Academic Affairs in the School of Dentistry at Oregon Health & Science University in Portland, Oregon.

Gwen Essex, RDH, MS, EdD is Health Science Clinical Professor and Director of Educational Technology for the University of California, San Francisco School of Dentistry. She earned her bachelor's degree in dental hygiene at UCSF and has been a member of the faculty at the UCSF School of Dentistry since 1996. Dr. Essex earned her master's degree in health science from San Francisco State University and a Doctorate in Learning and Instruction from the University of San Francisco. Dr. Essex focuses on the use of technology and adult learning theories in dental hygiene and dental education. She has practiced dental hygiene both in private office and academic faculty practice settings and has great insight into the significance of dental hygienists as educators for patients and dental team members.

CONTRIBUTORS

Gary C. Armitage, DDS, MS
Professor, Department of Orofacial Sciences
School of Dentistry
University of California
San Francisco, California

Cheryl A. Cameron, RDH, PhD, JD
Vice Provost for Academic Personnel
Office of the Provost
University of Washington
Seattle, Washington

Gina D. Evans, RDH, BS
Private Practice of Dental Hygiene
Seattle, Washington

Fritz Finzen, DDS
Health Sciences Clinical Professor
Department of Preventive and Restorative Dental Sciences
School of Dentistry
University of California
San Francisco, California

Peter M. Loomer, DDS, PhD
Clinical Professor, Department of Orofacial Sciences
School of Dentistry
University of California
San Francisco, California

CONTENTS

Background for the Study of Periodontology

The information addressed in the first group of chapters relates to background knowledge essential for dental hygienists. These chapters provide an understanding about what dental hygiene is and how diseases treated by dental hygienists affect patients. The following questions are asked and answered in Part I:

CHAPTER 1   How did dental hygiene develop as a profession?

CHAPTER 2   What are the anatomic characteristics of the periodontium and how does the host respond to changes?

CHAPTER 3   How many people have periodontal diseases and what risks are associated with them?

CHAPTER 4   What is the etiology of periodontal diseases?

1 Historical Perspectives on Dental Hygiene and Periodontology

Dorothy A. Perry
Based on the original work by Martha H. Fales

LEARNING OUTCOMES

- Describe the historical development of the profession of dental hygiene.
- Explain how we know that preventive oral health has been a concern throughout the ages.
- Define the roles and opportunities for the dental hygienist.

- Explain the effects of improved dental equipment and operatory design on working conditions for the dental hygienist.
- Describe the roles of the dental hygienist as defined by the American Dental Hygienists Association.

KEY TERMS

Administrator/manager
Advocate
Alfred C. Fones
American Dental Hygienists Association
Anthropology
Apprenticeship
Baltimore College of Dental Surgery

Barber-surgeons
Clinician
Educator
Expanded-duty dental hygiene skills
Gingivitis
Oral prophylaxis
Periodontics

Periodontitis
Periodontoclasia
Periodontology
Preceptor
Profession
Pyorrhea alveolaris
Researcher

History is a study of the past that unites recorded events with interpretations. This chapter provides a brief review of events that have brought together the professions of dentistry and dental hygiene with science. Dental hygienists provide oral health services today based on our rich history of education, research, and practice experiences. This panoramic view illustrates the need for dental hygienists to embrace a historical perspective and pursue lifelong learning to direct, modify, and expand their professional actions throughout their careers.

The dental profession owes a great deal to **anthropology**, the study of humanity. Anthropology provides insights into dental diseases that existed before there were written records. In 1948, Weinberger[1] described a study of prehistoric skulls with teeth that showed extensive dental caries, evidence of alveolar bone resorption, periapical abscesses, supernumerary teeth, and impacted teeth. This research showed that dental and periodontal diseases have plagued humans since the beginning of time.

ANCIENT EVIDENCE OF PERIODONTAL DISEASE AND ITS TREATMENT

Anthropologic expeditions to Mesopotamian sites in Iraq found relics used for dental care in gold vanity sets and cases, including ear scoops, tweezers, and toothpicks. One set found

in the Nigel Temple at Ur is estimated to have been used about 3000 BCE.

CLINICAL NOTE 1-1 Periodontal disease has been seen in skeletal remains since before recorded history.

The oldest written documents related to teeth are from about the same era and were found in the excavations of the Sumerian civilization in the Middle East. These are pictographic and cuneiform tablets and contain descriptions such as this:

"If a man's mouth has mouth trouble, thou shalt bray [grind finely] Lelium in well water, introduce salt, alum and vinegar therein, thou shalt leave it under the stars, in the morning, thou shalt wind a linen [strip] around his forefinger, without a meal thou shalt clean his mouth."[2]

Hippocrates (460-377 BCE), a Greek physician, was the first person known to prescribe a dentifrice. His cure was not something we would use today because it was a complex solution, including the head of a hare and three mice to be sieved and soaked in honey and white wine and then rubbed on the gums.[3] A twentieth century study of **periodontoclasia**, an early term for any destructive or degenerative disease of the periodontium, suggested that Hippocrates may have provided relatively effective periodontal treatment long before modern times.[4] Aristotle, who was born after Hippocrates (348-322 BCE), described "scrapers" used for teeth cleaning. Surviving examples show that these instruments were similar to modern scalers. Interestingly, Aristotle did not think that women had as many teeth as men.[1]

> **CLINICAL NOTE 1-2** The earliest known toothbrushes were fiber chew sticks.

Fiber sticks were the earliest known toothbrushes. They were the size of pencils and were hammered or flattened on one end to separate the fibers. Such sticks were recorded in Babylonian, Chinese, Greek, and Roman literature. All were made from trees or bushes with bark containing a cleansing substance plus aromatic fumes that acted as an astringent, like a kind of dentifrice. Early Mohammedans called their sticks "siwaks," which were made of arrak (*Salvadora persica,* the toothbrush tree).[5] In Greece and Italy, sticks came from the mastic tree (*Pistacia lentiscus,* the toothpick tree). In Saudi Arabia, the sticks are called "miswaks" (Figure 1-1).

THE MIDDLE AGES

An early written record of dental calculus, still commonly called tartar, is from Albucasis (936-1013 CE), a Moorish surgeon from Spain. His treatise, *De Chirurgia,* described removing foreign substances from teeth using a set of 14 scrapers he designed. He recognized the relationship between calculus and tooth loss, writing, "sometimes on the surface of the teeth, both inside and outside, as well as under the gums, are deposited rough scales of ugly appearance and black, green or yellowish in color; thus corruption is communicated to the gums and so the teeth are in process of time denuded."[6]

The writings of Johannes Aranculus (1412-1484) related diet to oral health and disease. He defined rules for oral hygiene, including avoiding desserts and sweets such as honey, not biting on hard things, and avoiding "substances that can set the teeth on edge." He also warned against eating onions but with no

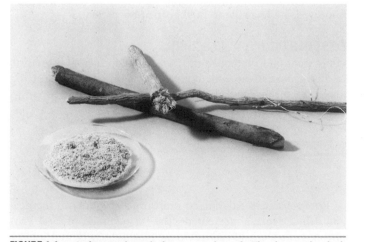

FIGURE 1-1 ■ **A chew stick made from a tree branch.** The chew stick, which has a frayed end, was made from sticks about 6 inches long. The dish holds the ground wood substance that contains an abrasive. (Courtesy of Dr. Lawrence Wolinsky.)

particular explanation. Teeth were to be cleaned using a thin piece of wood, followed by rinsing with wine.[1]

THE DEVELOPMENT OF MODERN DENTISTRY

The era of modern dentistry began in Europe. Dentists were trained by **apprenticeship,** learning by watching and assisting an established dentist. Ambroise Paré (1517-1590) was the first apprentice permitted to take an examination and apply for membership in the prestigious College of Surgeons in Paris, a privilege reserved for physicians. He extracted teeth, opened dental abscesses, set fractured jaws, and was recognized by medical colleagues for his professional work.[7]

Andreas Vesalius (1514-1564), a Flemish anatomist, and Bartolommeo Eustachio (1520-1574), an Italian anatomist, were responsible for early anatomic studies of the teeth. In the following century, Anton van Leeuwenhoek (1632-1723), a Dutch naturalist, discovered dentinal tubules when looking through his invention, the microscope. He also examined tartar scrapings from teeth and identified microorganisms in the mouth.[7]

> **CLINICAL NOTE 1-3** Pierre Fauchard is considered the father of modern dentistry.

Pierre Fauchard (1678-1761) is called the father of dentistry because of his powerful influence on progress in the profession. He was self-educated but developed systematic methods for dental practice. His classic text, *Le Chirurgien Dentiste,* was first published in 1728. Fauchard recognized the importance of oral health and described cleaning by "rubbing the teeth from below upwards and from above downwards outside and inside with a little sponge" dipped in warm water and brandy, followed by use of toothpick between the teeth.[8] Dentistry was touted as an important part of surgical practice by John Hunter (1728-1793), a surgeon and anatomist in London. He recognized that dental caries were initiated on the outside of the tooth on surfaces where food collected.[7]

The Pilgrims brought physicians, an apothecary, and three barber-surgeons to America in 1638. The **barber-surgeons** provided bloodletting and tooth extraction services along with shaving and hair treatments. It is not clear who was the first dentist to practice in the American colonies. Men such as Woofendale, Mills, Baker, Flagg, Greenwood, and Paul Revere were among the early dentists. However, their methods were only slightly removed from those of the barber-surgeons.[7]

ESTABLISHING FORMAL DENTAL EDUCATION: 1800 TO 1900

During the early 1800s, dentists began to understand that knowledge of anatomy, pathology, and physiology was required for practice. They further believed that the apprentice method (working and learning in the office of a **preceptor,** a clinician-teacher) was inadequate because no one person was competent to teach all scientific and technical subjects required of dentistry. Medicine was already firmly established as a healing profession, and many believed that dentistry should be a branch of medicine. So, the establishment of dentistry as an independent profession faced great challenges both from the apprentice-trained dentists and the better established medical practitioners.[9]

In 1939, Stillman reflected that to be a **profession,** dentistry had to combine science and technological arts, not merely create "prostheses."[10] When the first dental school was established, the faculty had little medical education and faced this challenge. There was also dissention among dentists of the time; those dealing with caries and fillings tended to view dentistry as a trade, and those who focused on periodontal tissues described dentistry as a healing profession.[10]

CLINICAL NOTE 1-4 The first dental school opened in 1840.

The first dental school was officially opened in 1840 as the **Baltimore College of Dental Surgery** with five students in the first class. The lack of respect for dentistry within the medical profession was slowly overcome and, in 1867, Harvard University established a dental department. At Harvard's first dental school graduation, its president, Oliver Wendell Holmes, referred to dentistry as a "branch of the medical profession to which this graduating class has devoted itself . . . yours is now an accepted province of this great and beneficent calling . . . medicine."[7] Between 1840 and 1867, 13 more dental schools were established. Some were short-lived, but others eventually affiliated with universities.

INTERRELATIONSHIP OF EARLY PERIODONTICS TO DENTAL HYGIENE

Periodontal diseases are as old as human civilization. Descriptions of early attempts at treating them were recorded, but in general, periodontal diseases were assumed to be incurable. In 1845 John M. Riggs first publicly called attention to this disease in the United States. He asserted that it was a curable disease and that with proper surgical treatment (by this he meant cleaning of the periodontal pockets), 90% of the cases could be cured. His opinion became widely accepted and periodontal disease became known as Riggs' disease. Curettage beyond the confines of the periodontal pocket to "stir up a healing reaction" was his original contribution to therapy.[11]

Leonard Koecker, a nineteenth century surgeon-dentist in London, was acknowledged to have successfully treated advanced cases of periodontal disease with conservative techniques. He is considered the first periodontist. His treatment to cure periodontoclasia, as it was called at the time, was very controversial. However, Riggs adopted these techniques and demonstrated them in public clinics. When dentists saw the results, these treatments became accepted.[4]

F.H. Rehwinkel renamed periodontoclasia **pyorrhea alveolaris** in a report he presented to the American Dental Association (ADA) in 1877. This name was never totally accepted because it was descriptive of only one aspect of pathology, bone loss. However, pyorrhea became a commonly used term that is still used today.[4]

CLINICAL NOTE 1-5 Periodontal disease has been known by many names including "pyorrhea," which is sometimes used today.

DEVELOPMENT OF THE PROFESSION OF DENTAL HYGIENE

Late in the 1800s, dental journals began to include articles about disease prevention and patient education. D.D. Smith of Philadelphia emphasized systematic change in the oral environment surrounding the teeth to prevent disease and demonstrated these techniques to colleagues. Smith had a profound influence on **Alfred C. Fones,** the founder of the role of the dental hygienist. Fones attended a meeting of the Northeastern Dental Society in 1898 at which Smith described his system of periodic **oral prophylaxis** (cleaning of the teeth). The treatment required patients to return at intervals of a few weeks for office treatment and to perform daily home care as they were instructed. Fones visited Smith's office three times to observe the practice. He then implemented this system in his own office for 5 years. Fones recognized that the procedures took an inordinate amount of his practice time. Smith believed that prophylaxis was too important to be delegated, but Fones disagreed and sought to develop an assistant to provide this care.[12]

FIRST DENTAL HYGIENIST
In 1906, Fones taught his dental assistant cousin, Irene Newman, to instruct and treat his patients to maintain their mouths in a clean state. His customized educational program was presented publicly at the National Dental Association Meeting in Cleveland in July 1911. The first dental hygiene education program included these elements:

- Drawings and books for the study of dental anatomy
- Extracted teeth with penciled markings to be removed with orangewood sticks and wet pumice
- Observation using a hand mirror while Fones cleaned Newman's teeth
- Fones becoming Ms. Newman's patient and instructing her as he observed in the hand mirror

All these procedures were repeated many times prior to treating patients in Fones' practice.

Newman's first patients were children and she only polished teeth. Later, she began to scale teeth with instruments but was only permitted to remove gross deposits. Fones found that her services saved him a great deal of chair time, and as her skills improved she was able to further treat his patients.[12]

FIRST DENTAL HYGIENE SCHOOLS
Fones went on to establish the first school for dental hygienists in Bridgeport, Connecticut, in 1913. His school graduated hygienists for 3 years before colleges and universities began to train dental hygienists in 1916 (Figure 1-2).

CLINICAL NOTE 1-6 Dental hygiene began as a profession in 1913.

Robin Adair of Atlanta, an oral surgeon with both medical and dental degrees, presented "The Introduction of Oral Prophylaxis into Dental Practice" to the Florida State Dental Society in June 1911. He described his system of regular dental cleanings for patients in his practice in which he first provided the treatment himself and then employed a "dental nurse." He

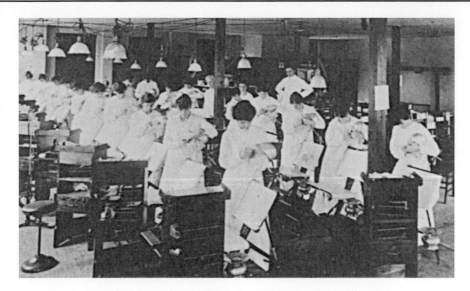

FIGURE 1-2 ■ Dr. Fones' first class of dental hygiene students appears here as they worked on manikins in 1913. Notice the white uniforms copied from nursing; students did not wear caps until they were awarded the privilege. (From Motley WE. *History of the American Dental Hygienists' Association 1923-1982.* Chicago, IL: American Dental Hygienists' Association; 1986.)

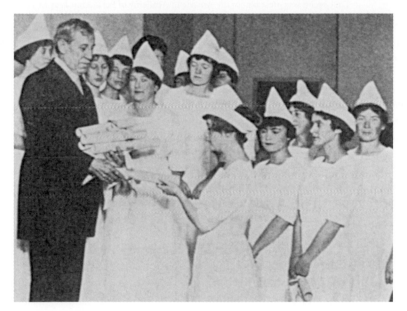

FIGURE 1-3 ■ Mr. Thomas Forsyth, one of the founders of the Forsyth Dental Infirmary, delivered diplomas to the Forsyth dental hygiene class of 1918. The class members were reported to be wearing the latest fashion in professional caps. (From Motley WE. *History of the American Dental Hygienists' Association 1923-1982.* Chicago, IL: American Dental Hygienists' Association; 1986.)

interviewed 150 applicants before selecting an experienced nurse to train for the position. He required that she assist him at the chair, read everything published on preventive dentistry, and practice on her family and friends before treating office patients. Adair performed the initial treatment and had the dental nurse finish. He reported that his patients were delighted and even sent out cards notifying his patients of the dental nurse and her skills.

Adair opened the fourth dental hygiene program in 1917 in Atlanta but graduated only 17 students. His untimely death in an automobile accident, which resulted in closure of the school, was a great loss to the development of dental hygiene.[13]

LICENSURE AND REGULATION

Professional demonstrations and communication, and the success of Fones' school in Bridgeport, followed by other dental hygiene education programs, led to regulation and licensure for dental hygienists. Dentists were first granted licenses by public agencies in 1841. The license verified that the individual was duly trained in the profession. By 1889, all states had adopted

laws that eliminated the preceptorship training so that all dentists had formal education. Connecticut was the first state to regulate dental hygiene practice, extending licensure and verification of educational credentials to hygienists in 1915. New York, Massachusetts, and Maine adopted laws regulating dental hygiene practice in 1917. The pattern of regulating dental hygiene practice in the United States followed the establishment and location of dental hygiene educational programs.[13]

SCHOOL PROGRAMS FOR CHILDREN

It was the general consensus during the period from 1900 to 1930 that a clean tooth would not decay. Because of this philosophy, many school dental health education programs were established to teach toothbrushing and promote prevention. Some of these community programs had benefactors who financed clinics for the dental treatment of children. Three of these programs also educated dental hygienists in their clinics: Guggenheim and Eastman, in New York State, and Forsyth, in Boston (Figure 1-3). Dental hygienist graduates from these programs had little experience treating adult patients. In contrast,

Fones' original educational program included instruction about permanent teeth and pyorrhea alveolaris, described as a curable disease requiring an exacting and painstaking treatment technique.[11]

Many public elementary school dental hygiene programs were initiated in the first half of the twentieth century because the greatest cause of student absence was recognized to be toothache. New York State had the most highly developed programs and required dental hygienists to have teaching credentials for the public schools. Boston also had many school dental clinics located throughout the city. School clinics were located directly in school buildings in Flint, Michigan. It was well into the 1930s before techniques for restoring primary teeth were generally taught and practiced by dentists, so these school clinics, staffed by dentists and hygienists, mostly extracted primary teeth, restored erupted permanent first molars, and cleaned children's teeth.[13]

RECOGNITION OF PERIODONTICS AS A SPECIALTY

Only a small percentage of the dentists of the early 1900s accepted the philosophy of treatment and prevention of periodontal diseases. Most believed that they were unable to cure or control periodontal disease and considered areas of pus around the teeth to be the foci of infection. Pyorrhea alveolaris was commonly accepted as a systemic disease that should be treated by physicians.[14] However, some dentists were interested in retaining the teeth. In 1914, two women dentists, Grace Rogers Spaulding of Detroit and Gillette Hayden of Columbus, Ohio, formed the American Academy of Periodontology in Cleveland. This new group adopted the name "periodontoclasia" for the ancient gum disease. There was considerable resistance to acceptance of the name, but these women dentists were accustomed to not being readily accepted. In fact, it has been suggested they became periodontists to establish their place separate from other women being educated as dental hygienists. However, except for Riggs and his followers in 1845 and the new periodontists, most dentists chose to treat periodontal diseases with surgical extraction of teeth. This remained the treatment of choice until the 1920s.

The first textbook devoted to periodontal disease, *A Textbook of Clinical Periodontia*, was written by Paul Stillman and John Oppie McCall of New York City and published in 1922. Early periodontists were dentists who were interested in periodontal disease and studied these references. The first periodontal specialty programs were established in the 1940s. Many early periodontists developed their own scalers, as had other early dental and medical practitioners (Figure 1-4).[15]

> **CLINICAL NOTE 1-7** Many early dentists designed their own instruments.

INSTRUMENTS FOR EVALUATING AND TREATING PERIODONTAL DISEASES

The most important assessment instrument now used by dental hygienists and dentists is the periodontal probe. It began to be used in the 1950s for measuring probing depths and, for the first time, periodontal destruction was quantified. Periodontal probes vary in design and are often named after the dentist or

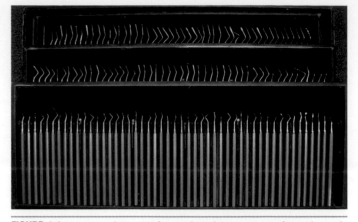

FIGURE 1-4 ■ A complete set of periodontal instruments from the early twentieth century. Each instrument has a slightly different angulation and blade configuration to make it adaptable to a particular area on a specific tooth. These instruments belonged to Dr. Robert M. Leggett, who graduated from the University of California, San Francisco, in 1910 and practiced until 1960. Dr. Leggett was president of the American Academy of Periodontology in 1935. (Courtesy of Dean Charles N. Bertolami, DDS, DMedSc, New York University, School of Dentistry.)

school where they were developed—the Marquis probe, the Michigan probe, the Goldman-Fox probe, and the World Health Organization (WHO) probe, to name a few. The WHO probe is associated with an international system for evaluating periodontal treatment needs, known as the Community Index of Periodontal Treatment Needs (see Chapter 3 for an explanation).[16] Periodontal probes permit the accurate evaluation and recording of periodontal status, as described in Chapter 8. The importance of identifying pocket depths, treating pockets, and maintaining records of periodontal conditions over time is standard practice today.

In the early 1960s, powered scalers that used sonic or ultrasonic frequencies became available for calculus removal. These instruments have been proven through extensive research to remove calculus, subgingival plaque, and endotoxins as effectively as hand scalers and curettes.[17] For additional information on the development of the periodontal instruments, see the section "Development of Modern Periodontal Instruments" in Chapter 13.

DEVELOPMENTS IN THE TREATMENT OF PERIODONTAL DISEASES

John Riggs is credited with originating and publicly describing treatment for the cure of inflammation of the gums, now called **gingivitis**, and absorption of the alveolar process, known as "scurvy of the gums," now called **periodontitis**. Riggs' treatment in 1845 emphasized calculus removal, subgingival curettage, and the reduction of inflammation-related tooth mobility. He believed that the cause of treatment failure was lack of thoroughness.[18]

UNDERSTANDING THE CAUSES OF PERIODONTAL DISEASES

Several reports from the 1880s presented bacteriologic theories of the etiology of periodontal diseases. In 1894, G.V. Black, considered the father of American dentistry, published an article on periodontal disease, which he called "phagedenic pericementitis." He concluded that the disease process was a "purely local affectation of an infectious character" related to the "glands of the periodontal membrane." Black is considered among the early leaders in the science of dentistry, although he was not educated beyond attendance at a country school. During his lifetime, he was awarded four honorary degrees: medical doctor, doctor of dental surgery, doctor of science, and doctor of laws.[18]

CLINICAL NOTE 1-8 Periodontal disease was first associated with bacterial infection in the nineteenth century.

T.B. Hartzell, the author of many articles on periodontal disease and its treatment, considered streptococcal infection to be an etiologic factor. In 1935, he expressed with great certainty that dentists should use the microbial principles of Pasteur and Dulaux. He called periodontoclasia, or pyorrhea alveolaris, a "germ ferment disease," in which the destruction of the periodontal membrane and surrounding bone and tissues resulted from bacteria. This idea led to enormous progress for dentistry as a learned profession and elevated it in the minds of medical colleagues, who at that time still tended to view dentistry as a trade.[19]

Occlusion and Periodontal Diseases

The issue of occlusion and its contribution to the etiology of periodontal disease has been controversial and widely discussed for decades. In 1917, P.R. Stillman wrote about possible damage to supporting tissues as a result of inharmonious relationships and stresses.[10] Harold K. Box of Toronto wrote extensively about this topic.[4] Currently, occlusion is thought to be a contributor to the periodontal disease process, but not a causative agent; it is described in Chapter 11.

CLINICAL NOTE 1-9 Occlusal relationships contribute to periodontal disease but do not cause it.

Systemic Influences on Periodontal Diseases

Around 1918, dentistry became concerned with the relationship of nutrition to periodontal disease. Percy Howe, whose major research related to dental caries, provided much valuable information about the effects of dietary deficiencies on the condition of the tissues that support the teeth. By 1939, dental practitioners were beginning to look for other causative factors and were going beyond the treatment of symptoms.[19]

CLINICAL NOTE 1-10 Periodontal diseases are related to systemic illnesses.

DEVELOPMENTS IN TREATMENT

Arthur D. Black, the son of G.V. Black and a renowned dental educator at Northwestern Dental School in Chicago, advocated surgical resection of diseased gingiva and bone tissue. Dr. A.W. Ward developed surgical instruments and created an adherent antiseptic and sedative cement to cover the cut tissues during healing. This material eliminated one objectionable feature of

TABLE 1-1	Percentage of Dental School Curriculum Assigned To Periodontics 1934-1987	
YEAR	**PERIODONTICS EDUCATION (%)**
1934*	*
1941	2.10
1950	4.25
1976	6.00
1987	7.10

*Not listed separately, included in operative dentistry.
(From Solomon ES, Brown WE. Dental school curriculum: a 50 year update. *J Dent Educ.* 1988;52:149–151.)

gum surgery, the painful and unsightly wound. Ward's periodontal pack is still used today, although not extensively.[19]

PERIODONTAL EDUCATION IN SCHOOLS OF DENTISTRY

The acceptance of the scientific basis for treating periodontal diseases resulted from its adoption in dental schools. However, this was a gradual process. The 1935 ADA survey of education reported that periodontal diagnosis and treatment were not adequately taught in dental schools. Six years later, the Horner Report on Dentistry stated that **periodontology**, the science of **periodontics**, accounted for only 2.1% of the curricular time in dental schools. Twelve years later, in 1954, the curriculum time had doubled to 4.25%.[20] The development of curriculum guidelines was initiated in 1985 by the joint efforts of the ADA Council on Dental Education and the American Association of Dental Schools, renamed the American Dental Education Association, or ADEA, in 2000. Subsequent to that, Solomon and Brown[21] reported in 1987 that periodontics accounted for 7.1% of clinical science hours in dental curricula (Table 1-1). The 2008-2009 ADA survey listed the mean hours of instruction in periodontics across dental schools to be 321 hours, or 8.4% of the total clinical science hours of instruction.[22]

SPECIALTY PROGRAMS IN PERIODONTOLOGY

Specialty training programs in periodontics arose in the 1940s in dental schools that had faculty members who were conducting research in the specialty: McCall, Prichard, and Schluger at Columbia University; Miller, Bunting, Jay, and Hard at the University of Michigan; and Glickman at Tufts University. The ADA recognized periodontology as a specialty in 1947 and a board to certify specialists was created in 1950.[20]

CLINICAL NOTE 1-11 Specialty programs in periodontology began in the 1940s.

GROWTH OF RESEARCH

Research in the 1960s verified that periodontal diseases were infectious (see Chapter 4). More recent research goals include identifying the pathogenic bacteria, clarifying host-bacteria interactions, understanding the pathologic process more fully, and determining the role of genetic and environmental factors in the natural history of periodontal disease.[23]

In 1984, a renowned teacher and researcher in periodontology, Sigurd Ramfjord, commented that a lag existed between the publication of research findings and their application in clinical practice. He was very concerned that dentists were routinely placing restorations subgingivally, although this placement had been known for more than 20 years to be a periodontal hazard.[24]

DENTAL HYGIENE IN DENTAL EDUCATION PROGRAMS

A simple comparison of the curriculum guidelines for periodontics published in the *Journal of Dental Education* in 1985 and 1992 highlighted recognition of the collaborative role in working with dental hygienists. In 1992, for the first time, behavioral objectives recommended that dental students be taught to "consult with and refer to dental hygienists those patients needing nonsurgical periodontal therapy and supportive periodontal treatment (more commonly known as maintenance care or recall)."[25,26] In addition, the 1992 article noted that dental hygienists may "be used in appropriate areas of the training program."[26]

The success of fluoridation in the prevention of caries has also had an effect on the emphasis of prevention in dental schools. National reports have demonstrated a decline in decay rates and a reduction in smooth surface caries in fluoridated areas. However, there are great disparities among communities. In response, dental school faculties have recognized the need for greater emphasis on prevention and oral health for children.[24]

The practice community requires general dentists and periodontists to maintain detailed periodontal records to provide evidence of evaluation and treatment of periodontal disease, to provide the best care for their patients, and to protect against malpractice suits. Complete evaluation of every patient includes periodontal assessment and must be performed to meet the expectations of patients. Confusion arises because the measurements used today do not evaluate disease activity, only the presence of gingival and bone changes related to disease processes. Research will eventually provide a means of identifying active disease, but until then, clinical attachment loss, probing depth, bone loss measured on images, and gingival bleeding continue to serve as measures of periodontal diseases.[17] For further explanation of the assessments required for periodontal diseases, see Chapter 8.

Microbiologists have sought to identify the principal pathogenic organisms associated with periodontal diseases for some time. The research is complicated, but presumptive evidence shows that there are identifiable pathogenic organisms associated with a variety of periodontal diseases. However, it is increasingly clear that the host response to infection is also a major determinant in the development of clinical disease. Pathogenic organisms are described in Chapter 4, host response is described in Chapter 2, and their role in disease development is described in Chapters 6 and 7. Control and prevention of periodontal diseases remain challenging both in research and in practice for the dental hygienist.[16]

ROLE OF DENTAL HYGIENISTS IN PERIODONTICS: 1913 AND BEYOND

Testimonies from the leading proponents of dental hygienists in the early 1900s reflected the attributes of the dentists who promoted the new profession. These individuals had great concern for the oral health of their patients, and they recognized the limitations of periodontal care at the time. They also realized that there was a cost-effective way to maintain the oral health of their patients. They recognized early on that individual preventive care was time-consuming. Many also had a strong belief in social causes, particularly promoting oral health in children. This belief led to the employment of dental hygienists in education programs in public schools, along with the introduction of dental hygiene services to private dental practices. Figure 1-5 shows an example of a school-based dental health program. From 1913 to 1923, the first 10 years of the existence

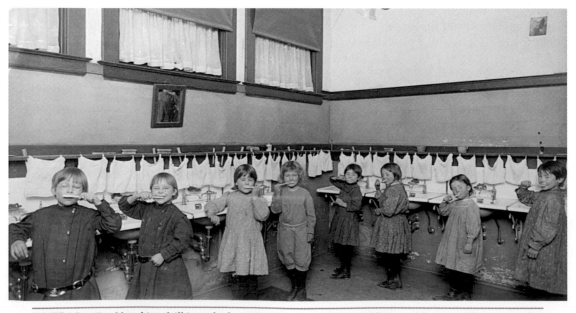

FIGURE 1-5 ■ **Toothbrushing drill in early the 1900s.** (Courtesy of Pemco, Webster, and Stevens Collection. Museum of History and Industry, Seattle, WA.)

of dental hygiene, 11 programs were initiated to teach dental hygienists. A professional society, the **American Dental Hygienists' Association (ADHA)**, was established, and a professional journal was published, the *Journal of the American Dental Hygienists' Association*. By 1923, the new dental hygiene schools had graduated 969 students and 24 states had established licensure systems for dental hygienists.[13]

CLINICAL NOTE 1-12 Dental hygienists play a significant role in the treatment and prevention of periodontal diseases.

From 1924 to 1935, much emphasis was placed on dental hygiene care in children's programs because of the extensive poverty during the Great Depression and rampant childhood caries. The Children's Bureau, housed in the U.S. Department of Labor in Washington, DC, provided grants to the Bureaus of Maternal and Child Health to educate mothers throughout the United States about child care, including oral health (Figure 1-6). In addition, conferences provided local physicians and dentists with information about the needs of children who were seen in their offices. During the depression era many of these programs hired dental hygienists, as did more than 100 city health departments. The Social Security Act of 1935 provided traineeships in public health for many dental hygienists. Numerous public health dental hygienists who earned advanced degrees through the support of the Maternal and Child Health programs went on to found and chair new dental hygiene programs.[13]

CHANGES IN DENTAL HYGIENE PRACTICE

The literature provides little information about the activities of the early dental hygienists in private practice. We do know that they were all women and that their patients and employers appreciated them. However, they had minimal job security, earned low wages, and were required to perform many service functions, such as housework in dental offices, which could be demeaning. Many women left the profession when they married and established families. Figure 1-7 shows a museum display of a dental office typical of the ones where the first dental hygienists would have worked.

A 1956 report on dental hygiene graduates, licensure, and practice, authored by Walter J. Pelton, Chief of the Division of Dental Resources of the U.S. Public Health Service, reported that the cumulative number of graduate dental hygienists was 15,649. These dental hygienists were on average 35.9 years old and 78.2% practiced full time. Of those working at the time of the study, 68.6% were employed by private dentists and 26.5%

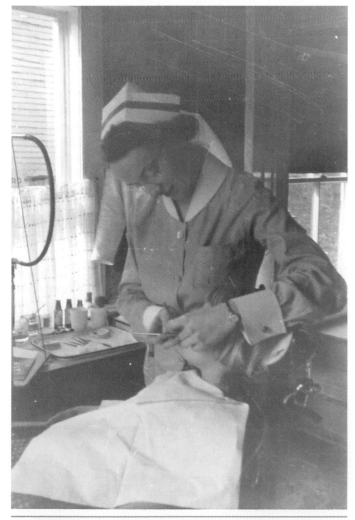

FIGURE 1-6 ■ Dr. Martha Fales examining a clinic patient in 1941.

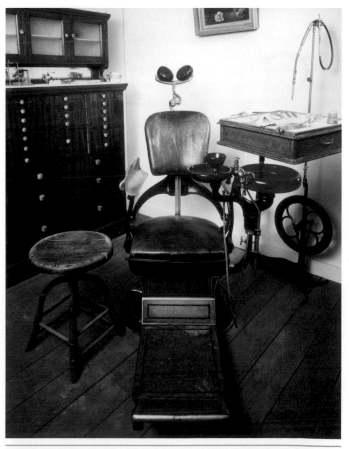

FIGURE 1-7 ■ Dental offices from the Victorian era and extending into the early twentieth century were dark and formal in appearance. This is an example of a dental unit and cabinetry from this period. There was no electricity in this office; note that the drill was powered by a foot pedal. The chair is adjustable but does not recline. The operator stool is too low to be used during treatment. (Photo by Howard Gishe and used courtesy of Museum of History and Industry, Seattle, WA.)

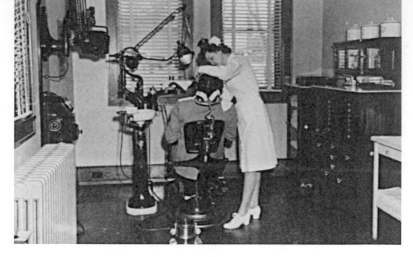

FIGURE 1-8 ■ **The typical appearance of a dental hygiene operatory from the 1940s.** Dental hygienists routinely worked standing at the side of the patient who was seated but not reclined. (From Motley WE. *History of the American Dental Hygienists' Association 1923-1982.* Chicago, IL: American Dental Hygienists' Association; 1986.)

were employed by government agencies. An additional 4.9% were employed by other sources, including 2% who worked in dental and dental hygiene schools. The remuneration as reported in this survey could explain why many women chose not to make dental hygiene a career at that time. Gross annual earnings for 1953-1954 were $3658 in private practice, $3484 in public health positions, and $4400 in education positions, about $300 per month, slightly more for educators.[27]

A report by the Survey Research Laboratory of the University of Illinois for the ADHA in 1981-1982 summarized the demographic and socioeconomic base of the dental hygiene profession 30 years later. Their composite showed that the average dental hygienist in the early 1980s was 29 years old, female, possessed an associate of arts degree, had 10 years of experience in private practice, was married, shared a joint income, and lived in a small urban or suburban community. This dental hygienist treated between 6 and 10 patients a day, allowed 30 to 35 minutes for each visit, worked between 30 and 40 hours per week, and was paid on a daily basis totaling approximately $15,000 per year, about $1250 per month or $300 per week.[28]

The 2002-2003 Survey of Allied Dental Education reported that approximately 148,000 dental hygienist jobs existed in the United States, the majority in dental practices. By 2011 there were over 177,000 dental hygienist positions, more than 170,500 in dentist's offices.[29] To meet this demand for dental hygienists, there were 309 accredited dental hygiene programs: 178 in community or junior colleges, 37 in technical colleges, 33 in allied health sciences schools, 23 in dental schools, 21 in university settings, and 17 in other types of institutions. In 2009, 6777 dental hygienists graduated, 81.9% received associate's degrees on graduation, 12.3% received bachelor's degrees, and the remainder earned certificates or diplomas.[30] Dental hygienists were employed mostly in private dental practices and earned an average of $33.16 per hour, approximately $68,980 per year.[29] Although there was considerable variation, the ADHA reported that in 2009, 55% of dental hygienists were 40 to 59 years of age and 35% were 39 or younger. They also reported that 98% were female and 87% were white non-Hispanic. Respondents also related that 42% worked 31 hours per week or more, 27% worked 21 to 30 hours, and 30% worked 20 or fewer hours per

week.[31] The average dental hygienist had 14.9 years of experience and had worked in the current dental office for an average of 7.3 years.[32]

CARE DELIVERY TECHNIQUES IMPROVE

These surveys highlight the statistical changes that have occurred in dental hygiene; the physical changes have also been dramatic. Early graduates followed the nursing education pattern because many people considered teaching and nursing the only acceptable career paths for women. Thus, early dental hygiene graduates wore starched white uniforms, white stockings, and caps. Dental hygiene and dentistry were practiced standing up by the side of the dental chair (Figure 1-8).

It was not until the advent of four-handed dentistry in the early 1960s, in which dentist and dental assistant work while seated at the head of the reclined patient, that operating stools for dentists and dental assistants were introduced. This development necessitated dramatic changes in dental school clinic and operatory arrangements. The more relaxed and comfortable physical advantages of sit-down dentistry were quickly recognized by dental hygienists. They, too, learned to practice sitting down, both in training programs and in private practice (Figure 1-9). The next major physical change in practice patterns was the introduction of the fully reclining (contoured) dental chair. This type of chair permitted dentists and dental hygienists to work while seated and promoted the use of the reclined Trendelenburg position for the patient. This position kept the patient's brain lower than the heart, which precluded fainting while providing good access, light, and visibility (Figure 1-10).[13]

There are also tremendous advances in the variety of automated equipment and technology available today, which has dramatically changed and improved dental hygiene practice.[33] Augmented safety features of protective eyewear were incorporated in the 1960s and the routine use of latex gloves started in the 1980s. State-of-the-art equipment choices[34] include the following:

- Computer-controlled local anesthesia delivery systems
- Intraoral cameras
- Automated and voice-activated periodontal probing systems
- Digital radiography

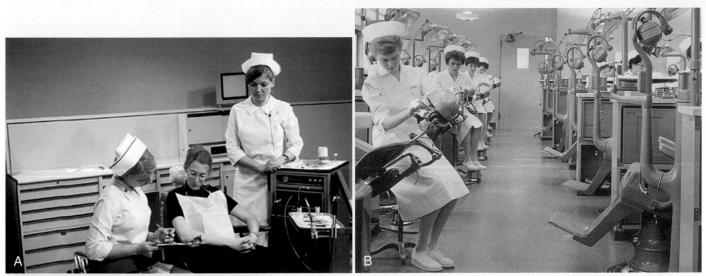

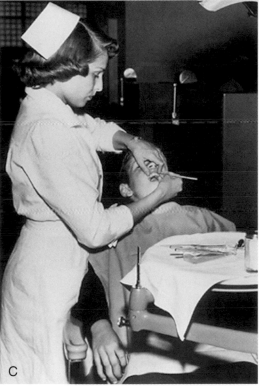

FIGURE 1-9 ■ **Dental hygiene education in the 1960s. A,** Dr Phyllis Beemsterboer (seated) and a classmate are interviewing a clinic patient. Typically dental hygiene students in the 1960s were trained to work seated next to the patient. **B,** Preclinical instruction was often on typodonts at the chairside. The dental hygiene students perched on stools and rested their feet on the foot control for the handpiece. Note that students wore no protective eyewear, masks, or gloves. **C,** This dental hygiene student is treating her patient while standing up. Dental chairs and equipment from earlier decades slowed the transition to working while seated because they did not accommodate a comfortable position. Note that the dental hygienist wears no protective eyewear, mask, or gloves.

- Video-based counseling and educational systems with flat panel monitors
- Phase-contrast microscopy
- Chairside laboratory tests for malodor and anaerobic periodontal pathogens
- Periodontal endoscopes and other calculus-detecting fiberoptic probes
- Computer- and web-based periodontal risk calculators
- Ultrasonic and air polishing devices with built-in sterile irrigation systems, fiberoptic illumination systems, and thin, probelike microultrasonic inserts
- Wrist blood pressure cuffs
- Magnification loupes with illumination
- Ergonomic hygiene stools and ergonomic dental chairs with built-in back massagers

EXPANDING ROLE OF THE DENTAL HYGIENIST

The late 1960s and early 1970s was a time of concern about the growing population and the availability of health care for all. One consequence was a significant increase in the number of dental hygiene programs in the United States, from 35 in 1956 to 61 in 1966 to 173 in 1976[13] to 309 in 2010.[30] During this time the federal government funded experimental programs to train dental hygienists in additional skills to treat patients with periodontal conditions and provide restorative services. Specific duties varied across the country, but they included local anesthesia administration, placement and carving of amalgam restorations, placement and finishing of composite restorations, placement and removal of periodontal sutures and periodontal packs, and gingival curettage. These skills, or combinations of

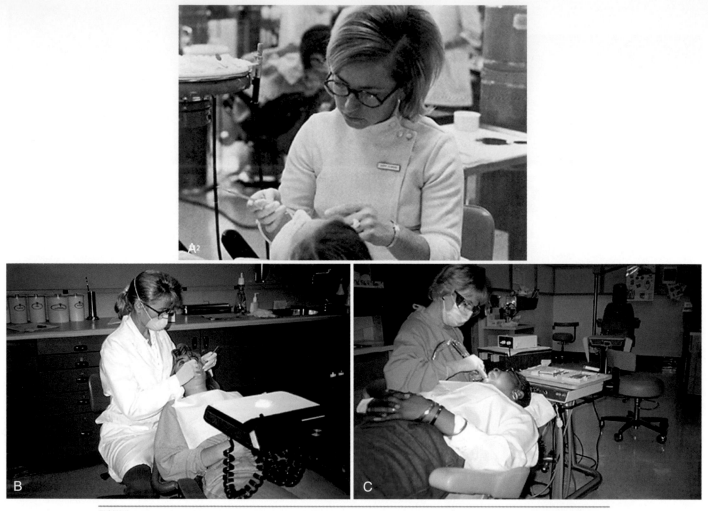

FIGURE 1-10 ■ **Dental hygiene practice then and now. A,** 1970. This dental hygienist is still a student (no cap). She is seated during treatment with the patient slightly reclined. Dental hygienists were encouraged to wear eyeglasses to protect themselves from splatter, but no other protective equipment was used. **B,** 1990. This dental hygienist is seated with the patient comfortably reclined. She is wearing eyeglasses, gloves, and a mask for protection. Note that the white uniform and cap has given way to a lab coat with long sleeves. The patient is not wearing protective eyewear. **C,** 2000. Dr. Dorothy Perry is seated treating a patient in a clinic setting. The patient is fully reclined, and the dental hygienist is comfortably at the side wearing goggles, a mask, a gown, and gloves. The patient has protective eyewear also. Equipment, which is mobile so that the hygienist can move around the head of the patient for better access, includes an ultrasonic scaler.

them, became known generally as **expanded-duty dental hygiene skills.**

> **CLINICAL NOTE 1-13** Dental hygiene practice has expanded to included important skills such as the administration of local anesthesia.

The federal government also supported the Teaching Expanded Auxiliary Management grant program in the 1970s. This program provided funds to dental schools for programs that emphasized management and behavioral skills of dental students who would graduate and employ auxiliaries in clinical practice, including dental hygienists. Although grant funding ended in 1978, many practice management courses were continued.

DENTAL HYGIENE PRACTICES

In 1986, Colorado passed a law allowing dental hygienists to provide many services without the supervision of dentists.[35] Between 1987 and 1990 a research demonstration project in California tested the possibility of specially trained dental hygienists practicing independently of dentist supervision.[36] Documented educational requirements and practice experiences resulted in 1998 legislative approval for the graduates of the Health Manpower Pilot Project to become registered dental hygienists in alternative practice (RDHAP).[37] All licensed dental hygienists in California are now able to gain this additional education and become licensed as RDHAPs. There is also considerable interest in the advanced dental hygiene practitioner, a mid-level hygienist who could assist the dental hygiene workforce in having a greater effect on meeting the oral health needs of the population.[38] Models now exist in Alaska with the dental health aide therapist and in Minnesota with the dental therapist and advanced dental therapist programs.[39]

RESPONSIBILITIES OF THE PROFESSION OF DENTAL HYGIENE

Currently, many dental hygienists are contributing to the improved periodontal health of the nation in general dental practices, specialty dental practices, public health practices, nursing homes, and a variety of educational programs—dental hygiene and dental, continuing education courses, and research. They enjoy recognition of their skills; adequate compensation; respect from the community, patients, coworkers, and employers; professional associations including the ADHA; and personal challenges in providing patient care. Dental hygiene provides a wide range of practice options and these options are growing. There are interesting and potentially powerful patient education opportunities through the now vast public use of mobile devices, social networking, and apps to keep patients connected to the dental hygienist and to their oral health.

CONCLUSION

Now, almost 100 years after the first dental hygiene graduates started to treat periodontal diseases and maintain the oral health of patients in dental practices, the profession enjoys new momentum and the challenge of addressing health care disparities. Dental hygiene and dental care should include not only therapy for all but also the application of proven preventive techniques. This approach could result in the prevention of oral diseases for the entire population. Dental hygiene has truly expanded to include all the roles articulated by the ADHA, a broad and encompassing view of the profession of dental hygiene as depicted in Figure 1-11.

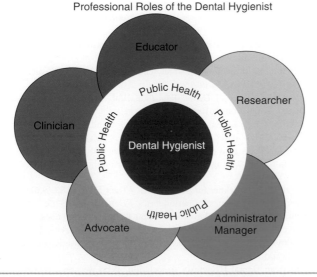

Professional Roles of the Dental Hygienist

FIGURE 1-11 ■ Professional roles of the dental hygienist. (Used with permission from the American Dental Hygienists' Association, 2012.)

DENTAL HYGIENE CONSIDERATIONS

- The study of anthropology and historical documents reveals that dental health and dental diseases have been of concern since the beginning of recorded history.
- Dentists' concerns about providing teeth cleaning and preventive care led to the creation of the dental hygienist.
- Dental hygienists received formal education and licensure beginning in 1913 in Connecticut.
- Over the decades, dental hygienists have been employed less in public health and school settings and more in private practice settings.
- Many technologic advances have improved dental hygiene practice, including ergonomically designed equipment, ultrasonic scalers, and automated probing devices.
- The American Dental Hygienists' Association has defined the professional role of dental hygiene broadly to encompass many aspects of oral health care.

★ CASE SCENARIO

You have been practicing as a licensed dental hygienist for 6 months in the office of Dr. Lamb. The first patient of the day looks at you funny as you escort her into your treatment area, and asks, "Why didn't you just go to dental school? Your mother told me you were at the top of your class and did really well on all of your exams."

1. How would you educate this patient as to your role in providing her oral health care?
   A. Explain the educational requirements and preventive focus of the dental hygienist.
   B. Explain to the patient that dental school training is heavily involved with restorative dentistry and surgical skills.
   C. All of the above.
2. How would you describe your role in the practice?
   A. The dental hygienist cleans teeth.
   B. The dental hygienist assists the dentist with patient care.
   C. The dental hygienist is a licensed professional who is trained to provide oral health care, prevention, and education.
   D. Call the dentist into your operatory to explain to the patient that you are a licensed professional and what duties you will be performing.
3. What is unique about the role of the dental hygienist?
   A. You are licensed.
   B. You do more than assist with procedures.
   C. You have had education and training.
   D. You specialize in treating and preventing diseases of the periodontium.

STUDY QUESTIONS

Answers and rationales to these questions can be obtained from your instructor.

MULTIPLE CHOICE

1. Who was the first individual to recognize the relationship between tooth loss and calculus?
   A. Albucasis
   B. Aranculus
   C. Aristotle
   D. Hippocrates
   E. Vesalius

2. Periodontal lesions are characterized by all of the following EXCEPT one. Which one is the EXCEPTION?
   A. Pockets
   B. Periodontal infection
   C. Periodontal pockets
   D. Periodontal disease
   E. Probe measurements

3. There is growing concern about the increase in population and the need for health care for all. This has resulted in a decrease in the number of dental hygiene programs in the United States.
   A. Both statements are true.
   B. Both statements are false.
   C. The first statement is true, and the second statement is false.
   D. The first statement is false, and the second statement is true.

4. The first dentist to practice in the United States was
   A. Mills.
   B. Revere.
   C. Greenwood.
   D. Woofendale.
   E. Never determined.

5. Dental hygienists are now able to provide a broader array of patient care services, including expanded duties in many states, because the profession of dental hygiene has grown and expanded its scope of practice over the decades.
   A. Both the statement and the reason are correct and related.
   B. Both the statement and the reason are correct but NOT related.
   C. The statement is correct, but the reason is NOT correct.
   D. The statement is NOT correct, but the reason is correct.
   E. NEITHER the statement NOR the reason is correct.

6. The American Dental Hygienists' Association was first established for dental hygienists. It has helped define the roles of the dental hygienist in dentistry.
   A. Both statements are true.
   B. Both statements are false.
   C. The first statement is true, and the second statement is false.
   D. The first statement is false, and the second statement is true.

7. Which early periodontist was an advocate for avoiding placing restorations subgingivally?
   A. Miller
   B. Bunting
   C. Glickman
   D. Ramfjord

8. The first school of dental hygiene was established in Bridgeport, Connecticut, in what year?
   A. 1867
   B. 1877
   C. 1913
   D. 1917

SHORT ANSWER

9. Why does studying the history of periodontology lead to a better understanding of dentistry and dental hygiene?

10. Keeping in mind the explosion of knowledge and the rapid transmission of scientific findings today, describe how the dental hygienist can evaluate what is important to know.

Please visit **http://evolve.elsevier.com/Perry/periodontology** for additional practice and study support tools.

REFERENCES

1. Weinberger BW. *An Introduction to the History of Dentistry in America. Vol 2.* St. Louis, MO: CV Mosby; 1948:14, 215.
2. Guerini V. *A History of Dentistry from the Ancient Times Until the End of the Eighteenth Century.* Philadelphia, PA: Lea & Febiger; 1909.
3. Hippocrates. *De Morbis Mulerum.* Lib II. 606.
4. Leonard HJ. The historical background of periodontology. *J Periodontol.* 1940;11:67, 70, 73.
5. Ring ME. *Dentistry: An Illustrated History.* St. Louis, MO: Avery/CV Mosby; 1985:71, 303.
6. Albucasis A. *De Chirurgia.* Channing S, trans. Oxford, England: Oxford University Press; 1778:181–183.
7. Bremner MDK. *The Story of Dentistry.* 2nd ed. New York, NY: Dental Items of Interest Publishing; 1946:52, 68, 85.
8. Fauchard P. *Chirurgien Dentiste.* Lindsay L, trans. New York, NY: Milford House; 1969:28.
9. Hollinshead BS. *The Survey of Dentistry.* Washington, DC: American Council on Education; 1961:240.
10. Stillman PR. The past and future of periodontia. *J Periodontol.* 1939;10:31–36.
11. Fones AC. *Mouth Hygiene.* 2nd ed. Philadelphia, PA: Lea & Febiger; 1921:166–172, 276.
12. Fones AC. The origin and the history of the dental hygiene movement. *J Am Dent Assoc.* 1920;13:1816.
13. Fales MJH. *History of Dental Hygiene Education in the United States, 1913-1975* [dissertation]. Ann Arbor: University of Michigan; 1975.
14. Yuretskyy W. An historical review of oral prophylaxis. *J Periodontol.* 1939;10:81–87.
15. McCall JO. The evolution of the scaler and its influence on the development of periodontia. *J Periodontol.* 1939;10:69–81.
16. Burt BA, Eklund SA. *Dentistry, Dental Practice and the Community.* 4th ed. Philadelphia, PA: Saunders; 1992:66–67, 114, 125.
17. Plemons JM, DeSpain Eden B. Nonsurgical therapy. In: Rose LF, Mealey BL, eds. *Periodontics: Medicine, Surgery, and Implants.* St. Louis, MO: Elsevier Mosby; 2004:237–262.
18. Merritt AH. The historical background of periodontology. *J Periodontol.* 1939;10:7–25.
19. Bryan AW. Progress in the recognition of etiologic factors of periodontal diseases. *J Periodontol.* 1939;10:25–30.
20. Hollinshead BS. *Dentistry in the United States.* Washington, DC: American Council on Education; 1960:246, 247, 315.
21. Solomon ES, Brown WE. Dental school curriculum: a 50-year update. *J Dent Educ.* 1988;52:149–151.
22. *2008/2009 Survey of Dental Education.* Vol 4. Chicago, IL: American Dental Association; 2010:12–20.
23. Sklar G, Carranza, FA. The historical background of periodontology. In: Newman MG, Takei HH, Klokkevold PR, et al, eds. *Carranza's Clinical Periodontology.* 11th ed. St. Louis, MO: Elsevier Saunders; 2012:2–9.
24. Ramfjord SP. Changing concepts in periodontics. *J Prosthet Dent.* 1984;52:781-786.
25. Curriculum guidelines for periodontics. *J Dent Educ.* 1985;49:611-615.
26. Curriculum guidelines for periodontics. *J Dent Educ.* 1992;56:773-778.
27. Pelton WJ, Pennell E, Vavra H. Section 8: Dental Hygienists. In: *Health Manpower Sourcebook.* Bethesda, MD: Public Health Service, U.S. Dept of Health Education and Welfare, Division of Public Health Resources; 1957: publication 263-1957.
28. American Dental Hygienists' Association. Who we are: a report on the survey of dental hygiene issues: attitudes, perceptions and preferences. *J Dent Hyg.* 1982;56:13–19.

29. U.S. Department of Labor, Bureau of Labor Statistics. Occupations, employment and wages. http://www.bls.gov. Accessed December 16, 2011.

30. American Dental Association. *2009-10 survey of allied dental education.* Chicago, IL: ADA Survey Center; 2011:7–8.

31. American Dental Hygienists' Association. 2009 dental hygiene job market and employment survey. http://www.adha.org. Accessed December 16, 2011.

32. Brown JL, Schaid K, Wagner BS, et al. A look at allied dental education in the United States. *J Am Dental Assoc.* 2005;136:797–804.

33. Wilkins EM. Patient reception and ergonomic practice. In: *Clinical Practice of the Dental Hygienist.* 11th ed. Philadelphia, PA: Lippincott Williams & Wilkins; 2013:88–99.

34. Slim LH, Rutledge CR. Nonsurgical periodontal therapy then and now: changes since the early 1980s. *Access.* 2005;19:32–38.

35. Thomas RD. On their own. *RDH.* 1994;14:14–26.

36. Perry DA, Freed JR, Kushman JE. The California demonstration project in independent practice. *J Dent Hyg.* 1994;68:137–142.

37. American Dental Hygienists' Association. Congratulations to California RDHAPs. *Access.* 1999;13:41.

38. American Dental Hygienists' Association. Advanced dental hygiene practitioner. http://www.adha.org. Accessed December 16, 2011.

39. American Dental Association. New class of DHATs. http://www.ada.org. Accessed December 16, 2011.

CHAPTER

2

Periodontium: Anatomic Characteristics and Host Response

Dorothy A. Perry and Phyllis L. Beemsterboer

LEARNING OUTCOMES

- Identify the tissues of the periodontium.
- Describe the anatomy and clinical characteristics of the tissues of the periodontium.
- Differentiate among the three types of oral epithelial surfaces: keratinized, parakeratinized, and nonkeratinized.
- List the functions of the periodontal ligament.
- Describe clinically normal gingivae in terms of color, size, contour, texture, and consistency.
- Describe the interactions of the major elements in the host response.
- Define the protective roles of gingival fluid and saliva.

KEY TERMS

Alveolar bone	Embrasure	Lamina propria
Alveolar process	Fenestration	Lysis
Alveoli	Fiber bundles	Macrophage
Antibody	Free gingiva	Melanin
Antigen	Free gingival groove	Mucogingival junction
Attached gingiva	Gingiva	Oral epithelium
Attachment apparatus	Gingival crevicular fluid	Oral mucosa
Basal lamina	Gingival ligament	Papillae
Cementoenamel junction	Gingival margin	Parakeratinized epithelium
Cementum	Hypersensitivity (allergic) reactions	Periodontal ligament
Chemotaxis	Immune system	Phagocytize
Col	Immunoglobulin	Physiologic mesial migration
Complement	Immunology	Rete pegs
Cytokine	Interdental gingiva	Sharpey's fibers
Dehiscence	Junctional epithelium	Stippled
Dentogingival unit	Keratinization	Sulcular epithelium
Effector molecule	Lamina dura	Tooth root proximity

Gingival and periodontal diseases are infectious diseases by nature. The changes these infections bring to the periodontal tissues can best be understood with a basic background in the unique anatomy of the periodontium and knowledge of the response the human body undertakes to protect itself. As will be further explained in Chapter 4 on microbial plaque biofilm and Chapters 6 and 7 devoted to gingival and periodontal diseases, the effects and damage caused by these microbe-induced diseases are complex. They can result in irreversible changes to the normal architecture, loss of teeth, loss of function, and changes in appearance.

This chapter is divided into two parts. The first part presents a basic description of the normal periodontium. This description provides the reader with an understanding of the environment affected by gingival and periodontal diseases. The second

part is an introduction into the rapidly growing area of host response, immunology. A basic understanding of these processes will inform the dental hygienist why tissue destruction occurs. The second part also provides a brief description of the protective influences that exist in the periodontium.

ANATOMIC CHARACTERISTICS OF THE PERIODONTIUM

The periodontium is defined simply as the tissues that surround, support, and attach to the teeth. These include the gingiva, periodontal ligament, cementum, and alveolar bone.[1] These tissues support the teeth and oral structures. Maintaining the health and function of the periodontium is the most significant factor in the longevity of the dentition.

GINGIVA

The gingiva is the visible component of the periodontium inside the mouth. It is described as coral pink,[2] pink,[3] or pale pink.[4] In clinical appearance the color can vary and can appear much darker when melanin pigmentation is present. The gingiva is distinguished from the **oral mucosa** at the **mucogingival junction**. This line indicates the transition from the loosely attached and movable oral mucosa to the **attached gingiva**, which is more firmly attached to the bone by collagen fibers. The attached gingiva is the portion that extends coronally from the mucogingival junction. The width of the attached gingiva varies from individual to individual and from tooth to tooth in the same mouth. The range of widths is 1 to 9 mm,[5] with an average of 3.5 to 4.5 mm in the maxilla and 3.3 to 3.9 mm in the mandible. There is usually a thinner band of attached gingiva in the posterior regions. The palatal attached gingiva blends into the palatal gingiva without demarcation.[2]

> **CLINICAL NOTE 2-1** There is no absolute minimum width of the attached gingiva required for periodontal health.

Frenum and muscle attachments are present in the gingiva, and those located coronally in the attached gingiva are associated with narrower widths of attached gingiva. The gingiva is keratinized or parakeratinized (discussion follows) tissue on the oral surface, and it is commonly **stippled**. Nonstippled gingiva is also seen in healthy mouths.[2,6] The degree of keratinization varies throughout the epithelium in the mouth, with the palatal gingiva being the most keratinized and the cheek the least. The tongue is also covered with keratinized epithelium. The location of the **gingival margin**, the edge of the gingiva next to the teeth, in fully erupted healthy teeth is 0.5 to 2 mm coronal to the **cementoenamel junction** of the teeth (Figure 2-1).[3]

The **free gingiva**, or free marginal gingiva, surrounds the tooth and creates a cuff or collar of gingiva extending coronally about 1.5 mm. The surface of the free gingiva next to the tooth forms the gingival wall of the sulcus.[2] The free gingiva may be distinguished from the attached gingiva by a **free gingival groove**, a slight depression on the gingiva corresponding to the depth of the sulcus. This groove varies from tooth to tooth, occurring about 50% of the time, most commonly in the mandibular anterior and premolar areas.[6] The free gingiva on buccal and lingual surfaces is often described as ending in a knife-edged tip next to the tooth surface; microscopically the coronal termination of the free gingiva appears more rounded (Figure 2-2).

The **papillae** are gingivae that fill the **embrasures**—proximal spaces created below the contact areas of the teeth. They are also referred to as the **interdental gingiva**. The papillae between anterior teeth are commonly described as pyramidal.[4] When the papilla is broad, as is often the case between posterior teeth, there is a nonkeratinized area called the **col**. This area is a slight depression of tissue between the buccal and lingual interdental papillae. It indicates a fusion of two papillae to cover a wide space. The col is not usually present between anterior teeth. When adjacent teeth do not contact each other, whether they

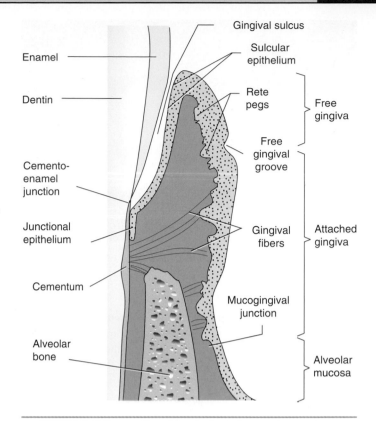

FIGURE 2-1 ■ Cross section of the gingiva and supporting structures.

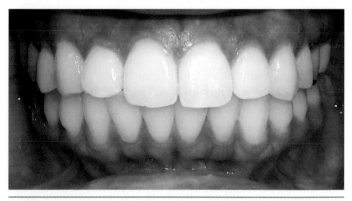

FIGURE 2-2 ■ Clinical presentation of normal gingiva showing knife-edged interdental papillae and free gingival margin. The mucogingival junction is clearly demarcated on the mandible.

are anterior or posterior teeth, attached gingivae form between the teeth and the papillae and col are absent.[2]

The gingival epithelium is joined to the underlying connective tissue by a **basal lamina**, 300 to 400 Å thick. The basal lamina is joined to the connective tissue by fibrils. The connection between the free and attached gingiva and the underlying connective tissue occurs in ridges of epithelium called **rete pegs.**[2]

Epithelium

The surface tissue of the oral cavity is made up of stratified squamous epithelium, primarily consisting of cells called keratinocytes, but also including Langerhans cells, Merkel cells, and melanocytes. The function of the epithelium is to protect the underlying structures while allowing some selective interchange with the oral environment.[2]

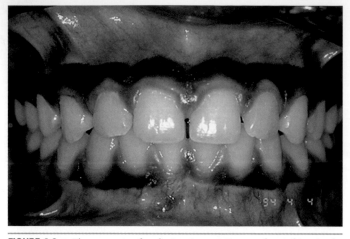

FIGURE 2-3 ■ The presence of melanin pigmentation can be striking in the normal gingiva.

CLINICAL NOTE 2-2 An example of selective interchange is the absorption of drugs through the epithelium. Smokeless tobacco and other drug users place drugs directly on the epithelium, and the active ingredients diffuse very quickly through the tissue and into the bloodstream.

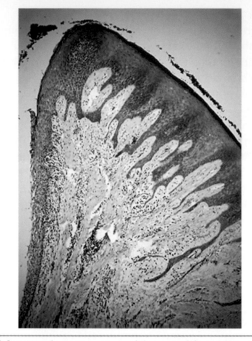

FIGURE 2-4 ■ **Histologic appearance of the normal free gingiva and sulcus.** Rete pegs are seen subjacent to the oral epithelium but not the sulcular epithelium. (Courtesy of Dr. Gary C. Armitage.)

The process of keratinization occurs as the keratinocyte migrates from the basal layer to the surface. The cells become increasingly flattened, develop keratohyaline granules in the subsurface, and produce a superficial layer that is similar to skin where no cell nuclei are present. In some cases, the epithelium shows signs of being keratinized, yet the cells of the superficial layers retain their nuclei. This surface is called a parakeratinized epithelium. If no signs of keratinization are present, the epithelial surface is considered nonkeratinized.[3] Keratinized, parakeratinized, and nonkeratinized gingivae are all found in the oral cavity.

Langerhans cells are considered to be part of the phagocytic system, and Merkel cells contain nerve endings and are associated with tactile sensitivity. Melanocytes are located in the basal layers of the epithelium and contain substances that convert to melanin. Melanin is phagocytized and remains within the cells of the epithelium, giving a pigmented appearance to the epithelium.[2] Figure 2-3 is an example of a normal gingiva with extensive melanin pigmentation.

Oral or Outer Epithelium

The oral epithelium is also called the outer gingival epithelium.[4] It is composed of the attached gingiva, the papillae, and the outer surface of the free gingiva. It covers the crest of the gingiva, the free gingiva, and the attached gingiva. This can be clearly seen in Figure 2-2. Microscopic rete pegs project into the connective tissue below. The oral epithelium's function is protective, and the epithelium is typically parakeratinized.[2]

Sulcular Epithelium

The sulcular epithelium is the thin nonkeratinized, or parakeratinized, epithelium extending from the outer epithelium into the gingival sulcus. It may be parakeratinized near the opening to the oral cavity. The sulcular epithelium is found

from the height of the gingiva along the inner surface of the sulcus extending to the junctional epithelium; it forms the gingival wall of the sulcus (Figure 2-4). In a healthy state, the epithelium lining the sulcus is smooth and intact; there are no rete pegs projecting into the connective tissue. The sulcular epithelium is also permeable and gingival crevicular fluid, made up of the components of the serum and other cells, is secreted through it into the sulcus.

The healthy sulcus is generally 1 to 3 mm deep. However, the sulcus depth determined clinically by measurement with a periodontal probe may be considerably different than the histologic sulcus depth. Probe measurements are subject to variation as a result of several influences: the probe insertion pressure, the ability of the probe tip to penetrate tissue, and the accuracy of the clinician reading the probe measurements.[5] For this reason, Löe and colleagues[3] suggested that the use of the term *sulcus depth* in reference to probe readings is misleading. A more accurate term would be *probing depth* or *probable depth* of the gingival sulcus.

Sulcular or Gingival Crevicular Fluid. Gingival crevicular fluid, also referred to as sulcular fluid or simply gingival fluid, flows from the underlying connective tissue into the sulcus. The amount of flow is related to the permeability of the connective tissue capillaries beneath the surface of the sulcular epithelium. The fluid escapes from the capillaries and seeps out between the epithelial cells into the sulcus. The amount of fluid flow is small, considered to be minimal to none in the healthy state.[4] Gingival fluid is believed to perform several functions: cleansing the sulcus, improving epithelial cell adherence to the tooth surface, and possessing antimicrobial and immune properties.[2,6]

Junctional Epithelium

The junctional epithelium separates the periodontal ligament from the oral environment. It is composed of nonkeratinized,

TABLE 2-1	Gingival Fiber Bundle Groups	
NAME	**PATH/LOCATION OF FIBERS**	**MAJOR FUNCTION**
PRINCIPAL GINGIVAL FIBER GROUPS		
Dentogingival	Radiate from the cementum into free gingiva and attached gingiva	Support the gingiva
Alveologingival	Radiate from periosteum into attached gingiva	Attach gingiva to underlying bone
Dentoperiosteal	Course from cementum, near cementoenamel junction, across to alveolar crest	Anchor tooth to bone and protect periodontal ligament
Circular	Encircle entire tooth coronal to alveolar crest	Support free gingiva
Transseptal	Span interdental space, with ends inserted into cementum of teeth	Maintain relationship between teeth
SECONDARY GINGIVAL FIBER GROUPS		
Periostogingival	Course from periosteum of alveolar bone and spread into connective tissue	Attach gingiva to bone
Interpapillary	Found in papillae, coronal to transseptal fiber bundles	Support papillary gingiva
Transgingival	Formed between teeth, coronal to cementoenamel junction	Support marginal gingiva
Intercircular	Run from distal, facial, and lingual surfaces of one tooth, around adjacent tooth, and insert on mesial surface of tooth beyond adjacent tooth	Maintain arch form
Semicircular	Course from mesial surface to distal surface of same tooth	Support free gingiva
Intergingival	Run mesiodistally in connective tissue immediately beneath gingival epithelium	Support attached gingiva

stratified, squamous epithelial cells that adhere organically to tooth structure, and its function is considered to be protection of the attachment of the tooth to the surrounding tissues. It forms a layer that is 15 or 20 cells thick at the coronal end and narrows to a few cells thick at the apical termination. Its length in the healthy state ranges from 0.25 to 1.35 mm.[4,6] This epithelium continually renews itself, and its most coronal portion determines the histologic base of the gingival sulcus.[7,8] The attachment of the junctional epithelium to the root surface is enhanced by fibers from the connective tissue. This attachment supports the free marginal gingival and it is considered to be a functional unit, called the **dentogingival unit.**[2,6]

Gingival Connective Tissue

The connective tissue beneath the gingiva is called the **lamina propria.** The lamina propria is made up of two layers: the papillary layer that is immediately beneath the epithelium, which consists of papillary projections between the rete pegs, and the reticular layer, which extends to the periosteum.[6] Approximately 60% of the lamina propria is made up of connective tissue that is composed of collagen fibrils that form discrete **fiber bundles.**[8] Other elements include cells such as fibroblasts, undifferentiated mesenchymal cells, mast cells, and macrophages as well as blood vessels and nerves.[3]

The fiber bundles are known as the **gingival ligament.**[8] These are not individual fibers, but fiber bundles, although they are commonly referred to as fibers. Their functions include protecting and supporting the junctional epithelium, maintaining the tone of the attached gingiva, and protecting the periodontal ligament. There are five principal fiber groups and six minor groups. All bundles are discrete, although fibrils often intertwine so that the gingival ligament supports its components. The bundles are best described by their orientation and attachment. These characteristics suggest the function of the specific bundle, although all are interdependent and no doubt share functions. The gingival fiber bundles are very important

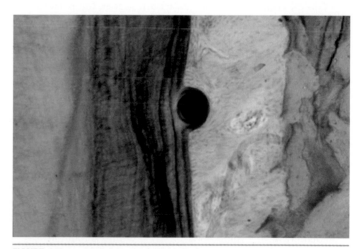

FIGURE 2-5 ■ Histologic appearance of the dentin, cementum, periodontal ligament, and alveolar bone. The cementum is dark pink and appears striated. The round structure in the cementum is a cementicle. (Courtesy of Dr. Gary C. Armitage.)

because they provide the most coronal connective tissue attachment for the teeth. Both principal and secondary fiber bundles have been described. Their locations and functions are listed in Table 2-1.

PERIODONTAL LIGAMENT

Teeth are not attached rigidly to the bone in humans and other mammals. The periodontal ligament provides a suspensory cushion in the 0.4- to 1.5-mm space between the surface of the tooth and the bone. The periodontal ligament is a connective tissue complex primarily filled with fiber bundles and cells.[8] The cells in the ligament perform an important formative function for the tissues; they generate a pericementum for the cemental surface of the root and a periosteum for the bone.[9] Unusual formations of cementum, called cementicles, can also occur in the periodontal ligament (Figure 2-5). These develop from calcified material in the periodontal ligament or from traumatically displaced bits of cementum or bone.[10]

The specific functions of the periodontal ligament include the following[8,10]:

- Tooth anchorage
- Fibrous tissue development and maintenance
- Calcified tissue development and maintenance
- Nutritive and metabolite transport
- Sensory functions, including touch, pressure, pain, and proprioception (displacement sensitivity)

Fiber Bundles

The fiber bundles in the periodontal ligament are made of collagen, arranged in bundles, and are spread throughout the periodontal ligament with the other cellular, vascular, and nerve tissues. In addition to attaching the tooth to the bone, they are believed to transmit occlusal forces to the bone, resist occlusal forces (the "shock absorber" effect), and protect the vessels and nerves from injury.[10]

Five principal fiber bundles in the periodontal ligament are summarized in Table 2-2. The principal fiber bundles are attached to the cementum with brush like fibers called **Sharpey's fibers**, course from the cementum across the periodontal ligament, and terminate in the alveolar bone as Sharpey's fibers.[8,10]

In addition to the principal fiber bundles, small collagen fibers that run in all directions in the periodontal ligament have been identified. These are referred to as the indifferent fiber plexus; their function is unknown. Less well formed collagen

bundles and immature forms of elastin are also observed in the periodontal ligament, mostly in association with blood vessels.[8]

Physiologic Mesial Migration or Drift

Physiologic mesial migration is normal tooth movement and is probably the result of wear of proximal and occlusal tooth surfaces. The movement is gradual, totaling no more than 1 cm during a lifetime. Physiologic mesial migration is considered an adjustment process that allows the dentition to retain balance among its complex structures. The cells of the periodontal ligament probably mediate the changes needed in the bone and the cementum to permit movement and maintain balance.[8] Migration occurs in conjunction with gradual remodeling of the alveolar bone, bone resorption by osteoclastic activity is increased in areas of pressure along the mesial surfaces, and new bone is deposited by osteoblasts in areas of tension along the distal surfaces.[2]

> **CLINICAL NOTE 2-3** Physiologic migration occurs throughout life in both mesial and occlusal directions.

CEMENTUM

The cementum covering the root surfaces of the teeth is a calcified structure formed by cementoblasts; it varies in thickness from 20 to 50 μm near the cementoenamel junction to 50 to 200 μm at the apex.[9] Once the cementoblasts are encased in cementum during the formation process, they are called cementocytes.

The cementum anchors the teeth, maintains occlusal relationships,[8] and provides a seal for the dentinal tubules.[4] It contains extrinsic fibers called Sharpey's fibers, which are the embedded portions of the fiber bundles that attach to the roots of the teeth (Figure 2-6).

> **CLINICAL NOTE 2-4** There are no vascular or nerve connections in the cementum so it cannot transmit pain sensations. This is why the cementum is not sensitive to scaling procedures.

TABLE 2-2	Periodontal Ligament Fiber Bundle Groups	
PERIODONTAL LIGAMENT BUNDLE GROUP	**PATH AND LOCATION OF FIBERS**	**MAJOR FUNCTION**
Alveolar crest	Runs from cementum, just apical to cementoenamel junction, to crestal bone	Retains tooth in socket; opposes lateral forces
Horizontal	Directly across periodontal ligament space	Attaches root surface to alveolar bone
Oblique	Courses in oblique direction across periodontal ligament space and into alveolar bone	Largest group of fiber bundles; transfers occlusal stresses to bone
Apical	Runs from apex of root into alveolar bone, both apical and lateral to root apex	Probably suspensory because it does not occur in erupting teeth
Interradicular	Spreads apically into bone, from furcation	Probably suspensory and protection of interradicular bone; present only in multirooted teeth

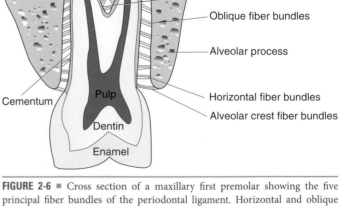

FIGURE 2-6 ■ Cross section of a maxillary first premolar showing the five principal fiber bundles of the periodontal ligament. Horizontal and oblique fibers are present throughout the periodontal ligament, not limited to the lateral portions of the root.

Labels: Apical fiber bundles; Interradicular fiber bundles; Oblique fiber bundles; Alveolar process; Horizontal fiber bundles; Alveolar crest fiber bundles; Cementum; Pulp; Dentin; Enamel

As reported by Carranza,[10] Schroeder described five types of cementum: acellular afibrillar cementum with no cementocytes and no fibers, acellular extrinsic fiber cementum with no cementocytes but with densely packed bundles of Sharpey's fibers, cellular mixed stratified cementum containing intrinsic fibers that may contain cells, cellular intrinsic fiber cementum containing cells but no extrinsic fibers, and intermediate cementum made up of cellular remnants in a calcified matrix.

Hydroxyapatite makes up about 50% of the inorganic components of cementum, which compares to 97% of enamel, 70% of dentin, and 65% of bone.[10] Incremental lines are readily seen in cementum, suggesting the dynamic nature of cementum, with alternating periods of apposition and periods of rest (Figure 2-7). A summary of the elements of cementum is presented in Table 2-3.

ALVEOLAR PROCESS

The **alveolar process** is the support system for the teeth. The alveolar process is similar to bone elsewhere in the body,[9] and it is an extension of the bone from the body of the mandible and the body of the maxilla. The alveolar bone lines the sockets of the teeth and provides bony support for the sockets. The walls of the sockets are called the **lamina dura** when viewed on radiographs. They may also be referred to as the cribriform plate on the basis of the histologic appearance of a dense plate of bone with many small holes perforating it. The dense plate of bone appears radiographically as a radio-opaque line around the roots of the teeth (Figure 2-8).[4,9] The term *cribriform plate* simply means a plate of bone with many perforations to permit the passage of blood vessels and nerves. The tooth sockets are called the alveoli.[10] The alveolar process is composed of three components:

1. The alveolar bone, the bone comprising the cribriform plate encompassing the alveoli, and adjacent cancellous bone
2. The compact bone, which makes up the facial and lingual cortical plates of bone
3. The trabecular and cancellous bone between the cortical plates surrounding the alveoli[8]

CLINICAL NOTE 2-5 The alveolar process functions as a unit, as indicated by its gradual resorption when teeth are lost.

The alveolar process is dependent on the teeth; the crest of the alveolar process follows the cementoenamel junction of the teeth. It is actually 2 to 3 mm apical to the cementoenamel junction and 0.5 to 1.5 mm apical to the epithelial attachment to the tooth in a state of periodontal health. The alveolar process is in a constant state of remodeling. This remodeling

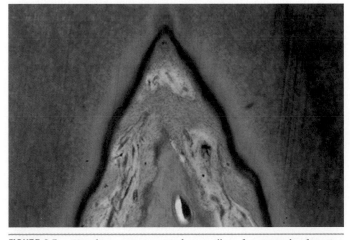

FIGURE 2-7 ■ Histologic appearance of a maxillary first premolar furcation area. Note the orientation of the periodontal ligament to the cementum (*dark line*). The interradicular alveolar bone appears as a triangular structure at the bottom of the illustration. The round lumen in the alveolar bone is a channel filled with a blood vessel. (Courtesy of Dr. Gary C. Armitage.)

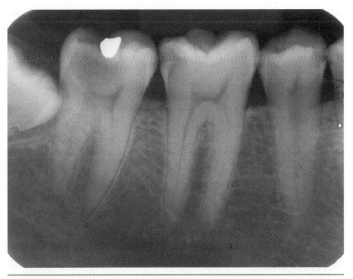

FIGURE 2-8 ■ Radiographic appearance of normal alveolar bone showing the lamina dura, trabecular bone, and periodontal ligament space. The cribriform plate appears as a distinct white line around the roots of the teeth. Note the presence of caries in the teeth and a small restoration, as well as a partially erupted third molar.

TABLE 2-3 Types of Cementum

TYPE OF CEMENTUM	LOCATION ON ROOT SURFACE	FIBERS	CEMENTOCYTES
Acellular afibrillar	Near cementoenamel junction	No	No
Acellular extrinsic fiber	Coronal third of root	Sharpey's fibers	No
Cellular mixed stratified	Apical third of root and furcations	Sharpey's fibers and intrinsic fibers	Yes
Cellular intrinsic fiber	Areas of resorption	Intrinsic fibers	Yes
Intermediate cementum	Near junction of cementum and dentin	No	Remnants

accommodates the physiologic tooth migration, bone apposition, and resorption that are constantly occurring at a slow rate.[6]

Alveoli

The **alveoli** are the tooth sockets. They are lined by the cribriform plate, which has thousands of pores through which the tooth and periodontal ligament are supplied with nerves and blood vessels. Each root of a multirooted tooth has its own alveolus.[8]

The bone lining the alveoli contains Sharpey's fibers, connections of the fiber bundles. It is referred to as a *bundle bone* because of the presence of many fibrils entering into the bone. This type of bone exists elsewhere in the body in locations where tendons or ligaments attach to bone.[10]

Compact Bone

Compact bone makes up the cortical plates on the facial and lingual sides of the jaws. This bone is dependent on the alignment of the teeth because it follows the contour of the root surfaces. The height and thickness of the compact bone are determined by this alignment, the angulation of the roots to the bone, and occlusal forces.[10]

Cancellous Bone

Cancellous bone lies between the cortical plates and the alveolar bone, connecting them. It is also known as spongiosum. In general, there is less spongiosum in the mandible than in the maxilla. The cancellous bone of the alveolar process blends into the spongiosum of the mandible and maxilla without demarcation.[8]

Variations in Normal Structure

There are three variations of the normal bone structure that are nonpathologic and of importance to periodontal health: **dehiscences**, **fenestrations**, and **tooth root proximity**. These configurations have consequences when the alveolar process is affected by periodontal disease. Therapeutic efforts are often modified to protect these areas and they can alter the prognosis for treatment.

Dehiscences. A dehiscence is a resorbed area of bone over the facial surface of the root. It can occur in patients with labially inclined roots.[8]

Fenestrations. A fenestration is an opening, or window, in the bone covering the facial surface of a root[8] or a boneless window between two adjacent roots that almost touch (Figure 2-9).[10]

Root Proximity. Teeth sometimes erupt in the alveolar process with roots that are very close together, termed *root proximity*. This can be due to poor alignment of teeth in the arch so that roots rest close together or from the roots of multirooted teeth being unusually widely spread out. There is some evidence that having roots close together near the coronal part of the root structure is related to having more severe periodontal attachment loss.[11]

Attachment Apparatus

The periodontal ligament, cementum, and alveolar bone are commonly referred to collectively as the **attachment apparatus**.

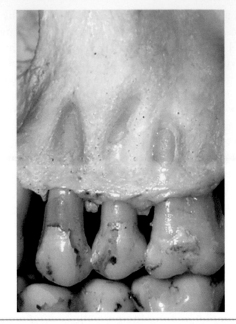

FIGURE 2-9 ■ Variations of normal alveolar bone include fenestrations and dehiscences. The defects on these roots are fenestrations. If the bone were missing over the root surface so that it did not look like a window, the defect would be a dehiscence.

BLOOD AND NERVE SUPPLY

Branches of the inferior and superior alveolar arteries supply blood to the periodontium. The superior alveolar artery supplies the maxilla and the inferior alveolar artery supplies the mandible. Branches of these vessels extend coronally from the apices of the teeth into the central alveolar bone and over the periosteum, terminating by penetrating into the periodontal ligament and alveolar bone. Other branches course along the surface of the alveolar bone and terminate in many capillary loops in the gingival connective tissue next to the epithelium.[6]

The nerve supply is from the trigeminal nerve and is sensory in nature. Branches of the nerves terminate in the periodontal ligament, the connective tissue, and on the surface of the alveolar bone. Nerve endings receive stimuli for pain (nociceptors) and position and pressure (proprioceptors).[6]

CLINICAL CONDITION OF THE PERIODONTAL TISSUES

It is primarily the gingival structures that are assessed to determine clinical signs of health or disease. These are also the areas that must be kept free of bacterial plaque biofilms, through personal and professional care, to maintain or restore periodontal health. Descriptions of the gingiva must note the clinical condition and either describe these structures as healthy or differentiate particular areas from those of normal appearance. Descriptions should include the color, size, shape or contour, texture, and consistency of the gingiva. The clinical characteristics of a healthy gingiva are presented in Table 2-4.

Color

The healthy gingiva is uniformly light pink or coral pink. Variations in color are produced by the vascular supply, the thickness and degree of keratinization, and the presence of melanin.[2,4,6] The mucogingival junction should be a clearly demarcated line, and the tissue apical to that line, the alveolar mucosa, should

TABLE 2-4	Characteristics of Healthy Gingiva		
CHARACTERISTIC	**FREE GINGIVA**	**ATTACHED GINGIVA**	**ALVEOLAR MUCOSA**
Color	Pink, light pink, or coral pink No redness May have melanin pigmentation	Pink, light pink, or coral pink No redness May have melanin pigmentation	Variations of red No red or white areas that are distinct from surrounding mucosa May have melanin pigmentation
Texture	Smooth, matte appearance May be stippled	Smooth, matte appearance May be stippled	Shiny No stippling
Size	No evidence of swelling	No evidence of swelling	No evidence of swelling

Shape	Knife-edged adaptation to tooth
	   surfaces
	
	Papillae should fill interproximal
	   spaces
		Continuous band of pink tissue
		   from apical edge of free
		   gingiva to mucogingival
		   junction
		Varies in thickness
			Smooth and flat to underlying bone

Consistency	Firm because of underlying
	   dense collagen
	Resilient when touched
		Firm because of underlying
		   dense collagen
		Resilient when touched
			Firm because of underlying bone
			
			Easily movable
			Not resilient

be bright red and shiny. The increased redness in alveolar mucosa is caused by increased vascularization, a nonkeratinized epithelium, and a less organized system of collagen fibrils. The alveolar mucosa should blend without demarcation into the vestibule or floor of the mouth. There is no mucogingival junction on the palate because all the tissue of the palate is keratinized masticatory mucosa.

Melanin pigmentation may be present. Melanin, a non–hemoglobin-derived brown pigment,[7] is the product of melanocytes in the gingiva. It is seen more often in black and Asian individuals than in whites.[8] The amount of pigmentation may vary greatly. It is uniform in some individuals but appears blotchy or irregular in others. Clinically, melanin pigmentation represents normal variations in the color of the gingiva (see Figure 2-3).

Texture

The stippled outer texture of the gingiva should provide a matte appearance (not shiny) when dried. The free gingiva should be smooth and the attached gingiva may appear stippled, resembling an orange peel. Stippling reflects protuberances of connective tissue into the epithelium, called rete pegs, and both stippled and nonstippled gingivae are keratinized.[4,7] Stippling varies with age. It appears in children at approximately 5 years of age, increases in adulthood, and becomes less pronounced in old age.[2]

Size

The gingiva should not be enlarged; its size should equal the total of its cellular elements and vascular supply.[2] Clinically, size is assessed by the presence or absence of swelling or other enlargement. As the gingiva responds to the collection of inflammatory infiltrate within, it swells and appears shiny because the natural stippling is lost.

Shape or Contour

The shape of the gingiva depends on the size and alignment of the teeth. The marginal gingiva should follow a scalloped line

around the crowns and lie flat to the tooth. This contour is sometimes referred to as knife-edged.[2,4] In general, papillae should fill the interdental spaces. The contour can be influenced by the shape, size, and position of the teeth and the relationship of the tooth contact areas.

Consistency

The consistency, or tone, of a healthy attached gingiva is firm because of the tight attachment of the fiber bundles in the underlying connective tissue to the bone and cementum.[4] It should be resilient[2,4,7] when gently touched by the back of an instrument. The free gingiva should also be firm in texture, not soft or spongy.

Sulcus Depth

The normal clinical sulcus depth, when measured by a periodontal probe, is 1 to 3 mm.[3] Measurements vary from clinician to clinician depending on pressure exerted on the probe and angulation of entry into the sulcus. The sulcular epithelium is intact in the healthy state, not ulcerated, and should not bleed on gentle probing.[2-4,7]

AGING AND THE HEALTHY PERIODONTIUM

Over a lifetime, various changes occur that are reflected in the tissues of the periodontium. The gingiva has been described as thinning with decreased keratinization of the epithelium, flattening of the rete pegs, and altered cell density. Connective tissue is reported to become more dense and coarse with age. The periodontal ligament reflects fewer cells and has a more irregular structure. Cementum becomes thickened by up to 10 times its width in youth as a result of continued apposition over the lifetime. Alveolar bone develops a less regular surface and collagen fiber insertion becomes less orderly.[12]

In a thoughtful review, Needleman[12] reported that on a purely biologic or physiologic basis, aging has negligible effects on the course of periodontal disease and its treatment. It is important to note that as individuals age other physiologic phenomena occur, such as loss of dexterity and reduced eyesight, and these changes may considerably alter the patient's ability to participate in the treatment of periodontal disease, thus affecting its outcome.

CLINICAL NOTE 2-6 The dental hygienist must consider the overall effects of aging when working with periodontal patients and perhaps modify suggested therapies, but not because the disease process itself is different.

HOST RESPONSE

Each person reacts to disease processes with a range of responses that is mediated by that individual's ability to react to assault by bacteria, viruses, tumor growth, injury, and a myriad of other influences. The **immune system** is responsible for the body's reaction, called the host response. **Immunology** is the study of the immune system and host response.

The development of disease in the healthy periodontium depends on both the microbial assault from dental plaque biofilms, which is described in Chapter 4, and the host response. The amount and type of pathogenic bacteria present in disease alone does not explain the variation seen in the degree of individual response. However, the contribution of the microbial population to periodontal disease cannot be minimized because infectious agents must be present for the disease to occur.[13-15] This section provides a brief introduction into the complex discipline of immunology so that the student can begin to understand how reactions of the human body are related to the etiology and pathogenesis of periodontal disease. Not only does microbial interaction with the individual patient play an important role in the development of disease, but the immune responses alone can manifest as disease processes in gingival and periodontal tissues. The actions of microbes and cells in the host cause inflammatory reactions, resulting in clinical inflammation. Inflammation is protective in that it leads to destruction of bacterial assault, but the complex immune system defenses can also lead to tissue alteration and destruction in the host. The consequences of inflammatory response can damage and destroy periodontal tissues, often leading to irreversible changes in the architecture of the periodontium.

The host response acts to wall off infections, localizing them to the specific tissues—in this case, the periodontal tissues. These attempts to isolate the effects of the microbial assault are also likely to result in some local tissue destruction, which in turn results in what we know as periodontal disease.[13] Simply put, in periodontal disease the bacterial plaque and its products infect the root surfaces. The inflammatory response attempts to get the infected roots away from the rest of the body. This response is an extremely complex set of events and is the focus of much investigation. An introductory knowledge is most easily gained by understanding the host response components and their actions. These components consist of the inflammatory cells—**antibody, antigen, complement**—and the **hypersensitivity (allergic) reactions**. Figure 2-10 shows examples of inflammatory periodontal changes resulting from various influences.

CLINICAL NOTE 2-7 It is important to note that the tissue destruction seen in periodontal disease results mainly from the host response. It is caused by the complex set of reactions that occur in the immune system.

INFLAMMATORY CELLS

Inflammatory cells are attracted to areas of the body by stimuli such as trauma or microbial influences; this signaling process is called **chemotaxis.** Cells such as polymorphonuclear leukocytes (PMNs or neutrophils), macrophages, lymphocytes, and plasma cells are chemotactically attracted to areas of tissue damage. In periodontal disease, the inflammatory cells are attracted to the gingiva, connective tissue, periodontal ligament, and bone. Once concentrated at the area of stimulus, the cells perform several functions; they **phagocytize** (ingest and neutralize) bacteria, they consume bacterial components, and they remove damaged tissues. Inflammatory cells also secrete products that affect the permeability of blood vessels, cause cell disintegration (referred to as **lysis**), or cause the destruction of alveolar bone by inducing osteoclastic activity. Some of these cells, such as certain lymphocytes, divide to increase their numbers in a process called blastogenesis, thus cascading their effects. The following is a brief description of some of the cells involved in these inflammatory reactions.[16]

Lymphocytes

Lymphocytes recognize foreign molecules, which are functionally called antigens. Cells, usually **macrophages,** take up antigens and present them to the lymphocytes for destruction. The recognition of antigens by lymphocytes is specific; they react to an individual antigen and then retain a memory so that the antigen is recognized again months or years later.

There are three types of lymphocytic cells–T lymphocytes, B lymphocytes, and killer or natural killer (NK) cells. T lymphocytes are derived from the thymus, have several subsets, and are active in cell-mediated (humoral or antibody-mediated) immune responses. They occur as helper T cells, which assist B cells in the production of antibody (protein that binds and disables antigen), or as cytotoxic T cells, which stimulate cytotoxic activity in other cells such as macrophages. The B lymphocytes are derived from the liver, spleen, and bone marrow. They serve as receptor sites for antigens and are the precursors of plasma cells. Helper T cells stimulate B cells to differentiate into plasma cells, and plasma cells produce antibodies. In addition, B cells stimulate other T cells so that the immune response grows. Antigen processing by macrophages leads to the development of NK cells. The NK cells produce antibodies and a variety of products to stimulate microbicidal effects of the immune response, and they are effective against viruses and tumor cells.[16]

Polymorphonuclear Leukocytes

PMNs, also called neutrophils, are attracted to periodontal lesions, particularly acute lesions, by chemotaxis. They make up about 70% of the circulating leukocytes.[16] PMNs phagocytize (digest) microorganisms and contain destructive substances that are very important in periodontal infections. PMNs contain granules that are filled with enzymes such as collagenase or

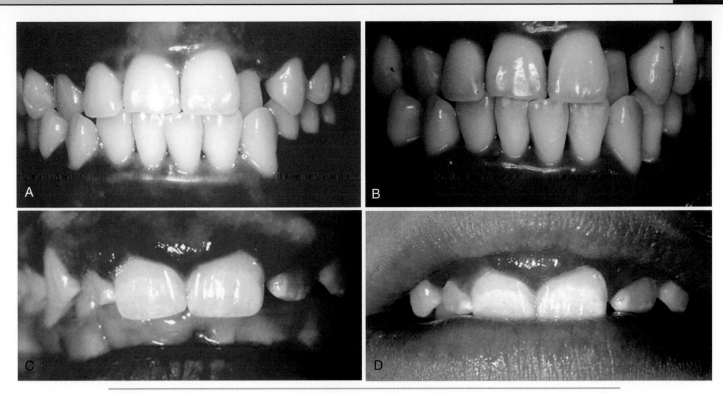

FIGURE 2-10 ■ Inflammatory responses of the gingiva. A, Dental plaque biofilm–induced gingivitis caused the inflammatory response seen here, including intense redness from capillary proliferation and inflammatory response in the tissue. The shiny appearance of the marginal gingiva is caused by swelling. The tissue was spongy and soft when touched gently. The tissue also bled very easily when probed, and the patient stated that the gingiva bled when he brushed his teeth. **B,** After dental hygiene treatment consisting of oral hygiene instructions, scaling, and root planing, the tissue responded well. This photograph was taken 1 week after treatment. The redness is reduced and the tissue no longer bleeds when probed by the dental hygienist or when the patient brushes. There is still some shininess to the tissue but the stippling is returning. **C,** Inflammation occurs for reasons other than the presence of dental plaque biofilms (see Chapter 6). This child demonstrated inflammation of the marginal gingiva primarily around the anterior teeth. **D,** Further observation of the child revealed that he did not fully close his lips much of the time. The inflammation resulted from constant drying of the marginal gingiva, a condition referred to as "mouth breathing." This condition did not resolve with plaque removal.

elastase. These enzymes are released and cause tissue destruction when the PMN cells degranulate. Abnormalities in PMNs can lead to more severe periodontal disease if the cells are unable to perform their functions or lack specific granules.

Mast Cells

Mast cells are important in mediating the inflammatory response. Their stimulation results in increased vascular permeability, which advances the inflammatory response.[16]

Macrophages

Macrophages are scavenger cells with important phagocytic activity. They can engulf and digest a wide variety of bacteria. Macrophages differentiate from monocytes, another type of white blood cell, when they leave the bloodstream and complete their differentiation in the tissues.[16] The functioning of macrophages is stimulated by the complement reaction (see later discussion). They are protective in that they phagocytize bacteria, but they produce enzymes and other substances that may play a significant role in collagen destruction, which leads to the loss of periodontal tissues.

Auxiliary Cells

Many cells can become involved in the immune response because they react to **cytokines**, which are released by the lymphoid cells and phagocytes. These cells include basophils, eosinophils, and platelets. Mast cells and basophils contain histamine and other substances important in hypersensitivity reactions. When these cells are activated, histamine and other substances that mediate hypersensitivity reactions are released and may enhance collagen destruction and bone resorption. Both eosinophils and platelets also produce a variety of mediating substances.[2]

EFFECTOR MOLECULES

The human body responds to tumor cells, bacteria, or their expressed products by plasma cell production of antibodies (immunoglobulins). First, antigens, the foreign molecules of the invading cell or substance, are recognized and then **effector molecules** are stimulated as part of systems that eliminate foreign substances. There are many effector molecules present in the complex immune system. Three of the most well understood and important molecules—antibodies, complement, and cytokines—are briefly described.

Antibodies

Antibody (**immunoglobulin**) production is a complex process involving macrophages processing antigens and presenting the fragments to T cells, which interact with B cells that differentiate into plasma cells, which produce the antibodies. Antibodies are found in blood, tissue fluids (e.g., gingival fluid), and secretions, and make up about 20% of serum protein. Antibodies are highly specific and sensitive. Human immunoglobulins (Ig) are divided into nine distinct classes on the basis of structural differences: IgG1, IgG2, IgG3, IgG4G, IgM, IgE, IgD, IgA1, and IgA2. The structural differences are responsible for variation in effects.[18]

Antibody responses appear to play an important role in periodontal disease. A strong antibody response is often seen in periodontal disease, the extent of the antibody response is positively related to the clinical severity of the disease in many cases, and the antibody response diminishes when the disease is treated.[14] The relationship is complex and research will further elucidate the significance of the role of antibodies in periodontal disease.

Complement

Complement is made up of proteins and glycoproteins that account for about 5% of the proteins in human serum. It has many functions, including bacteriolysis (destruction of bacteria) and promotion of the immune response. Proteins are not antibodies, so their concentration is not affected by immunization, as is the case with immunoglobulins. Complement reacts in concert with IgG and IgM, causing lysis and functional alteration of cell walls, which encourage phagocytosis. Bacteria can help protect themselves from this effect by developing a coating. Complement also mediates the degranulation of mast cells, which causes the release of histamine and other substances that increase permeability of small blood vessels. Increased permeability permits migration of PMNs and increased phagocytic activity in the area. The complement reaction occurs in a sequenced and cascading way; once begun, the reaction continues until it is complete. This allows for tremendous amplification of the immune response to a relatively small insult by antigen. The reaction also leads to a variety of effects that can result in destruction of periodontal tissues.

Cytokines

Cytokines are substances produced by the stimulated immune cells. They provide the communication between cells that mediates the complex interactions between cells and cellular elements. Cytokines assist in the development and regulation of immune effector cells (e.g., increasing the number of T cells so that their effects increase), cause cell to cell communication, and are themselves effector molecules. This is a very complex communication system. Many cytokines have been identified; they have effects on all cells of the immune system, act on many target cells, and play a major role in both the pathogenesis of disease and healing.[15]

Cytokines used to be named for their action, such as MAF (macrophage-activating factor) or OAF (osteoclast-activating factor). Cytokines are more commonly referred to as interleukins (IL), describing their communication function with leukocytes. They are referred to by number, such as IL-1 and IL-2. Other cytokines are named for their specific function, such as lymphotoxin or interferon. Interferon is of special interest because of its antiviral properties. Cytokines, specifically lymphotoxin, are found in large amounts in response to

plaque bacteria antigens in periodontal disease. Lymphotoxin is important because it can stimulate bone and cartilage resorption, leading to the destructive changes seen in periodontal disease. Cytokines can also have general cytotoxic effects on host cells when plaque bacteria antigens are present for long periods.

Figure 2-11 presents a diagrammatic scheme of the complex interrelationships among the major components of the host response in the periodontal pocket affecting the epithelium, the connective tissue, and the alveolar bone.

HYPERSENSITIVITY (ALLERGIC) REACTIONS

Allergic reactions are usually protective in nature. They are reactions to foreign bacteria, viruses, or other substances. They may also cause tissue destruction by triggering overreactions called hypersensitivity reactions. Tissue damage can occur in a host who has been sensitized by one exposure to a substance and then challenged again by the same substance. There are four types of hypersensitivity reactions: anaphylaxis or type I, cytotoxic or type II, immune complex or type III, and cell-mediated (delayed) or type IV. Types I, II, and III are immediate reactions and occur within minutes or hours; they are the more likely reactions to affect the periodontal tissues. Type IV reactions are delayed and can occur days later or beyond.

Histamine is released in type I hypersensitivity reactions. This can be a generalized or localized reaction. The generalized histamine release can lead to serious life-threatening consequences, as can be seen in individuals with food or drug allergies. A localized reaction can result in increased tissue destruction in an area such as the periodontium. Histamine is found in higher concentrations in chronically inflamed gingivae than in healthy gingivae. Histamine causes many actions, including increased capillary and venule permeability, which attracts more immune cells to an area and increases the inflammatory response.

Cytotoxic reactions, or type II hypersensitivity responses, result in the breakdown of tissue or blood cells. They are the products of antibodies that react directly to antigens tightly bound to the surfaces of cells. These reactions are not seen in gingival or periodontal disease but are manifested in other oral diseases such as pemphigus, where antibodies react directly with epithelial cell membranes.

Immune complex (Arthus) reactions, or type III hypersensitivity reactions, occur when high levels of antigen persist in an area without being eliminated. The reaction occurs around small blood vessels and activates complement, and can cause extensive localized tissue damage. An example of a type III or Arthus reaction is the wheal and flare response seen in skin tests for tuberculosis.

Cell-mediated, delayed, or type IV hypersensitivity reactions are related to the reaction of antigens with the surface of T lymphocytes. Once sensitized to an antigen, these lymphocytes can undergo blastogenesis, or transformation, resulting in mitotic division and greatly increasing the number of immunocompetent (reactive) cells sensitized to the specific antigen. These reactions explain why, on a second exposure to an allergic agent such as a bee sting, the reaction can be greatly increased and possibly become life-threatening.

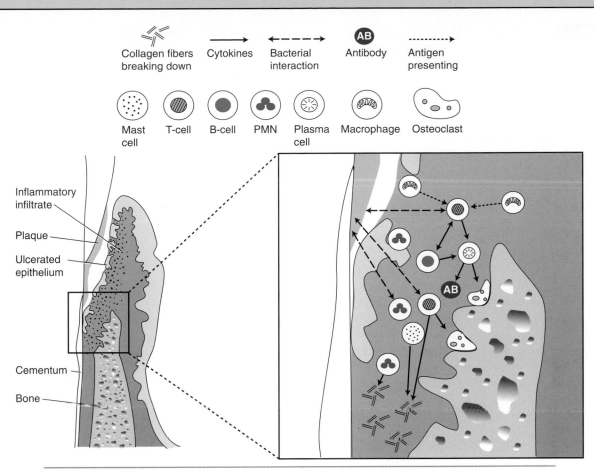

FIGURE 2-11 ■ Effects and interactions of cells in the immune response. PMNs are attracted to the site to phagocytize bacteria and neutralize toxic substances. Mast cells degranulate and produce substances that affect collagen destruction. Macrophages are phagocytic and present antigens to T cells and B cells to amplify the immune response. T cells produce cytokines, which regulate the immune response. B cells proliferate and mature to become plasma cells. Plasma cells produce antibodies that provide both local and systemic immune responses. Antibodies also alter bacteria so they can be phagocytized. Cytokines and bacterial interactions mediate this cascading cellular response. (Courtesy of Randal W. Rowland, MS, DMD, MS.)

The host response aspects of periodontal diseases are expanding areas of inquiry in dentistry. As these complex interactions are better understood, the disease process, particularly why it affects individuals differently, will become clearer. As understanding grows, the therapies to be discussed in later chapters in this book will also be refined and made more patient-specific.

CLINICAL NOTE 2-8 It is important to appreciate the significance of the host response. In treating periodontal disease, therapeutic scaling and root planing of one quadrant of teeth appears to invoke healing in untreated areas. This phenomenon is seen is clinical trials where untreated areas of the mouth show significant improvement in the course of the study.[16] It is thought that the stimulation of the host response against plaque antigens results in the unforeseen healing in untreated areas.[17]

OTHER PROTECTIVE RESPONSES IN THE ORAL ENVIRONMENT

The normal function of the oral epithelium is protective in nature, acting as a very effective barrier to mechanical and microbial assault. The host response acts to wall off infections when they do occur. The presence and amount of gingival fluid and the ameliorating effects of saliva affect the interface between the surface of the tissues and the host. These two substances play a protective role in the host[18] and are briefly described here.

Gingival or Sulcular Fluid

Gingival or sulcular fluid is considered an inflammatory exudate because it is present in much larger amounts when the gingiva is inflamed than when in the healthy state. It also increases with normal physiologic functions, such as the mastication of coarse foods, toothbrushing, increases in female sex hormones, smoking, and after periodontal surgery.

The sulcular epithelium permits migration of molecules into the gingival sulcus, although in very small amounts. The resulting fluid contains enzymes, cellular elements, electrolytes, and compounds such as glucose. Leukocytes, white blood cells (primarily PMNs), are excreted, making up about 92% of the cellular content of the fluid. These cells appear extravascularly in the connective tissue, travel across the epithelium, and are expelled into the sulcus. It is presumed that these cells protect against the extension of plaque biofilm into the sulcus.[18]

Saliva

Saliva exerts several major protective influences in the oral environment. These include lubrication, physical protection, cleansing, buffering, remineralization of teeth, and antibacterial actions.[19] Saliva contains organic elements that can cause structural damage to oral organisms, antibodies to inactivate bacteria so they can be engulfed by leukocytes, and enzymes to inhibit tissue breakdown. Saliva has an important buffering action to maintain the pH level in the mouth, thus reducing the demineralization of teeth. It contains coagulation factors to hasten blood coagulation and protect wounds from bacteria and minerals to restore tooth structure through remineralization. It also exhibits a major influence on plaque formation and maturation.[18]

Saliva is an extremely complex substance whose functions are far from fully understood. An increased incidence of both caries and periodontal disease is seen in people who have xerostomia (reduced salivary function or dry mouth), a condition that may occur for many reasons.[18]

◎ DENTAL HYGIENE CONSIDERATIONS

- Understanding the anatomic characteristics of the periodontium is essential background for providing assessments of disease, therapy, and evaluation of healing.
- Architecture of the alveolar bone is related to clinical characteristics of the periodontium.
- A normal healthy gingiva is predictable in color, texture, size, shape, and consistency.
- The immune system plays an important role in periodontal health and healing.
- Gingival crevicular fluid and saliva are protective of periodontal health.

✷ CASE SCENARIO

Mr. Marshall, a 40-year-old patient, arrives for your dental hygiene care. You have never met Mr. Marshall before and in reviewing his medical history, you see that he had multiple abdominal surgeries as a child. He states that he has an allergy to latex from the multiple exposures to the surgeon's gloves during these surgeries.

1. What type of allergic reaction has the patient developed?
   A. Anaphylaxis or type I reaction
   B. Cytotoxic or type II reaction
   C. Immune complex or type III reaction
   D. Cell-mediated or type IV reaction
2. The protective responses of the oral environment will protect Mr. Marshall from an allergic reaction because they assist in providing a barrier to microbial assault.
   A. Both the statement and the reason are correct and related.
   B. Both the statement and the reason are correct but NOT related.
   C. The statement is correct, but the reason is NOT correct.
   D. The statement is NOT correct, but the reason is correct.
   E. NEITHER the statement NOR the reason is correct.
3. You should not use latex products on Mr. Marshall or wear latex gloves to treat him because the cells sensitized to latex have produced many reactive cells also sensitive to the latex antigen.
   A. Both the statement and the reason are correct and related.
   B. Both the statement and the reason are correct but NOT related.
   C. The statement is correct, but the reason is NOT correct.
   D. The statement is NOT correct, but the reason is correct.
   E. NEITHER the statement NOR the reason is correct.

STUDY QUESTIONS

Answers and rationales to these questions can be obtained from your instructor.

MULTIPLE CHOICE

1. The attachment apparatus is made up of
   A. lamina dura and alveoli.
   B. periodontal ligament fiber bundles.
   C. elements of the junctional epithelium.
   D. periodontal ligament, cementum, and alveolar bone.
   E. Sharpey's fibers, cementum, and periodontal ligament fiber bundles.
2. The window of bone in healthy bone structure covering the surface of the root is called a dehiscence. The dehiscence is a significant structure in periodontal disease.
   A. Both statements are true.
   B. Both statements are false.
   C. The first statement is true, and the second statement is false.
   D. The first statement is false, and the second statement is true.
3. Cells attracted to areas of the body by stimuli such as microbial influence or trauma are referred to as
   A. cytokines.
   B. blood cells.
   C. chemotactic cells.
   D. inflammatory cells.

4. Inflammatory cells perform all of the following functions EXCEPT one. Which one is the EXCEPTION?
   A. Lyse cells
   B. Phagocytize bacteria
   C. Remove damaged tissue
   D. Reduce osteoclastic activity

5. B lymphocytes come from the liver, spleen, and bone marrow. B lymphocytes are important in the antigen-antibody response.
   A. Both statements are true.
   B. Both statements are false.
   C. The first statement is true, and the second statement is false.
   D. The first statement is false, and the second statement is true.

6. The term *probing depth* is more accurate than the term *sulcus depth* for the clinician because the latter term is for histologic description only.
   A. Both the statement and reason are correct and related
   B. Both the statement and reason are correct but NOT related.
   C. The statement is correct, but the reason is NOT correct.
   D. The statement is NOT correct, but the reason is correct.
   E. NEITHER the statement NOR the reason is correct.

7. The periodontal ligament fiber group that runs from the cementum to the crestal bone is termed
   A. alveolar crest.
   B. apical.
   C. horizontal.
   D. interradicular.
   E. oblique.

8. The presence of gingival fluid will increase
   A. after mastication of soft foods.
   B. before periodontal surgery.
   C. with inflammation.
   D. after menopause.

SHORT ANSWER

9. Describe the color, size, shape, texture, and consistency of the normal gingiva.
10. List the protective effects of saliva.

Ⓔ Please visit **http://evolve.elsevier.com/Perry/periodontology** for additional practice and study support tools.

REFERENCES

1. *Dorland's Medical Dictionary*. 32nd ed. New York, NY: Elsevier; 2011.
2. Fiorellini JP, Kim DM, Guzin Uzel N. Anatomy of the periodontium. In: Newman MG, Takei HH, Klokkevold PR, et al, eds. *Carranza's Clinical Periodontology*. 11th ed. St. Louis, MO: Elsevier Saunders; 2012:12–32.
3. Löe H, Listgarten MA, Terranova VP. The gingival structure and function. In: Genco RJ, Goldman HM, Cohen DW, eds. *Contemporary Periodontics*. St Louis, MO: Mosby; 1990:3–32.
4. Wilkins EM. *Clinical Practice of the Dental Hygienist*. 10th ed. Philadelphia, PA: Lippincott Williams & Wilkins; 2009:208–222.
5. Armitage GC. Clinical recognition and assessment of chronic inflammatory periodontal disease. In: *Biologic Basis of Periodontal Maintenance Therapy*. Berkeley, CA: Praxis; 1980:1–32.
6. Ryder MI. Anatomy, development and physiology of the periodontium. In: Rose LF, Mealey BL, Genco RJ, et al, eds. *Periodontics: Medicine, Surgery and Implants*. St. Louis, MO: Elsevier Mosby; 2004:3–18.
7. Vernino A, Gray J, Hughes E. *The Periodontic Syllabus*. 5th ed. Philadelphia, PA: Lippincott Williams & Wilkins; 2007.
8. Hassell TM. Tissues and cells of the periodontium. *Periodontol 2000*. 1993;3:9–38.
9. Fiorellini JP, Kim DM, Guzin Uzel N. Clinical Features of Gingivitis. In: Newman MG, Takei HH, Klokkevold PR, et al, eds: *Carranza's Clinical Periodontology*. 11th ed. St. Louis, MO: Elsevier Saunders; 2012:76–83.
10. Terranova VP, Goldman HM, Listgarten MA. The periodontal attachment apparatus structure, function, and chemistry. In: Genco RJ, Goldman HM, Cohen DW, eds. *Contemporary Periodontics*. St. Louis, MO: Mosby; 1990: 33–54.
11. Vermylen K, DeQuincey GNT, Wolffe GN, et al. Root proximity as a risk marker for periodontal disease: a case-controlled study. *J Clin Periodontol*. 2005;32:260–265.
12. Needleman I. Aging and the periodontium. In: Newman MG, Takei HH, Klokkevold PR, et al, eds. *Carranza's Clinical Periodontology*. 11th ed. St Louis, MO: Elsevier Saunders; 2012:28–33.
13. Genco RJ. Host responses in periodontal diseases: current concepts. *J Periodontol*. 1992;63;338–355.
14. Rowland RR. Immunoinflammatory responses in periodontal diseases. In: Rose LF, Mealey BL, eds. *Periodontics: Medicine, Surgery, and Implants*. St. Louis, MO: Elsevier Mosby; 2004:85–98.
15. Offenbacher S. Periodontal diseases: pathogenesis. *Ann Periodontol*. 1996;1:821–878.
16. Kaldahl WB, Kalkwarf KL, Patil KD, et al. Evaluation of four modalities of periodontal therapy: mean probing depth, probing attachment level and recession changes. *J Periodontol*. 1988;59:783–793.
17. Ebersole JL, Taubman MA, Smith DJ, et al. Effect of subgingival scaling on systemic antibody responses to oral microorganisms. *Infect Immun*. 1985;48:534–539.
18. Bulkacz J, Carranza FA Jr. Defense mechanisms of the gingiva. In: Newman MG, Takei HH, Klokkevold PR, et al, eds. *Carranza's Clinical Periodontology*. 11th ed. St. Louis, MO: Elsevier Saunders; 2012:66–71.
19. Drisko CH. Non-surgical pocket therapy: pharmacotherapeutics. *Ann Periodontol*. 1996;1:491–566.

Epidemiology of Periodontal Diseases

Dorothy A. Perry

LEARNING OUTCOMES

- Define epidemiology.
- Explain the relationship of this discipline to the identification and treatment of gingival and periodontal disease.
- Compare and contrast the plaque, calculus, bleeding, and periodontal indices that are used to quantify conditions in the oral cavity.
- Explain how population scoring systems are applied to the diagnosis and treatment of disease.

- Describe the national prevalence data relating to tooth loss and gingival and periodontal disease.
- Explain how national prevalence data are used to understand the status of periodontal health in the United States.
- List the major risk factors and determinants that are related to periodontal disease.
- Describe the disease prevalence trends revealed for gingival and periodontal disease.
- State the prevalence of aggressive periodontitis.

KEY TERMS

Calculus index
Calibrated
Case-control studies
Cohort studies
Community Index of Periodontal
  Treatment Needs (CIPTN)
Cross-sectional studies
Epidemiologic research
Epidemiology

Generalization
Gingival fluid flow
Gingival Index (GI)
Incidence
Indexes or indices
Miller Index of Tooth Mobility (MI)
Periodontal Disease Index (PDI)
Periodontal Screening and Recording
  (PSR)

Plaque Index of Silness and Löe (PI I)
Prevalence
Risk factors
Russell's Periodontal Index (PI)
Sample
Severity
Simplified Oral Hygiene Index (OHI-S)
Sulcus Bleeding Index (SBI)
Volpe-Manhold Index (VI)

EPIDEMIOLOGY

Epidemiology is the study of health and disease and associated factors in human populations. It also includes how the states of health and disease in the population are influenced by heredity, biology, physical environment, social environment, and personal behavior.[1] Epidemiology measures disease in several ways:

- Prevalence of disease, the number of individuals or sites with disease present in a given population at one time
- Incidence of disease, the rate of occurrence of new disease in a population over a given period of time
- Severity of disease, the level of disease, and risk, the probability that a site will become diseased
- Risk factors, which are exposures, behaviors, and characteristics associated with disease[2]

Epidemiologic research differs from clinical research in that entire groups are the focus of study, not individuals, and that persons without the disease are included in studies to assess the risk of having the disease among the members of a population.[1] It is important to understand that prevalence alone, simply counting the number of individuals in a given population with disease, is not sufficient to understand gingival and periodontal disease in the population.

Epidemiologic research uses relatively simple calculations to assess disease in a population. Prevalence is computed by dividing the number of persons with the disease by the number of persons in the population (P = number with disease/number in population).

Incidence is computed by dividing the number of new cases of the disease by the number of persons at risk in the population (I = number of new cases/number at risk).[2]

These calculations are based on evaluations of lots of individuals who make up the population being studied. Common types of experimental designs used in epidemiologic research, cross-sectional studies, cohort studies, and case-control studies,[2] are described in Box 3-1.

BOX 3-1   Types of Epidemiologic Studies

Cross-Sectional

These studies assess the presence or absence of disease at a particular point in time. An entire population or a defined subset (sample) that is representative of the population is examined to determine the prevalence of disease (extent present in the population).

Cohort

This type of study identifies a population to examine over time. Typically the individuals in the population are disease-free at the beginning and are monitored for the onset of disease. These studies help assess incidence of disease (numbers of new cases) and associated risk factors (characteristics or behaviors that make the disease more likely to develop).

Case-Control

These studies compare individuals with disease and those without the disease. They identify characteristics that are associated with the disease but cannot assess prevalence or incidence.

When patients are treated in the clinical setting, it is clear that periodontal diseases are complex interactions of bacterial infection, host response, and patient behaviors. Epidemiologic research:

- Demonstrates how much of a population is affected by periodontal disease
- Describes the severity of the disease in a group of individuals
- Identifies characteristics or behaviors likely to be found in persons with the disease

However, to make these observations about populations, researchers must define what constitutes gingival and periodontal disease. This is done by clinical assessment of a group within the population using scales or indices. All individuals within the population can be assessed or just a **sample**. Ideally, sample individuals are selected by identifying members of the group at random (there are computer programs called random number generators that can do this) so as not to select all individuals with some common characteristic. For example, if you chose to study everyone in the population whose last name began with "B," you might be selecting many individuals who are related; thus your data could be affected by family characteristics. If you selected randomly from all members of the population, familial characteristics would be spread out over the entire group and much less likely to affect your results. Sample selection is a very important characteristic of epidemiologic research and every study describes the process used.

CLINICAL NOTE 3-1 Epidemiologic studies provide information about entire populations including incidence, severity, risk of getting the disease, and associated risk factors.

Once the sample is selected, the individuals must be examined for clinical characteristics of disease using **indexes** or **indices.** The data then describe a general picture of the disease in the population. For example, periodontal disease can be defined as having probe depths of greater than 4 mm in at least one site in the mouth, so you can determine how many people in the population have that characteristic. It can also be defined

as having one or more probe depths of 7 mm or having the gingival tissue bleed when probed in one or more sites. Therefore, it is important to understand the definition of disease in the study. As you will see, a study that defines periodontal disease as bleeding at one site will provide a very different picture of disease than one that defines it as one or more 7-mm probe depths in the same population. In addition, you might want to know what percentage of the population with periodontal disease (as you have defined it) uses tobacco and compare that to the number of those in the population who use tobacco but do not fit your definition of periodontal disease.

The examiner or team of examiners is trained to apply the indices to members of a population. This means the examiners are **calibrated**, or standardized, so that what one examiner would interpret as a 4-mm probing depth, all would interpret the same way. It is impossible to have 100% agreement among examiners at all times, but with training they can agree most of the time. This agreement is essential for the information collected to be meaningful, and so that the data can be accurately interpreted. Imagine the difficulty if one examiner probed 7 mm and another probed 5 mm in the same pocket and the definition of periodontal disease is 6 mm. That patient might not be accurately classified as with or without the disease. The calibration process permits the epidemiologic data to provide meaningful information.

Another important point about epidemiologic research is related to the population of individuals to be examined. It is impossible to examine every person in large epidemiologic studies, so representative samples are selected. This can be done through random selection of subjects as mentioned earlier, or very sophisticated sampling techniques using subsets of the population. In either of these cases, the results found in the sample can be generalized to a much larger group of the population, but rarely to everyone in the world. This is referred to as **generalization** of results. As an example, in the past epidemiologic studies of heart disease were conducted solely on men, so although the findings could be generalized to men, there was real concern about applying the findings to women. These studies now include women because treatment effects or risk factors need to be assessed on the basis of differences, such as gender, in populations. Also, an epidemiologic study of an American population might not be at all representative of the population in Mexico, China, or any other country because there are many cultural differences that influence health.

CLINICAL NOTE 3-2 Epidemiologic research provides a general picture of the health of the population.

Although it is complex, epidemiologic research gives us important insights into health problems. It is very important for dental hygienists to understand the number of people in the population with periodontal disease, how severe it is, and what behaviors or characteristics are associated with the disease.

Epidemiologic data do not provide absolute values for a population, and studies differ in their findings as a result of differences in population, examiners, or measuring scales. However, well-designed, well-run epidemiologic studies provide us with much information that is distinct from information gained from clinical studies. Epidemiology provides a general understanding of the disease occurring in patients. For example, we know that periodontal disease occurs in a relatively small but significant percentage of the U.S. population, so not everyone seeking dental hygiene treatment has periodontal disease. However, it is also important to remember that in clinical practice, when a patient with periodontal disease requires dental hygiene care, the disease affects 100% of that person. Dental hygiene care is dictated by the specific findings for that person, not general population findings.

> **CLINICAL NOTE 3-3** The dental hygienist must treat the specific disease presented by individual patients.

The following section describes important epidemiologic indices to help the dental hygienist understand the common measurements used to define periodontal disease. Current data will be briefly reviewed to describe the overall periodontal health of U.S. populations. Several risk factors associated with more severe disease will be described, and other population study data will be presented.

REVIEW OF IMPORTANT INDICES

Epidemiologic data are collected with well-defined measuring systems known as indices. These indices have defined scales, are easily applied to populations of individuals, and measure some specific aspect of the disease or condition of interest—in this case, signs of periodontal disease.

Several indices have been used to evaluate the periodontal status of populations. In each case, the units of measurement are defined with upper and lower limits. This section explains what it means to say that the population had a mean (average) plaque index of 2 or that 7% of the population had severe periodontal disease characterized by one or more deep pockets. It is important to consider the scoring system used when interpreting research results because they are all different. For a detailed discussion of all indices, see Wilkins.[3]

PLAQUE DEBRIS INDICES

Plaque is an important quantity to define because it is the etiologic agent in periodontal disease. Screening populations for the presence of plaque determines whether all the people have plaque, how much, and how it relates to other signs of disease. Sometimes plaque is measured by a simple scale, presence (scored as 1) or absence (scored as 0). If all plaque caused periodontal disease, this approach might be sufficient. However, plaque is clearly associated with gingivitis.[4,5] Thus, the quantity of plaque provides a picture of oral hygiene (e.g., where the accumulation is greatest and how good or poor oral hygiene practices are in a given population) and can indicate the presence of gingivitis. It does not correlate well with periodontal disease.

PLAQUE INDEX OF SILNESS AND LÖE[5]

The **Plaque Index of Silness and Löe** (Pl I) places the most significance on the amount of plaque at the gingival margin because of the importance of the proximity and relationship of plaque in that location to gingival inflammation, which is

measured clinically by bleeding. This index, which has been used in many studies, can be used to measure all teeth or selected teeth in a study, or it can be applied to selected surfaces of the teeth. The following criteria are used for scoring:

0 = The gingival area of the tooth is free of plaque when the tooth surface is tested by running a probe across at the gingival margin; if no soft material adheres, then the area is free of plaque.

1 = No plaque is observed in situ by the unaided eye, but plaque is visible on the point of a probe after the probe has been moved over the tooth surface at the entrance of the gingival crevice.

2 = The gingival area is covered by a thin to moderately thick layer of plaque that is visible to the naked eye.

3 = The accumulation of soft matter is heavy, and it fills the crevice produced by the gingival margin and the tooth surface.

The tooth score is determined by adding the scores for the measured surfaces on each tooth and dividing this number by the number of surfaces. The whole mouth score is determined by adding the tooth scores and dividing this number by the number of teeth. These data can be evaluated by tooth, by groups of teeth, or over individuals in the population. In a population with an average plaque score of 2, a moderate level of plaque is present in most individuals. Alternatively, if a tooth has a plaque score of 1, little plaque is present and the plaque cannot be seen by the naked eye.

Simplified Oral Hygiene Index of Greene and Vermillion[6]

The **Simplified Oral Hygiene Index** of Greene and Vermillion (OHI-S) has both a debris index (DI-S) for plaque and a **calculus index** (CI-S). The scores can be used singly to provide a plaque index or a calculus index, or they may be combined to provide an oral hygiene index.

The DI-S, the plaque portion of the index, is a numeric assessment of plaque and other debris on the teeth. As representative of the entire dentition, six selected teeth are scored: the buccal surfaces of the maxillary first molars, the lingual surfaces of the mandibular first molars, and the labial aspects of the maxillary and mandibular left central incisors. Scoring criteria are as follows:

0 = No debris or stain on the tooth surface.

1 = Soft debris covering as much as one third of the tooth surface or extrinsic stain without debris

2 = Soft debris covering one third to two thirds of the tooth surface.

3 = Soft debris covering more than two thirds of the surface.

The debris score for the individual is obtained by adding the scores for all surfaces and dividing by the number of surfaces scored. An average score across the population can be determined by adding the debris scores for each individual and dividing by the number of individuals.

> **CLINICAL NOTE 3-4** When interpreting plaque scores, a DI-S score of 2 has a considerably different meaning than a Pl I score of 2. If an individual has an average DI-S score of 2, two thirds of the tooth surfaces are covered with plaque. In contrast, a Pl I score of 2 means that there is a thin to moderately thick layer of visible plaque at the gingival margin.

CALCULUS INDICES

Calculus is a significant factor associated with periodontal disease, although it is not an etiologic agent (see Chapter 5). It has been measured in many epidemiologic studies, and the amount of calculus present is significant to the practice of the dental hygienist. Knowing the extent of calculus formation in the population helps to explain why so much practice time is spent removing it.

Calculus Index of the OHI-S[6]

Selected teeth are scored using the calculus index, the CI-S. A score of 2 on the CI-S indicates a considerable quantity of supragingival calculus, some subgingival calculus, or both. The criteria are as follows:

0 = No calculus.
1 = Supragingival calculus covering up to one third of the tooth surface.
2 = Supragingival calculus covering one third to two thirds of the tooth surface, or flecks of subgingival calculus.
3 = Supragingival calculus covering more than two thirds of the surface, or a continuous heavy band of subgingival calculus.

To determine the OHI-S score (the combined score of DI-S and CI-S), the mean scores on both indices for all subjects are added and then divided by the total number of subjects. These OHI-S scores are higher, ranging from 0 to 6. A score of 6 is the highest score possible on the DI-S—3, the highest possible score on the DI-S, plus the highest score possible in the CI-S, 3. A combined OHI-S score does not indicate how much is due to debris or how much is due to calculus being present. An OHI-S score of 3 could indicate heavy calculus accumulation, heavy debris accumulation, or a combination. For this reason, it is often helpful to consider both components of the OHI-S score rather than combining them.

CLINICAL NOTE 3-5 The OHI-S provides a very gross measure of plaque and calculus. A score of 1 on the CI-S means very heavy supragingival calculus and some subgingival calculus.

Volpe-Manhold Probe Method of Calculus Assesment[7]

The **Volpe-Manhold Index** scoring system measures only supragingival calculus. It was designed to measure the mandibular incisors but has also been applied to other teeth. A periodontal probe with millimeter markings is used to bisect each of the three parts of the lingual surface of the incisor (mesial lingual, distal lingual, and direct lingual), and a measurement of the height of calculus is made for each of the three parts of the lingual surface. Scores for the direct lingual, mesial lingual, and distal lingual surfaces are averaged (added together and divided by three) to provide a tooth score. Tooth scores are averaged (added up and divided by the number of teeth measured) to provide a score for the individual. The score can be interpreted as indicating the approximate height of calculus, in millimeters, on the measured surfaces.

CLINICAL NOTE 3-6 Calculus indices are used in studies of the efficacy of tartar control products.

INDICES OF GINGIVAL DISEASE OR BLEEDING

Indices of gingival disease are assessments of bleeding of the gingiva. Bleeding is important to monitor because it is associated with inflammation. Bleeding on probing is the most common sign used in clinical practice to monitor gingival health, and bleeding is associated with periodontal destruction.

Gingival Index of Löe and Silness[8]

The Gingival Index of Löe and Silness (GI) is an evaluation of each of four sides of the tooth: mesial, distal, lingual, and facial. The index is scored by visual inspection of the gingiva and by gentle probing, stroking, or a sweeping motion into the sulcus. A score is assigned to each surface, and an average score is assigned to the tooth. GI scores for areas of the mouth, for selected teeth, or for the full mouth are computed by adding the tooth scores and averaging that number by the number of teeth examined. The following criteria are used for scoring:

0 = Absence of inflammation (no bleeding, color change, or texture change).
1 = Mild inflammation characterized by slight color change, little change in texture, and no bleeding on probing.
2 = Moderate inflammation characterized by redness and swelling of the gingiva and accompanied by bleeding on probing.
3 = Severe inflammation characterized by significant redness and hypertrophy (swelling), a tendency to bleed spontaneously, and ulceration.

With this index, a score of 2 indicates bleeding on probing. In general, a tooth score, individual score, or population score greater than 1 suggests some level of moderate inflammation characterized by bleeding on probing.

Sulcus Bleeding Index[9]

The **Sulcus Bleeding Index** (SBI) is also a measure of bleeding on probing. Like the GI, measurements are taken at four points around each tooth: the mesial, distal, buccal, and lingual surfaces. A probe is gently inserted in the sulcus areas across a quadrant and withdrawn. The gingival units are scored 30 seconds after probing to allow time for bleeding to become visible, which is important in evaluating less inflamed tissue. The scoring units are as follows:

0 = Healthy appearance with no bleeding on probing.
1 = Healthy appearance, with no color or contour change, but bleeding on probing.
2 = Bleeding on probing and color change in tissue, but no swelling.
3 = Bleeding on probing, color change, and slight swelling of the gingival unit.
4 = Bleeding on probing and obvious swelling, with or without color change.
5 = Spontaneous bleeding, bleeding on probing, color change, and significant swelling, with or without ulceration.

The SBI differentiates among the more severe signs of inflammation, including significant swelling and color change. It has been argued that the most important distinction is when the tissue bleeds, so the usefulness of identifying grades of inflammation beyond that point depends on the purpose of the study.

INDICES OF PERIODONTAL DISEASE

Indices of periodontal destruction measure factors beyond gingival changes, including bone loss around the teeth. They have been used to estimate periodontal health for individuals, communities, and populations. More recent national data have relied on millimeter measures of periodontal probing depth and attachment loss rather than on an encompassing index of periodontal disease. Millimeter data are more easily translated and understood by clinicians than index scores. However, important data have been collected with index scores. Two important indices are described here.

Russell's Periodontal Index[10]

Russell's Periodontal Index (PI) was designed in the 1950s and 1960s. It is a progressive scale that assigns a numeric score to each tooth. This scale is weighted more toward bone loss than toward gingival inflammation. The score for each tooth is added and averaged by all teeth examined in the individual, providing a score for each person. Population scores are determined by averaging the scores of individuals. The criteria for scoring are as follows:

0 = Negative, with no inflammation or loss of function.
1 = Mild gingivitis, with inflammation in the free gingiva, but not circumscribing the tooth.
2 = Gingivitis, with inflammation circumscribing the tooth, but normal probing depths.
6 = Gingivitis, with pocket formation; the gingival sulcus is deepened, function is normal, and there is no drifting.
8 = Advanced destruction, with loss of masticatory function; the tooth may be loose, may sound dull on percussion, and may be depressible in the socket.

The higher scores, 6 and 8, indicate the progressive nature of the scale, weighting it on bone loss so that it does not tell much about attachment loss, probe depth measurements, or gingival condition. However, it was developed early in the 1950s, and it provided important information that was not previously quantified. A PI score of 6.5 or 7 indicates extensive periodontal destruction, but not the amount of probing depth or attachment loss.

Periodontal Disease Index of Ramfjord[11]

The Periodontal Disease Index of Ramfjord (PDI) evaluates the gingival condition and measures both probe depths and attachment loss. It is designed to evaluate six teeth that have been demonstrated to be representative of the entire dentition:

#3, the maxillary right first molar
#9, the maxillary left central incisor
#12, the maxillary left first premolar
#19, the mandibular left first molar
#25, the mandibular right central incisor
#28, the mandibular right first premolar

Gingivitis. Scoring is determined on the following scale:
0 = Negative.
1 = Mild gingivitis involving the free gingiva.
2 = Moderate gingivitis involving the free and attached gingiva.
3 = Severe gingivitis with hypertrophy and hemorrhage.

Periodontal Disease. When one tooth has probing (pocket) depths that meet the following criteria, the gingivitis score is disregarded and only the periodontal disease portion of the index is used for that tooth:

4 = Pocket depths on two or more of the surfaces of the tooth measure up to 3 mm apical to the cementoenamel junction.
5 = Pocket depths on two or more of the surfaces of the tooth measure 3 to 6 mm apical to the cementoenamel junction.
6 = Pocket depths on two or more of the surfaces of the tooth measure more than 6 mm apical to the cementoenamel junction.

The scores for each of the six teeth are added and then averaged to provide a score for the individual. Individual scores can be averaged to compute a population score.

OTHER INDICES

A number of other indices have been developed and used. This section describes four of the most important, all of which have different goals.

Community Index of Periodontal Treatment Needs[12]

One of the most significant indices used in epidemiologic research is the Community Index of Periodontal Treatment Needs (CIPTN), which was developed by the World Health Organization. This index assesses the periodontal treatment needs in the community, not simply the level of disease. A specially designed periodontal probe is used for this assessment. It is a color-coded probe with a black band extending from 3.5 to 5.5 mm. It has a rounded ball tip 0.5 mm in diameter, which helps to prevent excessive penetration of the probe tip into the connective tissue. Excessive penetration leads to overestimation of pocket depths. Ten teeth are examined, two in each posterior sextant and one in each anterior sextant. The teeth examined are numbers 2, 3, 8, 14, 15, 18, 19, 25, 30, and 31. There are routines for scoring substitute teeth in the case of missing teeth. However, if a sextant has only one tooth, it is considered and scored as part of the next sextant. The worst finding for each tooth is coded, and the worst finding for the sextant is the treatment category for that sextant. Individual tooth codes are as follows:

> 0 = No signs of inflammation or pocketing.
> 1 = Gingival bleeding after probing.
> 2 = Supragingival or subgingival calculus present.
> 3 = Pathologic pockets of 4.0 to 5.5 mm.
> 4 = Pathologic pockets of 6 mm or more.

After the codes are assigned to teeth, the treatment categories are assigned per sextant on the basis of the highest score for each sextant. The treatment categories are as follows:

> 0 = No treatment (code 0 only).
> I = Improvement in oral hygiene (code 1 only).
> II = Category I + scaling (codes 2 and 3).
> III = Categories I + II + complex periodontal treatment (codes 2, 3, and 4).

This information can be expressed as the percentage of subjects in each treatment category or as the percentage of sextants needing specific treatment. For example, if 85% of the population is scored as category II, the population is in need of scaling, oral hygiene instruction, and treatment for deeper pockets, so the services of both the dental hygienist and the general dentist are required.

A study by Lang[13] suggested a weakness in the CIPTN system: it may overestimate the need for treatment. This highlights the difference in focus between the epidemiologist and the clinician in private practice. CIPTN treatment categories suggest the need for the population to be brought to a complete state of health. This individualized dental care model is used in the United States and in many other countries. However, when dealing with different populations and limited resources, the epidemiologist may choose to target individuals who are at greatest risk for tooth loss. The need for treatment does not equate to access to care. It is unrealistic to expect that certain populations—for example the Sri Lankan tea workers studied by Anerud and colleagues,[14] who have no oral hygiene practices and no dentists—would receive treatment at the level of industrialized populations.

> **CLINICAL NOTE 3-10** CIPTN provides a picture of the periodontal health of a population.

Gingival Fluid Flow[15]

Another important index is the measurement of gingival fluid flow from the sulcus. This index is primarily used in periodontal research studies to identify early inflammation. An increase in the flow of crevicular fluid is one of the first measurable changes in the inflammatory process of the periodontium. Fluid is measured on filter paper strips placed within the sulcus. The measurement is made on a calibrated machine called a Periotron (IDE Interstate, New York). Comparisons of fluid flow can be made over time in a study population to estimate changes in the amount of inflammation present, or the information can be used in a cross-sectional comparison study of a larger population. Gingival or sulcular fluid flow has also been used as a measurement to define the level of inflammation present for

subjects to qualify to participate in clinical studies such as case-control studies.

Periodontal Screening and Recording[3]

The Periodontal Screening and Recording (PSR) system was developed by the American Academy of Periodontology and the American Dental Association. This screening system enables the clinician to identify which patients need a full examination and which patients require only a screening examination in the private practice setting. The utility of the PSR system in practice has not been established.

The World Health Organization CIPTN probe is used to assess PSR scores. The probe is inserted around all areas of all teeth in the sextant, and the periodontium is examined for inflammation, plaque, and calculus. Sextants are graded individually, and only the worst score for the sextant is recorded. The sextant evaluation is coded in the following manner:

> 0 = The colored section of the probe is completely visible in the deepest probe depth of the sextant—no calculus, defective margins, or bleeding (no bleeding on probing).
> 1 = The colored section of the probe is completely visible in the deepest probe depth of the sextant—no calculus or defective margins, but bleeding after probing (bleeding on probing).
> 2 = The colored section of the probe is completely visible in the deepest probe depth of the sextant—supragingival or subgingival calculus or defective margins present (calculus or other irritants present).
> 3 = The color-coded section of the probe is only partly visible in the deepest probe depth in the sextant (indicating at least one 3.5- to 5-mm probe depth); calculus, defective restorations, and bleeding may or may not be present (deeper probe depths, calculus, irritants, and bleeding may be present).
> 4 = The color-coded section of the probe completely disappears into the deepest probe depth in the sextant, indicating at least one pocket of 6 mm or deeper (deep probing depths).
> * = An asterisk is added to any of the preceding sextant codes if any notable features, such as furcation involvement, pathologic mobility, mucogingival defect, or marked recession, are identified.

The highest score in any sextant for the individual patient determines the case management. If any score of 3 or 4 is identified, a complete, full-mouth periodontal examination should be performed. General management guidelines are associated with the sextant codes. Codes 0 and 1 require plaque control and preventive care. Code 2 indicates plaque control, prevention, calculus removal, and correction of defective restorations. Codes 3 and 4 require complete assessment and a periodontal treatment plan. Regardless of code, any sextant that has an abnormality asterisk (code *) requires a specific treatment plan.

> **CLINICAL NOTE 3-11** The PSR is a screening examination with criteria for identifying patients who need a complete evaluation. It is not a substitute for a thorough examination in the practice setting.

Miller Index of Tooth Mobility[16]

Miller described the system that is most commonly used to quantify tooth mobility, which is named after him, the **Miller Index of Tooth Mobility** (MI). It is used both in epidemiologic studies and in the clinical assessment of individual patients. Two metal instrument handles arc placed on either side of the tooth to be tested, and the tooth is moved in a facial-lingual direction. It is not advisable to assess mobility with the fingers because the soft pads may not provide enough resistance to detect slight mobility. The mobility grading scale is 0 to 3 as follows:

0 = No movement when force is applied.
1 = Barely distinguishable tooth movement.
2 = 1-mm movement in any direction.
3 = >1-mm movement in any direction, or tooth is depressible or can be rotated in the socket.

This index is often modified with plus or minus signs or identified with roman numerals. However, the more subtle the distinctions used (e.g., 1+, 2−, 2), the less reproducible and meaningful the scale becomes. Think about the significance of a score of 2 compared with a 2−; the difference would be very slight.

CLINICAL NOTE 3-12   A practical way to apply Miller's index is practiced by Dr. Jack Taggart:
- If the tooth is not mobile, then it is not mobile and should be scored a 0.
- If you think it is mobile, score it 1.
- If you are sure it is mobile, score it 2.
- If it is depressible in the socket, score it 3.

NATIONAL PREVALENCE DATA

The National Health and Nutrition Examination Study (NHANES-III)[17] was a series of studies designed to characterize the health and nutrition status of the population of the United States. It provided evidence about the oral health of the population. The data described here were collected and published between 1999 and 2004 and are the most recent national data. This was a cross-sectional study that provided an overview of the periodontal health of adults in the United States, a snapshot in time rather than a long-term study designed to evaluate changes over time.

GINGIVITIS[18]

Gingivitis was very commonly found in the population in the NHANES-III survey. It was defined in adults as bleeding on probing at one or more sites. However, the prevalence did vary by gender and by race and ethnicity. It was more prevalent in males than in females, and more commonly found in Mexican Americans than in non-Hispanic blacks or non-Hispanic whites. It was also recognized that individuals from low socioeconomic groups and those with less than a 12th-grade education had more gingivitis.

CLINICAL NOTE 3-13   NHANES data indicated that more than 50% of the U.S. adult population had gingivitis.

PERIODONTAL DISEASE[19]

Periodontal disease was also measured in the NHANES-III study. Overall, 8.52% of the adult population of the United States between the ages of 20 and 64 had periodontal disease.

The definition of periodontal disease used in the study was having one or more sites with 3 mm or more of attachment loss and 4 mm or more of pocket depth. Moderate disease was defined as having at least two teeth with 4 mm of interproximal attachment loss or 5 mm or more of pocket depth at interproximal sites. Severe disease was defined as having at least two teeth with 6 mm or more of interproximal attachment loss and one tooth or more with 5 mm or more of pocket depth.

Percentage with Disease

The percentage of adults with periodontal disease varied from 3.84% in younger adults aged 10 to 34 to 10.41% in adults aged 35 to 49 years. For adults aged 50 to 64 years, the percentage increased slightly to 11.88%.

Gender

The prevalence of periodontal disease was higher in males than in females, with 10.65% of men having the disease compared to 6.40% of women.

Socioeconomic Status

The prevalence of periodontal disease among individuals living below the federal poverty level (a complex guideline, but generally an earned income of $22,350 for a family of four in 2012) was 13.95%, compared with 5.96% for those more than 200% above the poverty level.

Education Level

For those with less than a high school education, the percentage with periodontal disease was 17.33%, compared with 5.78% for those with more than a high school education.

Race and Ethnicity

Among Mexican Americans, 13.75% of the population was affected by periodontal disease, compared with 16.81% for the non-Hispanic black population and 5.82% for the non-Hispanic white population.

Smoking History

Smokers also had a higher prevalence of periodontal disease. The percentage of those with periodontal disease was 5.94% for those who had never smoked, 7.61% for former smokers, and 14.74% for current smokers.

Senior Adults Aged 65 or Over[20]

The same general trends regarding the prevalence of periodontal disease were reported in older adults. Overall, 10.20% of those aged 65 to 74 presented with disease and 11.03% of those 75 and over. It was more commonly found in males than females, more than twice as commonly found in those living below the federal poverty level than those above, more common in those with less than a high school education, more common in Mexican Americans and non-Hispanic blacks than in non-Hispanic whites, and more common in current smokers than those who had never smoked or who had quit smoking. It was also noted that periodontal disease was more severe in older people, men, poor people, minority populations, those less educated, and smokers.

> **CLINICAL NOTE 3-14** It is possible to conclude that a considerable portion of the population has moderate to severe periodontal disease.[18-20] Evidence also makes clear that the prevalence of periodontal disease is higher in older populations, males, minority groups, the poor, people who are less educated, and smokers.

RISK FACTORS AND OTHER DETERMINANTS

Several determinants and risk factors are related to periodontal disease. These risk factors are more prevalent in groups or populations with periodontal disease than those without. It is important to keep in mind that these determinants and risk factors are associated with periodontal disease, but they do not necessarily cause disease.

Gender

There are differences seen in the amount of periodontal disease between groups divided by gender and age. As a group, men are more likely than women to have periodontal diseases.[17,18,19] However, men tend to go to the dentist less often and have poorer oral hygiene, which may explain the gender differences noted in epidemiologic studies. It is also known that disease worsens as populations age, as reported in cross-sectional studies. This may better reflect a lifetime accumulation of disease effects rather than more disease or more severe disease.[1]

Socioeconomic Status

Members of lower income groups tend to have more periodontal disease. They also tend to have less dental insurance coverage, be less educated, and visit the dentist less often than wealthier and better educated people.[1,19] The differences noted here may exist because people with more education tend to have better paying jobs, which may lead to better access to dental care. Epidemiologic research does not answer these questions; it simply describes the population.

Tobacco Use

Tobacco use is also associated with the extent and severity of periodontal diseases.[19,20] Tobacco use, primarily smoking, has been associated with increased levels of periodontal disease in adults[19] and seniors.[20] Smoking is clearly a major risk factor in periodontitis. The reaction to and biologic events associated with smoking are complex and can be described briefly as follows[1]:

- Smokers have a higher prevalence of periodontal pathogenic species in the plaque (Chapter 4).
- Smoking suppresses the vascular reaction, resulting in a masking of the signs of gingival inflammation (Chapter 5).
- Smoking suppresses bleeding in periodontal disease (Chapter 5).
- Smoking may reduce granulocyte function, contributing to the decreased inflammatory signs noted in smokers (Chapter 5).

Systemic Disease

Certain systemic conditions are also associated with an increased risk of periodontal disease:

- It has been shown that diabetic individuals, particularly those with insulin-dependent diabetes, are two to three times as likely to have more pocketing, more calculus, and more tooth loss than similar groups of individuals without diabetes.[1]
- The presence of periodontal disease is considered to be associated with cardiovascular disease.[21,22]
- Low-birth-weight babies are more prevalent in women with periodontal disease.[23]
- Obesity has been suggested as a potential risk factor for periodontal disease in the young population.[24]
- Alcohol consumption has also been targeted by some as a modifiable risk factor for periodontal disease in adults.[25]

> **CLINICAL NOTE 3-15** Oral infections such as periodontal disease are not isolated from the rest of the body, and epidemiologic data provide clues to better understanding of the disease and the effects on the body.

TRENDS IN DISEASE PREVALENCE

It is difficult to compare the results of epidemiologic studies directly. They have different populations and were scored with different tools, indices, and examiners. However, the trends in the epidemiologic data suggest that 10% or more of the population has periodontal disease and that the proportion increases with age and other variables. The American Academy of Periodontology, in its position paper, suggested that the amount of periodontal disease in the U.S. population is somewhere between 5% and 20%, with a much higher percentage having slight or moderate disease levels.[1] One recent analysis of the NHANES data using different criteria reported that 47.2% of adults aged 30 or more had periodontitis.[26] Data from the 1987 survey of employed persons clearly showed that edentulism is decreasing, gingival bleeding is very common, and calculus is present in most adults and almost all seniors.[27] Figures 3-1, 3-2, and 3-3 provide evidence of these population

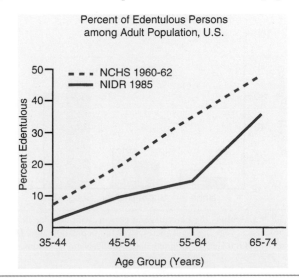

FIGURE 3-1 ■ Edentulousness. The percentage of edentulous persons among the U.S. adult population increases with age. (Used by permission from Oral Health of United States Adults, National Findings, 1987.)

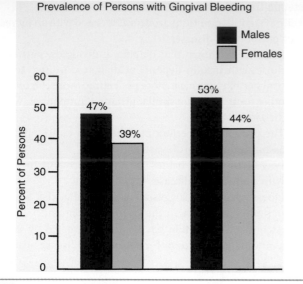

FIGURE 3-2 ■ Gingival bleeding. The prevalence of persons with gingival bleeding is very high. (Used by permission from Oral Health of United States Adults, National Findings, 1987.)

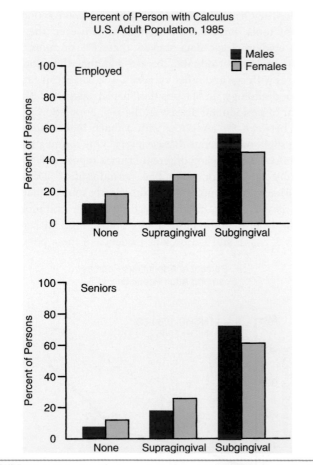

FIGURE 3-3 ■ Calculus. The percentage of persons with calculus in the U.S. adult population is very high and increases as the population ages. (Used by permission from Oral Health of United States Adults, National Findings, 1987.)

characteristics. All of these analyses suggest a significant role for the dental hygienist in meeting the treatment needs of the population.

◎ DENTAL HYGIENE CONSIDERATIONS

- Epidemiology teaches us an understanding of the amount and distribution of disease in the population and provides insight into the factors associated with disease.
- Recent data suggest that much of the periodontal treatment needed by most individuals can be provided by the dental hygienist.
- Collaboration with dentists and periodontists, proper assessment of individual needs, calculus and plaque removal, prevention education, and appropriate referral are essential to provide comprehensive dental hygiene care that will restore most patients to periodontal health.
- As noted by Löe,[28] "Modern dentistry has changed the face of America." Individuals have more teeth and healthier teeth, less tooth decay, and less periodontal and gingival disease. This change is a significant accomplishment for the dental hygienists, dentists, and periodontists in the United States.

✶ CASE SCENARIO

In an epidemiologic study of periodontal disease, the dental hygienist identified a population of 100 individuals but could only examine a randomly selected sample of 50 of them due to time and resource constraints. All individuals were to be examined within 2 weeks while they were visiting the local dental clinic. The dental hygienist planned to probe all teeth in each subject and set the definition of disease at one probing depth of 4 mm or more. Both men and women were to be included in the study and were in equal proportion in the population of 100. The dental hygienist was also interested in identifying risk factors, so subjects were questioned regarding gender, age, socioeconomic status, and smoking habits. A total of 10 individuals in the sample had a history of smoking.

1. What kind of study was planned?
   A. Cohort
   B. Case-control
   C. Cross-sectional
2. The data collected on the 50 subjects can be generalized to which population?
   A. The 50 individuals selected
   B. The entire population of the community
   C. The entire population of the dental clinic
   D. The population of 100 from whom the sample was selected
3. Based on the results of the study, 20% of the population would be expected to have periodontal disease because 10 of the examined subjects met the criteria for periodontal disease.
   A. Both the statement and the reason are correct and related.
   B. Both the statement and the reason are correct but NOT related.
   C. The statement is correct, but the reason is NOT correct.
   D. The statement is NOT correct, but the reason is correct.
   E. NEITHER the statement NOR the reason is correct.

4. Men and women were found to have periodontal disease at the same rate in this population because
   A. there were gender differences in the results of this study.
   B. men and women have periodontal disease at the same rate in all populations.
   C. men and women had periodontal disease at the same rate in the population of this study.
   D. men and women had periodontal disease at the same rate in the sample, and the result was generalized to the study population.

5. Because 10 individuals in the sample had a history of smoking, how many individuals in the population from which the sample was taken would you expect to have a history of smoking?
   A. 10
   B. 15
   C. 20
   D. Cannot be determined

STUDY QUESTIONS

Answers and rationales to these questions can be obtained from your instructor.

MULTIPLE CHOICE

1. What is the reported percentage of the U.S. adult population that suffers from severe periodontal disease?
   A. 5% to 20%
   B. 5% to 35%
   C. 10% to 45%
   D. 10% to 55%

2. Epidemiologic studies have shown that periodontal disease is present in a significant portion of the older population. They have also shown that the percentage of the population with periodontal disease decreases with age.
   A. Both statements are true.
   B. Both statements are false.
   C. The first statement is true, and the second statement is false.
   D. The first statement is false, and the second statement is true.

3. All of the following are associated with a greater incidence of periodontal disease EXCEPT one. Which one is the EXCEPTION?
   A. Race
   B. Smoking
   C. Coffee drinking
   D. Economic status

4. Periodontal disease is associated with a systemic diseases because it has never been demonstrated through epidemiologic research studies.
   A. Both the statement and the reason are correct and related.
   B. Both the statement and the reason are correct but NOT related.
   C. The statement is correct, but the reason is NOT correct.
   D. The statement is NOT correct, but the reason is correct.
   E. NEITHER the statement NOR the reason is correct.

5. Indices of periodontal disease can measure all of the following conditions EXCEPT one. Which one is the EXCEPTION?
   A. Cause of disease
   B. Extent of disease
   C. Severity of disease
   D. Incidence of disease

6. The most commonly used index for measuring gingival disease or bleeding is the
   A. GI of Löe and Silness.
   B. Volpe-Manhold Index.
   C. Plaque Index of Silness and Löe.
   D. OHI-S of Greene and Vermillion.

7. All of the following statements about smoking and smokers are true EXCEPT one. Which one is the EXCEPTION?
   A. Smoking suppresses vascular reactions.
   B. Smoking increases bleeding in periodontal disease.
   C. Smokers have more species of periodontal pathogens.
   D. Smokers have more calculus deposits than nonsmokers.
   E. Smokers have deeper periodontal pockets than non-smokers.

8. Evidence from large studies on oral health has shown a decrease in the prevalence of gingivitis in the United States. This decrease is suggested to be a result of fluoridation, a more educated population, and more available dental care.
   A. Both the statement and the reason are correct and related.
   B. Both the statement and the reason are correct but NOT related.
   C. The statement is correct, but the reason is NOT correct.
   D. The statement is NOT correct, but the reason is correct.
   E. NEITHER the statement NOR the reason is correct.

SHORT ANSWER

9. Describe the technique for determining tooth mobility with the Miller Index of Mobility.
10. List five conditions associated with increased incidence of periodontal disease.

Please visit **http://evolve.elsevier.com/Perry/periodontology** for additional practice and study support tools.

REFERENCES

1. Burt B. Research, Science and Therapy Committee of the American Academy of Periodontology. Position paper: epidemiology of periodontal diseases. *J Periodontol.* 2005;76:1406–1419.
2. Hujoel P. Fundamentals in methods of periodontal disease epidemiology. In: Newman MG, Takei HH, Klokkevold PR, et al, eds. *Carranza's Clinical Periodontology.* 11th ed. St. Louis, MO: Elsevier Saunders; 2012:55–64.
3. Wyche CJ. Indices and scoring methods. In: Wilkins EM, ed. *Clinical Practice of the Dental Hygienist.* 11th ed. Philadelphia, PA: Lippincott Williams & Wilkins; 2013:312–335.
4. Loe H, Theilade E, Jensen BS. Experimental gingivitis in man. *J Periodontol.* 1965;36:177–187.
5. Silness J, Löe H. Periodontal disease in pregnancy, II: Correlation between oral hygiene and periodontal condition. *Acta Odontol Scand.* 1964;22:121–125.

6. Greene JC, Vermillion JR. The simplified oral hygiene index. *J Am Dent Assoc.* 1964;68:7–12.
7. Manhold JH, Volpe AR, Hazen SP, et al. In vivo calculus assessment, II: a comparison of scoring techniques. *J Periodontol.* 1965;36:299–304.
8. Löe H. The gingival index, the plaque index, and the retention index systems. *J Periodontol.* 1967;38:610–616.
9. Muhlemann HR, Son S. Gingival sulcus bleeding: a leading symptom in initial gingivitis. *Helv Odontol Acta.* 1971;15:107–113.
10. Russell AL. A system of classification and scoring for prevalence surveys of periodontal disease. *J Dent Res.* 1956;35:350–359.
11. Ramjford SP. Indices for prevalence and incidence of periodontal disease. *J Periodontol.* 1959;30:51–55.
12. Ainamo J, Barmes D, Beagrie G, et al. Development at the World Health Organization (WHO) community index of periodontal treatment needs (CIPTN). *Int Dent J.* 1982;32:281–291.
13. Lang NP. Epidemiology of periodontal disease. *Arch Oral Biol.* 1990;35(suppl):9S–14S.
14. Anerud A, Löe H, Boysen H. The natural history and clinical course of calculus formation in man. *J Clin Periodontol.* 1991;18:160–170.
15. Bulkacz J, Carranza FA. Defense mechanisms of the gingiva. In: Newman MG, Takei HH, Klokkevold PR, et al, eds. *Carranza's Clinical Periodontology.* 11th ed. St. Louis, MO: Elsevier Saunders; 2012:66–70.
16. Miller SC. *Textbook of Periodontia.* 3rd ed. Philadelphia, PA: Blakestone; 1950.
17. Centers for Disease Control and Prevention. National health and nutrition examination survey. http://www.cdc.gov. Accessed April 2012.
18. National Institute of Dental and Craniofacial Research, National Institutes of Health and the Division of Oral Health, Centers for Disease Control and Prevention. Periodontal diseases. In: *Oral Health US, 2002.* Rockville, MD: Dental, Oral and Craniofacial Data Resource Center; 2002; section 3:21–23.
19. National Institute of Dental and Craniofacial Research. Periodontal disease in adults (age 20-64). http://www.nidcr.nih.gov/datastatistics. Accessed January 2012.
20. National Institute of Dental and Craniofacial Research. Periodontal disease in seniors (age 65 and over). http://www.nidcr.nih.gov/datastatistics. Accessed January 2012.
21. Friedewald VE, Kornman KS, Beck JD, et al. American Journal of Cardiology; Journal of Periodontology. The American Journal of Cardiology and Journal of Periodontology editors' consensus: periodontitis and atherosclerotic cardiovascular disease. *J Periodontol.* 2009;80:1021–1032.
22. Lockhart PB, Bolger AF, Papapanou PN, et al. American Heart Association Rheumatic Fever, Endocarditis, and Kawasaki Disease Committee of the Council on Cardiovascular Disease in the Young, Council on Epidemiology and Prevention, Council on Peripheral Vascular Disease, and Council on Clinical Cardiology. Periodontal disease and atherosclerotic vascular disease: does the evidence support an independent association? *Circulation.* 2012;125:2520–2544.
23. Offenbacher S, Katx V, Fertik G, et al. Periodontal infection as a risk factor or preterm low birth weight. *J Periodontol.* 1996;67(suppl): 1103–1113.
24. Al-Zahrani MS, Bissada NF, Borawski EA. Obesity and periodontal disease in young, middle-aged and older adults. *J Periodontol.* 2003;74: 610–615.
25. Pitiphat W, Merchant AT, Rimm EV, et al. Alcohol consumption increased periodontitis risk. *J Dent Res.* 2003;82:509–513.
26. National Institute of Dental Research. Oral Health of United States adults: the National Survey of Oral Health in U.S. Employed Adults and Seniors, 1985–1986: national findings. *Bethesda, MD: U.S. Department of Health and Human Services, Public Health Service, 1987:3–31*; NIH publication; no. 87–2868.
27. Eke PI, Dye BA, Wei L, Thornton-Evans GO, Genco RJ. Prevalence of periodontitis in adults in the United States: 2009 and 2010. *J Dent Res.* 2012;91:914–920.
28. Loe H. Periodontics of tomorrow. *Dent Clin North Am.* 1988;32:395–405.

Microbiology of Periodontal Diseases

Peter M. Loomer
Based on the original work by Dorothy J. Rowe

LEARNING OUTCOMES

- Describe the development of supragingival and subgingival plaque biofilms.
- Compare the composition of supragingival and subgingival plaque biofilms.
- Describe the role of saliva in pellicle formation.
- Define the mechanisms for bacterial plaque biofilm adherence to tooth surfaces.
- Describe the influence of bacterial surface components (e.g., capsules, appendages) on bacterial colonization and coaggregation.
- Discuss plaque biofilm microbial succession in terms of oxygen and nutrient requirements and bacterial adherence.

- Compare the nonspecific and specific plaque hypotheses.
- Describe and classify the specific bacteria associated with the major periodontal infections: gingivitis, chronic periodontitis, localized aggressive periodontitis, generalized aggressive periodontitis, and necrotizing ulcerative gingivitis and periodontitis.
- Define the bacterial characteristics that contribute to their virulence.
- Describe the significance of dental plaque biofilm to dental hygiene practice.

KEY TERMS

Adherence	Glycocalyx	Pellicle
Aerobe	Gram-positive and gram-negative	Red complex bacteria
Anaerobe	Lipopolysaccharide	Salivary glycoproteins
Bacterial coaggregation	Microbial succession	Specific plaque hypothesis
Dental plaque biofilm	Microbiota	Subgingival plaque biofilm
Endotoxin	Material alba	Supragingival plaque biofilm
Facultative anaerobic organism	Nonspecific plaque hypothesis	Virulence
Gingival crevicular fluid	Orange complex bacteria	
Glucan	Pathogenicity	

The presence of dental plaque is essential in the initiation and progression of gingivitis and periodontitis. A critical role of the dental hygienist is the instruction of patients in proper oral hygiene practices to remove plaque as a preventive measure against periodontal disease and dental caries. Studies evaluating the relationship between oral hygiene and periodontal disease have shown that poorer plaque control correlates to a greater prevalence and severity of periodontal disease.[1] With improved oral hygiene practices, however, there is less plaque and therefore decreased gingival inflammation and disease.

In the mid-1960s, researchers began to recognize the significance of plaque in the disease process. Experiments showed that when patients did not clean their teeth, and plaque was allowed to accumulate over time, inflammation of the gingival tissues occurred.[2] When plaque control was resumed, the inflammation decreased and the tissues returned to a healthier state.[3] Thus, dental plaque biofilms play critical roles in the etiology of periodontal diseases, and a thorough understanding of their composition and mechanisms of formation is essential in the diagnosis and treatment of periodontal diseases.

GENERAL CHARACTERISTICS OF PLAQUE FORMATION

Dental plaque biofilms are defined as accumulations of microbes on the surface of the teeth or other solid oral structures, not easily removed by rinsing. Dental plaque biofilms are different than material alba, which is loosely adherent bacteria and tissue debris that can be easily removed by the mechanical action of a strong water spray. A dental plaque biofilm is a complex, naturally occurring organized dense film of microorganisms bound in **glycocalyx** (the sticky polysaccharide matrix they produce) and other organic and inorganic products. The glycocalyx contains a network of channels and canals within the biofilm that allow for exchange of nutrients among various microbes and for the removal of their waste products. The complex biofilm structure also provides some protection for its resident microorganisms from invasion by outside intruders including other bacteria, antimicrobial drugs, and antiseptic rinses. Thus, both the nutritional and protective roles of the biofilm help it to thrive. For this reason, physical removal of dental plaque biofilms by daily brushing, interproximal cleaning, and periodic professional cleaning are essential for maintaining and restoring gingival and periodontal health.[1]

Colonization (accumulation) of plaque biofilms onto the supragingival and subgingival tooth surfaces is a complex procedure. It requires understanding of the bacterial characteristics and the oral environment.

BACTERIAL CHARACTERISTICS

Dental plaque biofilm consists mostly of bacteria. One mm³ of plaque biofilm, weighing about 1 mg, may contain more than 10^{10} bacteria, of which there may be several hundred species. Plaque biofilm is not a random accumulation of assorted types of bacteria but a specific and complex arrangement based on bacterial characteristics.[4] To help understand how plaque biofilm forms, this section reviews some important microbiologic concepts that are used to classify or describe bacteria.

MORPHOTYPES
Bacteria can be classified based on their shape, also referred to as morphotype. They may be:
- Cocci—round in shape
- Bacilli—rod like or elongated in shape
- Spirochetes—spiral in shape

CELL WALL CHARACTERISTICS
The cell walls of bacteria may contain structures and compounds that help them survive and cause damage to the patient's tissues. Bacteria are classified by laboratory procedures as either **gram-positive** or **gram-negative** based on a staining technique that causes gram-positive organisms to stain violet (purple) and gram-negative ones to stain safranin (red). The structures of these cell walls are presented in Figure 4-1.

Characteristics of Gram-Positive Bacteria
As seen in Figure 4-1, the capsule is the outer surface component of gram-positive bacteria. The glycocalyx (sticky extracellular matrix, or slime layer) is a loose, gel-like polysaccharide substance around the bacteria that is important in bacterial **adherence** (attachment) to the tooth surface and aggregation.

Characteristics of Gram-Negative Bacteria
An important feature of gram-negative bacteria is that the outer membrane of the cell wall is composed of proteins, called receptors, that are important in adherence and contain complex lipopolysaccharides. **Lipopolysaccharides** (LPSs), also known as **endotoxins,** are released when the cell wall is disrupted. They are highly potent destructive substances that can damage host

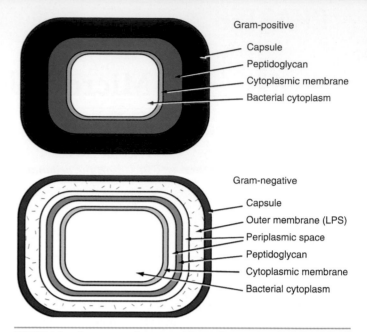

FIGURE 4-1 ■ **Structures of gram-positive and gram-negative bacterial cell walls.** Note the larger glycan layer in the gram-positive cell wall. The outer membrane of the gram-negative cell wall contains lipopolysaccharide (endotoxin). (Courtesy of Dr. P.W. Johnson.)

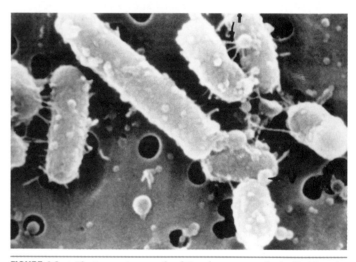

FIGURE 4-2 ■ Electron micrograph of *Porphyromonas gingivalis.* Note the fimbriae (pili) extending from the cell surface, an important virulence factor. (Courtesy of Dr. T. E. Bramanti.)

tissue directly or cause tissue damage through the activation of host inflammatory responses. Vesicles (often called microvesicles or blebs) are surface structures containing parts of the outer membrane and, hence, contain LPSs. Most bacteria that are pathogens in periodontal diseases are gram-negative.

Cell Surface Appendages
Cell surface appendages are important in the attachment of bacteria to tooth surfaces and to each other through bacterial adherence. Fimbriae, or pili, are small proteins that are attached to the external surface of both gram-negative and gram-positive bacteria. They mediate the adherence process to hydroxyapatite. Figure 4-2 shows an example of pili on bacterial cell surfaces. Flagella are long, fine, wavy filamentous structures that are used for bacterial movement. Bacteria may have single or multiple

flagella, arranged at either or both ends or distributed around the cell.

OXYGEN ENVIRONMENT

Bacteria are also classified on their ability to grow in the presence or absence of oxygen. Bacteria that require oxygen for growth are called aerobes. In contrast, anaerobes are bacterial species that do not need oxygen to grow. Facultative anaerobic organisms can grow in both aerobic and anaerobic environments. The subgingival pocket of a tooth is considered to be an anaerobic environment.

BACTERIAL METABOLISM

All bacteria need nutrients to grow, but their requirements and waste products vary. Many gram-positive organisms, such as *Streptococcus mutans,* are fermentative, or saccharolytic. This means they obtain their energy by breaking down complex organic compounds, such as sugars, to smaller end products, such as lactic acid. Many gram-negative organisms, including those that are pathogens in periodontal disease, are known as nonfermentative, or asaccharolytic. They tend to use proteins for energy and growth.

CLASSIFICATION OF PERIODONTAL BACTERIA

Bacteria are classified based on their characteristics, some of which have been described here. Box 4-1 contains the classification of common periodontal bacteria based on these characteristics.

ORAL MICROBIAL ECOSYSTEMS

The oral cavity is composed of several unique environments, or ecosystems, in which microorganisms thrive. The five major ones are the tongue, the buccal mucosa, saliva, the supragingival tooth surfaces, and the subgingival tooth surfaces.

Dorsum of the Tongue

The dorsum of the tongue has a highly irregular surface consisting of several types of sensory papillae and foramen. The majority of the microorganisms on the tongue are gram-positive members of the *Streptococcus* family, including *Streptococcus salivarius* and *Streptococcus sanguis*. Many gram-negative bacteria associated with halitosis (bad breath) and periodontal disease are also found in the normal oral microbiota of the tongue, including *Porphyromonas gingivalis*. Some studies have attributed as much as 50% of bad breath to plaque biofilm on the dorsum of the tongue.[4]

CLINICAL NOTE 4-1 Cleaning the surface of the tongue with scrapers or by brushing helps remove plaque biofilm and reduce oral malodor.

Oral Mucosal Surfaces

The oral mucosal surfaces include all the other oral soft tissues: the buccal mucosa, the floor of the mouth, and the hard and soft palates. The mucosal surfaces are either covered with keratinized epithelium or nonkeratinized epithelium. Streptococci are the predominant type of bacteria on these surfaces.

BOX 4-1   Classification of Bacterial Species Associated With Chronic Periodontitis

Gram-Negative Bacteria
Rods
Nonmotile
Facultative
   Actinobacillus actinomycetemcomitans
   Capnocytophaga ochraceus
   Eikenella corrodens
Anaerobic
   Porphyromonas gingivalis
   Prevotella intermedia
   Tannerella forsythia
   Fusobacterium nucleatum
   Leptotrichia buccalis
Motile
Facultative
   Campylobacter (Wolinella) rectus
Anaerobic
   Selenomonas
Cocci
Anaerobic
   Veillonella alkalescens
Spirochetes
Anaerobic, Motile
   Treponema denticola
Gram-Positive Bacteria
Rods
   Irregular morphologic features
Facultative
   Actinomyces israelii and *Actinomyces naeslundii*
   Corynebacterium matruchotii
Anaerobic
   Eubacterium
Straight rod
   Facultative
   Lactobacillus
Cocci
Facultative
   Streptococcus
Anaerobic
   Peptostreptococcus micros

Saliva

Saliva represents a unique and changing environment for microorganisms that is protective in nature. It contains shed gingival tissue cells and plaque biofilm from other locations in the oral cavity. Saliva is involved in the removal of biofilms from within the oral cavity because of fluid movement in the mouth. In addition, antimicrobial proteins in saliva help regulate microbial attachment to oral cavity surfaces.

CLINICAL NOTE 4-2 Cleaning teeth and maintaining young, nonpathogenic plaque biofilm is significant for older and immunocompromised individuals because aspiration into the lungs of pathogenic microbiota from biofilm has been found to cause aspiration pneumonia.

Tooth Surfaces

On the basis of their relationship to the gingival margin, tooth-adherent plaque biofilms are classified as supragingival or subgingival. Supragingival plaque biofilm is deposited on the

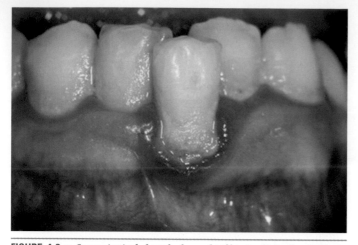

FIGURE 4-3 ■ Supragingival dental plaque biofilm is clinically visible in large masses. Note the yellowish accumulations on the facial and interproximal surfaces of these mandibular teeth. The dark ring appearing on the facial side of the incisor is plaque that has absorbed pigment from oxidized blood products and is mineralizing into calculus. The redness of the tissue is directly related to the pathogenicity of the plaque, which has caused an intense inflammatory response.

clinical crowns of the teeth, whereas subgingival plaque biofilm is located in the gingival sulcus or periodontal pocket. Small amounts of supragingival plaque biofilm are difficult to detect clinically without placing a disclosing solution or dye on the teeth, or scraping the tooth surfaces with an instrument. As plaque accumulation grows, it becomes visible as a white-yellow mass, as seen in Figure 4-3. Supragingival plaque biofilm forms in sites that are protected from the normal cleansing action of the tongue, cheek, and lips. This includes surfaces along the gingival margin of the tooth and the occlusal pits and fissures. Subgingival plaque biofilm can only be seen when it is removed from the pocket with an instrument. Plaque biofilm deposits also form on orthodontic appliances and permanent and temporary restorations, including implants, fixtures and restorations, fixed and removable partial dentures, and full dentures. It is extremely important to instruct patients on how to clean all these surfaces well.

SUPRAGINGIVAL PLAQUE FORMATION

The development of dental plaque is a complex and dynamic process. In-depth, detailed discussions of this subject are reviewed by Liljemark and Bloomquist,[3] Kolenbrander and London,[5] Jakubovics and Kolenbrander,[6] and Teughels et al.[7] Plaque forms in stages as described next.

STEP 1: PELLICLE FORMATION

After a tooth is cleaned, proteins from the saliva, termed salivary glycoproteins, selectively attach to the tooth surface, forming an amorphous and tenacious film called pellicle. Toothbrushing does not remove pellicle; only polishing the teeth with an abrasive agent will remove it. However, pellicle re-forms on the clean tooth surface within minutes. Pellicle is important because it influences the subsequent colonization of bacteria on the tooth surface. For example, certain proteins in saliva that form part of the pellicle can enhance the ability of specific microorganisms, such as *Actinomyces* species, to bind

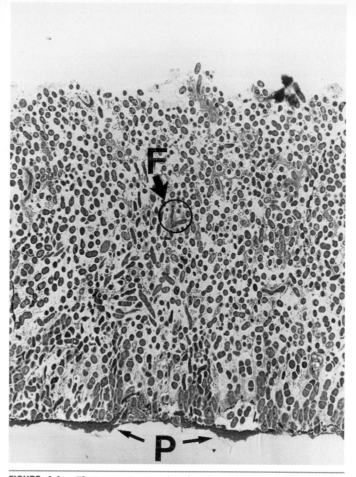

FIGURE 4-4 ■ Electron micrograph of 1-day-old supragingival plaque. Coccal forms predominate, exhibiting differing sizes and morphologic features. Note the pellicle (P) at the plaque-crown interface and a branching filament (F). (Used with permission from Listgarten MA, Mayo HE, Tremblay R. Development of dental plaque on epoxy resin crowns in man. *J Periodontol.* 1975;46:10–26.)

to tooth surfaces. Not all of the bacteria available in the saliva can attach to the pellicle, only those with binding sites for pellicle constituents.

STEP 2: INITIAL BACTERIAL COLONIZATION OF PELLICLE

Bacterial cells are continually transported to the pellicle-coated tooth surface by saliva. However, the only ones that colonize are those that attach to the pellicle. They stick through specific receptor mechanisms, or are in some other way physically retained. Otherwise, salivary flow, chewing forces, and oral hygiene procedures would eliminate or remove them from the oral cavity. Bacteria are also retained in pits and fissures, tooth surface irregularities, and other areas that are relatively sheltered from oral cleaning mechanisms. Oral bacteria vary significantly in their ability to adhere to different surfaces, and their prevalence at specific oral sites reflects this ability. For example, *S. mutans* and *S. sanguis* preferentially colonize supragingival plaque, whereas *S. salivarius* is present in high proportions on the tongue and in the saliva, but in low proportions on teeth.

The initial plaque biofilm that forms on the pellicle is composed of mainly gram-positive, coccal, facultative anaerobic bacteria, largely streptococci, as seen in Figure 4-4. The first

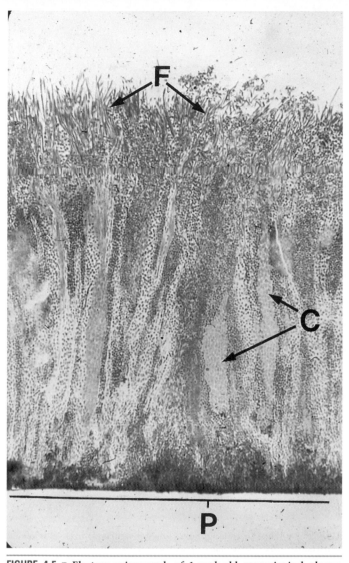

FIGURE 4-5 ■ **Electron micrograph of 1-week-old supragingival plaque.** Note the microcolonies of cocci (C) extending outward from the pellicle (P) and the numerous filaments (F) attached to the plaque surface. (Used with permission from Listgarten MA, Mayo HE, Tremblay R. Development of dental plaque on epoxy resin crowns in man. *J Periodontol.* 1975;46:10–26.)

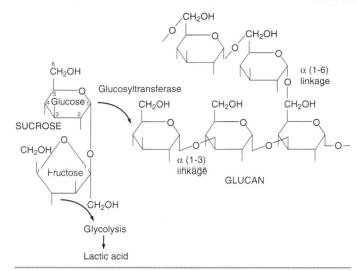

FIGURE 4-6 ■ **Chemical reaction of the synthesis of glucan from sucrose catalyzed by the enzyme glucosyltransferase.** This is a complex process that results in the production of glucan, the sticky material on the surface of bacteria that permits binding to pellicle and bacterial aggregation. (Courtesy of D.L. Del Carlo.)

Extracellular Polysaccharides

A variety of oral bacteria, such as *S. mutans, S. sanguis, Streptococcus mitis,* and *S. salivarius,* have the capability to produce metabolic products from sucrose, such as extracellular polysaccharide polymers. These products serve as either an energy source or as material to help retain the bacteria in the plaque. As shown in Figure 4-6, by the action of the bacterial enzyme glucosyltransferase, sucrose is cleaved into a highly branched glucose polymer, or **glucan,** whereas the fructose moiety (fructans) is available as an energy source. The accumulation of one type of glucan (mutan), which is insoluble, results in increased bacterial attachment of organisms such as *S. mutans,* which bind to glucan molecules. Furthermore, it may help entrap other microorganisms and thus promote the accumulation of cohesive bacteria.

The protein matrix is made up of salivary glycoproteins, which promote bacterial adherence when adsorbed to the tooth surface, permitting plaque biofilm to grow. There is also a small amount of lipid present in plaque and lipopolysaccharide from gram-negative cell walls. The concentration of inorganic components, primarily calcium and phosphate, is low in early plaque, but increases significantly as plaque is transformed into calculus.

Bacterial Coaggregation

Plaque biofilm accumulation also results from the **bacterial coaggregation** to previously attached cells. Certain bacteria adhere to other bacterial species and thus form complex aggregations. Filament-shaped bacteria at the salivary or outer plaque surfaces often become coated with cocci, presenting a "corncob" appearance, so called because of the resemblance to an ear of corn, as shown in Figure 4-7. Corncob formation is restricted to species with mutually attractive surface molecules that can bind to each other. The complex is composed of a central filament surrounded by cocci, usually a type of *S. sanguis.* The filaments could be either the facultative gram-positive *Actinomyces* species and *Corynebacterium matruchotii* or the anaerobic

organisms adhere and form a monolayer of cells, either individually or in small groups. During the next few hours, the attached bacteria proliferate and form small colonies. These microcolonies of cocci usually form a series of columns that extend out from the pellicle, as seen in Figure 4-5. Bacilli and filament-shaped bacteria are usually aligned perpendicular to the tooth surface, often attached to the surface of the predominantly coccal flora. As the colonies expand, they meet and join together to form a continuous bacterial mass.

STEP 3: GROWTH AND MATURATION OF PLAQUE

As plaque biofilm matures, there is an increase in mass and thickness as a result of the growth of the attached bacteria. Maturation of plaque also requires that different types of bacterial cells attach to each other. The material in the plaque between the bacteria is called the intermicrobial matrix and is composed of salivary material, gingival exudate, and microbial substances such as polysaccharides.

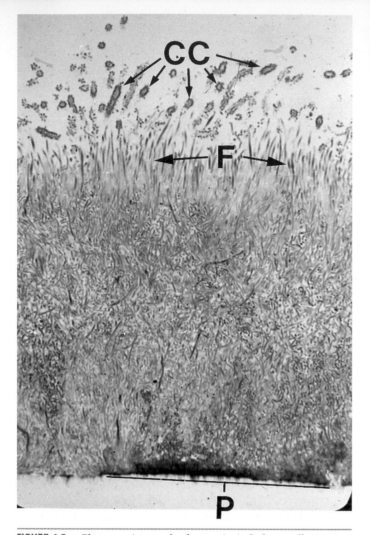

FIGURE 4-7 ■ **Electron micrograph of supragingival plaque adhering to a periodontally compromised tooth.** A dense, predominantly filamentous mass (F) is adherent to the enamel surface, and corncob formations (CC) extend from the surface. These complexes consist of filamentous bacteria surrounded by adherent cocci. P, Pellicle. (Used with permission from Listgarten MA. Structure of the microbial flora associated with periodontal health and disease in man. *J Periodontol.* 1976;47:1–18.)

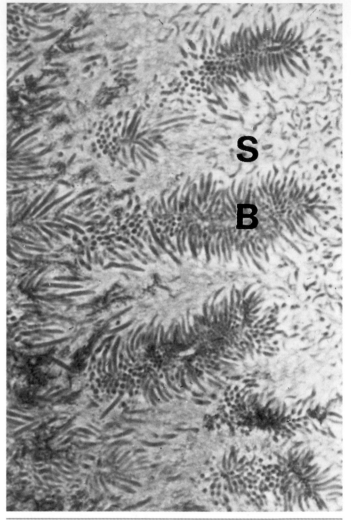

FIGURE 4-8 ■ **Electron micrograph of subgingival plaque from an inflamed periodontal pocket.** Test tube brush formations (B), composed of gram-negative rods attaching to filamentous bacteria, are surrounded by spirochetes (S). (Used with permission from Listgarten MA. Structure of the microbial flora associated with periodontal health and disease in man. *J Periodontol.* 1976;47:1–18.)

gram-negative *Fusobacterium nucleatum*. Other bacteria can aggregate together to form structures that resemble test tubes or bristle brushes, as seen in Figure 4-8. These coaggregates consist of a central axis that is composed of a filamentous bacterium and bristles that are composed of gram-negative rods. Interbacterial coaggregation may be the only means whereby some organisms adhere to plaque. There are many other coaggregating pairs of organisms. Generally, early colonizers coaggregate with streptococci or *Actinomyces* species, whereas late colonizers primarily coaggregate with *Fusobacteria* species, which bridges these coaggregations with early colonizers.

In another type of bacterial aggregation, one organism acts as a bridge between two other bacteria that do not interact. For example, some strains of *S. sanguis* aggregate with both *Actinomyces naeslundii* genospecies 2 and *Prevotella loescheii*, which do not coaggregate with each other. These multibacterial interactions may be an important mechanism for the attachment of new organisms within plaque biofilm and for the ability of organisms to resist the forces that would remove them.

Microbial Succession

As plaque ages, its composition changes; this process is referred to as **microbial succession.**[5,8] The initial colonizers proliferate and alter the environment at the tooth surface, thereby enabling new and different bacterial species to inhabit the developing plaque biofilm. After the first day of plaque growth, the proportion of gram-positive streptococci decreases and *Actinomyces* and *Veillonella* strains become more prominent. During the next 3 weeks of undisturbed plaque formation, cocci continue to decrease in relative numbers, particularly because of the increase in filamentous bacteria. These filamentous forms actually invade the plaque and replace many of the streptococci in the deeper levels of the biofilm. As the plaque increases in thickness, further changes occur in the environment. Plaque becomes anaerobic when it is allowed to grow undisturbed. The level of oxygen decreases as a result of oxygen consumption by facultative organisms, and this lower oxygen level allows the growth of anaerobes. Thus, the more mature plaque biofilm harbors increasing numbers of anaerobic organisms, such as spirochetes and gram-negative rods. At this point, no additional bacterial species can join the plaque, although the absolute numbers of bacteria may continue to increase. The mature supragingival plaque has a greater variety of bacterial shapes, including gram-negative and anaerobic bacteria. However, the most important difference between mature and immature plaque biofilm is that the maturation process gives supragingival plaque the potential to invade the subgingival space and to cause localized gingival disease.

CLINICAL NOTE 4-3 Removing supragingival plaque helps reduce gingival inflammation of the marginal tissues and prevent bacterial plaque biofilm from growing subgingivally.

SUBGINGIVAL PLAQUE FORMATION

Subgingival plaque formation is initiated by the presence of mature supragingival dental plaque biofilm. The bacterial composition of subgingival plaque is partly influenced by bacteria in the adjacent supragingival plaque. However, the microbiota in subgingival plaque are generally more anaerobic, gram-negative, motile, and asaccharolytic (using proteins rather than sugars for nutrients) than supragingival plaque.

SUBGINGIVAL ENVIRONMENT

The maturation of supragingival plaque is accompanied by inflammation in the gingiva. Because inflamed gingiva is less closely adapted to the tooth surface, the formation of supragingival plaque moves apically into the gingival crevice. In addition, edema causes gingival enlargement, such that the swollen gingival margin now covers supragingival biofilm, making it subgingival and permitting the growth of anaerobic organisms. This newly created subgingival space, which is protected from normal oral cleansing mechanisms, facilitates further maturation of plaque biofilm.

The subgingival environment is bathed in fluid from the plasma in blood vessels, rather than in saliva. Inflammation in response to plaque organisms causes an increase in capillary permeability, which allows the plasma to escape. When the fluid leaks into the gingival crevice it is referred to as gingival crevicular fluid (GCF). Inflammation increases GCF flow along with gingival bleeding, resulting in the presence of serum-derived proteins that provide excellent sources of nutrients for the bacteria in the biofilm.

MICROBIOLOGIC COMPOSITION

The composition and structure of subgingival plaque is very different from that of adjacent supragingival plaque for several reasons. The limited access to the oral cavity allows the most finicky anaerobic bacteria to grow and restricts the addition of salivary bacteria. Also, the subgingival area is not subject to the mechanical forces that tend to dislodge bacteria from the clinical crowns of the teeth. Thus, the ability to adhere to the tooth or biofilm matrix is not important for survival, so motile organisms that are completely unattached to the plaque matrix can proliferate and survive.

There are a number of differences between subgingival plaque associated with the tooth and that associated with tissue, pockets, or the sulcular lining.

Tooth Surface

The structure of the tooth-adjacent biofilm is similar to that of the supragingival plaque, in particular that associated with gingivitis. Bacteria are densely packed and are adjacent to the pellicle covering the tooth surface. The microbiota is dominated by gram-positive filamentous bacteria, but gram-positive and gram-negative cocci and rods are also present. In the apical portion, fewer filamentous organisms are found, and the bacterial structure is dominated by gram-negative rods without any particular orientation.

Tissue-Associated Subgingival Plaque

The layers of biofilm closest to the soft tissues of the pocket contain a large number of flagellated motile bacteria and spirochetes that are not oriented in any specific manner. There is no defined intercellular matrix similar to that found in supragingival plaque. These motile bacteria are loosely adherent to the surface and the soft tissue walls are probably responsible for their retention. This loosely adherent mass is made up of late-colonizing bacteria that activate the host response, resulting in the most destructive processes seen in periodontal disease.

Comparisons of the general characteristics of supragingival and subgingival plaque biofilm are presented in Table 4-1.

PERIODONTAL MICROBIOTA

Early theories about the role of dental plaque in periodontal disease suggested that the severity of inflammation was directly related to the quantity of plaque in the mouth. These theories were based on the belief that plaque was a homogeneous bacterial mass and that all plaques in all mouths have equal potential to cause disease. This theory was called the nonspecific plaque hypothesis.[9]

With improvements in microbial research techniques, the experimental gingivitis model was used to show that plaque bacteria components change as gingivitis develops.[8] These findings led to the development of the specific plaque hypothesis. This theory is based on the belief that because of their presence or elevated levels in plaque biofilm, a combination of as many as a dozen microbial species are responsible for most cases of periodontitis.[9] Molecular biology laboratory techniques that identify genes have been developed to detect additional bacteria that may also play an important role in periodontitis. Box 4-2 presents a comparison of the specific and nonspecific plaque hypotheses.

SUBGINGIVAL HEALTH

The gingival crevice harbors microorganisms in both health and disease. In the state of health, the microbiota are relatively simple and sparse and reflect the bacterial types found in the early stages of biofilm formation. Most of the bacteria are gram-positive organisms and facultative anaerobic species.[10] Cocci, the predominant morphotype, compose almost two thirds of the microorganisms. Streptococci are of particular importance because several species adhere to the pellicle and produce extracellular polysaccharides from sucrose. These polysaccharides enhance further bacterial accumulation on the tooth. The gram-positive facultative anaerobic rods tend to be filamentous forms,

TABLE 4-1   Development of Supragingival and Subgingival Plaque Biofilms

SUPRAGINGIVAL PLAQUE BIOFILM	
Location	Clinical crowns of the teeth
Formation	Early stage
	Pellicle forms of salivary proteins on tooth surface
	Specific bacteria that are mostly gram-positive coccal forms bind to pellicle through adhesins on cell surfaces
	Monolayer of microorganisms occurs on tooth surface
	Bacteria proliferate into colonies over a few hours
	Colonies coalesce to form a mass
	Mature stage
	Bacteria increase in mass and thickness
	Aggregation occurs when glucan forms so bacteria can stick
	Aggregation increases mass of organisms and entraps others
	Biofilm produces its own energy
	Inorganic elements are low (increase as calcification occurs)
	Coaggregation (direct bacterial attachment) occurs
	Microbial succession occurs
	Deeper layers of biofilm become anaerobic, dominated by gram-negative forms and spirochetes
Inhibitors	Salivary components coat bacterial surfaces and inhibit binding
	Self-cleansing mechanisms of swallowing and salivary flow help wash bacteria away from teeth
SUBGINGIVAL PLAQUE BIOFILM	
Location	Within gingival sulcus or periodontal pocket
Formation	Initiated by presence of supragingival biofilm
	Influenced by specific microbial population in adjacent supragingival biofilm
	Biofilm grows apically
	Biofilm produces its own energy
	Tissue responses occur
	Inflammatory response
	Swelling
	Crevicular fluid flow
	Crevicular fluid provides nutrients
	Anaerobic microorganisms predominate
	Protected environment permits survival of motile organisms
	Asaccharolytic organisms predominate
	Dense colonies exist on tooth surface
	Loosely attached and motile forms (the most pathogenic organisms) reside on outer portion of biofilm close to tissue
Inhibitors	Crevicular fluid helps wash microorganisms out of pocket

BOX 4-2   Theories of Dental Plaque Biofilm

Nonspecific Plaque Hypothesis	Specific Plaque Hypothesis
• Homogenous plaque	• Microorganisms differ as plaque ages
• All microorganisms in plaque have pathogenic potential	• Disease is site-specific because of presence of specific microorganisms in those sites
• Inflammation related to age and quantity of dental plaque biofilm	• A limited number of pathogens responsible for disease
	• Quantity of plaque not significant in pathogenicity

such as *Actinomyces*. The proportions of various bacterial groups in health and disease are presented in Figure 4-9.

GINGIVITIS

The experimental gingivitis model of Löe was used to describe the changes that occurred when dental plaque was allowed to accumulate along the gingival margin of subjects for 10 to 21 days. All subjects went from a healthy state to having localized inflammation characterized by red edematous tissue. In addition, the composition of the microbial plaque biofilm changed from gram-positive cocci and rods and gram-negative cocci to a more complex ecosystem. First, there was a substantial increase in filamentous bacteria, such as *Actinomyces*. After that, the number of anaerobic and gram-negative species (*Veillonella* and especially gram-negative anaerobic rods such as *Fusobacterium* and *Prevotella intermedia*) increased, and motile rods and spirochetes appeared.[8,10]

Gingival inflammation can be initiated by any number of bacterial species if they are present in high numbers as a result of poor oral hygiene. Thus, the development of most cases of chronic gingivitis probably reflects a nonspecific infection. This is in contrast to a specific infection, in which a limited number of bacteria are known to create progressive periodontal lesions.

CHRONIC PERIODONTITIS

The continued presence and growth of pathogenic bacterial biofilm causes the inflammatory process to extend into the periodontal ligament, cementum, and alveolar bone, and leads to the loss of supporting bone and attachment of the gingiva to a tooth. In the early stages of periodontitis, the bacterial

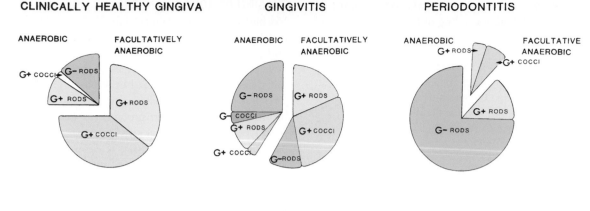

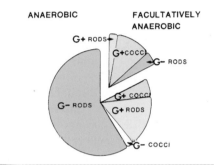

FIGURE 4-9 ■ The relative proportions of various bacterial groups from dental plaque biofilms associated with clinically healthy gingivae, gingivitis, chronic periodontitis, and juvenile periodontitis (now more properly termed *localized aggressive periodontitis*). (Used with permission from Carlsson J. Microbiology of plaque-associated periodontal disease. In: Lindhe J, ed. *Textbook of Clinical Periodontology.* 2nd ed. Copenhagen, Denmark: Munksgaard; 1989.)

components of the gingival pocket are similar to that of gingivitis, but these components become more complex as the biofilm matures and the disease progresses. Chronic periodontitis has a variety of clinical appearances in terms of probing depths, bleeding, and tooth mobility. Accordingly, the composition of the periodontal microbiota differs significantly from patient to patient and even from pocket to pocket in the same patient. In most cases these differences relate to the greater proportions of a limited number of organisms. In general, patients with chronic periodontitis have higher proportions of anaerobes, gram-negative organisms, and spirochetes; the predominant organisms are gram-negative anaerobic rods.[10]

A variety of microbial species, predominantly gram-negative species, have been implicated in the etiology of periodontitis. *P. gingivalis* seems to be the most important periodontal pathogen on the basis of its higher numbers and its possession of specific virulence factors (e.g., the production of LPSs) related to its cell wall,[11] as illustrated in Figure 4-1. Clinical studies of patients with chronic periodontitis that specifically evaluated the oral microbiota have revealed that certain groups of bacteria tend to be found in sites with disease. These have been called the red complex bacteria and the orange complex bacteria. These bacteria have been characterized as late colonizers and tend to reside in the biofilm closest to the soft tissue lining of the pocket. The red complex bacteria is composed of *P. gingivalis*, *Tannerella forsythensis*, and *Treponema denticola*.[12,13] The orange complex bacteria contribute to the pathogenesis but are considered less virulent in the periodontal disease process. They include *P. intermedia*, *F. nucleatum*, *Campylobacter* species,

Eubacterium nodatum, *Peptostreptococcus micros*, and others. The other complexes, referred to as yellow, green, blue, and purple, are earlier colonizers, and therefore they reside deeper in the biofilm (closer to the tooth surface), making them less associated with clinical disease.[14]

LOCALIZED AGGRESSIVE PERIODONTITIS

Localized aggressive periodontitis (LAP) is characterized by a rapid destruction of periodontal attachment over a short period of time. It usually involves destruction around the permanent incisors and first molars in otherwise healthy children or teenagers who exhibit relatively little dental plaque and gingival inflammation. The familial pattern of disease suggests a genetically determined susceptibility. Patients frequently have defective polymorphonuclear neutrophils (PMNs) that have impaired ability to migrate to and phagocytose bacteria, thereby increasing the individual's susceptibility to infection.[15] This disease is still commonly called localized juvenile periodontitis, although that is no longer the accepted term. A case illustrating this disease is presented in Chapter 7.

Gram-negative rods dominate the microbiota of patients with LAP, as is the situation in chronic periodontitis.[8] Commonly isolated microorganisms from patients with LAP include *A. naeslundii*, *F. nucleatum*, and *Campylobacter rectus*. In some populations, *A. actinomycetemcomitans* has been strongly implicated as one of the major pathogens.[10,15] This organism is found in higher numbers in the localized affected sites than in either healthy periodontal sites of patients with LAP or in adult patients with chronic periodontitis. The presence or absence of

A. actinomycetemcomitans in periodontal pockets must be determined by microbiologic sampling of the plaque.

CLINICAL NOTE 4-4 In some cases, patients who do not respond to conventional periodontal therapy may harbor certain virulent bacteria that can be identified by laboratory analysis of the biofilm. Once identified, appropriate antibiotics may be prescribed to treat the specific infection.

GENERALIZED AGGRESSIVE PERIODONTITIS

Similar to LAP, generalized aggressive periodontitis is characterized by a rapid destruction of periodontal attachment over a short period of time in otherwise healthy young adults, usually with little plaque and calculus. The destruction involves most, if not all, of the dentition. The subgingival microbiota in these patients is similar to those of other forms of periodontitis, with gram-negative rods predominating. Antibiotics, in conjunction with scaling and root planing, are often used for therapeutic management of this condition.

NECROTIZING ULCERATIVE GINGIVITIS AND PERIODONTITIS

Necrotizing ulcerative gingivitis (NUG) and necrotizing ulcerative periodontitis (NUP) are both forms of aggressive periodontitis. They are characterized clinically by necrotic ulcerative lesions of the interdental papillae, severe pain, rapid loss of supporting structures, and significant halitosis. NUG has a characteristic histopathologic profile; the outer surface bacteria of the supragingival biofilm are similar to the subgingival bacteria of periodontal lesions. A PMN-rich zone with a necrotic zone containing spirochetes and gram-negative rods characterizes it, and the adjacent connective tissue is infiltrated with spirochetes. NUG becomes NUP when the infection invades the deeper tissues and bone loss occurs.

NUG and NUP lesions harbor large numbers of spirochetes and *P. intermedia,* with gram-negative rods often accounting for more than 50% of the bacterial population. Examinations of NUG lesions have also identified high levels of *Fusobacteria* and *Selenomonas* species.[16]

VIRULENCE OF PERIODONTAL PATHOGENS

The virulence, or pathogenicity, of a microorganism is its ability to cause disease. The factors that contribute to the virulence potential of the major periodontal pathogens are varied and have been extensively discussed in classic reviews by Slots and Genco[11] and Listgarten.[17] In general, virulence is related to three factors: proximity to the tissue, ability to evade host defenses, and ability to destroy tissue.

PROXIMITY TO THE TISSUE

For a microorganism to be virulent, it must be established in close proximity to the periodontal tissue and it must be able to withstand the forces of saliva and gingival crevicular fluid flow capable of washing it away. Colonization is mediated by cell surface characteristics—for example, fimbriae and extracellular polysaccharides, such as glucan. Bacterial interactions are important for colonization and for the availability of nutrients.

EVASION OF HOST DEFENSES

Normally, the humoral and cellular defense systems as described in Chapter 2 are able to remove most microbes from the host and protect the tissues. However, periodontal pathogens have developed a variety of strategies to evade or overcome these self-defense mechanisms. For example, *P. gingivalis, Tannerella forsythia,* and *T. denticola* have enzymes (proteases) that degrade the host immune system proteins. *A. actinomycetemcomitans* produces a leukotoxin that kills or impairs PMNs that enter the periodontal pocket. *P. gingivalis* releases a factor that interferes with PMN movement to a site of infection.

TISSUE DESTRUCTION

The majority of the destruction of the periodontal tissues is a result of the inflammation produced by human host cells. This occurs in response to molecules released from bacteria, primarily the red and orange complexes of bacteria associated with periodontal diseases. Also, some bacterial products directly injure the host cells and tissues.

Direct Effects

Enzymes. The subgingival microbiota produce many enzymes that are capable of damaging host tissues. For example, *P. gingivalis* produces collagenase, the enzyme that degrades collagen in the tissues.

Toxins. Lipopolysaccharide, a gram-negative bacterial cell wall component, induces inflammatory reactions and stimulates osteoclast-mediated bone resorption. Another type of bone-resorbing toxin is released from *A. actinomycetemcomitans.* Toxins that affect fibroblasts and, hence, the synthesis and turnover of collagen are produced by *P. gingivalis, P. intermedia, A. actinomycetemcomitans,* and *Capnocytophaga.* In addition, several pathogens release volatile sulfides that inhibit both the synthesis of collagen and noncollagenous substances.

Indirect Effects

Some microbial products have the potential to activate immune inflammatory reactions, which in turn cause tissue destruction. For example, lipopolysaccharides from *P. gingivalis* and other gram-negative organisms stimulate the release of prostaglandin E2, interleukin-1β, and C-reactive protein from macrophages and fibroblasts. These have the potential to induce inflammation and bone resorption. The microbial components act as antigens, initiating the classic humoral and cellular hypersensitivity responses of the immune system and resulting in tissue destruction.

CLINICAL NOTE 4-5 Dental plaque biofilm has tremendous pathogenic potential. Its reduction and control are essential to achieve gingival and periodontal health. The dental hygienist plays a critical role in benefiting patients by reducing the amount of plaque biofilm and teaching patients how to control its regrowth.

PLAQUE CONTROL

A major focus of dental hygiene is educating patients about plaque biofilm control, primarily consisting of instructing individuals and school or community groups about both the importance and the techniques of toothbrushing and interproximal cleaning. Although our understanding of the role of biofilm in causing disease has evolved from a nonspecific to a specific species theory, the importance of plaque biofilm control has not changed. It is clear that thorough plaque removal should be performed daily to keep biofilm perpetually in the initial stages of formation. The bacteria that colonize on the pellicle in the first few hours of growth do not possess the same pathogenic potential as the bacteria that dominate once a biofilm has accumulated for more than 24 hours. Thorough mechanical cleaning of the teeth before the biofilm matures prevents the initiation of the disease process. The hygienist has an important role in educating patients about how plaque biofilm causes disease and how to effectively prevent or control disease by daily oral hygiene procedures. This role is crucial to the treatment of gingivitis and periodontitis and the long-term maintenance of oral health.

PERIODONTAL THERAPY

Subgingival plaque biofilm deep in periodontal pockets is inaccessible to home care procedures, making professional cleaning at regular intervals necessary to remove it, disrupt its formation, and keep it in a more immature state. Frequent recall intervals for professional plaque control procedures are effective because physical disruption of the plaque biofilm converts the pathogenic microbiota back to one more compatible with health. Studies have shown that antimicrobial agents, such as antibiotics and antiseptic rinses, are also more effective when given in conjunction with physical disruption of the plaque biofilm during professional debridement.

Our understanding of the role of dental plaque in the initiation and progression of periodontal diseases continues to evolve. For the dental hygienist, plaque biofilm assessment, removal, and control remain integral parts of professional practice.

◎ DENTAL HYGIENE CONSIDERATIONS

- Dental plaque biofilms are complex ecologic systems made up of many species of bacterial organisms.
- Bacteria are classified according to specific characteristics: morphotype, cell wall structure, oxygen environment, and metabolism.
- Different oral environments—mucosa, tongue, teeth—harbor different bacteria on the basis of specific bacterial characteristics.
- Supragingival plaque biofilm forms on pellicle composed of salivary proteins, exhibits a complex growth and maturation process, and becomes more pathogenic as it ages.
- Subgingival plaque biofilm is initiated from supragingival biofilms, contains more gram-negative anaerobic species, and is protected in the pocket, making it easy for loosely adherent motile forms to thrive near the pocket lining.
- Plaque biofilms differ among patients with gingival health, gingivitis, chronic periodontitis, localized aggressive periodontitis (LAP), generalized aggressive periodontitis, and necrotizing ulcerative gingivitis (NUG) and necrotizing ulcerative periodontitis (NUP).
- The virulence, or pathogenicity, of plaque biofilm is related to proximity to tissue, ability to evade host defenses, and ability to destroy tissue.
- The goal of dental plaque biofilm control is to keep biofilm in a perpetually immature state through home care procedures and professional care by the dental hygienist.

★ CASE SCENARIO

Mr. Hughes is a patient to whom you have been providing regular professional care (including scaling, root planing, and home care instruction) every 3 months for more than a year. His periodontal condition has improved markedly, so that the gingiva is no longer red and there is no bleeding except in the areas where he has deeper pockets. His plaque biofilm control is excellent and no supragingival plaque is present at his appointment. Mr. Hughes is very concerned about the expense of regular dental hygiene care and wishes to come in less often, no more than once per year.

1. Mr. Hughes needs to come in often for care (including plaque biofilm removal from his deeper pockets) because plaque biofilm matures and becomes more virulent as it ages.
   A. Both the statement and the reason are correct and related.
   B. Both the statement and the reason are correct but NOT related.
   C. The statement is correct, but the reason is NOT correct.
   D. The statement is NOT correct, but the reason is correct.
   E. NEITHER the statement NOR the reason is correct.

2. There are self-cleansing mechanisms in the mouth that help control the development of plaque biofilm. These mechanisms also cleanse deep pockets.
   A. Both statements are true.
   B. Both statements are false.
   C. The first statement is true, and the second statement is false.
   D. The first statement is false, and the second statement is true.

3. Why are some of Mr. Hughes' deeper pockets still bleeding?
   A. He has not removed the subgingival plaque biofilm.
   B. He has not removed the supragingival plaque biofilm between his teeth.
   C. Dental hygiene instrumentation primarily removes supragingival plaque.
   D. Brushing and interproximal cleaning devices primarily remove subgingival plaque.

4. Plaque biofilm regrows in the deep pockets in a more virulent form than supragingival biofilm because it is difficult to disrupt with home plaque control methods.
   A. Both the statement and the reason are correct and related.
   B. Both the statement and the reason are correct but NOT related.
   C. The statement is correct, but the reason is NOT correct.
   D. The statement is NOT correct, but the reason is correct.
   E. NEITHER the statement NOR the reason is correct.

5. Plaque biofilm that is regularly disrupted by home care procedures
   A. remains a less virulent form with more motile forms.
   B. remains a less virulent from with fewer gram-positive forms.
   C. remains a less virulent form with fewer gram-negative and motile forms.
   D. remains a more virulent form with fewer gram-negative and motile forms.

STUDY QUESTIONS

Answers and rationales to these questions can be obtained from your instructor.

MULTIPLE CHOICE

1. Plaque biofilm microbiota produces enzymes. Some of the enzymes produced by biofilm organisms enhance tissue destruction by activating the host immune response.
   A. Both statements are true.
   B. Both statements are false.
   C. The first statement is true, and the second statement is false.
   D. The first statement is false, and the second statement is true.

2. The scientific rationale for the dental hygienist to teach patients good plaque biofilm control is to
   A. keep plaque in a mature state.
   B. keep plaque in an immature state.
   C. enhance self-cleansing mechanisms in the mouth.
   D. remove pellicle from teeth so that bacteria cannot adhere.

3. Plaque biofilm should be removed by the patient at a minimum every
   A. 6 hours.
   B. 24 hours.
   C. 48 hours.
   D. 72 hours.

4. Understanding that plaque is a biofilm is significant because
   A. plaque biofilms are protective of the gingiva.
   B. it highlights the importance of mechanical removal.
   C. biofilm enhances the effectiveness of antimicrobial rinses.
   D. the quantity of plaque is more significant than the composition of the biofilm.

5. Gingivitis, which is considered to be a nonspecific infection, is a disease process that is unlikely to be progressive. Chronic periodontitis is likely caused by a limited number of organisms and is a disease process that is likely to progress.
   A. Both statements are true.
   B. Both statements are false.
   C. The first statement is true, and the second statement is false.
   D. The first statement is false, and the second statement is true.

6. The morphotypes of mature biofilm microbiota are different than those generally found in gram-positive biofilms because the environment becomes conducive to gram-negative and motile bacterial species.
   A. Both the statement and the reason are correct and related.
   B. Both the statement and the reason are correct but NOT related.
   C. The statement is correct, but the reason is NOT correct.
   D. The statement is NOT correct, but the reason is correct.
   E. NEITHER the statement NOR the reason is correct.

7. The most commonly found periodontal pathogen in chronic periodontitis is
   A. gram-positive cocci.
   B. orange complex bacteria.
   C. red complex bacteria.
   D. spirochetes.

8. Necrotizing ulcerative gingivitis is referred to as necrotizing ulcerative periodontitis when which event occurs?
   A. The infection is no longer painful to the patient.
   B. The infection invades the deeper tissues and bone loss occurs.
   C. The microbiota changes to fewer spirochetes and gram-negative rods.
   D. The ulcerative lesions dissipate.

SHORT ANSWER

9. Describe the effects of lipopolysaccharides (endotoxins).
10. Describe the importance of pellicle in the formation of dental plaque biofilm.

Please visit **http://evolve.elsevier.com/Perry/periodontology** for additional practice and study support tools.

REFERENCES

1. Wirthlin MR, Armitage GC. Dental plaque and calculus: microbial biofilms and periodontal diseases. In: Rose LF, Mealey BL, eds. *Periodontics: Medicine, Surgery, and Implants.* St. Louis, MO: Elsevier Mosby; 2004: 99–116.
2. Löe HE, Theilade E, Jensen SB. Experimental gingivitis in man. *J Periodontol.* 1965;36:177–187.
3. Liljemark WF, Bloomquist C. Human oral microbial ecology and dental caries and periodontal diseases. *Crit Rev Oral Biol Med.* 1996;7:180–198.
4. Loomer PM, Armitage GC. Microbiology of periodontal diseases. In: Rose LF, Mealey BL, eds. *Periodontics: Medicine, Surgery, and Implants.* St. Louis, MO: Elsevier Mosby; 2004:69–84.
5. Kolenbrander PE, London J. Adhere today, here tomorrow: oral bacterial adherence. *J Bacteriol.* 1993;175:3247–3252.
6. Jakubovics NS, Kolenbrander PE. The road to ruin: the formation of disease-associated oral biofilms. *Oral Dis.* 2010;16: 729–739.
7. Teughels W, Quirynen M, Jakubovics N. Periodontal microbiology. In: Newman MG, Takei HH, Klokkevold PA, et al, eds. *Carranza's Clinical Periodontology.* 11th ed. St. Louis, MO: Elsevier Saunders; 2012:232–269.
8. Theilade E, Wright WH, Jensen SB, et al. Experimental gingivitis in man, II: a longitudinal clinical and bacteriological investigation. *J Periodont Res.* 1966;1:1–13.
9. Loesche WH. Chemotherapy of dental plaque infections. *Oral Sci Rev.* 1976;9:65–107.
10. Slots J. Subgingival microflora and periodontal disease. *J Clin Periodontol.* 1979;6:351–382.
11. Slots J, Genco RJ. Black-pigmented *Bacteroides* species, *Capnocytophaga* species, and *Actinobacillus actinomycetemcomitans* in human periodontal disease: virulence factors in colonization, survival, and tissue destruction. *J Dent Res.* 1984;63:412–421.
12. Moore WEC. Microbiology of periodontal disease. *J Periodontol.* 1987; 22:335–341.
13. Socransky SS, Haffajee AD, Cugini MA, et al. Microbial complexes in subgingival plaque. *J Clin Periodontol.* 1998;25:133–144.
14. Socransky SS, Haffajee AD. Dental biofilms: difficult therapeutic targets. *Periodontol.* 2002;28:12–55.
15. Zambon JJ. *Actinobacillus actinomycetemcomitans* in human periodontal disease. *J Clin Periodontol.* 1985;12:1–20.
16. Loesche WJ, Syed SA, Laughon BG, et al. The bacteriology of acute necrotizing ulcerative gingivitis. *J Periodontol.* 1982;53:223–230.
17. Listgarten MA. Nature of periodontal diseases: pathogenic mechanisms. *J Periodontal Res.* 1987;22:172–178.

PART II

Foundations of Periodontal Therapy

The information addressed in the following chapters defines the disease process. The dental hygienist must be well grounded in the diseases and processes that affect patient care. The following questions are asked and answered in Part II:

5

Calculus and Other Disease-Associated Factors

Gwen Essex and Dorothy Perry

LEARNING OUTCOMES

- Describe the role of dental calculus and other disease-associated factors in the initiation and perpetuation of gingival and periodontal disease.
- Describe the formation and attachment of supragingival and subgingival calculus in the oral environment.
- Describe the distribution of calculus deposits.
- Compare the composition, distribution, and attachment of supragingival and subgingival calculus.

- Explain how anticalculus agents work in reducing calculus formations in humans.
- List the variety of factors that are linked to periodontal disease.
- Describe hygienic restorations.
- Explain the role of the dental hygienist in the recognition and provision of care for patients with disease-associated factors.

KEY TERMS

Acquired pellicle	Malocclusion	Risk indicator
Amalgam overhangs	Mouth breathing	Salivary duct calculus
Anatomic anomalies	Orthodontic appliances	Serumal calculus
Calculus	Overcontoured crowns	Subgingival calculus
First molar loss	Overcontoured restorations	Submarginal calculus
Food impaction areas	Pyrophosphate	Supragingival calculus
Lingual groove	Risk factor	Tartar

A thorough understanding of calculus, what it is and why it is important, places calculus removal in perspective in dental hygiene practice. A good deal of practice time is spent removing calculus and preventing its formation. Calculus removal has an important place in dental hygiene care because its presence tends to accelerate the progression of disease (frequently in localized areas), and it is a readily modifiable factor associated with improved periodontal health.[1] In addition, other irritating factors related to tooth placement and tooth replacement can also present complications in dental hygiene care by providing areas where plaque biofilms accumulate and are hard to control. These factors are very important in dental hygiene practice, and dental hygienists spend much of their work time addressing them.

CALCULUS

The removal of calculus occupies much of the treatment time of the dental hygienist. Perfecting the skills necessary to achieve calculus removal can take years. Calculus removal too often becomes the focus of dental hygiene care for this reason: anything that requires so much time and effort must be more

valuable than activities that require less treatment time. Calculus removal is important, but it is only part of dental hygiene care. Calculus is not a benign substance unrelated to the pathogenesis of gingival and periodontal disease, but it plays a much smaller part in these diseases than bacterial plaque biofilms. The dental hygienist may spend 90% of treatment time on calculus removal and 5% on plaque biofilm control, but must not lose sight of the significance of each. Calculus removal is passive treatment for the patient that is provided by a dental hygienist. Daily plaque control (interrupting the biofilm on the tooth surfaces), taught by the dental hygienist and performed by the patient, requires active daily participation. Daily plaque control allows the individual to maintain gingival health for a lifetime and concurrently limit calculus formation.

CLINICAL NOTE 5-1 Although calculus removal is significant, it is also important to educate patients regarding preventive measures.

TARTAR

Tartar is the common name, often used by patients, for dental calculus. Although introduced in the sixteenth century, and wrongly attributed with causation of malady,[2] the use of the term is likely to continue because it is often used in advertising. Products referred to as tartar control toothpaste and rinses are popular and reinforce the use of this term.

SIGNIFICANCE

Calculus is formed by the deposition of calcium and phosphate salts present in bacterial plaque. It has long been thought to be the cause of periodontal diseases due to its association with gingival infections and the improved gingival health observed following its removal. A thoughtful review by Mandel and Gaffar[3] reported that 11% of sites with calculus also had gingivitis, whereas 75% of tooth surfaces with plaque had gingivitis. This finding suggested that calculus may be a result of disease rather than the cause and that more strongly identified plaque bacteria biofilm is a causative factor.

Calculus does contribute to the development of disease, serving as a reservoir for bacterial plaque biofilm, the etiologic agent. Calculus has been shown to have nonmineralized areas appearing microscopically as channels that contain bacteria and other debris.[4] Colonies of bacteria inside the calculus are impossible to remove by any oral hygiene procedure and provide sheltered areas in periodontal pockets that keep plaque in close proximity to the tissues.

> **CLINICAL NOTE 5-2** Calculus is not itself the causative agent of periodontal diseases; its removal permits healing of periodontal tissues by reducing and eliminating the plaque bacterial biofilm that is always associated with mineral deposits.

It is also clear that even in young people, the presence of calculus is associated with increased levels of gingival disease. A study of Thai children aged 11 to 13 years showed a significant association among gingivitis, plaque status, and calculus accumulation, but no association between calculus status and caries.[5] An evaluation of data from 1285 young people aged 13 to 20 years who participated in the 1986-1987 national survey of the oral health of U.S. adolescents indicated that **subgingival calculus** is associated with both attachment loss and aggressive forms of periodontitis. The young people with measurable attachment loss had significantly more gingival bleeding and subgingival calculus than matched control subjects. Importantly, the aggressive periodontitis group had significantly more subgingival calculus than those with attachment loss, but no aggressive disease, suggesting an association between gingival disease and the presence of subgingival calculus.[6] (See Chapter 7 for a discussion of aggressive periodontitis.)

The role of the bacteria in relation to calculus formation is not completely understood. As oral biologic research continues to increase the understanding of this relationship, dental hygienists will be better able to help patients control calculus formation.

DEFINITION

Calculus is defined by its location relative to the gingival margin. It is either supragingival or subgingival.

Dental hygienists commonly describe patients as light, moderate, or heavy calculus formers, depending on the amount of

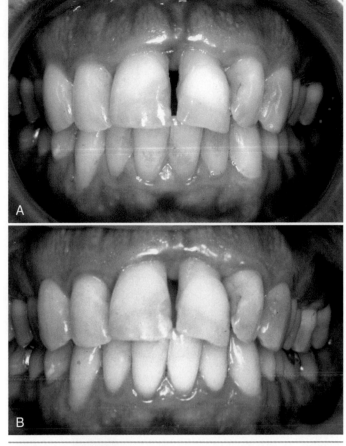

FIGURE 5-1 ■ The effects of plaque-associated calculus on periodontal tissues. Calculus removal results in reduction in the signs of inflammation and easier plaque control. **A,** Before nonsurgical calculus removal and periodontal therapy. **B,** After nonsurgical calculus removal and periodontal therapy.

supragingival calculus that forms between recall visits. This distinction is useful in terms of estimating treatment time, but not much else. Patients may have light, moderate, or heavy deposits of subgingival calculus that forms below the gingival margin, supragingival calculus alone, or both. Figure 5-1 highlights the effects of dental hygiene care on a patient with heavy deposits of subgingival calculus. Tissue tone and color improve and the calculus and plaque biofilm removal results in reduced inflammation, causing tissue shrinkage.

SUPRAGINGIVAL CALCULUS

Supragingival calculus is found on the clinical crowns of the teeth, above the margin of the gingiva.[7] It is readily visible as a yellowish-white accumulation, although it may darken with age. Figure 5-2 shows an extreme deposition of supragingival calculus.

Formation and Components

Supragingival calculus is tightly adherent to the teeth and may occur on any tooth in the mouth. Supragingival calculus is most abundant near the openings of salivary ducts such as the sublingual ducts (adjacent to the lingual surfaces of the lower anterior teeth) and the parotid ducts (near the buccal surfaces of the maxillary molars).

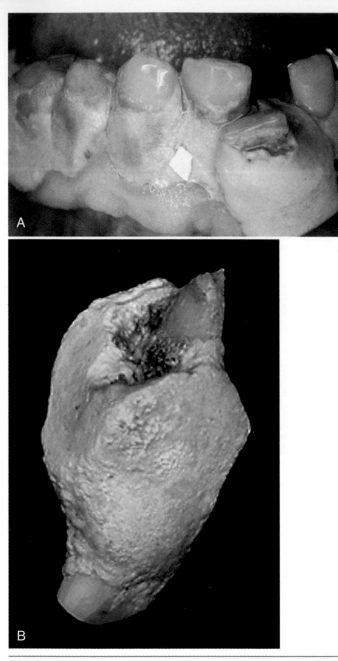

magnesium,[8] sodium, and potassium, and trace elements of fluoride, zinc, and strontium.[2]

The main crystal types in calculus are as follows:
- 58% hydroxyapatite ($Ca_{10}[PO_4]_6 \cdot OH_2$)
- About 21% octacalcium phosphate ($Ca_8[HPO_4]_4$)
- About 21% magnesium whitlockite ($Ca_3[PO_4]_2$)
- Approximately 9% brushite ($Ca[HPO_4] \cdot 2H_2O$)[8]

Brushite appears in large proportions, up to 50%, in young, recently deposited calculus. After a few weeks or months, the predominant crystal type becomes hydroxyapatite.[2]

The organic component of calculus makes up 15% to 20% of the dry weight of calculus. Half is protein from the bacterial cells, but it also includes carbohydrates and lipids from bacteria and saliva.[2] Carbohydrates make up 1.9% to 9.1% of the organic component of supragingival calculus, salivary proteins account for 5.9% to 8.2% of the mass, and there are trace amounts of lipids. Dental calculus, salivary duct calculus (calculi that can form and block the openings of major and minor salivary ducts, referred to as sialoliths, or salivary stones), and calcified dental tissues are all similar in organic composition, but subgingival calculus lacks the quantity of salivary protein.[8]

Attachment to the Tooth Structure

Attachment to the tooth surface occurs in relationship to bacterial plaque biofilm. Acquired pellicle is a layer of glycoprotein deposited from salivary and crevicular fluids that are strongly bound to the tooth surface.[9] Bacterial plaque biofilm formation begins on the pellicle with gram-positive coccoid organisms and then calcification occurs. After about 5 days, the plaque becomes filamentous and resembles decalcified mature calculus.[2] Pellicle can grow into microscopic pores and openings and form dendritic (finger-like) structures in the cementum. These structures are thought to increase the tenacity of calculus attachment.[2] Mechanical locking of calculus into tooth surface irregularities and close adaptation to tooth shape are also forms of attachment that can add to its tenacity.[8]

CLINICAL NOTE 5-4 Tooth morphology plays a role in the adherence of calculus, so a thorough knowledge of morphology is essential for dental hygienists to access grooves and concavities that can harbor calculus.

Mineralization in plaque can begin within 4 to 8 hours. Plaque may become 50% mineralized in 2 days and up to 90% mineralized after 12 days. Mineralization occurs more rapidly in some individuals and more slowly in others.[7] Supragingival calculus can form on occlusal tooth surfaces when the teeth are out of occlusion or in crossbite, as well as on both fixed and removable prosthetic devices.

SUBGINGIVAL CALCULUS

Subgingival calculus forms on root surfaces below the gingival margin and can extend into the periodontal pockets. Subgingival calculus is likely to be tenacious and is typically dark green or black, probably because of the organic matrix products of the subgingival plaque. The subgingival matrix of plaque biofilm contains blood products associated with subgingival hemorrhage. These matrix products have a dark pigment and differ

FIGURE 5-2 ■ A, Supragingival calculus can accumulate in huge amounts and may obliterate the structure of the teeth. The white area is food debris. **B,** Only the root tip and incisal edge of this tooth are visible because of the extensive calculus accumulation. The tooth simply fell out.

CLINICAL NOTE 5-3 Even patients with good plaque control can exhibit calculus formation on the buccal surfaces of maxillary molars and lingual surfaces of lower anterior teeth because these surfaces are bathed in fresh saliva from the opening of the adjacent salivary ducts.

In supragingival calculus formation, mineral crystals are deposited in an organic matrix of plaque microorganisms, glucans, glycoproteins, and lipids. The calculi (calcified nodules) are stratified, suggesting that supragingival calculus is deposited in layers. Inorganic mineral content makes up about 80% of supragingival calculus. The minerals are primarily calcium phosphate (75.9%), calcium carbonate (3.1%), traces of from supragingival calculus, where the organic matrix components come primarily from saliva and do not contain blood.[9] Subgingival calculus is commonly deposited in rings or ledges on root surfaces, but it may also appear on veneers. Subgingival calculus is also called **submarginal calculus** because of its location or **serumal calculus** because of the source of the mineral content.[7] Figure 5-3 shows a patient with subgingival calculus.

CLINICAL NOTE 5-5 Subgingival calculus is tenacious, and by definition, rarely directly visible, making sharp instruments and well-honed detection skills essential for the dental hygienist.

Formation and Components

Like supragingival calculus, subgingival calculus forms from mineralized plaque biofilm. Pellicle forms first, subgingival plaque is seeded or forms by extension of supragingival plaque biofilm, and then mineralization occurs. The mineral content is derived from crevicular fluid rather than from saliva, differentiating it from supragingival calculus.

The organic components of subgingival calculus are similar to those of supragingival calculus, but contain more calcium, magnesium, and fluoride because of the higher concentrations of these minerals in crevicular fluid.[2] There is no salivary protein present in subgingival calculus and, interestingly, the sodium content of subgingival calculus increases with the depth of the periodontal pockets.[8]

The pocket contents are composed of subgingival calculus adjacent to the root surface, attached plaque biofilm, and loosely attached or unattached bacteria. Bacterial cells become mineralized in the calculus, but do not form a solid mass; there are channels in which bacteria survive so that calculus is filled with bacteria that perpetuate the disease process.[4] As with supragingival calculus, there is a layer of attached plaque biofilm covering the calculus and loosely adherent bacteria next to the tissue in the pocket. Figure 5-4 shows the contents of the periodontal pocket, including calculus.

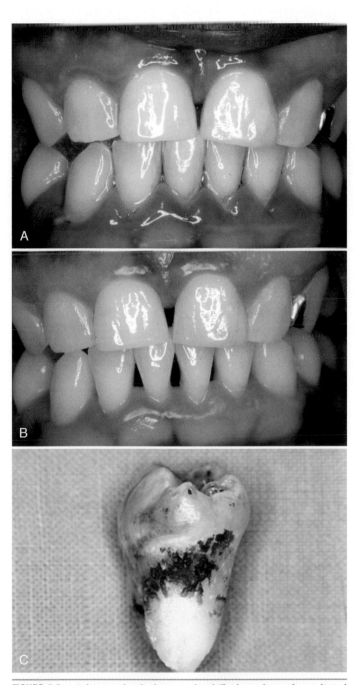

FIGURE 5-3 ■ Subgingival calculus may be difficult to detect from clinical appearance alone. Explorer examination is required for accurate assessment. **A,** This patient had heavy deposits of subgingival calculus that were not readily apparent by visual inspection, but the associated periodontal inflammation is obvious. **B,** After the dental hygienist scaled and root-planed the teeth to remove the subgingival calculus, the tissue health improved dramatically. **C,** This extracted molar is covered with a sheet of black subgingival calculus. This type of calculus becomes embedded in the cementum and is very difficult to remove.

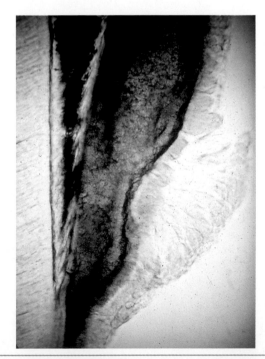

FIGURE 5-4 ■ **Histologic section of the contents of the periodontal pocket.** The calculus is immediately adjacent to the tooth root and crown and appears dark red. The enamel surface is dark blue and the dentin is light blue and appears striated because of the presence of dentinal tubules. Organized bacterial plaque biofilm is attached to the surface of the calculus and the unattached plaque is apparent as the less organized bacterial masses. There is no epithelium in the section. (Courtesy of Dr. Edward Green.)

Attachment to the Tooth Structure

Due to multiple means of attachment, subgingival calculus is tenacious and more difficult to remove than supragingival calculus. Pellicle attachment to cementum is the primary mechanism of subgingival calculus adherence. Deposits also form in and around microorganisms on the more irregular cemental surfaces, possibly caused by the loss of Sharpey's fibers, resorption lacunae, or arrested caries.[2] Crystals can grow deep into cemental irregularities. They appear morphologically similar to cementum (termed *calculocementum*)[8] and exhibit intercrystalline bonding.[2] Figure 5-5 shows a scanning electron micrograph of subgingival calculus adapted to a cemental surface and Figure 5-6 illustrates the microscopic appearance of calculus embedded in a root surface.

Unlike supragingival calculus, the location of subgingival calculus is not site-specific.[10] It is found anywhere throughout the mouth, and both radiographic examination and explorer detection are required to evaluate the extent and location of deposits. Radiographs alone tend to show mesial and distal deposits and underestimate the amount of calculus present because of technique-related artifacts. Overangulation of film,

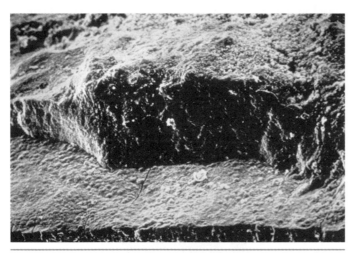

FIGURE 5-5 ■ Scanning electron micrograph of subgingival calculus attached to a cementum surface. The cementum is the flat surface on the lower portion of the micrograph. (Courtesy of Dr. John Sottosanti.)

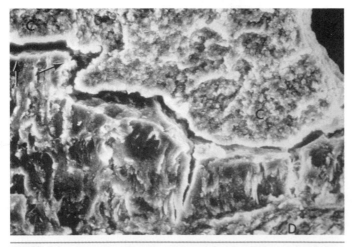

FIGURE 5-6 ■ Scanning electron micrograph of calculus embedded in cemental irregularities. The cementum surface is the lower portion of the micrograph, calculus above. (Courtesy of Dr. John Sottosanti.)

cervical burnout, and poor processing techniques limit the reliability of radiographic detection of subgingival calculus. Explorer detection provides the dental hygienist with buccal and lingual estimates of deposits, along with proximal estimates, but it is also subject to individual technique. It is advisable to use both radiographs and tactile skill to evaluate the amount of subgingival calculus present.

Distribution. Supragingival calculus appears most commonly on the mandibular incisors and maxillary molars, especially the first molar, and is related to the openings of the major salivary ducts. Subgingival calculus is more evenly distributed throughout the mouth.[10] It is a common mistake to assume that no calculus deposits occur around the maxillary anterior teeth. Although less frequent than other locations, both subgingival and supragingival calculus can occur there in as many as 10% of patients. Figure 5-7 shows the distribution of calculus found in a large population of patients.[11]

The course of calculus formation and its distribution in humans has also been described. An important study by Anerud and colleagues[12] compared 480 Sri Lankan male tea laborers, 14 to 31 years old, over a 15-year period with Norwegian men and boys, 16 to 30 years old, over a 20-year period. The researchers described the natural history of calculus formation with these data. Findings from Sri Lanka, a country with no dental care and in which toothbrushing was not performed, were compared with the clinical course of calculus formation in Norwegian subjects, who had optimum preventive dental care. Natural history refers to the course of calculus formation over time without any intervention, as in the case of the Sri Lankan subjects. The Norwegian subjects had ample opportunity to receive regular care in school clinics and private dental practices and represented the course of calculus formation tempered by regular, modern dental treatment. These data, summarized in Table 5-1, clearly showed the importance of calculus removal for long-term gingival health and emphasized the importance of maintenance therapy, including thorough calculus removal by the dental hygienist.

For reasons that are not completely understood, there is tremendous individual variation in calculus formation rates. Plaque has shown evidence of mineral precipitation occurring in 1 to 14 days, but it can occur as quickly as within 4 hours. Calcifying plaques may become up to 50% mineralized in 2 days and 60% to 90% mineralized in 12 days.[8] Heavy calculus formers have higher levels of calcium and phosphorus (from the saliva) in the plaque within a few days after a prophylaxis. In addition, differences in diet and in the composition of the microbial flora may contribute to formation rates. Mandel[2] reviewed a number of characteristics that may be related to an increased rate of calculus formation:

1. Elevated salivary pH
2. Concentration of calcium in saliva
3. Concentration of salivary bacterial protein and lipid
4. Lower individual inhibitory factors
5. Higher salivary urea and protein from the submandibular glands
6. Higher total salivary lipid levels

Light calculus formers have higher levels of parotid **pyrophosphate,** similar to the chemical found in tartar control toothpastes. It has been suggested that dental patients who are

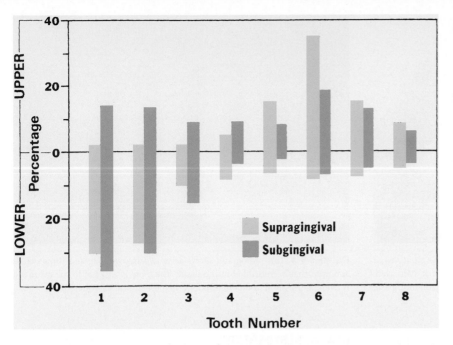

FIGURE 5-7 ■ Distribution of calculus by individual teeth. The percentage of individual teeth with supragingival and subgingival calculus is shown by tooth number and arch. Tooth #1 is the central incisor and tooth #8 is the third molar in each quadrant. Subgingival calculus forms on all teeth in the mouth, with greater formation in the mandibular anterior area. Supragingival calculus is most prevalent in the mandibular anterior and maxillary posterior areas but can also form on any tooth. (Adapted with permission from Schroeder HE. *Formation and Inhibition of Dental Calculus.* Vienna, Austria: H. Huber; 1969.)

TABLE 5-1 Calculus Formation in Adult Male Populations on the Basis of the Findings of Anerud, Löe, and Boysen[12]

	CALCULUS	SUPRAGINGIVAL	SUBGINGIVAL	TOBACCO EFFECTS	LOSS OF ATTACHMENT
Natural history: Sri Lankan tea workers with no dental care	All had some; amount increased over years	Formed early in life on maxillary molars and mandibular anterior teeth; continued to grow until age 25 or 30 years; was present on all teeth	Formed 6-8 years after eruption; continued to increase in extent and severity; leveled off at age 30 years	Smokers and betel nut chewers had more calculus than nonsmokers or nonchewers	Subgingival calculus associated with more attachment loss than teeth with no subgingival calculus
Clinical course: Norwegian men with regular dental care	Generally low levels over years	Found on maxillary molars and mandibular anterior teeth but at low levels; rarely found in other locations; did not increase in amount with age	Seen at low levels around age 20-29 years; no predilection for specific teeth; increased somewhat with age	Not associated with increased amounts of calculus	Accumulation of supragingival and subgingival calculus that were removed regularly had no effect on attachment loss

taking some medications, such as beta-blockers, diuretics, and thyroid supplements, form less supragingival calculus than comparable individuals who are not taking any medications.[13,14]

PATHOGENESIS

Supragingival calculus is porous and rough and provides an excellent lattice on which plaque can grow. It assists in maintaining the bacterial colonies close to the tissue, interfering with oral self-cleansing mechanisms, and making plaque biofilm removal more difficult for patients, if not impossible in some areas.[2,8]

Subgingival calculus is associated with the chronic nature and progression of periodontal diseases. Periodontal pockets virtually always contain subgingival calculus, even if in microscopic amounts.[8] Calculus provides a reservoir for bacteria and

endotoxins that are significantly related to the disease process. In addition, subgingival calculus covered by bacterial plaque biofilm is associated with greater disease progression than plaque alone.[2] Long-term studies clearly support the removal of all calculus to promote healing and prevent further loss of attachment.[15]

ANTICALCULUS AGENTS

A number of agents can reduce supragingival calculus formation. These agents work through inhibition of hydroxyapatite crystal growth by pyrophosphates or the analogue, diphosphonate.[2] Studies in the 1980s showed reduced supragingival calculus in several hundred subjects considered to be heavy calculus formers. In each of the studies, supragingival calculus was reduced by 26% after 2 months,[16] 37% after 6 months,[17] and 21.4% after 6 months,[18] respectively. All three studies found that

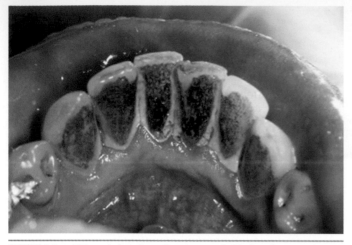

FIGURE 5-8 ■ This periodontal recall patient used chlorhexidine mouth rinse for 6 weeks. Heavy deposits of supragingival calculus and dark stain were evident at the 3-month recall appointment. Calculus (tartar control) toothpaste would reduce this accumulation considerably.

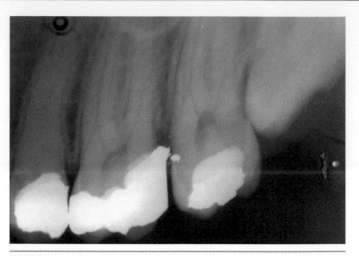

FIGURE 5-9 ■ This radiograph shows an amalgam overhang and some excess amalgam that is embedded in the tissue. The bone loss apical to the overhang is evident. This is all too common a finding on clinical examination.

pyrophosphate-containing dentifrices were safe and well tolerated by the oral soft tissues of the subjects. Only one comparison study of three types of pyrophosphate toothpastes reported slightly greater calculus reduction by one product over another. These products are quite safe to use because just one case of oral ulcers was reported among 118 subjects who used the products over a 3-month period.[19] Anticalculus toothpastes with fluoride have no negative effects on tooth remineralization and do not interfere with the inhibition of caries by fluorides.

It is important for the dental hygienist to educate patients about the realistic effects of these preparations. They are widely advertised, safe to use, reduce the formation of new supragingival calculus, and prevent caries (from fluoride in the preparations). However, they do not reduce the quantity of calculus already present in the mouth. Their effectiveness is limited to reduction in the formation of new supragingival calculus and they have no measurable effects on subgingival calculus.[7] It is important to understand that improved toothbrushing alone can reduce the formation of new supragingival calculus by as much as 50% on the lingual surfaces of the lower anterior teeth, so the benefits of these preparations are real but limited.[2]

These commercially available tartar control anticalculus toothpastes and mouthwashes may be helpful for periodontal patients who accumulate supragingival calculus and for patients using chlorhexidine mouth rinse, which is associated with dark staining and increased calculus deposition. Figure 5-8 is representative of a patient who forms heavy calculus and stain on the lower anterior teeth. The dental hygienist should be aware of the usefulness of these products, but should not expect them to provide complete calculus control or to replace needed instrumentation.

PLAQUE RETENTION FACTORS

Individual patient factors are clearly linked to periodontal health; such factors include the following:

- Overcontoured or worn dental restorations
- Food impaction areas
- Orthodontic bands and brackets

DENTAL RESTORATIONS

Dental restorations can significantly alter dental plaque growth, retention, and gingival health. Marginal discrepancies between the edges of the restorations and the remaining tooth surface, particularly those margins placed subgingivally, are associated with detrimental periodontal changes. Unfortunately, the fit of restorations is generally less than perfect. Studies show that up to 80% of restorations examined on radiographs exhibit marginal defects and that those larger than 0.2 mm are always associated with bone loss. In addition, 69% of fillings and 82% of bridges show evidence of ill-fitting margins.[20] Figure 5-9 is a posterior radiograph showing an extensive amalgam overhang.

Crown Contours and Margins

Overcontoured crowns, bridges, and other cast and ceramic restorations have been associated with gingival inflammation and periodontal disease. Plaque biofilm formation, the cause of inflammation, is enhanced by subgingival placement of fixed restorations for a variety of reasons, such as greater surface roughness of the materials, fit of the margin to the remaining tooth structure, and contour of the restoration.[21] One study of 831 private practice dental patients in North Carolina showed that crown margins placed subgingivally were almost always associated with increased gingival inflammation and probing depth (Figure 5-10) compared with uncrowned surfaces. This finding was true even in the case of subjects who had regular maintenance visits.[22]

Ragged subgingival margins of restorations are difficult for the dentist or dental hygienist to remove, even more than calculus. These ragged margins provide a sheltered place for plaque growth, much like subgingival calculus. Adequate patient plaque control is also more difficult on restorations than on smoother unrestored surfaces. Figure 5-11 shows an amalgam restoration that contributed to the progression of periodontal bone loss into the furcation area.[21]

All cast margins, even those that fit properly, leave at least a microscopically thin line of cement. This line is either next to the gingiva in the case of subgingival margins or open to the

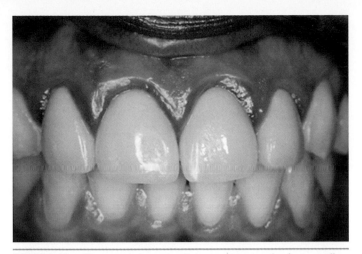

FIGURE 5-10 ■ These attractive cosmetic restorations on the four maxillary incisor teeth have caused inflammation in the gingival tissues. The margins of the restorations were placed subgingivally and impinge on the tissue. The patient is very happy with the cosmetic results, not concerned about the inflamed gingiva, and not willing to have the restorations replaced.

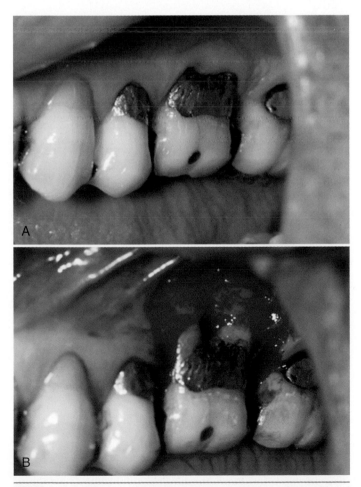

FIGURE 5-11 ■ Class V amalgam restorations can impinge on the periodontal tissues. **A,** A large restoration was placed on the buccal surface of tooth #3. **B,** The amalgam surface was rough and was extremely hard to contour. The deep furcation defect developed and, when the periodontal tissue was reflected during surgery, the amalgam was seen to extend directly into the furcation area. The surgery resulted in the creation of a wide open space that was a challenge for the patient to keep free of plaque biofilm. (Courtesy of Dr. Gary C. Armitage.)

oral environment if the margins are supragingival. The larger the gap, the more biofilm it can harbor, just like any ragged restoration margin. In addition, the cement is slowly dissolved by saliva, creating a space ideal for plaque growth. These observations suggest that the poorer the fit of the subgingival cast restoration margin, the more extreme the gingival reaction is likely to be. The contour of crown restorations is also significant. Bulbous rounded crowns can impinge on the embrasure space, making plaque control difficult and resulting in increased inflammation of the associated tissues.[21]

Kenney[23] recommended that adaptation of restoration margins be above the gingival margin, if possible, contours of restorations facilitate cleaning, proximal relationships between the teeth leave space for the gingiva and make cleaning easy, and restoration surfaces be as smooth as possible so that plaque accumulation is not enhanced.

Specifically, seven items should be kept in mind in relation to dental hygiene care[23]:

1. A healthy gingival sulcus is required before restorative treatment is performed so that the height of the gingiva in relation to the restoration margin can be determined.
2. Margins of restorations should be kept away from the gingiva.
3. Even properly fitting crown margins have a thin line of cement to which biofilms can readily adhere.
4. Temporary crowns should have margins that fit as well as possible and should be polished to minimize roughness. Figure 5-12 shows correctly contoured temporary crowns.
5. Restorations should preserve the embrasure space, particularly the interproximal embrasure, so that there is adequate room for the gingiva. The gingiva will fill the space after treatment, and there must be enough room for an adequate collagen attachment.
6. Crowns must be contoured to facilitate oral hygiene procedures, especially in furcation areas. In some cases, the height of the contour of the tooth will be reduced and grooves will be accentuated to allow access to the gingival margin for cleaning. This requirement is especially important in furcation areas. Crowns contoured to allow cleaning of furcation areas are shown in Figure 5-13.
7. Pontics of the older saddle design, overlapping the alveolar ridge on both sides, are impossible to keep clean. Newer designs that are bullet-shaped or spherical are preferable, and hygienic pontics that leave a 3-mm space between the bottom of the pontic and the gingiva should be used when possible. Figure 5-14 shows a hygienic pontic.

Amalgam Overhangs

Amalgam overhangs are one of the most common forms of poorly contoured restorations and they cause plaque traps, leading to increased gingival inflammation. Their major contribution to pathologic conditions is as a source of plaque biofilm retention and they complicate plaque control for patients. They are associated with increased plaque mass and with plaque colonized by likely periodontal pathogens (Figure 5-15).[24]

The prevalence of amalgam overhangs is startling. Data reviewed from a number of studies involving several thousand

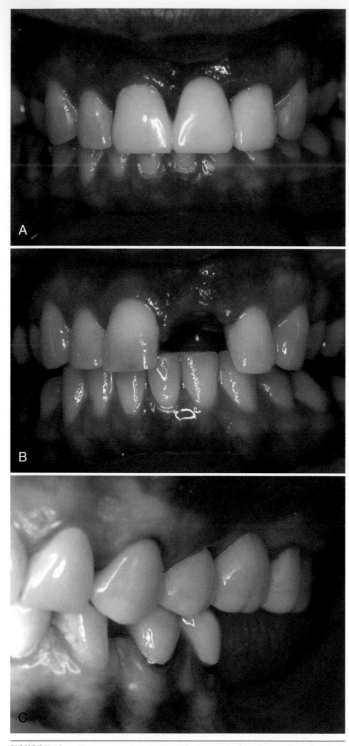

FIGURE 5-12 ■ Temporary crowns must be contoured to the teeth and permit access for oral hygiene procedures. **A,** Temporary three-unit bridge replacing tooth #9 leaves access for plaque biofilm control. **B,** The space closed by the restorative procedure shown in **A. C,** Temporary bridge replacing tooth #14. Note the contour of the distal abutment and the embrasure spaces designed to permit access for cleaning devices. (Courtesy of Dr. Mark Dellinges.)

subjects revealed that 25% to 76% of all amalgam-restored proximal surfaces had overhangs. Data also showed that 33% of adult dental patients had one or more overhanging amalgams. In addition, these studies reported that bone loss increased under overhangs by 0.16 to 0.87 mm, probing depth was increased by 0.2 to 0.67 mm, and attachment loss was increased

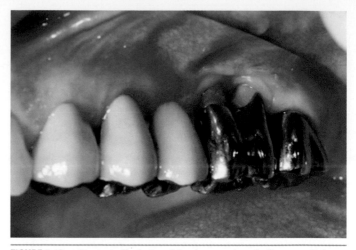

FIGURE 5-13 ■ Hygienically designed fixed restorations facilitate good plaque control for the periodontal patient. The shape of the crown on tooth #3 permits access to an exposed furcation area for easy cleaning. Although the pontics are not 3 mm away from the gingiva for cosmetic reasons, there is sufficient space to permit access for cleaning.

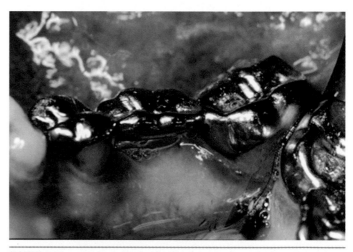

FIGURE 5-14 ■ Hygienically designed pontics, such as the one shown here, facilitate plaque control. This pontic is elevated off the gingiva, leaving space. The space permits the patient to clean under the pontic with floss or an interproximal brush. (Courtesy of Dr. Paulo Camargo.)

by 0.2 to 0.5 mm.[24] In a young dental patient population studied by Kells and Linden,[25] overhangs were present in 57% of patients aged 20 to 29 years, but in this young population they were not associated with increased bone loss.

> **CLINICAL NOTE 5-6** Recognition of overhanging amalgam restorations is a critical element in dental hygiene care. Pack[26] noted that overhangs exist in an alarming amount and that removal of the overhangs, scaling of the areas, and oral hygiene instruction result in significant improvements in oral health.

Amalgam finishing and overhang removal is a legally permitted duty for dental hygienists in many states. Certainly, evaluation of amalgam margins for possible overhangs is a responsibility of all dental hygienists because it is an important

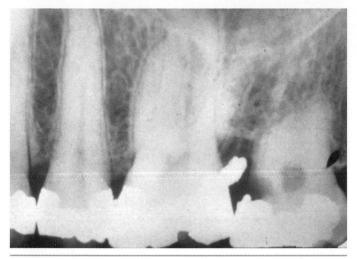

FIGURE 5-15 ■ This radiograph shows a very large overhanging amalgam restoration that has contributed to periodontal destruction on tooth #3 distal and tooth #2 mesial. It promotes growth and retention of plaque biofilm. This huge overhang would be very difficult to remove and recontour. Note the recurrent caries apical to the restoration on the second molar. The restorations on both the first and second molars were replaced.

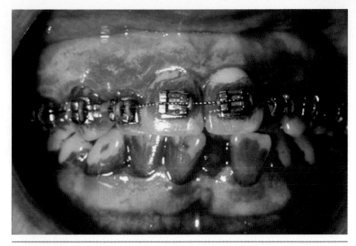

FIGURE 5-16 ■ Orthodontic appliances make plaque biofilm control more difficult. This young patient was not very motivated to brush anyway, and the appliances were a barrier to compliance. The plaque biofilm has been highlighted with disclosing solution staining it red and making it easy for the patient and clinician to see.

part of disease prevention and maintenance care. Overhangs are best detected by a combination of radiographic observation, evaluation of tissues adjacent to restorations, and clinical examination with explorers.[24-26] Small overhangs can be removed by hand instruments such as dental knives, ultrasonic instruments, rotary burs, or reciprocating polishers. If removed, large overhangs may leave poorly condensed amalgam with voids that will continue to act as reservoirs for plaque biofilms. To optimize periodontal health, poor restorations must be replaced.[26]

> **CLINICAL NOTE 5-7** Determine if your state's dental practice act permits dental hygienists to remove amalgam overhangs, because detecting and correcting overhangs can significantly simplify patient plaque control and improve tissue health.

REMOVABLE PARTIAL DENTURES

Many individuals have lost teeth as the result of periodontal disease, injury, or other conditions. Removable partial dentures make excellent functional and aesthetic restorative solutions for many individuals, although some think that fixed restorations are preferred for the periodontally involved dentition.[23] Partial dentures, complete dentures, and all other removable appliances can collect supragingival calculus. The dental hygienist should remove this calculus during the hygiene appointment by using powered or hand scalers and polishing. Partial denture wearers should also be instructed to clean the appliance daily at home with an accepted denture cleaner, denture brush, and clasp brush.

It is also important to know that natural teeth in function with removable partial dentures tend to have more and deeper periodontal pockets.[8,27] Increased susceptibility to caries is also associated with abutment teeth for partial dentures.[23] Clearly, excellent oral hygiene and caries prevention measures must be part of the dental hygiene care provided to these patients. In addition, regular recall maintenance appointments for

thorough examination, calculus removal, oral hygiene reinforcement, and caries prevention should be emphasized.[28]

CONDITIONS AFFECTING PERIODONTAL HEALTH

A number of dental conditions affect the periodontal health of patients who are routinely seen by dental hygienists. These include the following:

- **Orthodontic appliances**
- **Malocclusion**
- Unreplaced missing teeth
- **Mouth breathing**
- **Anatomic anomalies**
- Tobacco and alcohol use

ORTHODONTIC APPLIANCES

Orthodontic appliances have long been associated with increased plaque accumulation, gingivitis,[8] and caries susceptibility in children and adolescents.[29,30] Lang and Siegrist[31] reviewed studies evaluating the quantity and quality of plaque biofilm in adolescents undergoing orthodontic treatment. The quantity was less affected than the microbial composition and there was a shift to a more pathogenic plaque biofilm. In addition, molar bands were more highly associated with gingival inflammation than bonded brackets, suggesting that plaque retention in the sulcus was decreased by bonded attachments that did not enter the sulcus.[32] Little evidence implicates orthodontic therapy as a condition that causes severe periodontal consequences in the young population. Figure 5-16 shows plaque accumulation typical of young orthodontic patients.

Currently, more than 20% of orthodontic patients in the United States are adults. That percentage is expected to grow. Clinical evidence has shown that when adult periodontal patients undergoing orthodontic therapy received normal periodontal maintenance therapy at 3-month intervals, they were no more likely to have increased attachment loss than adolescents or adults without periodontal disease.[33]

MALOCCLUSION

Malocclusion is not a cause of periodontal disease; poorly aligned teeth can change embrasure spaces, complicate daily plaque control, and make dental hygiene care more challenging, but malocclusion is not an initiator of pathologic conditions. A 20-year study of 176 adolescents examined for malocclusion in their teen years and subsequently examined in their 30s showed no greater risk for periodontal disease characterized by bone loss in comparisons between men and women, or between lower socioeconomic groups and higher socioeconomic groups. However, subjects with crossbite, overjet, and crowding had higher gingival inflammation scores and more pocketing than the comparison group with no malocclusion.[34] Severe periodontal destruction was rare and most pocketing was in the 3.5- to 5.5-mm range, suggesting that dental hygiene care would be sufficient to control the disease process. Figure 5-17 shows a patient with malocclusion that contributes to the difficulty of plaque removal.

UNREPLACED MISSING TEETH

Unreplaced missing teeth can cause problems for periodontal patients. Missing teeth focus occlusal pressure on the remaining teeth and thus contribute to migration. Migration in periodontally involved dentitions usually occurs in a mesial direction and tilting or extrusion is common in the anterior areas. Premolars can drift distally.[35] Migrating teeth create spaces that complicate plaque control, and many patients find the extrusion and spreading of anterior teeth to be unsightly (Figure 5-18).

First Molar Loss

Too often, permanent first molars are lost in childhood or the teen years. If the molar is not replaced, a well-defined set of changes occurs in the dentition. First molar loss and other malocclusions and migrations have not been proven to initiate periodontal disease, but they are associated with gingival inflammation and pocket formation as the disease progresses.

The typical course of events after the loss of the permanent first molar is as follows[35]:

1. The second and third molars drift mesially and tilt, creating spaces and causing loss of the vertical dimension.
2. The mandibular premolars drift distally and can tilt.
3. The maxillary first molar extrudes into space on the mandibular arch.
4. The anterior overbite is increased, causing the lower anterior teeth to strike the maxillary incisors on or near the gingiva. Lower anterior teeth drift lingually, and the increased pressure results in splaying or spreading of the maxillary anterior teeth.

Although these changes are not primarily responsible for initiating periodontal disease, they create areas of food impaction and spaces that are difficult to clean. In addition to providing periodontal treatment, the dental hygienist must identify these problems, educate the patient about them, and encourage replacement of missing molars. Figure 5-19 shows the classic radiographic appearance of changes after premature loss of the first molar.

MOUTH BREATHING

Mouth breathing leads to localized gingival inflammation that is usually confined to the labial gingiva of the maxillary anterior teeth. The tissue becomes reddened and swollen and it bleeds easily. The surface of the gingiva is shiny.[36] Mouth breathing is

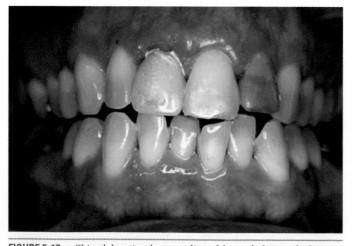

FIGURE 5-17 ■ This adult patient has crowding of the teeth that resulted in very tight and long contacts that altered the embrasure spaces. The inflammation is related to poor plaque biofilm control. Note the large deposit of subgingival calculus on tooth #8 facial and tooth #10 mesial. The subgingival calculus is very dark in color.

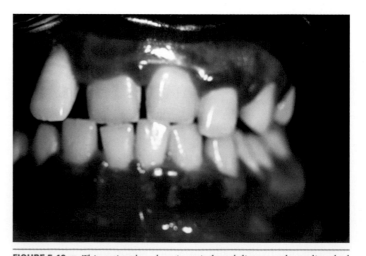

FIGURE 5-18 ■ This patient has chronic periodontal disease and was disturbed about the appearance of the anterior teeth. Significant migration has occurred as a result of loss of support.

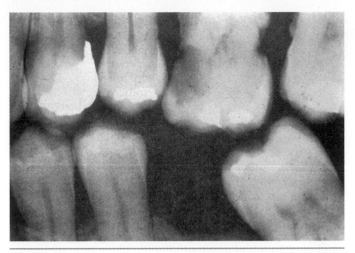

FIGURE 5-19 ■ Radiograph of the consequences of an unreplaced mandibular first molar. Drifting, extrusion, and plaque retention resulted in altered occlusion, caries, and periodontal disease.

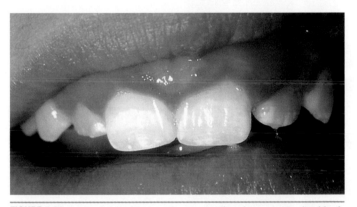

FIGURE 5-20 ■ Mouth breathing results in a swollen shiny gingiva that bleeds easily and appears reddened on clinical examination. The inflamed appearance is unrelated to the amount of plaque present and does not respond to improved plaque control measures.

also associated with higher levels of plaque and gingivitis.[30] The gingival inflammation does not respond to periodontal therapy: inflammation persists despite dental hygiene care and plaque biofilm control. The inflammation is thought to occur because of the constant drying of the tissues and the interference with natural protective factors in saliva; however, drying of tissue in laboratory animal studies has not reproduced the inflammation.[36] The best care for this condition is palliative, possibly placing petrolatum jelly over the tissue or using a saliva substitute product. Figure 5-20 is an example of the gingival effects of mouth breathing.

ANATOMIC ANOMALIES

The dental hygienist needs to be very knowledgeable about tooth and root anatomy so that long root surfaces that require instrument and plaque biofilm control and unusual variations of normal can be identified. These anatomic presentations have significant effects on gingival health. Figure 5-21 shows the effects on periodontal health that are commonly associated with the presence of a **lingual groove** (in this case on a maxillary lateral incisor) and highlights the technical difficulties of cleaning root surfaces in deep pockets.

TOBACCO AND ALCOHOL USE

Both tobacco and alcohol use, singly and in combination, have been convincingly related to the amount and severity of periodontal disease. In the past, these habits were not associated with increased disease because tobacco and alcohol users tend to have more plaque accumulation, so the differences in disease rates were attributed to poor control of plaque biofilms. Adding to the complexity of this, tobacco and alcohol are frequently used together; approximately 70% of alcoholics are heavy smokers compared with 10% of the population, and smokers are 1.3 times more likely to drink alcohol compared with nonsmokers. Smoking and excessive alcohol use frequently occur together and the combination greatly increases the risk of esophageal, throat, and other oral cancers. The relative risks of oral cancers are 7 times higher for smokers, 6 times higher for drinkers, and 38 times higher for those who both smoke and drink.[37]

> **CLINICAL NOTE 5-10** The dental hygienist must be aware that tobacco use is a **risk factor** for periodontal disease and that alcohol consumption is a **risk indicator**, meaning that patients who use these products are more likely to have disease than those who do not use them.

Tobacco Use

The use of all tobacco products—cigarette smoking, cigar smoking, and smokeless tobacco—has been strongly identified as a risk factor for periodontal disease. Studies have shown that smoking is associated with deeper pockets and more clinical attachment loss. In fact, the risk for severe periodontal disease is increased 2.8 times for those who smoke.[37] In addition, increased amounts of calculus and dental stains and the development of acute aggressive forms of periodontal disease are more common in smokers.[38] There is much compelling evidence that strongly supports the association between tobacco use and periodontal disease. Bergstrom and Eliasson[39] compared a group of Swedish periodontal patients with a random sample of city dwellers and determined that smokers were 2.5 times more likely to have periodontal destruction. In addition, among those with periodontal disease, the prevalence and severity of diseased sites were greater in smokers than in nonsmokers, although the subjects had similar amounts of plaque and gingivitis. Others have reported greater alveolar bone loss in smokers.[40] Haber and colleagues[41] compared smoking as a risk factor for periodontal disease in patients with insulin-dependent diabetes mellitus and in healthy subjects of similar age groups, 19 to 40 years old. The primary finding was that periodontitis was more severe and more prevalent among smokers than among nonsmokers, regardless of diabetic condition, although the prevalence and severity of disease were slightly higher among subjects with diabetes. The findings also indicated that young smokers, aged 19 to 30 years, were 3.9 times as likely to have periodontal disease characterized by attachment loss greater than 2 mm and at least one site of probing depth greater than 5 mm. Statistically, smoking accounted for 56% of the periodontal disease in the 19- to 30-year-old subjects and 32% of the periodontal disease in the 31- to 40-year-old group. Even former smokers had a higher

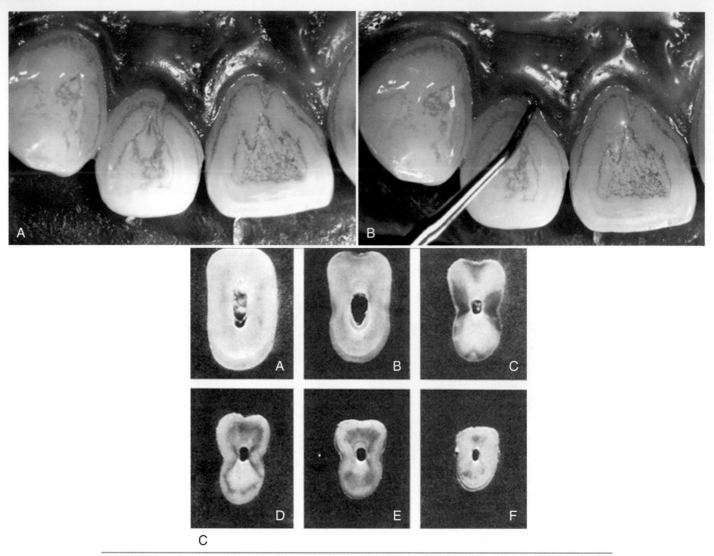

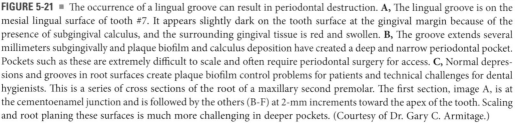

FIGURE 5-21 ■ The occurrence of a lingual groove can result in periodontal destruction. **A,** The lingual groove is on the mesial lingual surface of tooth #7. It appears slightly dark on the tooth surface at the gingival margin because of the presence of subgingival calculus, and the surrounding gingival tissue is red and swollen. **B,** The groove extends several millimeters subgingivally and plaque biofilm and calculus deposition have created a deep and narrow periodontal pocket. Pockets such as these are extremely difficult to scale and often require periodontal surgery for access. **C,** Normal depressions and grooves in root surfaces create plaque biofilm control problems for patients and technical challenges for dental hygienists. This is a series of cross sections of the root of a maxillary second premolar. The first section, image A, is at the cementoenamel junction and is followed by the others (B-F) at 2-mm increments toward the apex of the tooth. Scaling and root planing these surfaces is much more challenging in deeper pockets. (Courtesy of Dr. Gary C. Armitage.)

percentage of probing depths greater than 4 mm than those who had never smoked, but this finding was considerably less than that for current smokers.[41]

Haber and Kent[42] studied the extent of cigarette smoking among patients treated in periodontal offices compared with general dental offices. They reported that smokers were more often found in periodontal practices and that periodontal patients with moderate to advanced periodontal disease were 2.6 times more likely to be smokers. In addition, the frequency of current smoking was associated with increased disease severity. Figure 5-21 also represents an example of the calculus formation, stain accumulation, and periodontal attachment loss seen in a smoker.

The toxic effects of tobacco use, regardless of the form of tobacco, are recognized and are of importance to dental hygienists and patients. Research has suggested a number of tobacco-induced changes that may be responsible for the increased periodontal disease seen in tobacco users. The epithelial cells of the gingiva show increased keratinization and the buccal mucosa demonstrates altered oxygen consumption. There is also vasoconstriction of the gingival tissues so that they become ischemic, starved for blood and nutrients. Nicotine metabolites are also found in saliva and gingival crevicular fluid. Polymorphonuclear leukocytes in smokers have a reduced ability to phagocytize substances, and the vascular reaction to inflammation is reduced in smokers. Users of smokeless tobacco are not safe from these harmful effects. In fact, a specific type of tissue destruction is seen with the gingiva and bone underlying the location where smokeless tobacco rests in the mouths of users (Figure 5-22). It has been demonstrated that smoking

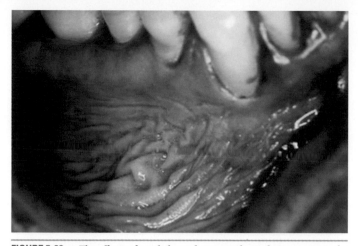

FIGURE 5-22 ■ **The effects of smokeless tobacco on the oral mucosa.** Note the wrinkled leukoplakia of the buccal mucosa caused by repeated placement of a smokeless tobacco plug. There is recession and staining on adjacent teeth, also associated with habitual use of smokeless tobacco.

has a negative effect on healing during periodontal therapy; pocket reduction and gain in clinical attachment are greatly reduced.[37]

An interesting study identified the presence of nicotine or cotinine, the metabolic byproduct of nicotine, on the root surfaces of recently extracted teeth from periodontal patients. The nicotine was absent from a sample that had been root-planed before extraction.[43] This observation suggests that nicotine can be removed during periodontal therapy, leaving tooth surfaces more compatible with wound healing. However, the nicotine would be quickly replaced by the next cigarette.

> **CLINICAL NOTE 5-11** Our understanding of the effects of tobacco is growing; it is no longer considered an innocuous social habit or one that affects only the heart and lungs. Educating dental hygiene patients regarding the negative impact of tobacco use is an essential preventive service provided by dental hygienists.

Alcohol Use

Until recently, alcohol use had been overlooked as a contributing factor to the severity of periodontal disease. In a review and analysis of studies by Grossi,[37] data showed that consumption of 3.5 drinks or more per week is associated with greater pocket depths, after adjustment for smoking and plaque control. Also, patients consuming five or more drinks per week were 65% more likely to have gingival bleeding and 36% more likely to have severe attachment loss compared with those who consumed fewer than five drinks per week.

Although some protective effects have been ascribed to moderate or social drinking, it is extremely important for the dental hygienist to be aware of these increased risks to periodontal health. The association between alcohol use and periodontal disease appears to be dose-dependent. It is important to be aware of social habits so that each patient's periodontal disease can be treated and patients can be referred for needed assistance.

✳ CASE SCENARIO

You met Mr. Sanchez 6 months ago when he came to your practice for routine care. You were surprised at the heavy accumulation of supragingival calculus on his teeth, which was generalized throughout his mouth. You carefully removed it and provided him with oral hygiene instructions about brushing and flossing every day. Three months later he returned for a recall appointment and most of the supragingival calculus had re-formed. The gingival tissues were not reddened and inflamed, and there was little bleeding on probing. Mr. Sanchez assured you that he was conscientious about brushing and flossing. You reminded him about his home care regimen and encouraged him to brush and floss daily.

1. Mr. Sanchez is likely
   A. a light calculus former.
   B. a heavy calculus former.
   C. eating a lot of refined carbohydrates.
   D. not being honest about his home care routine.
2. The home care instructions you are likely to provide Mr. Sanchez at this appointment include
   A. more brushing and flossing instruction.
   B. a hard toothbrush to remove more plaque biofilm.
   C. use of a metallic instrument to scrape off his own calculus.
   D. products containing anticalculus agents that include pyrophosphates.
3. You are likely to recommend a shorter recall interval for Mr. Sanchez because the calculus can trap plaque and cause gingival inflammation.
   A. Both the statement and the reason are correct and related.
   B. Both the statement and the reason are correct but NOT related.
   C. The statement is correct, but the reason is NOT correct.
   D. The statement is NOT correct, but the reason is correct.
   E. NEITHER the statement NOR the reason is correct.

STUDY QUESTIONS

Answers and rationales to these questions can be obtained from your instructor.

MULTIPLE CHOICE

1. Supragingival calculus is primarily composed of
   A. calcium carbonate.
   B. calcium phosphate.
   C. glycoproteins.
   D. magnesium.

2. Calculus is a major causative factor in the formation of periodontal disease. Subgingival calculus covered with plaque does not contribute to greater disease progression.
   A. Both statements are true.
   B. Both statements are false.
   C. The first statement is true, and the second statement is false.
   D. The first statement is false, and the second statement is true.

3. Anticalculus toothpastes reduce the formation of new supragingival calculus due to which agent?
   A. Calcium
   B. Fluoride
   C. Pyrophosphate
   D. Stannous ions

4. Amalgam restoration discrepancies are detrimental to periodontal health because they serve as a sheltered place for plaque and calculus growth.
   A. Both the statement and reason are correct and related.
   B. Both the statement and reason are correct but NOT related.
   C. The statement is correct, but the reason is NOT correct.
   D. The statement is NOT correct, but the reason is correct.
   E. NEITHER the statement NOR the reason is correct.

5. All of the following statements regarding calculus removal are true EXCEPT one. Which one is the EXCEPTION?
   A. It is the most critical aspect of dental hygiene care.
   B. It reduces the retention of plaque bacterial biofilm.
   C. It must be done on a regular basis.
   D. It requires technical skill.

6. Routine plaque control can be complicated for the periodontal patient by poorly aligned teeth. Orthodontic therapy will cause severe periodontal disease in children and teenagers.
   A. Both statements are true.
   B. Both statements are false.
   C. The first statement is true, and the second statement is false.
   D. The first statement is false, and the second statement is true.

7. All of the following characteristics may be related to calculus formation EXCEPT one. Which one is the EXCEPTION?
   A. Concentration of calcium in saliva
   B. Concentration of salivary bacterial protein
   C. Higher salivary pH
   D. Higher levels of pyrophosphate

8. Smoking and the use of tobacco products are considered risk
   A. indicators.
   B. effects.
   C. factors.
   D. mediators.

SHORT ANSWER

9. Why is dental hygiene care often focused on calculus removal more than other aspects of preventive dentistry?
10. Why is subgingival calculus often dark in color?

Please visit **http://evolve.elsevier.com/Perry/periodontology** for additional practice and study support tools.

REFERENCES

1. Greenwell H, Armitage GC, Mealey BL. Local contributing factors. In: Rose LF, Mealey BL, eds. *Periodontics: Medicine, Surgery, and Implants.* St. Louis, MO: Elsevier Mosby; 2004:117–130.
2. Mandel ID. Dental calculus (calcified dental plaque). In: Genco RJ, Goldman HM, Cohen DW, eds. *Contemporary Periodontics.* St. Louis, MO: Mosby; 1990:135–146.
3. Mandel ID, Gaffar A. Calculus revisited: a review. *J Clin Periodontol.* 1986;13:249–257.
4. Tan B, Gillam DG, Mordan NJ, et al. A preliminary investigation into the ultrastructure of dental calculus and associated debris. *J Clin Periodontol.* 2004;31:364–368.
5. Pattanaporn K, Navia JM. The relationship of dental calculus to caries, gingivitis, and selected salivary factors in 11- to 13-year old Thai children in Chiang Mai, Thailand. *J Periodontol.* 1998;69:955–961.
6. Albandar JM, Brown LJ, Brunelle JA, et al. Gingival state and dental calculus in early-onset periodontitis. *J Periodontol.* 1996;67:953–959.
7. Wilkins EM. Calculus. In: Wilkins EM, ed. *Clinical Practice of the Dental Hygienist.* 11th ed. Philadelphia, PA: Lippincott Williams & Wilkins; 2013:296–304.
8. Hinrichs JE. The role of calculus and other predisposing factors. In: Newman MG, Takei HH, Klokkevold PR, Carranza FA, eds. *Carranza's Clinical Periodontology.* 11th ed. St. Louis, MO: Elsevier Saunders; 2012:217–231.
9. Haake SK, Newman MG, Quirynen M, et al. Microbiology of periodontal diseases. In: Newman MG, Takei HH, Klokkevold PR, et al, eds. *Carranza's Clinical Periodontology.* 11th ed. St Louis, MO: Elsevier Saunders; 2006:134–169.
10. Corbett TL, Dawes C. A comparison of the site-specificity of supragingival and subgingival calculus deposition. *J Periodontol.* 1998;69:1–8.
11. Spolsky V. The epidemiology of gingival and periodontal disease. In: Carranza FA, Newman MG, eds. *Clinical Periodontology.* 8th ed. Philadelphia, PA: WB Saunders; 1996:61–81.
12. Anerud A, Löe H, Boysen H. The natural history and clinical course of calculus formation in man. *J Clin Periodontol.* 1991;18:160–170.
13. Turesky S, Breuer M, Coffman G. The effect of certain systemic medications on oral calculus formation. *J Periodontol.* 1992;63:871–875.
14. Breuer MM, Mboya SA, Moroi H, et al. Effects of selected beta-blockers on supragingival calculus formation. *J Periodontol.* 1996;67:428–432.
15. Ramfjord SP. Long-term assessment of periodontal surgery versus curettage or scaling and root planing. *Int J Technol Assess Health Care.* 1990;6:392–402.
16. Mallatt ME, Beiswanger BB, Stookey GK, et al. Influence of soluble pyrophosphate on calculus formation in adults. *J Dent Res.* 1985;64:1159–1162.
17. Zacherl WA, Pfeiffer HJ, Swancar JR. The effect of soluble pyrophosphates on dental calculus in adults. *J Am Dent Assoc.* 1985;110:737–738.
18. Kazmierczak M, Mather M, Ciancio S, et al. A clinical evaluation of anticalculus dentifrices. *Clin Prev Dent.* 1990;12:13–17.

19. Kohut BE, Rubin H, Baron HJ. The relative clinical effectiveness of three anticalculus dentifrices. *Clin Prev Dent.* 1989;11:13–16.

20. Leknes KN. The influence of anatomic and iatrogenic root surface characteristics on bacterial colonization and periodontal destruction: a review. *J Periodontol.* 1997;68:507–516.

21. Sorensen JA. A rationale for comparison of plaque-retaining properties of crown systems. *J Prosthet Dent.* 1989;62:264–269.

22. Bader JD, Rozier RG, McFall WT Jr, et al. Effect of crown margins on periodontal conditions in regularly attending patients. *J Prosthet Dent.* 1991;65:75–79.

23. Kenney EB. Restorative-periodontal inter-relationships. In: Carranza FA, ed. *Glickman's Clinical Periodontology.* 7th ed. Philadelphia, PA: WB Saunders; 1990:924–955.

24. Brunsvold MA, Lane JJ. The prevalence of overhanging dental restorations and their relationship to periodontal disease. *J Clin Periodontol.* 1990;17:67–72.

25. Kells BE, Linden GJ. Overhanging amalgam restorations in young adults attending a periodontal department. *J Dent.* 1992;20:85–89.

26. Pack ARC. The amalgam overhang dilemma: a review of causes and effects, prevention, and removal. *N Z Dent J.* 1989;85:55–58.

27. Tuominen R, Ranta K, Paunio I. Wearing of partial dentures in relation to periodontal pockets. *J Oral Rehabil.* 1989;16:119–126.

28. Wilkins EM. Care of dental prostheses. In: Wilkins EM, ed. *Clinical Practice of the Dental Hygienist.* 11th ed. Philadelphia, PA: Lippincott Williams & Wilkins; 2013:447–462.

29. Wilkins EM. The patient with orthodontic appliances. In: Wilkins EM, ed. *Clinical Practice of the Dental Hygienist.* 11th ed. Philadelphia, PA: Lippincott Williams & Wilkins; 2013:436–446.

30. Wagaiyu EG, Ashley FP. Mouthbreathing, lip seal, and upper lip coverage and their relationship with gingival inflammation in 11–14 year-old school-children. *J Clin Periodontol.* 1991;18:698–702.

31. Lang NP, Siegrist BE. Mechanical plaque retention factors. In: Genco RJ, Goldman HM, Cohen DW, eds. *Contemporary Periodontics.* St. Louis, MO: Mosby; 1990:170–183.

32. Alexander SA. Effects of orthodontic attachments on the gingival health of permanent second molars. *Am J Orthod Dentofac Orthop.* 1991;102:337–340.

33. Boyd RL, Leggott PJ, Quinn RS, et al. Periodontal implications of orthodontic treatment in adults with reduced or normal periodontal tissues versus those of adolescents. *Am J Orthod Dentofac Orthop.* 1989;100:191–199.

34. Helm S, Petersen PE. Causal relation between malocclusion and periodontal health. *Acta Odontol Scand.* 1989;47:223–228.

35. Carranza FA. Periodontal response to external forces. In: Newman MG, Takei HH, Klokkevold PR, et al, eds. *Carranza's Clinical Periodontology.* 11th ed. St. Louis, MO: Elsevier Saunders; 2012:151–159.

36. Carranza FA, Hogan EL. Gingival enlargement. In: Newman MG, Takei HH, Klokkevold PR, et al, eds. *Carranza's Clinical Periodontology.* 11th ed. St. Louis, MO: Elsevier Saunders; 2012:84–96.

37. Grossi SG. Effects of tobacco smoking and alcohol use on periodontal disease. In: Rose LF, Mealy BL, Genco RJ, Cohen WJ, eds. *Periodontics: Medicine, Surgery and Implants.* St. Louis, MO: Elsevier Mosby; 2004:869–880.

38. Carranza FA, Klokkevold PR. Acute gingival infections. In: Newman MG, Takei HH, Klokkevold PR, et al, eds. *Carranza's Clinical Periodontology.* 11th ed. St. Louis, MO: Elsevier Saunders; 2012:97–103.

39. Bergstrom J. Cigarette smoking as risk factor in chronic periodontal disease. *Commun Dent Oral Epidemiol.* 1989;17:245–247.

40. Bergstrom J, Eliasson S. Cigarette smoking and alveolar bone height in subjects with a high standard of oral hygiene. *J Clin Periodontol.* 1987;14:446–469.

41. Haber J, Wattles J, Crowley M, et al. Evidence for cigarette smoking as a major risk factor for periodontitis. *J Periodontol.* 1993;64:16–23.

42. Haber J, Kent RL. Cigarette smoking in a periodontal practice. *J Periodontol.* 1992;63:100–106.

43. Cuff MJA, McQuade MJ, Scheidt MJ, et al. The presence of nicotine on root surfaces of periodontally diseased teeth in smokers. *J Periodontol.* 1989;60:564–569.

Gingival Diseases

Gwen Essex and Dorothy A. Perry
Based on the original work by Edward J. Taggart

LEARNING OUTCOMES

- Define the types of gingivitis.
- Relate the clinical signs and symptoms of gingivitis to the pathogenesis of each stage of disease.
- List the similarities and differences in the clinical presentation, treatment, and healing of dental plaque biofilm–induced gingivitis and other gingival conditions.
- Identify the medications that can cause gingival hyperplasia in patients.

- Describe examples of bacterial, viral, and fungal infections that affect the gingiva.
- Define necrotizing ulcerative gingivitis.
- List the relatively common systemic conditions that have gingival manifestations.
- Describe the role of the dental hygienist in the treatment of gingivitis.

KEY TERMS

Dental plaque biofilm–induced gingivitis	Gingival diseases of specific bacterial origin	Hyperplasia
Foreign body reactions	Gingival diseases of viral origin	Nonplaque biofilm–induced gingival lesions
Gingival diseases modified by malnutrition	Gingival fluid flow	Pregnancy tumor
Gingival diseases modified by medications	Gingival manifestations of systemic conditions	Recession
		Stage I gingivitis
Gingival diseases modified by systemic factors	Gingivitis	Stage II gingivitis
	Gingivitis associated with dental plaque biofilm only	Stage III gingivitis
Gingival diseases of fungal origin		Stage IV gingivitis
		Traumatic lesions

The dental hygienist plays a crucial role in the treatment of gingivitis and in the prevention of its recurrence. Diseases of the gingival tissues range from common forms, such as dental plaque biofilm–induced gingivitis, to rare but potentially life-threatening forms, such as squamous cell carcinoma or acute leukemia. The dental hygienist may be the first member of the health care team to identify these lesions and bring them to the attention of the patient and other dental health professionals.

A description of the gingival tissues in health is presented in Chapter 2. To review, in health, the gingival epithelium is usually described as pink or coral pink, with significant variation based on the presence of melanin in the tissue, which is a genetic characteristic. The attached gingiva is tightly bound to the underlying connective tissue and is not movable. The surface epithelium of the attached gingiva is often stippled, shows no signs of inflammatory color changes, and the papillae fill the interdental spaces completely. The marginal gingiva reaches the tooth surface in a knife edge pattern, and there are measurable sulcus depths of less than 3 mm. The gingival epithelium

consists of a keratinized oral epithelium, a keratinized or parakeratinized sulcular epithelium, and a junctional epithelium that forms the attachment to the root surface. Beneath the gingival epithelium, there is dense connective tissue coronal to the alveolar bone. This tissue is laced with bundles of collagen fibers. The normal appearance of healthy gingiva is shown in Figure 6-1.

GINGIVITIS

Gingivitis is inflammation of the gingival tissues. It occurs in a periodontium with no attachment loss or in a periodontium with attachment loss that is not progressing. Gingivitis manifests as color change (redness), edema (swelling of the tissues), exudate (drainage of gingival fluid from the sulcus), and a tendency to bleed readily (hemorrhage in response to gentle periodontal probing or tooth brushing).[1] In addition, there may be changes in gingival contour, loss of tissue adaptation to the teeth, and an increased flow of gingival crevicular fluid.[2] Gingivitis is perhaps the most common human disease and among

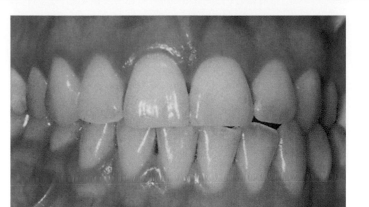

FIGURE 6-1 ■ Normal gingiva. The clinical appearance of healthy gingiva: tissue is pink and uniform in color, stippling can be seen, and the papillae fill the interdental spaces.

the easiest to treat and control. However, gingivitis is painless and often unrecognized. Many patients are unaware that they have it, even though their gums bleed, and, because it is so common, dentists and dental hygienists frequently do not emphasize its importance. Perhaps the best approach that dental hygienists and dentists can take is to inform their patients that they have a disease—gingivitis—and that it is easily treated and cured. When the balance between disease and health is understood, patients often cooperate with dental hygiene care and improve their daily oral hygiene practice to cure the disease.

> **CLINICAL NOTE 6-1** Even though gingivitis is so commonly seen, it is important to recognize, document, and discuss it with your patients and provide appropriate treatment.

PATHOGENESIS OF GINGIVAL DISEASE

Pathogenesis refers to the events in the development and progression of a disease. The pathogenesis of gingivitis is best explained by describing the histologic events as they relate to clinical signs. Extensive research on the pathogenesis of gingivitis, obtained by observing people and animals when bacterial plaque was allowed to accumulate, has explained most of the events in the development of gingival inflammation. With this knowledge, scientists have classified the development of gingival inflammation into three separate stages:

1. Initial stage
2. Early stage
3. Established stage[3]

Research has also defined a fourth stage, characterized by the extension of inflammation into the alveolar bone, which is the stage of periodontal breakdown, or advanced stage.[4] The fourth stage is the point at which the gingival disease has progressed to periodontal disease.

> **CLINICAL NOTE 6-2** It is critical to treat gingivitis because it can progress to periodontal disease.

Stage I Gingivitis (Initial or Subclinical Stage)

Stage I gingivitis, the initial stage, occurs in the first few days of contact between microbial plaque and the gingival tissues.

This stage is an acute inflammatory response that is characterized by dilation of the blood vessels and increased blood flow. The polymorphonuclear leukocytes (PMNs, or neutrophils) attach to the vessel walls and begin to migrate into the surrounding connective tissues. PMNs (white blood cells with multilobulated nuclei) are the principal defense in acute inflammation. They phagocytize (engulf) bacteria, their products, and other products of destroyed tissue. Small amounts of plasma also leak into the surrounding tissues, causing edema in the tissues. PMNs amass in the connective tissue and migrate through the sulcular epithelium into the plaque, forming exudate. Exudate from early gingival inflammation, composed mostly of serum, is referred to as gingival fluid flow. The gingival fluid is clear, not yellow (like pus), because few cells are present. A significant number of lymphocytes appear in the gingival connective tissues. These are almost all T lymphocytes, the type that do not cause tissue damage but maintain a homeostatic (stabilizing) response to bacterial infection.[5] In addition, there are epithelial cell changes and collagen degradation caused by activation of the host immune system. These first tissue reactions to plaque infection are not visible in the gingival tissues because they do not cause obvious clinical changes. This initial inflammatory response with no outwardly observable clinical signs is a subclinical infection.[4]

Stage II Gingivitis (Early Stage)

Stage II gingivitis is referred to as early gingivitis. Lesions begin to form 4 to 7 days after plaque has accumulated in the gingival sulcus. The T lymphocytes increase in number and are localized in the connective tissue under the epithelium of the gingival sulcus. The inflammatory exudate increases; it may appear white or yellow. Clinically, the tissues appear slightly red and swollen. The increase in gingival fluid flow (exudate) reaches its peak 6 to 12 days after clinical redness is observed. The perivascular collagen fibers in the connective tissues are destroyed by the inflammation and replaced by blood plasma and inflammatory cell infiltrate. Collagen fibers that attach the underlying connective tissue to the gingival epithelium are also destroyed and gingival stippling, if present, begins to disappear, causing the gingiva to appear shiny. The junctional epithelium begins to lengthen against the root surface and it is disrupted by the migrating PMNs and lymphocytes. The gingival tissues tend to bleed when gently probed and often do so when a patient brushes and flosses. Cellular changes occur in the connective tissue fibroblasts, leading to their destruction, probably related to interaction with the lymphoid tissues. The early stage of gingivitis may continue for 21 days or longer. It is the earliest clinical evidence of gingivitis.[4]

> **CLINICAL NOTE 6-3** Asking patients about any bleeding that occurs during home care can be an effective means of beginning the discussion about gingivitis and its treatment.

Stage III Gingivitis (Established Stage)

After 15 to 21 days, the gingival inflammation reaches the established stage, called stage III gingivitis.[4] In established gingivitis, there is a distinct change in the type of white blood cells seen in histologic specimens. Plasma cells, usually associated with an intense antigen-antibody response, are present. T and

B lymphocytes are found in equal amounts, indicating that tissue destruction by the inflammatory reaction is taking place. B lymphocytes are related to cell surface immunity and release lymphokines that accelerate the tissue destruction in inflammation. More connective tissue collagen is destroyed and the junctional epithelium begins to thicken and extend apically on the root surface and deep into the underlying connective tissues. This activity represents a conversion of the junctional epithelium into one correctly described as pocket epithelium. The clinical probing depth increases for two reasons: the periodontal probe penetrates more deeply through the junctional epithelium into the connective tissue by about 1 mm because of the loss of collagen, and edema in the tissues moves the gingival margin coronally, increasing the probe readings.

The blood vessels proliferate into capillary loops that reach nearly to the basement membrane of the epithelium, permitting more seepage of serum into the tissues and through the sulcular epithelium. That change, along with the increased presence and activity of inflammatory cells, causes visible pus formation. Capillary proliferation also causes the gingiva to appear red. In extreme cases of congested blood cells in the gingiva, the tissue appears blue, or cyanotic, because of the presence of many oxygen-depleted red blood cells. In combination, these changes result in red, swollen, and shiny gingivae that may also exhibit noticeable pus formation and gingival exudate.

The established gingivitis lesion may persist unchanged for months or years. The condition is reversible when plaque is regularly removed, permitting the tissues to return to normal. When healing occurs, there is no residual tissue destruction.[2]

Stage IV Gingivitis (Advanced Stage)

Stage IV gingivitis is the advanced stage of gingivitis. The inflammatory processes have extended beyond the gingiva and into the other periodontal tissues.[4] The extension of disease into the bone, referred to as periodontitis, is described in Chapter 7. The pathogenesis of the stages of gingivitis is summarized in Table 6-1.

HEALING OF THE GINGIVA AFTER TREATMENT

The sequence of healing events is the reverse of those described for the pathogenesis. Healing of gingivitis begins in the connective tissues. The inflammatory cells are replaced by fibroblasts, which lay down a firm extracellular matrix of collagen. With maturity, these fibers become functionally oriented and produce a dense subgingival connective tissue. This connective tissue does not permit penetration of the periodontal probe tip, thus reducing the clinical periodontal probing depth. The gingival color returns to pink as the proliferation of inflammatory cells resolves, and stippling reappears when serum no longer leaks into the tissues to cause edema.

In some cases, stable gingivitis transforms into progressive disease. This change results in advanced lesions with bone destruction, progressing from gingivitis to periodontitis.[5] Periodontitis is discussed in Chapter 7.

Gingivitis has been classified into a number of categories on the basis of the clinical manifestations of the disease, etiology, association with systemic diseases, association with medications, or other causes. The gingiva mirrors the effects of many factors beyond disease-associated causes, including allergies and injuries. The classification of gingival diseases and conditions is complex and is presented in Box 6-1.[5,6] The major elements of gingival diseases and conditions are described and illustrated in the remainder of this chapter.

Recession of the Gingiva

Recession of the gingiva refers to the location of the margin of the tissue, not its condition. Recession can occur in gingivitis, or it can be associated with clinically healthy tissue. Gingival recession, which is common, increases with age. It can be localized to one tooth or extend to any number of teeth. It has been reported to be present in 8% of children and 100% of adults by the age of 50 years. Etiologic factors associated with recession are as follows[7]:

- Gingival abrasion related to faulty toothbrushing technique
- Tooth malposition (rotated, tilted, or displaced teeth)

TABLE 6-1 Correlation of Clinical Signs to the Pathogenesis of Gingivitis

STAGE	CLINICAL SIGNS	PATHOLOGIC EVENTS
Initial (stage I)	None (subclinical infection)	Blood vessels dilate Polymorphonuclear leukocytes migrate into connective tissue Plasma leaks into connective tissue Gingival fluid flows from pockets T lymphocytes predominate
Early (stage II)	Gingiva reddens Stippling disappears Exudate may appear Bleeding on probing usually occurs	T lymphocytes increase Cells congregate under sulcular epithelium Gingival fluid flow increases Collagen is destroyed Lengthened junctional epithelium is disrupted Fibroblasts are destroyed
Established (stage III)	Gingiva is reddened Gingiva may appear blue-red Probing depths increase Pus forms Tissue swells	Capillaries proliferate T and B lymphocytes occur in equal numbers Extensive collagen destruction occurs Junctional epithelium thickens Rete pegs extend into connective tissue Plasma cells infiltrate Edema increases
Advanced (stage IV)	Similar to stage III	Destructive changes extend into bone and other periodontal tissues

---

BOX 6-1 Classification of Gingival Diseases and Conditions Defined at the 1999 International Workshop for Classification of Periodontal Diseases and Conditions

Gingival Diseases
A. Dental plaque–induced gingival diseases
  1. Gingivitis associated with dental plaque only
    a. Without other local contributing factors
    b. With local contributing factors
  2. Gingival diseases modified by systemic factors
    a. Associated with the endocrine system
      1) Puberty-associated gingivitis
      2) Menstrual cycle–associated gingivitis
      3) Pregnancy-associated
        a) Gingivitis
        b) Pyogenic granuloma
      4) Diabetes mellitus–associated gingivitis
    b. Associated with blood dyscrasias
      1) Leukemia-associated gingivitis
      2) Other
  3. Gingival diseases modified by medications
    a. Drug-influenced gingival diseases
      1) Drug-influenced gingival enlargements
      2) Drug-influenced gingivitis
        a) Oral contraceptive–associated gingivitis
        b) Other
  4. Gingival diseases modified by malnutrition
    a. Ascorbic acid deficiency gingivitis
    b. Other
B. Non-plaque-Induced Gingival Lesions
  1. Gingival diseases of specific bacterial origin
    a. *Neisseria gonorrhoeae*–associated lesions
    b. *Treponema pallidum*–associated lesions
    c. *Streptococcus* species–associated lesions
    d. Other
  2. Gingival diseases of viral origin
    a. Herpesvirus infections
      1) Primary herpetic gingivostomatitis
      2) Recurrent oral herpes
      3) Varicella zoster infections
    b. Other
  3. Gingival diseases of fungal origin
    a. *Candida* species infections
      1) Generalized gingival candidiasis

    b. Linear gingival erythema
    c. Histoplasmosis
    d. Other
  4. Gingival lesions of genetic origin
    a. Hereditary gingival fibromatosis
    b. Other
  5. Gingival manifestations of systemic conditions
    a. Mucocutaneous disorders
      1) Lichen planus
      2) Pemphigoid
      3) Pemphigus vulgaris
      4) Erythema multiforme
      5) Lupus erythematosus
      6) Drug-induced
      7) Other
    b. Allergic reactions
      1) Dental restorative materials
        a) Mercury
        b) Nickel
        c) Acrylic
        d) Other
      2) Reactions attributable to
        a) Toothpastes, dentifrices
        b) Mouth rinses, mouthwashes
        c) Chewing gum additives
        d) Foods and additives
      3) Other
  6. Traumatic lesions (e.g., factitious, iatrogenic, accidental)
    a. Chemical injury
    b. Physical injury
    c. Thermal injury
  7. Foreign body reactions
  8. Not otherwise specified

NOTE: Necrotizing ulcerative gingivitis is classified under periodontal disease (see Chapter 7) because it is most commonly associated with attachment loss and bone changes.

Modified from Armitage GC. Development of a classification system for periodontal diseases and conditions. *Ann Periodontol.* 1999;4:10-6.

- Gingival ablation (friction from other soft tissues)
- Gingival inflammation
- Abnormal frenum attachment

Recession is of clinical significance in dental hygiene care because root surfaces exposed through recession can decay and cemental surfaces can wear away, leaving the root surface sensitive. Also, these surfaces can be more difficult for the patient to clean.

CLINICAL NOTE 6-4 Asking patients with gingival recession about root sensitivity and offering desensitizing treatments will assist patients in performing necessary plaque control without discomfort.

Dental Plaque–Induced Gingival Disease

Gingivitis occurs very commonly in all levels of society, rich or poor, industrial or agricultural. The most obvious symptom is bleeding gums. So many people live with this condition that

they are often not aware that it is a disease. Many patients will tell the dental hygienist that they believe that everyone's gums bleed, or they always expect their gums to bleed when they brush their teeth. Despite this common assumption, it is true that the gingiva becomes inflamed as a result of the presence of dental plaque. The following section describes gingivitis and factors that contribute to the disease.

Gingivitis Associated with Dental Plaque Biofilm Only. The most common form of gingivitis found in the general population is **gingivitis associated with dental plaque only,** also called plaque-associated gingivitis, or gingivitis. This disease is directly related to the presence of bacterial plaque on the tooth surface.[1]

Clinically, gingivitis causes a reddened gingival margin (with pocket formation as a result of gingival swelling and edema), hypertrophy, and deepened penetration of the periodontal probe on clinical evaluation. The surface of the gingiva may appear glazed or smooth, and stippling (when present in health) usually disappears. Microscopically, there is an increase in

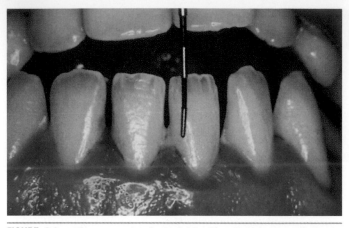

FIGURE 6-2 ■ Plaque-associated gingivitis. The clinical signs of plaque-associated gingivitis are an intense inflammatory response at the gingival margin and bleeding in response to gentle probing. The marginal gingiva is very red around the lower anterior teeth, and slight bleeding is evident at the gingival margin after probing.

capillaries along the gingival margin and the epithelium lining the gingival sulcus is ulcerated. This ulceration results in a tendency to bleed when a periodontal probe is placed in the gingival crevice. Bleeding in response to gentle probing is the major clinical indicator of gingivitis. Another common feature of chronic gingivitis is a clear gingival fluid flow, or exudate, which appears to increase with the severity of the gingivitis. Figure 6-2 shows the typical appearance of dental plaque–induced gingivitis.

Gingivitis appears to be directly related to the amount of plaque biofilm on the tooth surface and the amount of time that the plaque is allowed to remain undisturbed. The bacterial plaque biofilm is considered nonspecific because it is not associated with any specific type of microorganisms. The mature plaque biofilm found in long-standing gingivitis has a large percentage of gram-negative bacteria. This change from gram-positive plaque associated with health, or healthy plaque, to predominantly gram-negative plaque, or pathogenic plaque, is characteristic of gingivitis.

Distribution of Gingivitis. Plaque-associated gingivitis may be further classified by its location and the degree of involvement in the dentition. It may be localized to a few teeth or generalized throughout the mouth. It may be limited to the interdental papilla, spread along the entire gingival margin, or involve all of the attached gingival tissues. By definition, gingivitis does not involve the periodontal attachment tissues and there is no loss of connective tissue attachment to the tooth and no loss of supporting bone.

Describing the Gingival Condition. Gingival tissue descriptions should be recorded in the patient's chart. The location and extent of gingivitis should be noted. The terms commonly used to describe the tissues include the following[6]:

- Extent of involvement
- Localized
- Generalized
- Tissues affected
- Marginal
- Papillary
- Degree of inflammation
- Slight

- Moderate
- Severe

These descriptors can be combined, depending on the extent and severity of the gingivitis. It is also helpful to describe the color, shape, and shininess of the tissues, such as in the following examples:

- "Localized inflammation, redness, and swelling on the buccal and lingual posterior sextants."
- "Generalized severe inflammation, tissues intensely red, with rounded, shiny marginal and papillary gingiva; bleeds easily on probing."

These clinical descriptors reflect the histologic changes that have occurred and permit the dental hygienist to evaluate changes in the clinical appearance at subsequent appointments.

Gingivitis is reversible. In the experimental setting, the signs and symptoms of gingivitis disappeared in approximately 1 week when good plaque control was reinstituted. It is important for the dental hygienist to understand that adequate removal of dental plaque on a daily basis, along with the appropriate periodic recall to remove calculus and other irritants, cures gingivitis and prevents it from recurring.[8] Evidence of complete resolution of gingival inflammation is illustrated in Figure 6-3. The importance of regular maintenance appointments, or recalls, is described in Chapter 17.

Many other conditions can lead to gingival inflammation. These are much less common than plaque-associated gingivitis, but they are important to recognize. The dental hygienist must distinguish between common gingivitis and conditions with other causes because treatment and healing results differ.

Plaque Biofilm–Induced Gingivitis Modified by Local Contributing Factors. Although bacterial plaque biofilm–induced gingivitis may occur with the accumulation of dental plaque biofilm alone, there are often tooth-related factors that modify or predispose to a localized gingivitis. Such factors include dental restorations, orthodontic appliances, and malposed, or crowded, teeth. These factors, called plaque traps, usually act to retain plaque and serve to make oral hygiene practices more difficult and less effective. They do not cause the gingivitis, but ordinary daily cleaning practices that may be adequate in other places in the mouth are not sufficient to remove enough plaque biofilm in these places and therefore do not prevent inflammation from occurring. Figure 6-4 shows examples of gingivitis that has occurred in response to plaque biofilm accumulation and local contributing factors.

Gingival Diseases Modified by Systemic Factors. Many systemic factors act to modify the manner in which the individual's immune system responds to the assault of accumulated dental plaque biofilm. Some conditions that alone do not cause gingivitis may act to intensify it, resulting in **gingival diseases modified by systemic factors**. For example, circulating corticosteroids associated with stress change the environment and may result in the formation of a more pathologic plaque biofilm.[9] Changes in the endocrine system, such as hormonal changes during puberty, the menstrual cycle, or pregnancy, are frequently, but not always, associated with inflammatory changes in the gingiva. These conditions may not heal completely through local therapy, but the dental hygienist can help patients with these conditions improve the health of the gingiva.[5] The following section describes the more commonly

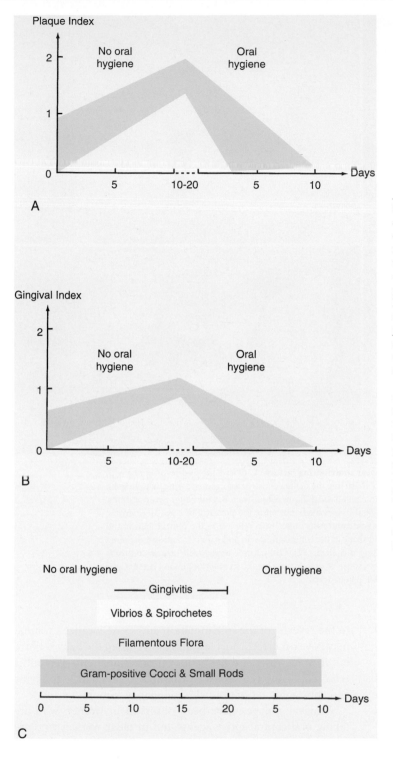

FIGURE 6-3 ■ **The effects of experimental gingivitis on healthy young adults. A,** Accumulation of plaque and debris when no oral hygiene procedures were performed. The Plaque Index scores for subjects at the beginning of the experiment ranged from 0 to just under 1. This score indicates that no plaque was visible in any of the subjects. After 10 to 21 days, all subjects had plaque indices above 1 and approaching 2, indicating visible plaque. The shaded area shows the range of plaque scores for subjects. Oral hygiene was reinstituted at day 21 and plaque scores returned to near 0. In some subjects, the score returned to 0 in as little as 3 days, but other subjects took as long as 10 days to achieve a score of 0. **B,** The Gingival Index scores measuring redness and bleeding also increased for all individuals during the experiment. The shaded area shows the range of scores among subjects. Scores approached 1, indicating clinical redness (gingivitis), after 10 to 21 days with no oral hygiene. When oral hygiene procedures were reinstituted at day 21, scores returned to baseline levels or below. This finding suggests that all individuals are susceptible to plaque biofilm–induced inflammation and that this condition is reversible. **C,** Plaque-induced inflammation is associated with changes in the microflora of the plaque. The graph shows that gram-positive cocci and small rods persisted in the plaque found at the gingival margin throughout the experiment. However, gram-negative forms, mostly filamentous forms, vibrios, and spirochetes, appeared after the plaque had accumulated for several days. These forms disappeared rapidly when plaque control was reinstituted at day 21. This finding indicates that different floras are associated with gingival health and disease. (From Löe H, Theilade E, Jensen SB. Experimental gingivitis in man. *J Periodontol*. 1965;36:177-187.)

seen gingival changes associated with these fluctuations in hormone production.

Endocrine-Influenced Gingival Disease. Gingivitis is often influenced by steroid-type hormones produced by the endocrine glands. These include the hormones associated with puberty and pregnancy. The use of birth control medications, particularly the early high hormone content preparations, is associated with gingival changes. When female hormone levels are increased, there is an increase in some subgingival bacteria, such as *Bacteroides* species, possibly causing the increased gingival inflammation.[10] There are estrogen receptors in the gingival tissues and serum concentrations of female sex hormones during pregnancy influence the gingival tissues.[11] Estrogen may also regulate cellular proliferation, keratinization, and vascular proliferation and fragility in the gingival tissues.[12] The extent of hormone-related changes also depends on the level of plaque biofilm control.[13] Poor plaque control aggravates the condition, underscoring the importance of proper home care and regular dental hygiene care.

Several changes in the gingiva have been associated with pregnancy. As hormone levels increase during the second trimester of pregnancy, gingival inflammation may increase significantly. This increase occurs even with good plaque control, but it may be substantial when plaque control is marginal or

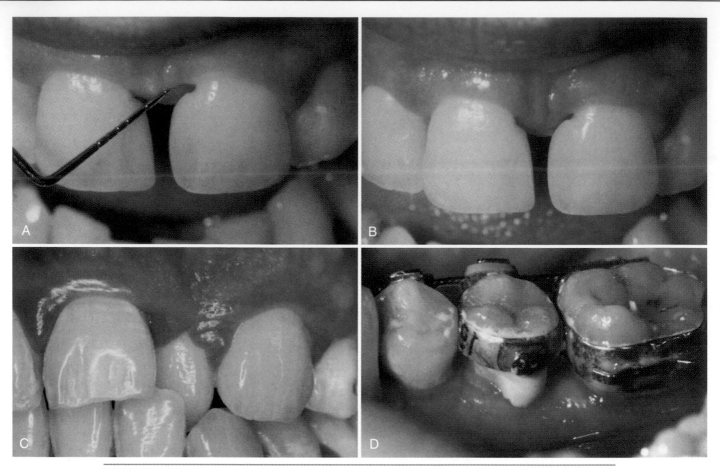

FIGURE 6-4 ■ **Plaque-induced gingivitis modified by local contributing factors. A,** Overcontoured restorations with probe retracting tissues. In an effort to minimize the large diastema, the dentist constructed cosmetic veneers to help fill the space on the mesial surfaces of the central incisors. This created a significant plaque trap. **B,** Overhanging restorations, probe removed. After the probe was withdrawn, the gingival tissues bled, indicating the presence of stage II gingivitis. **C,** Malposed teeth. The maxillary lateral incisor is in crossbite and rests lingually in relation to the central incisor and canine. This occlusion resulted in alterations in the size and shape of the embrasure spaces and papilla, creating a sheltered space for plaque biofilm and making brushing and flossing a challenge. **D,** Orthodontic appliances. Plaque control is poor in this patient and was made more difficult by the presence of orthodontic bands. In addition, excess cement was left protruding over the gingival margin, creating a terrible plaque trap.

poor. The gingiva may become dark red and hyperplastic and may bleed excessively. Figure 6-5 shows an example of pregnancy gingivitis. Changes may increase as the pregnancy progresses.[14] Most pregnancy-related gingivitis improves or resolves with good home care and removal of local irritants. Sometimes it does not heal completely until after the baby is born and hormone levels return to normal.

CLINICAL NOTE 6-5 The term *pregnancy gingivitis* may be misleading to some pregnant patients, because it suggests that the gingivitis will resolve after delivery. Without adequate plaque control, the gingivitis will persist.

Another striking feature in some pregnant women is the presence of a specific type of gingival lesion, a **pregnancy tumor.** This lesion is not really a tumor, such as a neoplasm, but a localized area of pyogenic granulation tissue. The tissues are highly inflamed, bleed easily, and may cause teeth to be mobile and possibly migrate out of the way. As in other types of gingival enlargement, poor plaque biofilm control is related

to the severity of the inflammation and some localized trauma may have occurred. Most lesions resolve when the baby is born, but in some cases, surgical removal of residual enlargement is required. Figure 6-6 shows an example of pregnancy gingivitis and commonly referred to as a pregnancy tumor.[5]

Gingival changes have been observed in women who are taking oral contraceptive agents and in older women who are taking hormone replacement therapy to mitigate symptoms associated with menopause. In general, changes include an increase in gingival inflammation that appears out of proportion to the amount of supragingival plaque present. This condition clearly does not occur in all women. Two mechanisms may cause this significant response:

1. There may be an increase in some pathogenic bacteria, such as *Porphyromonas gingivalis* and *Actinobacillus actinomycetemcomitans.*
2. There may be an increase in prostaglandin E, a mediator of inflammation.

Both circumstances increase the inflammatory response. However, hormone drugs can be important to a woman's health, and their benefits may greatly outweigh any potential

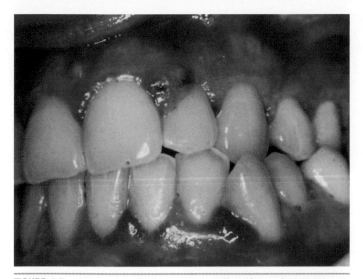

FIGURE 6-5 ■ **Pregnancy gingivitis.** Hormonally influenced gingivitis was seen in this 27-year-old woman who was 7 months pregnant and had poor plaque control. The gingival margin was intensely red and swollen. This tissue was extremely painful, making oral hygiene practices more difficult and causing the patient to consume a soft diet, which resulted in more plaque growth and accumulation. Dental hygiene care improved the condition, but it did not completely resolve until after the baby was born.

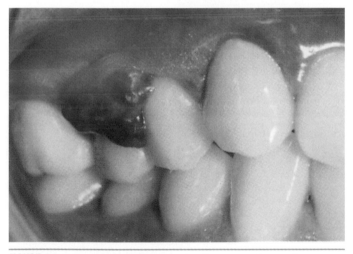

FIGURE 6-6 ■ **Pregnancy tumor.** Occasionally, a pyogenic granuloma, commonly called a pregnancy tumor, will appear during pregnancy. Improved oral hygiene and regular dental hygiene care improved the condition. Many small "tumors" resolve after delivery. In this case, the granuloma was large, and although it shrank after the baby was born, it had to be surgically removed.

side effects to oral health. For example, evidence suggests that osteoporosis associated with menopause may be a risk factor for periodontal disease.[15] Reducing osteoporosis through the use of hormone supplements or other drugs is far more critical than the potential increase of gingival inflammation.

Gingival Diseases Modified by Medications. A variety of medications can cause changes in the gingival tissues, resulting in **gingival diseases modified by medications.** Most commonly, the antiseizure medication phenytoin, which is often used to control the seizures that occur with various forms of epilepsy, has long been associated with gingival **hyperplasia** (overgrowth). The gingival tissues may become fibrotic and enlarged. Studies have shown that the enlargement is caused by changes in the epithelial cells and the fibroblasts, which create

a denser connective tissue. These changes can be seen even in tissue cultures of cells grown in the laboratory. There is also some evidence that an increase in bacterial plaque causes a concurrent increase in gingival overgrowth in patients taking phenytoin.[16] Therefore, in patients taking this medication, excellent plaque control is necessary to prevent or slow the formation of enlarged gingiva.

Medication-induced gingival enlargement results in gingival contours that enhance plaque accumulation and make plaque biofilm removal more difficult. Patients often have heavy calculus formation and increased levels of inflammation because of plaque biofilm retention. Treatment of this type of gingival enlargement requires good home care, regular scaling and root planing and, often, reduction of the enlargements with surgical **gingivectomy** procedures.

Some cardiac medications also cause overgrowth of gingival tissues. These include nifedipine and verapamil, which are commonly used to control blood pressure and reduce the recurrence of heart attack in patients who have had already had one or more. Both of these agents are classified as calcium channel blockers. These medications are commonly prescribed and dental hygienists will see more patients with this type of gingival enlargement with our aging population. As with phenytoin, there is some evidence that excellent plaque control helps to control the symptoms of hyperplasia and gingivitis. Regular dental hygiene care is important to limit the effects of these drugs to the gingiva. Figure 6-7 shows examples of drug-induced gingival enlargement.

Another medication that causes gingival overgrowth is cyclosporine, the major drug used for immunosuppression in transplant patients. This medication may also be used to treat multiple sclerosis.[17] Unlike phenytoin- or nifedipine-induced hyperplasia, which is usually limited to the gingiva, cyclosporine can cause excessive accumulation of connective tissue in many other tissues of the body. Most transplant patients take cyclosporine, so this drug is increasingly found in dental patients. In addition, patients with heart, liver, and kidney transplants are taking both cyclosporine and nifedipine. In these cases, gingival enlargement may be extreme. The dental hygienist should remember that many of these patients have complicated medical histories and the patient should be questioned carefully about the reason for taking these medications. These patients usually require consultation with their physician before undergoing any dental therapy, including dental hygiene treatment. Figure 6-8 shows gingival enlargement that occurred subsequent to the use of cyclosporine.

Gingival Diseases Modified by Malnutrition. Although relatively rare in developed countries, serious nutritional deficiencies modify the body's response to dental plaque biofilms. Many vitamin deficiencies can produce changes in the oral tissues, referred to as **gingival diseases modified by malnutrition.** These vitamins include A, B_1, B_2, B_6, and C. The deficiency of ascorbic acid (vitamin C) has been the most studied. Vitamin C deficiency causes scurvy, a severe condition resulting in defective collagen formation and maintenance. The gingiva becomes very hemorrhagic and swollen, and the condition rapidly progresses to advanced periodontitis characterized by extensive bone loss and extremely loose teeth.[18,19] Severe vitamin C deficiency is rare today; relatively small

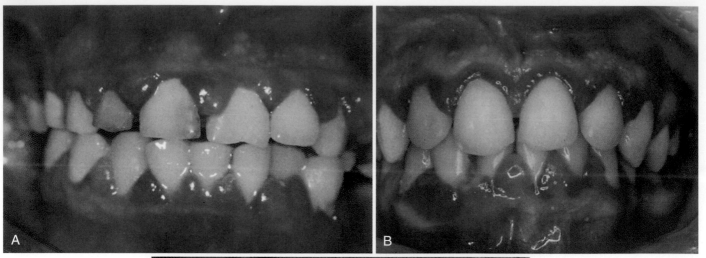

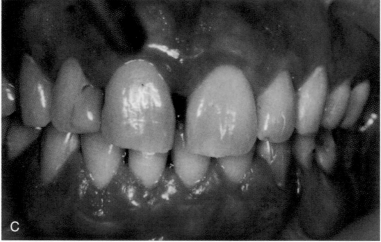

FIGURE 6-7 ■ **Drug-induced gingival enlargement. A,** Gingival enlargement often results from drug treatment with phenytoin, a drug commonly used to control seizures. This 23-year-old white male had significant gingival enlargements complicated with intense gingivitis caused by poor plaque biofilm control. The condition had been treated 1 year earlier by surgical excision of the excess tissue (gingivectomy). The overgrowth returned gradually during the following months. **B,** Another example of phenytoin-induced enlargement, also termed *Dilantin hyperplasia,* occurred in this young adult male. Gingivectomy was performed and the enlargement recurred in just a few months. (Courtesy of University of California, San Francisco, Division of Periodontology.) **C,** Gingival enlargement has been noted with the use of the drug nifedipine to treat heart disease and hypertension. This 50-year-old man had been taking nifedipine for 2 years. Note the swollen and shiny interdental papillae particularly on the mandibular anterior teeth. The tissue improved with dental hygiene care but significant enlargement remained.

amounts of ascorbic acid, largely found in citrus fruits, prevents it. However, sailors on long sea voyages in the seventeenth and eighteenth centuries experienced these symptoms quite commonly. As this nutritional deficiency became understood, the British navy stowed limes on its sailing ships to provide the crews with a source of vitamin C. The British sailors would suck the limes and thus became known as "limeys." Figure 6-9 shows an example of gingival disease associated with severe malnutrition.

Nonplaque Biofilm–Induced Gingival Lesions

Dental plaque biofilm is not the only cause of changes in the gingiva. Many systemic infections caused by specific bacteria, such as those found in gonorrhea and syphilis, may have gingival signs and symptoms. Fungal infections such as *Candida* infection and histoplasmosis may also be manifested in the gingival tissues. Perhaps the most common condition noted

in the gingival tissues, usually in young people, is caused by the virus herpes simplex. Some of these conditions require antimicrobial or antiviral interventions or, in the case of many viruses, usually run their course. Some of the most common nonplaque biofilm–induced gingival lesions seen by the dental hygienist are described in the following sections. These are often seen in the dental office because the patients think the infections are of dental origin. In addition, the dental hygienist may be able to help the patient by treating overlying gingivitis.

Gingival Diseases of Specific Bacterial Origin. Many common bacterial infections can occur in the mouth, causing gingival diseases of specific bacterial origin. An example of concern to parents is streptococcal infection of the throat and oral tissues (including the gingiva) in young children. Figure 6-10 shows an example of this condition. Sexually transmitted diseases such as meningococcal gonorrhea or syphilis have oral

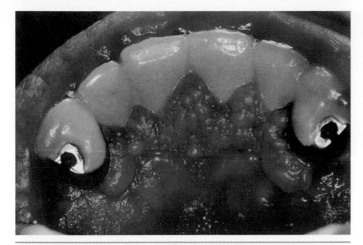

FIGURE 6-8 ■ **Drug-induced gingival enlargement.** Gingival enlargement occurred in this 54-year-old man who had undergone kidney transplantation. He was taking cyclosporine to prevent organ rejection and verapamil to control his blood pressure. The lesions developed over a period of 2 years. The bulbous, rounded, bubbly surface of the gingiva is a classic sign of drug-induced gingival enlargement. Verapamil also caused dry mouth in this patient, making him susceptible to tooth decay around the crown margins. Gingivectomy could remove this excess tissue; however, it would expose the crown margins and increase the risk of root caries. No gingivectomy was performed.

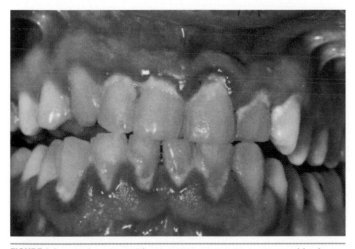

FIGURE 6-9 ■ **Malnutrition.** This severe gingivitis was seen in an older, homeless female patient who had consumed an extremely restricted diet for many months, noticeably deficient in vitamin C. There was intense redness of the gingiva and thick exudate. The teeth had grade I and grade II mobility (teeth could be moved 1 to 2 mm in the buccal-lingual direction).

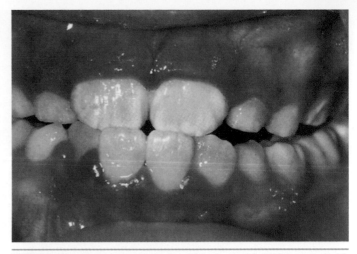

FIGURE 6-10 ■ **Streptococcal infection.** This 6-year-old child presented with a history of high fever and sore throat. Oral examination revealed an acute gingivitis, especially around the erupting incisors. Laboratory culture confirmed streptococcal infection that resolved with appropriate antibiotic therapy.

manifestations. These examples are less commonly seen in dental offices. However, the following section describes one disease that was extremely common until about 30 years ago; it is less common now but is still seen and treated by dental hygienists.

Necrotizing Ulcerative Gingivitis. Necrotizing ulcerative gingivitis (NUG) is a disease that has been described over the centuries and is characterized by the rapid onset of pain and development of necrotic ulcerative lesions of the gingiva.[5] NUG is a periodontal condition that can occur with no bone loss but that has a specific, identifiable bacterial component. It is common enough that cases are sometimes seen in general dental practices. NUG is related to excessive stress; for example, outbreaks have been reported after examination periods at colleges and universities. Historically, this relationship to stress is

shown by the common name for NUG, "trench mouth." This condition was widespread among soldiers in the trenches during World War I, probably because of stress, filthy living conditions, and poor oral hygiene. NUG is extremely painful. Patients report the sudden onset of burning mouth and inability to eat. The disease most commonly begins in the interdental papillae. After a few days, the tips of the papillae appear punched out and covered by a white necrotic pseudomembrane. This covering is referred to as a pseudomembrane because the white biofilm covering the punched-out papillae is simply a collection of PMNs trapped in the fibrin clot. The attached gingival tissues are usually inflamed. There is often a distinctive breath odor that has been termed *fetor oris* that is unique to this disease. These clinical signs are usually all that is needed to make the diagnosis. Figure 6-11 shows examples of NUG.

A significant feature of NUG infection is the presence of two microorganisms, a fusiform bacillus and a spirochete. These so-called Vincent's organisms (the disease was originally called Vincent's angina) appear to be present in all cases of NUG. Authorities believe that spirochetes may play an important role in the infection, but a direct causative effect has not been proven.[20] Occasionally, patients develop a fever. Antibiotics such as penicillin and metronidazole are useful in the treatment of NUG but are recommended only if the patient has systemic symptoms of fever and severe malaise.

The treatment for NUG is to debride plaque completely from the tissues and begin a home regimen of excellent plaque control. Although the gingival tissues are tender, careful scaling with curettes or ultrasonic scalers can be performed, usually over the course of two or more appointments. Patients obtain relief after the scaling treatment and postoperatively by rinsing with a dilute solution of hydrogen peroxide and warm water. Repeated bouts of NUG may cause permanent gingival deformation and leave the patient at higher risk for periodontal disease. Untreated, this disease may lead to bone loss and become necrotizing ulcerative periodontitis (NUP).

The relationship between NUG and NUP is not clear. The periodontal disease might be a consequence of extension of the gingival infection into the deeper tissues, or it may be a

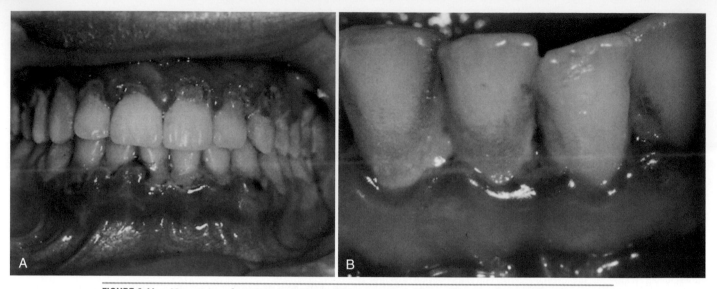

FIGURE 6-11 ■ Necrotizing ulcerative gingivitis. A, Lesions seen in a 20-year-old male college student characterized by punched-out papillae covered by a pseudomembrane. This is a severe case and the pseudomembrane, consisting primarily of necrotic tissue, extends across the facial marginal gingiva. The patient exhibited fetor oris that could be smelled when the patient entered the room. **B,** Close-up view of the pseudomembrane and cratering of papillae in the lower anterior area of another male college student. The patient had been under severe stress and smoked two packs of cigarettes per day. This condition is extremely painful so patients will not brush or floss, contributing to plaque biofilm accumulation and worsening the disease. (Courtesy of University of California, San Francisco, Division of Periodontology.)

separate entity. Until this is better understood, NUG and NUP are grouped under the single category of necrotizing periodontal diseases.[5]

Gingival Diseases of Viral Origin. Gingival diseases of viral origin may resemble plaque-induced gingivitis. However, these conditions have been studied much less extensively. One viral infection in particular, herpesvirus infection, is important to understand because it is highly contagious, very common, and can easily be transmitted to the dental hygienist. The primary form of herpetic infection is described here. There are also secondary forms of the infection that occur around the mouth. These secondary lesions are commonly called cold sores or fever blisters. These are also highly contagious but do not resemble gingivitis. For further information regarding secondary herpetic infections and the various types of herpesviruses, consult an oral pathology text.

Primary Herpetic Gingivostomatitis. Primary herpetic gingivostomatitis, or primary herpesvirus infection, is a common condition, although it is not technically a gingival disease. It must be differentiated from NUG because the symptoms are similar. This disease is more likely than NUG to occur in younger children and adolescents, but it is also seen in young adults or middle-aged patients. There are several signs that the dental hygienist may note that differentiate primary herpesvirus infection from NUG. The following symptoms are present during a primary herpesvirus infection, but not found with NUG:

- Elevated temperature
- Greater malaise
- Vesicle formation

The vesicles associated with herpesvirus coalesce to form ulcerative lesions on the gingiva or oral mucosa. This appearance contrasts with the punched-out interdental papillae found

in NUG. Although the patient may have strong breath odor because of poor plaque control, the distinctive fetor oris of NUG is absent. Figure 6-12 shows an example of primary herpetic infection.[20]

Gingival Diseases of Fungal Origin. Fungal organisms have been associated with gingival conditions. Although several fungi species can infect the oral tissues, the most common is *Candida albicans*. It is quite common to observe erythematous and fragile gingival and mucosal tissues under dentures in the mouths of patients who have worn prostheses for long periods of time. These gingival diseases of fungal origin are caused by an overgrowth of *C. albicans* and must be treated with antifungal therapies, antiseptic therapies, or both.

Candidiasis of the Gingiva. Fungal infections may occur on the gingiva and other oral tissues. The most common are caused by the yeast organism *C. albicans*. There have been reports of *Candida* isolated from the gingiva of otherwise healthy patients with periodontitis.[21] *Candida* infections have also been associated with some of the signs of gingival disease observed in patients with pronounced immunosuppression, such as those with human immunodeficiency virus (HIV) infection. The gingival conditions caused by *Candida* range from initial signs of redness at the gingival margin, called linear gingival erythema, to severe redness with white patches on the gingiva. The white patches are accumulations of organisms and debris that easily rub off the gingiva, exposing ulcerated tissue. Although the exact mechanism for this infection is still under investigation, it has been suggested that HIV infection may alter the lymphocyte response to *C. albicans*.[22] It is important to remember that individuals who are immunosuppressed for any reason, including organ transplant patients, are at risk for oral fungal infections. Figure 6-13 shows an example of *Candida* infection associated with HIV.

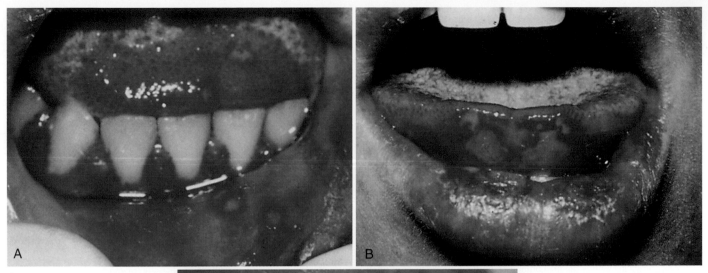

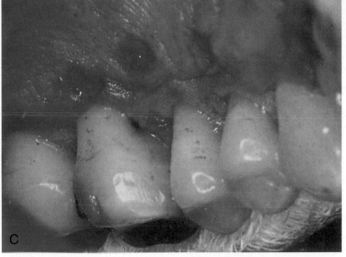

FIGURE 6-12 ■ **Primary herpetic gingivostomatitis. A,** Lesions on the attached gingiva and oral mucosa characterize this disease. The lip ulcers and inflamed gingiva in this 14-year-old female patient were extremely painful. (Courtesy of Joseph A. Regezi, DDS, MS.) **B,** The vesicles of the herpetic lesions can coalesce to form large ulcers as seen under the tongue of the same patient. Notice the cracked dry mucosa on the lip. Patients with this condition will not eat or drink anything nor brush the teeth because it is so painful. (Courtesy of Joseph A. Regezi, DDS, MS.) **C,** Secondary herpetic infections or posttreatment herpetic infection are also seen in the dental office. One week after scaling and root planing, this patient was seen with small, painful vesicles on the gingiva adjacent to the area that was treated. The condition resolved without further treatment. Herpes lesions shed virus into the saliva and oral environment. Patients with either primary or secondary herpetic lesions should be rescheduled for dental treatment after the lesions have resolved to prevent spread of the lesions and inoculation of the dental hygienist. (Courtesy of University of California, San Francisco, Division of Periodontology.)

Gingival Lesions of Genetic Origin. Some individuals have gingival changes that seem to be genetically predisposed. Research into genetic diseases is a vastly growing discipline, and much more information will be available as human genome research continues. One condition that may be observed by the dental hygienist is gingival enlargement.

Gingival Enlargement. Gingival enlargement, historically termed *hyperplasia* or *hypertrophy*, is a pathologic overgrowth of the gingiva. It has a variety of causes, so its actual incidence in the population is not known. Gingival enlargement may be caused by excessive reactions to bacterial plaque biofilm, a variety of medications, or infections, or it may occur as a side effect of systemic diseases, as described earlier. Gingival hypertrophy related to plaque and other factors is important for the dental hygienist to recognize because there are several

important diseases that may be observed in the gingiva. These conditions do not completely heal with good plaque biofilm control; however, plaque biofilm control will improve the conditions and continued poor patient plaque biofilm control worsens most of these gingival conditions. A case of gingival enlargement is presented in Figure 6-14.

In all cases, when the oral tissues appear dramatically different from what would be expected with chronic plaque-associated gingivitis, the patient should be evaluated for possible systemic disease. If excessive gingivitis is seen, the patient should be treated appropriately and reevaluated in 2 to 4 weeks to ensure that the clinical situation has resolved. If it has not, the dental hygienist and dentist should consider further evaluation and possible referral of the patient to a specialist.

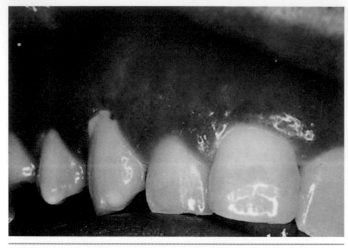

FIGURE 6-13 ■ *Candida* infection associated with HIV. This 35-year-old man had severe gingivitis with white membranous deposits. Note the mass of white material at the gingival margin on the buccal surface of the canine. Histologic smear of the white material revealed the characteristic hyphae found in these infections. The patient was treated with antifungal medication and good oral hygiene care and the condition resolved.

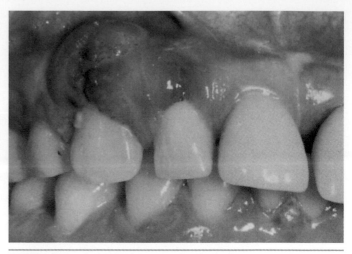

FIGURE 6-15 ■ Acute leukemia. A 35-year-old woman was seen for a severely swollen and painful gingiva that was intensely inflamed with granulation-type tissue. The pain was so severe that the patient could not brush her teeth and was reluctant to eat. In these cases, dental hygiene care will not produce normal healing, although it may slightly improve the oral condition.

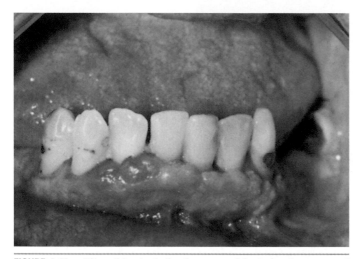

FIGURE 6-14 ■ Idiopathic gingival enlargement (gingival enlargement of unknown origin). These lesions were present in a 61-year-old male. A pebbled surface and enlarged papillae are seen between the lower right central and lateral incisors, creating a diastema. Periodontal probing depths were within normal limits.

Gingival Manifestations of Systemic Conditions. Certain systemic conditions can result in changes to the gingival tissues. Although rare compared with plaque biofilm–induced gingivitis, they are important and must be considered when evaluating a patient with gingival inflammation that does not appear to be consistent with the amount of plaque observed. The more common conditions are related to mucocutaneous disorders or dermatologic diseases. Others include blood dyscrasias. Only the gingival manifestations of systemic conditions that are occasionally seen in the dental office will be described in the following sections. For a further discussion of other systemic diseases, see Chapter 16.

Blood Dyscrasia–Associated Gingivitis. There are many blood dyscrasias and they are a significant health risk to the patient with the dyscrasia, but they are not often observed in the dental office. One condition, acute leukemia, is sometimes

first seen in the dental office because of the quick onset of gingival changes. These may be the first dramatic symptoms of the disease and will cause the patient, not knowing that the problem is medical, to seek dental treatment.

Acute Leukemia. Acute leukemia is a life-threatening disease that may initially be seen in the gingival tissues. This condition causes hemorrhagic and swollen gingival tissues, far more pronounced than would be expected from the amount of plaque and calculus present. The patient often reports that the tissues were normal until recently. The gums bleed easily and are swollen and tender. Sometimes the dental hygienist is the first health care provider to recognize that this is not dental plaque–induced gingivitis. Figure 6-15 shows an example of a gingival condition associated with acute leukemia.

Gingival Manifestations of Dermatologic Disease. Many other systemic diseases are manifested in the gingival tissues. The more common diseases are related to dermatologic diseases such as lichen planus and benign mucous membrane pemphigoid. These diseases must be recognized so that patients can receive appropriate therapeutic and palliative care.

Lichen Planus. Lichen planus is a chronic disease thought to be immune-related. It affects the skin and mucous membranes of middle-aged patients. Men and women are equally affected. It occurs in a variety of forms, ranging from the common asymptomatic reticular form, with keratotic lines called striae, to the more rare erosive and bullous forms in which portions of the lesions become ulcerated and painful.

The reticular form commonly affects the gingival tissues and usually appears as lacy white lines (Wickham's striae) with a bumpy appearance. There may be areas of white lesions alternating with raw reddened areas in the erosive form of lichen planus. The severity of this disease appears to be related to the stress level of the patient. Most studies suggest that this disease is caused by a cell-mediated immune reaction, although the mechanism is not known. Skin lesions are less common and appear as a rash of small, flat-topped papules that tend to itch. There is concern about the potential of the erosive form of lichen planus to transform into squamous cell carcinoma. For this reason, periodic observation of this chronic condition is warranted. Topical steroids have been used to control this disease during flare-ups, but no known cure has been developed.[23] Figure 6-16 presents an example of gingival changes associated with lichen planus.

Mucous Membrane Pemphigoid. Benign mucous membrane pemphigoid or, more correctly, cicatricial pemphigoid, is a chronic vesiculobullous disease that is seen as blistering and sloughing of the surface of the gingival epithelium. Although its cause is not known, it is considered an autoimmune reaction, similar to lichen planus. It is more common in older individuals and much more common in women than in men. These lesions

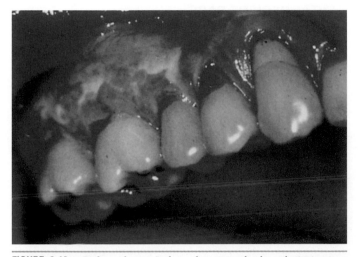

FIGURE 6-16 ■ Lichen planus. Lichen planus on the buccal gingiva in a 71-year-old woman appeared as a lacy, white, flat lesion. It was generally asymptomatic, with occasional flare-ups that the patient described as tender. Symptoms were relieved by topical steroid application. Good plaque control should be encouraged in these cases, even if the lesions are sore. (Courtesy of University of California, San Francisco, Division of Periodontology.)

may also appear on other oral tissues, such as the buccal mucosa and the inner surface of the lips, helping to distinguish them from common plaque-associated gingivitis. Symptoms of the gingival lesions range from mild discomfort to painfully raw bleeding areas because the epithelium actually strips away from the underlying connective tissue. This peeling of the epithelium when rubbed, known as the Nikolsky sign, may prevent the patient from performing any form of oral hygiene. Eating can be difficult and the patient may switch to a diet of soft foods to avoid having anything touch the painful gingival surface. Figure 6-17 shows examples of mucous membrane pemphigoid. Treatment is often palliative at best, but steroid therapy may help to relieve symptoms. Topical corticosteroids may bring gingival lesions under control and allow for better eating habits and plaque biofilm control. Chlorhexidine mouth rinses may help to control plaque accumulation and permit the topical steroids to lessen the intensity of these lesions.[23]

Desquamative Gingivitis. When cicatricial pemphigoid lesions are limited to the gingival tissues, the disease may be termed *desquamative gingivitis* or *gingivosis.* This condition is most often described as sloughing of the gingival epithelium, leaving a painfully raw, red surface. Figure 6-18 shows an example of desquamative gingivitis, or gingivosis. The etiology is suspected to be autoimmune, but desquamative gingivitis may also be caused by allergic reactions to drugs, food, or other substances.[24] As with other pemphigoid lesions, meticulous plaque control may help, but it is often difficult for the patient to perform because of the painful erosive lesions. The disease may continue for many years or, particularly in children, may disappear spontaneously. Topical and systemic steroid therapy may help to control the disease process.

Traumatic Lesions. Often, the gingival tissues are damaged by trauma. These traumatic lesions can be painful and be a surprise finding made by the patient. Common lesions seen in dental hygiene practice are burns from foods such as hot pizza

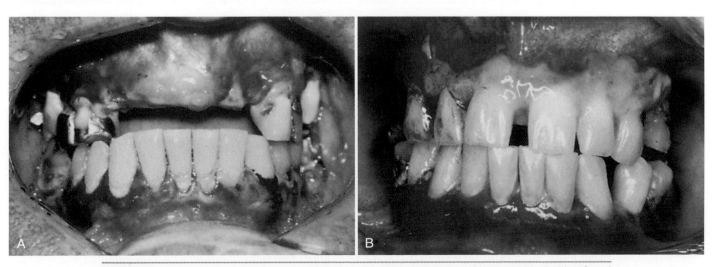

FIGURE 6-17 ■ Benign mucous membrane pemphigoid. A, This patient is an 81-year-old woman with a highly inflamed gingiva. The epithelium sloughed when rubbed with gauze, leaving a raw bleeding surface. The maxillary partial denture that replaced the anterior teeth may have irritated the tissue further. The patient had significant pain when eating and brushing her teeth, so plaque biofilm control was difficult. The condition improved with dental hygiene care. **B,** This 64-year-old woman had a painful and sloughing gingiva. Note that the areas she was able to brush have less severe inflammation. (Courtesy of Dr. Joseph A. Regezi.)

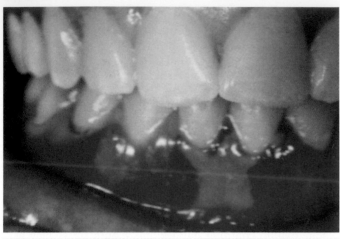

FIGURE 6-18 ■ Desquamative gingivitis. Desquamative gingivitis in this 14-year-old girl exhibited bullous lesions (splits in the tissue). Tissues were intensely inflamed and painful. In these cases, plaque control is important to reduce the inflammation. Oxygenating mouth rinses may also help relieve symptoms. (Courtesy of University of California, San Francisco, Division of Periodontology.)

or burritos, chemical burns from aspirin placed on the gingiva for pain relief, or cuts from chicken bones or hard bread crusts. Some interesting cases of advanced recession caused by trauma are illustrated in Figure 6-19.

Foreign Body Reactions. Damage to gingival tissue, similar to traumatic lesions, can be caused by foreign body reactions in or near the tissues. A relatively common lesion observed in dental practices is an acute gingival reaction to food impaction from food particles such as popcorn husks or apple skins. These are localized painful lesions with sudden onset. Often, a good dental history will reveal the source and removal of the foreign substance will bring immediate relief. Figure 6-20 shows an example of such an acute gingival reaction.

DENTAL HYGIENE CARE

Dental hygiene care is a critical part of the treatment of gingival conditions. In all the conditions described in this chapter, the dental hygienist can improve the patient's comfort and gingival health, even if the gingival condition cannot be cured.

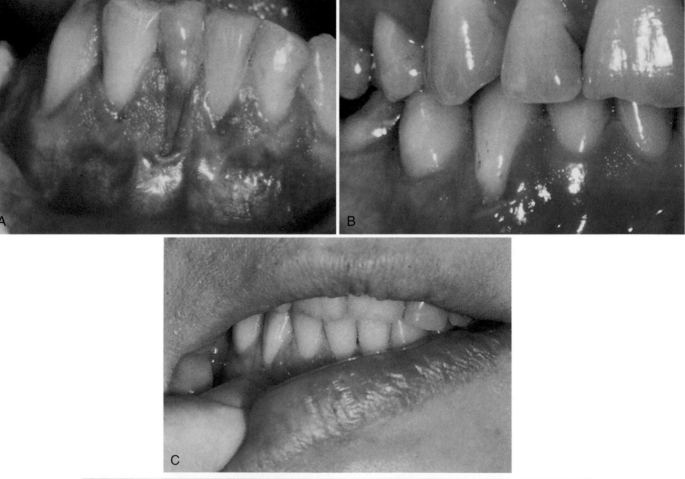

FIGURE 6-19 ■ Traumatic lesions of the gingiva. A, This patient had excessive gingival recession on the buccal surface of the mandibular central incisor. His deep overbite caused this recession by actually scraping away the gingival tissue every time the patient closed the teeth together. The condition stabilized with this amount of recession and has not changed for several years. **B,** The dental hygienist noted an area of unexplained localized gingival recession on the mandibular left canine. No cause could be identified. While questioning this patient, the hygienist noticed her nervous habit of scratching the tooth root with her fingernail. **C,** The cause of the recession was the repeated traumatic injury illustrated in this photograph.

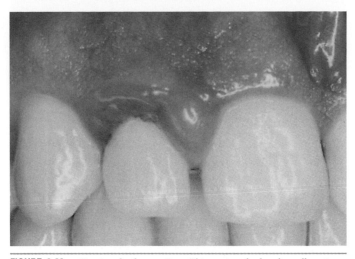

FIGURE 6-20 ■ Foreign body reaction. This patient had red swollen tissue localized to this one interproximal area. The papilla was very painful and bled with slight provocation. The dental history revealed that the swelling and soreness had started suddenly the previous weekend. Exploration of the area with a periodontal probe and a curette dislodged a popcorn husk embedded in the sulcus. When the husk was removed, the patient felt immediate pain relief and the lesion resolved in 2 days. Dental history revealed that the patient had been to the movie theater the previous weekend and had eaten popcorn.

Plaque biofilm–induced gingivitis may be one of the most common human diseases. It is certainly the most common periodontal disease.[25] The relationship between the accumulation of plaque biofilm and gingival inflammation has been well documented. Understanding this relationship is critical because gingival disease will develop in everyone if plaque is allowed to accumulate. No person is genetically resistant to plaque biofilm–induced gingivitis. The bacterial population of plaque biofilm–induced gingivitis appears to be nonspecific. The overall composition of the plaque biofilm in gingivitis is different from that in health, but no specific bacteria are known to be responsible. Therefore, the control and prevention of gingivitis are a primary responsibility of the patient and the dental hygienist, with therapy and home care aimed at reducing all the bacterial plaque biofilm on the tooth surfaces.

> **CLINICAL NOTE 6-6** Consistent disruption of plaque biofilm is necessary to treat and prevent gingivitis; therefore, allotting appointment time to patient education is essential for every patient and must continue throughout the treatment relationship.

Other gingival diseases or manifestations of systemic diseases can mimic dental plaque–induced gingivitis and may be exacerbated by poor plaque biofilm control and the presence of local irritants. For this reason, it is important to recognize unusual conditions and distinguish them from chronic gingivitis. Dental hygiene care will always consist of patient education and the removal of local irritants to promote healing. The level of responsibility, frequency, and results of treatment may vary, but the patient's condition can be improved with dental hygiene care.

◎ DENTAL HYGIENE CONSIDERATIONS

- Gingivitis has distinct stages that are defined by both histologic and clinical signs.
- Dental plaque biofilm–induced gingivitis heals completely without residual changes to the oral tissues.
- Gingival recession is related to inflammation, tooth position, trauma, and abnormal frenum attachment.
- Gingivitis can be localized or generalized.
- There are many contributing factors to gingivitis, including local tooth-related factors, systemic disease, medications, malnutrition, specific infections (e.g., bacterial, viral, or fungal), genetic factors, trauma, and foreign body reactions.
- Gingivitis that has contributing factors may not resolve completely with dental hygiene care alone, but oral health can be improved.
- The dental hygienist has a unique role in recognizing gingivitis, educating patients about the disease, and treating the condition.

★ CASE SCENARIO

Your first patient of the day, Ms. Coluzzi, is scheduled for a regular preventive maintenance appointment. She is a 32-year-old healthy female with no systemic disease and she has a history of regular dental visits. This is the first time you have treated her, and you observe that the buccal gingiva adjacent to both mandibular canines and first premolars appears red, rolled, and edematous. Further assessment reveals a layer of plaque present at the gingival margin in these areas and 2 mm of gingival recession. The areas exhibit slight bleeding when you assess them with a periodontal probe. She tells you that it always bleeds around the lower teeth, but she knows that everybody's gums bleed so she doesn't worry about it. During your oral hygiene instruction, the patient tells you that it is too uncomfortable to brush in those areas.

1. The most likely cause of the gingival inflammation you have noted is
   A. gingivitis.
   B. periodontitis.
   C. gingival recession.
   D. supragingival plaque biofilm.

2. Ms. Coluzzi is probably experiencing discomfort because the recession has exposed root surfaces that have become sensitive.
   A. Both the statement and the reason are correct and related.
   B. Both the statement and the reason are correct but NOT related.
   C. The statement is correct, but the reason is NOT correct.
   D. The statement is NOT correct, but the reason is correct.
   E. NEITHER the statement NOR the reason is correct.

3. Ms. Coluzzi has gingivitis around the mandibular teeth, and the tissues bleed when probed. Everyone has bleeding gums so this should not concern you.
   A. Both statements are true.
   B. Both statements are false.
   C. The first statement is true, and the second statement is false.
   D. The first statement is false, and the second statement is true.

4. The bleeding of Ms. Coluzzi's gingiva indicates a shift in the bacterial flora to one that is
   A. gram-positive.
   B. gram-negative.
   C. unchanged; there is no shift in the flora.
   D. gram-positive and gram-negative.

STUDY QUESTIONS

Answers and rationales to these questions can be obtained from your instructor.

MULTIPLE CHOICE

1. Which of the following is the clinical descriptor of swelling?
   A. Erythema
   B. Rubor
   C. Edema
   D. Hemorrhage
2. Which of the following may contribute to the development of gingivitis?
   A. Restorations
   B. Misaligned teeth
   C. Mouth breathing
   D. Pregnancy
   E. All of the above
3. Which statement below is correct?
   A. Gingivitis is defined by loss of support tissues.
   B. Gingivitis is generally very painful.
   C. Plaque control is critical in the resolution of gingivitis.
   D. Everyone older than 16 years has gingivitis.
4. Gingivitis is classified based on
   A. tissue color.
   B. histologic events.
   C. probing depths.
   D. necessary treatment.
5. Dental plaque biofilm–induced gingivitis may lead to periodontal disease. Like gingivitis, periodontal disease is curable.
   A. Both statements are true.
   B. Both statements are false.
   C. The first statement is true, and the second statement is false.
   D. The first statement is false, and the second statement is true.
6. What is the etiology of pregnancy gingivitis?
   A. Lack of home care due to increased patient fatigue
   B. The influence of hormones on oral tissues
   C. Vitamin deficiency due to nutritional needs of the fetus
   D. None of the above
7. It is the dental hygienist's responsibility to educate patients regarding gingivitis because
   A. patients can easily ignore gingivitis.
   B. gingivitis can be caused by changes in hormones.
   C. patients think that gingival bleeding resulting from toothbrushing is normal.
   D. all of the above statements are correct.

8. Which of the following diseases is considered the most prevalent?
   A. Gingivitis
   B. Periodontal disease
   C. Pregnancy gingivitis
   D. Hypertension

SHORT ANSWER

9. Why do patients sometimes think that gingivitis is normal?
10. What is the most essential aspect of treating a patient with gingivitis?

Please visit **http://evolve.elsevier.com/Perry/periodontology** for additional practice and study support tools.

REFERENCES

1. American Academy of Periodontology. *Proceedings of the World Workshop on Clinical Periodontology.* Chicago, IL: American Academy of Periodontology; 1989:1–2.
2. American Academy of Periodontology. The pathogenesis of periodontal diseases. *J Periodontol.* 1999;70:457–470.
3. Page RC, Schroeder HE. *Periodontitis in Man and Other Animals. A Comparative Review.* Basel, Switzerland: S Karger; 1982:5–45.
4. Fiorellini JP, Kim DM, Uzel, NG. Gingival inflammation. In: Newman MG, Takei HH, Klokkevold PR, et al, eds. *Carranza's Clinical Periodontology.* 11th ed. St. Louis, MO: Elsevier Saunders; 2012:71–75.
5. Armitage GC. Diagnosis and classification of periodontal diseases. In: Rose LF, Mealey BL, eds. *Periodontics: Medicine, Surgery and Implants.* St. Louis, MO: Elsevier Mosby; 2004:19–31.
6. Armitage GC. Development of a classification system for periodontal diseases and conditions. *Ann Periodontol.* 1999;4:1–6.
7. Fiorellini JP, Kim DM, Uzel, NG. Clinical features of gingivitis. In: Newman MG, Takei HH, Klokkevold PR, et al, eds. *Carranza's Clinical Periodontology.* 11th ed. St. Louis, MO: Elsevier Saunders; 2012:76–83.
8. Löe H, Theilade E, Jensen SB. Experimental gingivitis in man. *J Periodontol.* 1965;36:177–187.
9. Atkinson PT. *Refractory Adult Periodontitis: The Influence of Repressive Coping Style* [dissertation]. Ann Arbor, MI: Fielding Institute; 1998.
10. Kornman KS. Age, supragingival plaque, and steroid hormones as ecological determinants of the subgingival flora. In: Genco RJ, Mergenhagen SE, eds. *Host-Parasite Interactions in Periodontal Diseases.* Washington, DC: American Society for Microbiology; 1982:132–138.
11. Hugoson A. Gingival inflammation and female sex hormones: a clinical investigation of pregnant women and experimental studies in dogs. *J Periodontal Res Suppl.* 1970;5:1–18.
12. Vittek J, Hernandez JR, Wenk EJ, et al. Specific estrogen receptors in human gingiva. *J Clin Endocrinol Metab.* 1982;54:608–612.
13. Silness J, Löe H. Periodontal disease in pregnancy, II: correlation between oral hygiene and periodontal condition. *Acta Odontol Scand.* 1964;22:121–135.
14. Löe H, Silness J. Periodontal disease in pregnancy, I: prevalence and severity. *Acta Odontol Scand.* 1963;21:533–551.
15. Van Wowern N, Kausen B, Kollerup G. Osteoporosis: a risk factor in periodontal disease. *J Periodontol.* 1994;65:1134–1138.
16. O'Neil T, Figures K. The effects of chlorhexidine and mechanical methods of plaque control on the recurrence of gingival hyperplasia in young patients taking phenytoin. *Br Dent J.* 1982;152:130–133.
17. Hefti AF, Eshenaur AE, Hassell TM, et al. Gingival overgrowth in cyclosporine: a treated multiple sclerosis patient. *J Periodontol.* 1994;65:744–749.
18. Woolfe SN, Hume WR, Kenney EB. Ascorbic acid and periodontal disease: a review of the literature. *J West Soc Periodontol.* 1980;28:44–52.

19. Charbeneau TD, Hurt WC. Gingival findings in spontaneous scurvy: a case report. *J Periodontol*. 1983;54:694–697.

20. Listgarten MA. Electron microscopic observations of the bacterial flora of acute necrotizing ulcerative gingivitis. *J Periodontol*. 1965;36:328–339.

21. Rams TE, Slots J. *Candida* biotypes in human adult periodontitis. *Oral Microbiol Immunol*. 1991;6:191–192.

22. Lamster IB, Grbic JT, Mitchell-Lewis DA, et al. New concepts regarding the pathogenesis of periodontal disease in HIV infection. *Ann Periodontol*. 1998;3:62–67.

23. Regezi JA, Sciubba J, Jordan RCK. White lesions. In: *Oral Pathology: Clinical-Pathologic Correlations*. 4th ed. St. Louis, MO: WB Saunders; 2003: 75–109.

24. Nisengard RJ, Neiders M. Desquamative lesions of the gingiva. *J Periodontol*. 1981;52:500–510.

25. Page RC. Oral health status in the United States: prevalence of inflammatory periodontal diseases. *J Dent Educ*. 1985;49:354–364.

Periodontal Diseases

Dorothy A. Perry

LEARNING OUTCOMES

- Describe the pathogenesis of periodontitis.
- Define periodontal disease activity.
- List and describe the American Academy of Periodontology categories of periodontal diagnosis.
- Define clinical attachment loss and its relationship to periodontitis.
- Compare and contrast the following forms of periodontitis as to demographics and clinical and microbiologic characteristics:
  - Chronic periodontitis
  - Aggressive periodontitis
  - Prepubertal periodontitis

- Early-onset periodontitis
- Rapidly progressing periodontitis
- Refractory periodontitis
- Necrotizing ulcerative periodontitis
- Periodontitis as a manifestation of systemic disease
- Identify systemic diseases and genetic factors associated with periodontal disease.
- State the role of systemic antibiotic treatment, locally delivered controlled-release antibiotic treatment, and enzyme suppression treatment in periodontitis.
- Describe the role of the dental hygienist in treating periodontal disease.

KEY TERMS

Abscess	Gingival enlargements	Periodontitis
Acquired deformities	Intrabony pocket	Prepubertal periodontitis
Aggressive periodontitis	Necrotizing ulcerative gingivitis	Pseudopockets
Antibiotic therapy	Necrotizing ulcerative periodontitis	Rapidly progressing periodontitis
Bone loss	Pathogenesis	Refractory periodontitis
Chronic periodontitis	Pathogenicity	Risk factor
Clinical attachment loss	Periodontal abscess	Site specific
Developmental anomalies	Periodontal bone loss	Suprabony pocket
Enzyme suppression therapy	Periodontal disease	Suppuration
Episodic periodontal disease	Periodontal pocket	

Periodontal disease is an inclusive term describing any disease of the tissues surrounding the teeth, including gingival diseases and diseases of the supporting structures. This chapter describes forms of **periodontitis**, the periodontal diseases of the supporting tissues of the teeth.

Periodontitis is a set of diseases. It is characterized by inflammation of the supporting tissues of the teeth, specifically the periodontal ligament, cementum, and alveolar bone.[1] Unlike gingivitis, which is limited to the epithelium and gingival connective tissues, periodontitis results in loss of connective tissue attachment to the cementum on the tooth root. Loss of attachment creates a deepening of the gingival sulcus to form a periodontal pocket by migration of the junctional epithelium along the root surface. This is an inflammatory response that results in **bone loss**, recession, or both. Left unchecked, periodontitis continues to worsen and causes a weakened periodontium characterized by mobile teeth that are susceptible to **abscess**

formation. The disease can be uncomfortable and unsightly. Teeth do not function effectively and are lost; they simply fall out, or they are extracted if they become acutely infected or untreatable by periodontal or restorative dental methods.

> **CLINICAL NOTE 7-1** Periodontitis is a destructive disease involving tissue inflammation, elongated junctional epithelium, loss of connective tissue, and destruction of collagen fibers and bone. The clinical appearance includes pocket formation and inflamed tissues, and the loss of alveolar bone results in tooth mobility.

PERIODONTAL POCKET

The **periodontal pocket** is a pathologically deepened gingival sulcus. It occurs in all types of periodontal disease and presents similar histologic features as periodontitis progresses.

Clinically, the pockets in the various periodontal diseases are similar, but diseases are distinct in their etiology, natural history, progression, and response to therapy.

PATHOGENESIS OF PERIODONTAL POCKETS

Probing pocket depths can increase for two reasons:

1. Coronal movement of the gingival margin through swelling or deepening of the sulcus. The resulting pockets that form are classified as gingival enlargements and periodontal pockets. Gingival pockets reflect tissue enlargement often related to inflammation and systemic conditions and are not associated with bone loss.[7]
2. Periodontal pockets reflect a progressive deepening of the sulcus through tissue destruction and are associated with bone loss.[3]

Periodontal pockets are also classified as suprabony and infrabony, depending on their relationship to the adjacent alveolar bone. Suprabony periodontal pockets occur above the crest of the alveolar bone and intrabony pockets extend apically from the crest of the alveolar bone.

Inflammatory periodontal pocket lesions begin with bacterial challenge from plaque biofilms that lead to the destruction of surrounding connective tissues. The mechanisms associated with collagen loss in connective tissue are phagocytosis of collagen fibers and secretion of enzymes by both healthy cells and inflammatory cells. As a result of collagen loss apical to the junctional epithelium, the epithelial cells migrate apically and the coronal portion of the junctional epithelium detaches from the root surface as it becomes more engorged with inflammatory cells. As part of the inflammation process, the gingiva also swells from becoming engorged with increased amounts of cellular and serum elements, so it moves coronally on the tooth. The epithelial lining of the pocket loses its integrity so that leukocytes and products of the inflammatory response escape into the pocket space, and epithelial projections (rete pegs) spread from the pocket lining into the connective tissue.

This periodontal pocket harbors plaque biofilm that the patient cannot remove. It results in a disease cycle, as follows:

Biofilm → gingival inflammation → pocket formation → more biofilm formation[2]

CLINICAL NOTE 7-2 This periodontal pocket harbors a dynamic system of inflammation that includes both destruction and repair of tissues. Complete healing does not occur because the pathogenic plaque biofilm persists in the pocket and constantly stimulates both the destructive and healing processes.

Contents of the Pocket

The periodontal pocket contains subgingival plaque biofilm with many virulent bacteria, including motile forms that can survive in the sheltered pocket environment. It also contains metabolic products from the biofilm, which can be quite toxic, copious amounts of gingival fluid from the proliferating capillaries, and many cells. The pocket also contains calculus that has formed in the matrix of the plaque biofilm and adheres strongly to the teeth. Pus (accumulations of large numbers of dead cells and serum products) can also often be seen in periodontal pockets. The contents of the pocket are so virulent that they have been demonstrated to cause toxic effects in experimental animals even when the bacteria themselves have been filtered out.[3]

The contents of the pocket have effects on the root surfaces of the teeth. Lipopolysaccharides (endotoxins) from the organisms in biofilm penetrate cementum, where they interfere with epithelial adherence to the root surface.

CLINICAL NOTE 7-3 The rationale for scaling and root planing is endotoxin removal, calculus removal, and biofilm disruption.

PATHOGENESIS OF PERIODONTITIS

It is not known exactly when gingivitis ends and periodontitis begins. Clinical studies have not shown if and when this transition occurs from a gingival inflammation to one involving the deeper tissues. In periodontitis, the pathogenicity of periodontitis is the extension of inflammation into the attachment apparatus and development of periodontal pockets. As inflammation progresses, the sulcular epithelium increases in thickness and begins to infiltrate into the underlying connective tissue.

Pockets deepen because of the breakdown of collagen fibers in the gingival connective tissue by enzymes such as collagenase, which are released by some of the plaque bacteria and the host's inflammatory cells. The junctional epithelium elongates and then separates from the root surface at the coronal end. The plaque bacteria release a number of chemotactic substances that increase the flow of neutrophils into the gingival sulcus. The neutrophils react with bacteria, producing the suppuration (pus or exudates) often seen in progressing periodontal disease. Figure 7-1 shows the histologic events that occur in the periodontal pocket and crest of the bone.

Periodontitis begins with apical migration of the junctional epithelium and loss of alveolar crest bone. Bone is an active tissue undergoing continuous resorption and formation, so when bone resorption exceeds apposition, a net decrease in the amount of bone occurs. Loss of crestal alveolar bone through the inflammatory process is called periodontal bone loss. There is limited evidence that systemic bone thinning, such as seen in osteoporosis,[4] is related to increased alveolar bone loss and tooth loss.

When periodontal disease becomes established, both plasma cells and lymphocytes are present in the periodontal tissues. Plasma cells are important in antigen-antibody reactions, a major activity of the immune system. Antigen-antibody reactions activate a cascade of events that attract additional inflammatory cells to the periodontal tissues. These cells produce active molecules that cause additional destruction of the collagen fibers in the periodontal connective tissue. Lymphocytes, when stimulated by the bacteria in the plaque biofilm, release lymphokines, another class of active proteins. Lymphokines have many effects on the inflammatory system, including the production of chemical factors that activate osteoclasts and thus increase osseous resorption.[4] For a more complete description of the host response, review Chapter 2.

Other products of the interaction of bacterial plaque with inflammatory cells include prostaglandins, which stimulate bone resorption. In combination, these and other factors, such

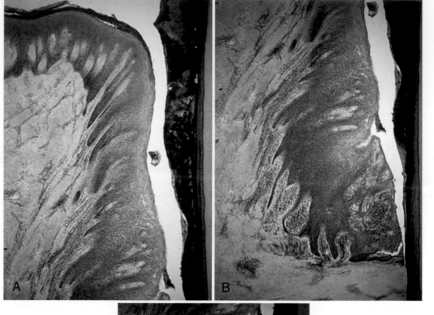

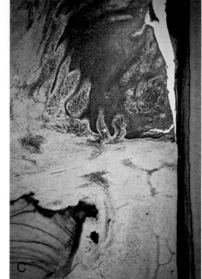

FIGURE 7-1 ■ The histology of a periodontal pocket. A, The coronal portion of the periodontal pocket is adjacent to a plaque biofilm and calculus-covered root surface. The sulcular epithelium is thickened, with exaggerated rete pegs extending into the underlying connective tissue. There is a dense inflammatory cell infiltrate under the sulcular epithelium and surrounding the blood vessels. **B,** The base of the same periodontal pocket shows the apical termination of the thickened junctional epithelium, which has separated from the root surface during specimen preparation. The epithelium precisely follows the contours of the root surface and calculus *(right).* A large amount of inflammatory cell infiltrate is seen within the thickened junctional epithelium. Microulcerations appear on the epithelium lining the pocket, and the dense infiltrate has replaced the collagen fibers in the connective tissue. **C,** A lower power view of the same specimen shows the crest of the alveolar bone and the periodontal ligament space. The inflammatory cells have migrated along the vascular channels into the periodontal ligament, spreading the infection. The structure on the lower left side is the crest of the alveolar bone. There is a single osteoclast seen in its resorption bay at the crest of the bone; the cell appears pale. (Courtesy of Dr. Gary C. Armitage.)

as activated complement, appear to cause bone loss in progressing periodontitis. Interestingly, understanding the mechanisms of bone resorption may provide a clue to new methods of periodontal disease treatment. For example, nonsteroidal anti-inflammatory drugs inhibit prostaglandins and current research suggests that these drugs may inhibit some of the bone loss seen in periodontitis.[5] However, in combination, these processes result in varying degrees of deepened pockets, tissue inflammation, bone loss, exposed furcations, and mobile teeth seen in periodontitis.[6]

DISEASE ACTIVITY

For many years, it was thought that periodontal disease was a constantly progressing infection characterized by nonspecific pathogens. As understanding of the specific plaque hypothesis increased, the concept of episodic periodontal disease emerged. This means that periodontal disease has episodic bursts of activity followed by periods of remission. During the active phase, bone and other periodontal tissues are lost and the pockets deepen. Active periods are associated with tissue bleeding and provide the opportunity for researchers to develop diagnostic tests. During the periods of quiescence (remission), the disease is static and pockets do not deepen.

It is also important to know that periodontal disease is site specific. It does not occur in all teeth at any given time, and some teeth in the mouth may be untouched by disease. This is likely related to differences in the pathogenicity of plaque biofilm in various sites around the mouth. Site specificity of disease activity can result in new disease sites, increased tissue damage in existing sites, or both.[7]

CLASSIFICATION OF PERIODONTITIS

Periodontitis occurs in a variety of forms. The American Academy of Periodontology has classified periodontitis into a number of general categories on the basis of etiology, clinical presentation, pathogenesis, progression, and response to therapy.[1] Seven categories of periodontitis are recognized, but they probably represent many different bacterial infections with similar symptoms. An additional category describes

BOX 7-1   Classification of Periodontal Diseases and Conditions[7]

I. Gingival diseases (complete listing is in Chapter 6)
II. Chronic periodontitis
   A. Localized (≤30% of involved sites)
   B. Generalized (>30% of involved sites)
III. Aggressive periodontitis
   A. Localized
   B. Generalized
IV. Periodontitis as a manifestation of systemic disease
   A. Associated with hematologic disorders
      1. Acquired neutropenia
      2. Leukemias
      3. Other
   B. Associated with genetic disorders
      1. Familial and cyclic neutropenia
      2. Down syndrome
      3. Leukocyte adhesion deficiency syndromes
      4. Papillon-Lefèvre syndrome
      5. Chédiak-Higashi syndrome
      6. Histiocytosis syndromes
      7. Glycogen storage disease
      8. Infantile genetic agranulocytosis
      9. Cohen syndrome
     10. Ehlers-Danlos syndrome (Types IV and VIII)
     11. Hypophosphatasia
     12. Other
   C. Not otherwise specified
V. Necrotizing periodontal disease
   A. Necrotizing ulcerative gingivitis (NUG) (described in Chapter 6)
   B. Necrotizing ulcerative periodontitis (NUP)
VI. Abscess of the periodontium
   A. Gingival abscess
   B. Periodontal abscess
   C. Pericoronal abscess
VII. Periodontitis associated with endodontic lesions
   A. Combined periodontal-endodontic lesions
VIII. Developmental or acquired deformities and conditions
   A. Localized tooth-related factors that modify or predispose to plaque-induced gingival diseases or periodontitis
      1. Tooth anatomic factors
      2. Dental restorations or appliances
      3. Root fractures
      4. Cervical root resorption and cemental tears
   B. Mucogingival deformities and conditions around teeth
      1. Gingival or soft tissue recession
        a. Facial or lingual surfaces
        b. Interproximal (papillary)
      2. Lack of keratinized gingiva
      3. Decreased vestibular depth
      4. Aberrant frenum/muscle position
      5. Gingival excess
        a. Pseudopocket
        b. Inconsistent gingival margin
        c. Excessive gingival display
        d. Gingival enlargement
      6. Abnormal color
   C. Mucogingival deformities and conditions on edentulous ridges
      1. Vertical or horizontal ridge deficiency
      2. Lack of gingiva or keratinized tissue
      3. Gingival or soft tissue enlargement
      4. Aberrant frenum/muscle position
      5. Decreased vestibular depth
      6. Abnormal color
   D. Occlusal trauma
      1. Primary occlusal trauma
      2. Secondary occlusal trauma

---

developmental or **acquired deformities** that are related to periodontitis. The classification categories are presented in Box 7-1.[8]

CHRONIC PERIODONTITIS

Chronic periodontitis is the most common form of periodontal disease. When most clinicians say periodontitis or periodontal disease, they are referring to chronic periodontitis. In this chapter, the terms are used interchangeably except when the term *chronic periodontitis* is used to differentiate one disease entity from another specific disease.

Chronic periodontitis may have its preclinical onset in adolescence and, unless halted by therapy, it appears to progress for the life of the individual. This disease is characterized by bone resorption that progresses slowly and predominantly in a horizontal direction. It is not usually significant clinically until about the age of 35 years; however, clinically significant pocketing and bone loss can occur at any age. Epidemiologic evidence suggests that periodontitis may occur more commonly among U.S. men than women, but this is not a consistent finding throughout the world. It may be explained by the fact that women visit the dentist more regularly in this country and therefore may benefit from more prevention and earlier treatment (see Chapter 3).

The severity of chronic periodontitis is directly related to the accumulation of plaque biofilm and calculus on the surfaces of the teeth. The rate of periodontal destruction varies depending on disease activity and the patient's resistance (host response). Chronic periodontitis is not associated with systemic disease or abnormalities in host defense.[9]

Chronic periodontitis is a prevalent disease that may be either localized or generalized and progresses intermittently until the teeth are lost by exfoliation or extraction. The progression of periodontitis appears to occur in episodic bursts of activity that cause attachment loss.[7] The disease progresses in the presence of pathologic dental plaque biofilm and attachment loss occurs when collagen fibers in the local pocket are destroyed. Disease activity halts when the host resistance controls the disease process through therapy or natural defenses. The severity of disease can be characterized as described in Table 7-1.

CLINICAL NOTE 7-4 The most reliable method of determining disease activity is to document the loss of periodontal attachment by measuring clinical attachment loss (CAL) over time. This measurement documents increases in the distance from the cementoenamel junction to the apical depth of the periodontal pocket. It requires successive measurements over weeks, months, or years and does not indicate if the disease is actively progressing at the moment the patient is examined, but gives a measure of progression over time.

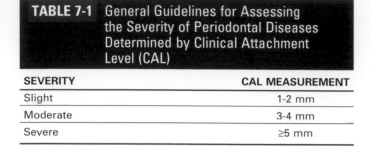

TABLE 7-1 General Guidelines for Assessing the Severity of Periodontal Diseases Determined by Clinical Attachment Level (CAL)

SEVERITY	CAL MEASUREMENT
Slight	1-2 mm
Moderate	3-4 mm
Severe	≥5 mm

CLINICAL ATTACHMENT LOSS

The defining element for classifying periodontal disease is not probing depth, but the level of attachment loss from the cementoenamel junction, which indicates bone loss. This concept is important for the dental hygienist to remember. Probing pocket depth (also called probe depth, probing depth, or pocket depth) is significant because the patient's ability to adequately clean deepened pockets is greatly reduced. In addition, deepened periodontal pockets usually require instrumentation of complex root anatomy, including flutes, grooves, and furcation areas. Cleansing of the root surfaces, both through instrumentation and patient home care practices, is more difficult, and the prognosis for the tooth may be altered. However, the degree of periodontal disease severity is directly related to the amount of periodontal ligament destroyed and the amount of bone lost, which indicate loss of physical support for the tooth. In the healthy state, the crest of alveolar bone does not begin exactly at the cementoenamel junction but 1 to 2 mm apical to it. Viewing radiographs is therefore an indispensable aid in assessing the severity of bone loss in periodontal disease. Figure 7-2 highlights the significance of clinical attachment loss in evaluating periodontal disease compared with probe depth measurements and Figure 7-3 shows the long-term effectiveness of dental hygiene care in maintaining teeth with significant attachment loss.

PLAQUE BIOFILM

Chronic periodontitis is considered a multibacterial disease. Subgingival plaque biofilms associated with periodontal pockets

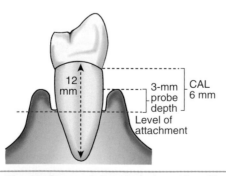

FIGURE 7-2 ■ **The significance of clinical attachment loss.** The typical root length is 10 to 12 mm, although there is significant variation among the teeth in the arch. Probing depth in the presence of attachment loss represents a more complete assessment of loss of support for the tooth than probing depth alone.

at diseased sites contain high levels of gram-negative anaerobic and motile organisms. Elevated levels of spirochetes are also present. Of the primary pathogens associated with periodontal diseases, *Porphyromonas gingivalis*, one of the red complex bacteria, is perhaps the most common species identified.[10] Other species commonly found in higher levels in chronic periodontitis include *Tannerella forsythensis*, *Treponema denticola*, *Prevotella* and *Fusobacterium* species, and *Actinomyces actinomycetemcomitans*. Our understanding of this extremely complex microbiology is growing through exciting research that will lead to improvements in both diagnosis and treatment for periodontal disease. For a further understanding of bacteria associated with plaque biofilms and periodontal disease, review Chapter 4.

The presence of specific pathogens is not always associated with the clinical presentation of chronic periodontal disease. A significant number of cases of chronic periodontitis have been reported without detection of *P. gingivalis* or other forms of periodontal pathogens in the pockets.[11] Thus, diagnosis of periodontal diseases through the analysis of bacterial plaque biofilm remains an adjunctive technique. Until it is better understood, clinical rather than bacteriologic diagnosis remains the primary method of classifying periodontal disease.

CLINICAL NOTE 7-5 The complex plaque biofilm in chronic periodontitis is considered a mixed infection. The goal of treatment is not eradication but control of the process. Antibiotics are not usually indicated. Usually, the infection can be replaced with a younger, less mature and established plaque that is associated with health. Less pathogenic plaque biofilm can usually be created by mechanical debridement through scaling and plaque removal procedures.

EPIDEMIOLOGY OF CHRONIC PERIODONTITIS

Most patients with periodontal diseases have chronic adult periodontitis. It affects 20% or more of the adult population in the United States (see Chapter 3). Although this is a very complex disease, the 1999 Consensus Report of the World Workshop[8] (sponsored by the American Academy of Periodontology) identified the following characteristics of chronic periodontitis:

- Most prevalent in adults, but it may appear in children and adolescents
- Periodontal destruction consistent with the amount of local factors
- Subgingival calculus frequently found
- Variable microbial pattern
- Slow to moderate progression, with periods of rapid progression
- Classified on the basis of extent and severity
- Associated with local predisposing factors
- May be modified by systemic diseases
- May be modified by factors such as stress and tobacco use

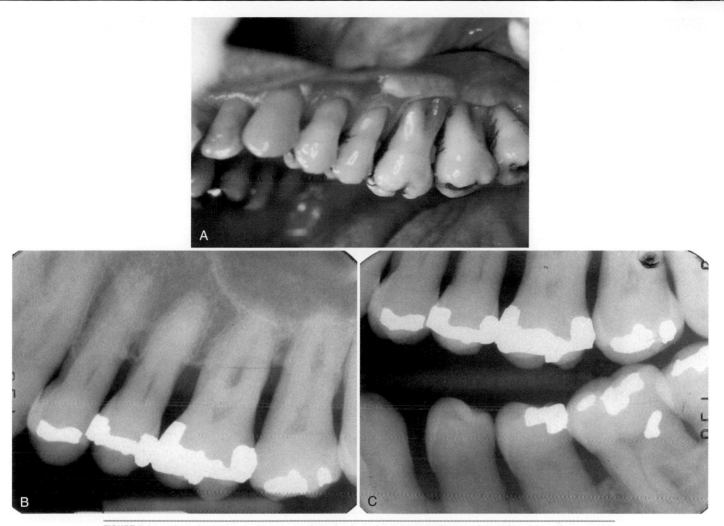

FIGURE 7-3 ■ Clinical attachment loss, not probing depth, is the primary indicator of periodontal bone loss. **A,** This patient is a 65-year-old man with advanced bone and attachment loss, but with minimal probing pocket depths of 2 to 3 mm in the maxillary right posterior sextant. The patient was treated 20 years ago with nonsurgical periodontal therapy. His condition has been stable for 20 years because of good personal oral hygiene and regular periodontal maintenance at 3- to 4-month intervals. The stain seen on the proximal root surfaces is due to daily use of 0.12% chlorhexidine mouth rinse. **B,** Periapical radiograph of the maxillary right posterior area of the same patient. Advanced bone loss and furcation involvement are seen in the first molar. **C,** Bitewing radiograph of the right side. The amount of bone loss is so extensive that the bone level cannot be seen in the bitewing radiograph. Therefore, periapical radiographs or vertical bitewings are required to assess the degree of bone loss adequately. (Courtesy of Dr. Calvin S. Lau.)

TREATMENT

Patients with a diagnosis of slight to moderate chronic periodontitis are often treated in the general dental practice, with the dental hygienist taking a major role in initial therapy. However, patients with a diagnosis of advanced periodontitis are best treated in a specialty periodontics practice. Although an important part of the treatment may be performed by the dental hygienist in the periodontist's office, the patient should be referred to a specialist for evaluation before any periodontal treatment is begun. With this approach, all signs of the disease will still be evident to assist the periodontist in complete diagnosis and treatment planning. Figures 7-4 to 7-6 show examples of slight, moderate, and severe periodontitis. A complete description of the dental hygiene treatment protocols for adult periodontitis is found in Chapter 10.

CLINICAL NOTE 7-6 Dental hygiene treatment of chronic periodontitis requires the following:
- Removal of local etiologic factors
- Patient education in personal plaque biofilm control
- Complete removal of all plaque and calculus from the root surfaces
- Control of associated factors such as overhanging margins and habits such as smoking

Increased attachment loss makes complete removal of calculus difficult and may require additional procedures, such as periodontal surgery.

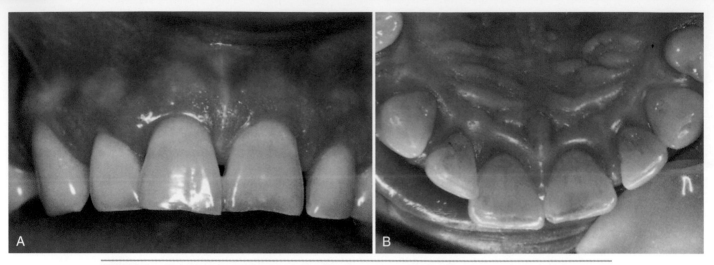

FIGURE 7-4 ■ **Slight chronic periodontitis. A,** The clinical appearance of the maxillary anterior shows normal-appearing gingiva, with little obvious attachment loss. **B,** The clinical appearance of the lingual view suggests inflamed gingiva, but attachment loss must be assessed by careful probing around the teeth.

PERIODONTITIS AS A RISK FACTOR FOR SYSTEMIC DISEASES

It has long been known that some systemic diseases alter the presentation and progression of periodontal disease (see Chapter 9). Evidence also suggests that periodontal disease may play a role as a risk factor in the development and management of serious systemic disease. In particular, periodontal infections have been implicated in cardiovascular disease, preterm and low-birth-weight infants, and bacterial pneumonia. In addition, it appears to be more difficult to control non–insulin-dependent diabetes in patients with severe periodontitis.[12] Although the exact mechanisms for these interrelationships have not been determined, our understanding of these increases in risk is growing.

PERIODONTITIS AND CARDIOVASCULAR DISEASE

Cardiovascular disease, including heart attack and stroke, annually accounts for almost half the deaths in the United States and most developed countries. Periodontal disease, along with other factors such as high cholesterol, smoking, diabetes, obesity, and sedentary lifestyle, appears to be associated with a significant increased risk for heart attack and death.[12,13] Poor periodontal health is a factor known to precede many heart attacks, and specific periodontal pathogens are associated with coronary heart disease.[14] With use of data from the third National Health and Nutrition Examination Survey conducted by the National Institutes of Health, scientists evaluated the relationship of periodontal conditions and history of heart attack in people 40 years of age and older. When other factors were controlled, the statistical evaluation of the data indicated a 14% increase in the odds of heart attack for every patient, with a 10% increase in sites with 3 mm or more of attachment loss.[13] These studies suggest that adverse health effects are related to chronic infections, which are mediated by inflammatory agents that trigger the development of atherosclerosis (plaque development) in the coronary arteries.[12]

PERIODONTITIS AND PRETERM BIRTH

Preterm birth (defined as a gestation of 36 weeks or less) and low birth weight (defined as birth weight less than 2500 g) are major public health concerns. The significance is that these conditions occur in about 10% of all births and are associated with many prenatal deaths. Evidence suggests that active periodontal disease may account for some of these outcomes, especially in the absence of other risk factors such as smoking.[15] It is clear that appropriate periodontal care and personal oral hygiene during pregnancy are extremely important.

CLINICAL NOTE 7-7 It has been shown that pregnant women with periodontal disease who are treated with scaling, root planing, and oral hygiene instruction have no greater risk for preterm or low-birth-weight babies than pregnant women without periodontal disease.[16]

PERIODONTITIS AND BACTERIAL PNEUMONIA

Bacterial pneumonia, a bacterial infection of the lung tissues, can be life-threatening, particularly in older or immunocompromised patients and those living in nursing home environments. This is a particularly important problem in nursing home populations because more antibiotic-resistant infections emerge, oral hygiene is often poor among these individuals, and approximately 25% of nursing home deaths are a result of pneumonia. Pneumonia occurs in the lower respiratory tract, which is usually sterile, but aspiration or spread of infectious agents can contaminate it and many virulent species associated with pneumonia reside in the periodontal plaque biofilm. Because oral hygiene in nursing home patients is generally very poor and decreases with the increase in age of the residents and the length of stay in the home, improving oral hygiene in these patients may also decrease the incidence of bacterial pneumonia.[17]

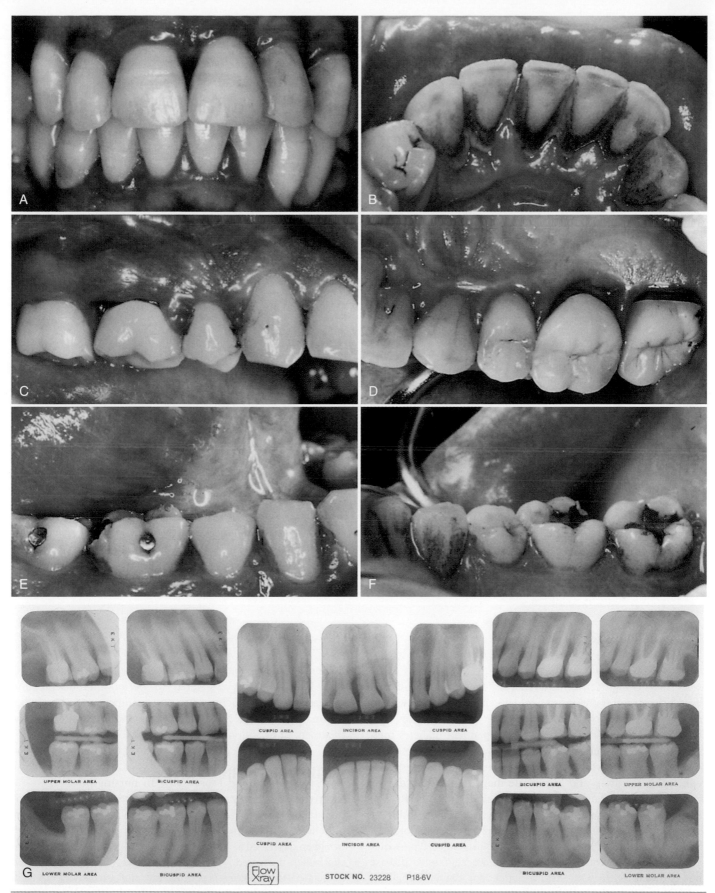

FIGURE 7-5 ■ **Moderate chronic periodontitis. A,** The facial view shows a swollen, shiny marginal gingiva, with missing interdental papillae. Recession is visible on the upper right canine and lateral incisor. However, the extent of the attachment loss cannot be assessed without radiographs and periodontal probing to determine clinical attachment loss. **B,** The mandibular lingual view shows heavy deposits of plaque and calculus, with intense inflammation and edema of the marginal gingiva. **C,** The maxillary right buccal view shows recession on the distal surface of the first molar, with gingival hyperplasia on the mesial papilla. The tissue has receded enough to expose the margin of the crowns. **D,** The maxillary right lingual view shows marked swelling of the marginal gingiva. Recession is indicated by the exposed crown margin on the molars. **E,** The mandibular right buccal view shows boggy interdental tissue. **F,** The mandibular right lingual view shows less obvious interdental swelling but heavy plaque, calculus, and stain accumulation. **G,** The full-mouth radiographs indicate 3 to 5 mm of mostly horizontal bone loss generalized throughout the mouth. The maxillary and mandibular right first molars show localized advanced bone loss, with furcation involvement.

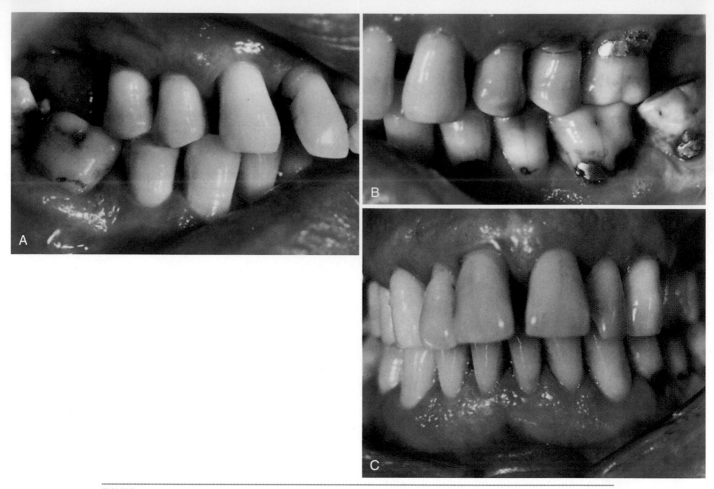

FIGURE 7-6 ■ Advanced chronic periodontitis. Advanced periodontitis presents the clinical characteristics of recession, plaque, calculus, inflammation, and drifting and missing teeth. It is not possible to assess the extent of the disease precisely without radiographs and full-mouth probing to determine clinical attachment loss. However, the clinical signs in this case suggest more severe bone loss because of the visible recession and furcations. The gingiva appears firm and stippled, masking the underlying inflammation. This masking is common in chronic periodontal disease. **A,** Right side. **B,** Left side. **C,** Anterior view.

PERIODONTITIS AND DIABETES

Diabetes has long been considered a risk factor for periodontal disease because it increases patient susceptibility to many types of infections. The exact mechanism for this is unclear. It is thought that in patients with insulin-dependent diabetes mellitus (IDDM) the periodontal ligament cells may be less able to respond to growth factors in the inflammatory response required to maintain and regenerate the periodontium during healing.[18] In addition, polymorphonuclear leukocytes (PMNs) in patients with diabetes have altered characteristics, and their adherence, chemotactic capacity, and phagocytosis potential are diminished.[12,16] Patients with IDDM, also called type 1 diabetes, tend to be younger and have more aggressive disease than patients with non–insulin-dependent diabetes mellitus (NIDDM), also called adult-onset or type 2 diabetes, so there are many systemic effects beyond those seen in the periodontium. However, when IDDM has a later onset, it is associated with increased clinical attachment, particularly in patients who smoke cigarettes.[19]

NIDDM is usually found in patients older than 50 years of age and is rarely seen in anyone younger than 40 years of age.

Evidence suggests that poor glycemic control among patients with NIDDM may be related to periodontal disease and increased clinical attachment loss. It is important to know that the management of NIDDM may be improved through the treatment of periodontal infections and their prevention.[17]

AGGRESSIVE PERIODONTITIS

Aggressive periodontitis is the appropriate term for those periodontal diseases that progress exceedingly rapidly with massive bone loss.[1,9] This is in contrast to chronic periodontitis, which has been described as attachment loss progression up to 1 mm/year when untreated.[19] Aggressive periodontal disease is often associated with younger people, but not exclusively. In fact, these diseases were long identified as localized and generalized juvenile periodontitis, or early-onset periodontal disease, and presented as localized or generalized in nature.[20] Aggressive forms of the disease in younger adults, up to about age 40, was also referred to as **rapidly progressing periodontitis.** These age distinctions do not distinguish among these diseases as once thought, but there may be a familial component indicating a

BOX 7-2 Types of Aggressive Periodontitis

Early-onset periodontitis
   Prepubertal periodontitis
   Juvenile periodontitis
      Localized juvenile periodontitis
      Generalized juvenile periodontitis
Rapidly progressing periodontitis
Refractory periodontitis

genetic association. Attachment loss progression does vary widely by individual, although there is a clear increase in progression with age.[21]

The microbiota associated with both aggressive periodontitis and chronic periodontitis appear to be quite similar, so it is difficult to describe a separate diagnosis on the basis of bacterial identification alone.[22] In fact, the interaction of different bacteria in subgingival plaque biofilm may be a more important factor in determining the progression of periodontal destruction than individual components. This finding reflects increased understanding of dental plaque as a biofilm (see Chapter 4).[23] In spite of the similarity in microbiota, it is possible to distinguish between aggressive periodontitis and chronic periodontitis on the basis of the progression of bone loss. It is also possible to distinguish among different forms of aggressive periodontitis on the basis of other factors, such as age of the patient at clinical detection, relative levels of certain bacterial species, presence or absence of possible defects in the immune response or other general health problems, and periodontal destruction that is greater than would be expected given the amount of local factors present.[21] Like chronic periodontitis, aggressive forms of the disease can be localized or generalized, which further helps characterize the disease (Box 7-2).

CLINICAL NOTE 7-8 Treatment of aggressive forms of periodontal disease requires control of the subgingival plaque biofilm. Therapy requires mechanical debridement with scaling and root planing and the use of adjunctive antibiotics. Periodontal surgery may also need to be performed to eliminate the infection and the deep bony defects in the periodontium.

Prepubertal periodontitis is a very rare form of aggressive periodontitis that may be localized or generalized and may affect both the primary and secondary dentitions. Usually, there is severe gingival inflammation, rapid bone loss, and early tooth loss. Deciduous teeth are often lost because of periodontal infection, and permanent teeth become infected as they erupt. These patients are likely to lose all their teeth in childhood. Many of these young patients have white blood cell defects that also leave them susceptible to other infections. Prepubertal periodontitis responds poorly to conventional treatment techniques, such as scaling and root planing. **Antibiotic therapy** may help. However, this adjunctive treatment usually slows but does not stop progression of the disease. Figure 7-7 presents a case of prepubertal periodontitis, Figure 7-8 presents the case of a young teenager with localized aggressive periodontitis and Figure 7-9 illustrates a generalized aggressive infection.

Aggressive periodontitis seen in young adults, usually between 20 and 30 years old, involves most of the teeth, but localized forms have been reported. Loss of bone and connective tissue usually occurs rapidly over a period of weeks or months. The loss can be so rapid that it is startling to the treating dental hygienist and dentist. Figure 7-10 shows an example of rapidly progressing aggressive periodontitis.

This disease may have a genetic component because a large percentage of affected patients have altered neutrophil chemotaxis. For reasons that are not understood, this progression of attachment loss may suddenly cease. Unfortunately, in most cases, the disease progresses until the teeth are lost if untreated. In fact, the disease process can only be slowed, not stopped, with treatment.

Refractory periodontitis is a term used to describe periodontal disease that is not responsive to appropriate treatment. In other words, thorough treatment and home care followed by continuing maintenance therapy does not arrest the progress of the disease.[9] The disease may occur at single or multiple sites around the dentition. Presumably, these sites continue to be infected with periodontal pathogens, regardless of which treatments have been tried. These individuals have been called "downhill patients." Data suggest that they may represent 8% to 14% of patients originally diagnosed as having advanced chronic periodontitis.[24] Refractory periodontitis is illustrated in Figure 7-11.

CLINICAL NOTE 7-9 Refractory periodontitis is periodontal disease that does not respond to therapy. It presents with a wide variety of symptoms and these patients have typically undergone multiple treatment regimens. This disease differs from recurrent periodontal disease in that it is a continuing process. The gradually deteriorating condition can be discouraging for both the dental hygienist and the patient.

A comparison of the major characteristics of chronic periodontitis and aggressive periodontitis is presented in Table 7-2, which provides a brief overview of the two types of periodontal disease.

It is also important to note that there are some necrotizing aggressive forms of disease termed **necrotizing ulcerative gingivitis** (NUG) and **necrotizing ulcerative periodontitis** (NUP). NUP is most likely an extension of the conditions seen in NUG and, because these conditions represent attachment loss, the term *gingivitis* is not sufficient to describe them. These diseases have been identified and described for centuries. Clinical characteristics of NUG and NUP are very foul mouth odor and destruction of the gingival papillae, leaving a punched-out appearance covered with a membrane of sloughing tissue. The condition is very painful and a number of predisposing conditions are related to these diagnoses: stress, poor oral hygiene, smoking, malnutrition, and immunocompromised status. Figure 7-12 reflects the typical clinical appearance of necrotizing periodontal disease.[25]

PERIODONTITIS AS A MANIFESTATION OF SYSTEMIC DISEASE

Periodontitis may present as a manifestation of systemic disease. There are a number of diseases that increase the severity and

Text continued on page 102

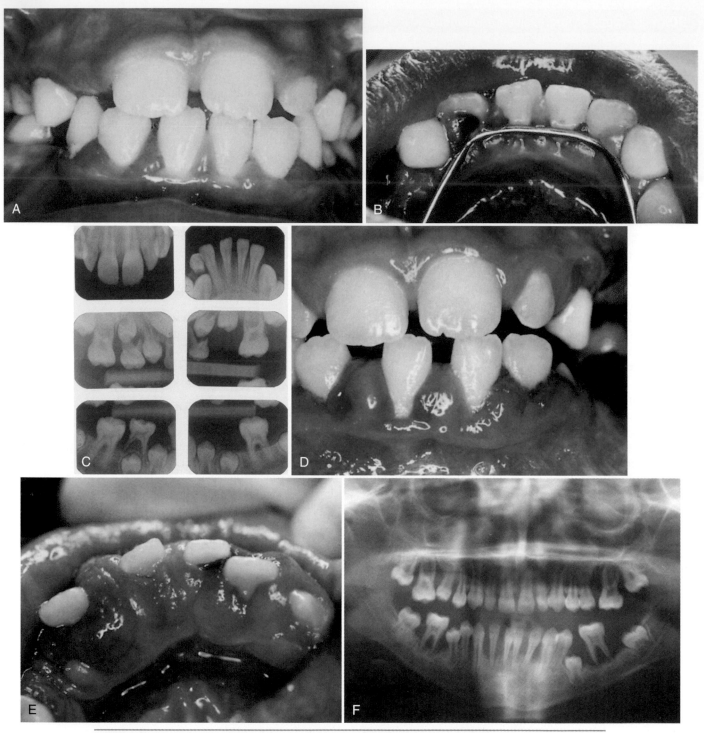

FIGURE 7-7 ■ Prepubertal periodontitis. Prepubertal periodontitis is an extremely rare disease characterized by advanced bone loss and premature tooth loss in children. This boy with prepubertal periodontitis had multiple periodontal procedures performed, including periodontal surgery and several courses of antibiotic therapy. The bone loss continued to progress, and many of these teeth were lost. **A,** At age 8 years, the clinical presentation of the anterior teeth showed erupting teeth with signs of gingival inflammation. Tissue swelling and redness were extensive, and there were heavy deposits of plaque. **B,** The mandibular lingual view showed granulation tissue growing over and around the mandibular space maintainer. **C,** Periapical radiographs at age 8 years showed erupting teeth and significant bone loss around both the permanent and deciduous molars. **D,** By age 10 years, the clinical presentation of the anterior teeth showed extreme hyperplastic tissue and tooth migration. **E,** The hyperplastic tissue condition was remarkable in the lower anterior area at age 10 years. **F,** The panographic x-ray film taken at age 10 years. Bone loss has proceeded to the apices of the permanent first molars. Treatment included multiple sessions of scaling and root planing, periodontal surgery, and antibiotic therapy. The prognosis for the teeth is poor, and this child became edentulous as a teenager.

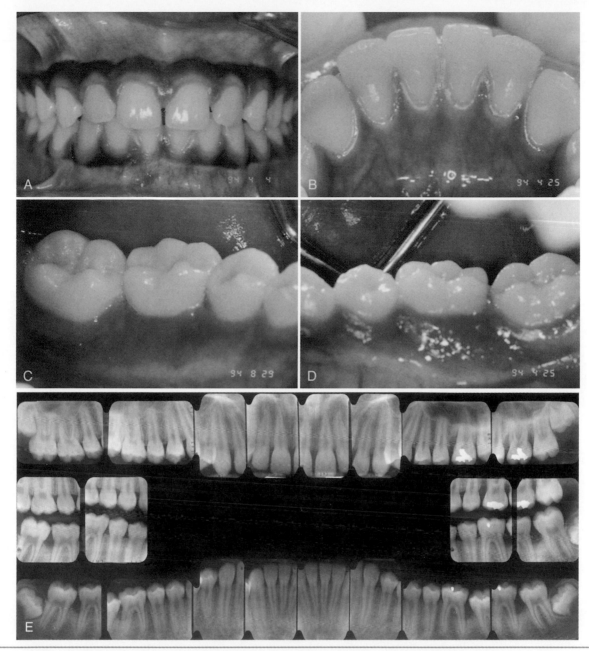

FIGURE 7-8 ■ **Localized juvenile periodontitis.** Localized juvenile periodontitis is an aggressive form of periodontal disease that is more common than prepubertal periodontitis, but it is still a rare disease. This 15-year-old male patient has deceptively normal-appearing gingiva. Plaque, calculus, and signs of inflammation were minimal. The patient had nonsurgical and surgical periodontal treatment and a course of tetracycline therapy. The condition was stabilized. **A,** Anterior view of the maxillary and mandibular teeth and gingiva. **B,** Lingual view of the mandibular anterior teeth. **C,** Lingual view of the right mandibular posterior teeth. **D,** Lingual view of the left mandibular posterior teeth. **E,** A full-mouth radiographic series showed moderate localized bone loss around both mandibular first molars and the maxillary left first molar. These were angular bony defects and did not represent horizontal bone loss because the bone level appeared normal on the other teeth. There was furcation involvement on both maxillary and mandibular first molars. The formation of the third molars appeared normal. (Courtesy of Dr. Lisa T. Grosso.)

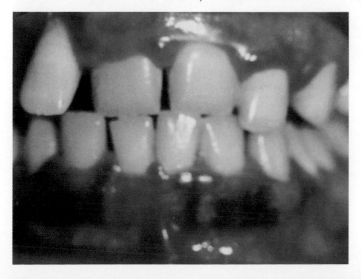

FIGURE 7-9 ■ **Generalized juvenile periodontitis.** Advanced generalized juvenile periodontitis can be characterized by mobile and drifting teeth, as seen in this 17-year-old female patient.

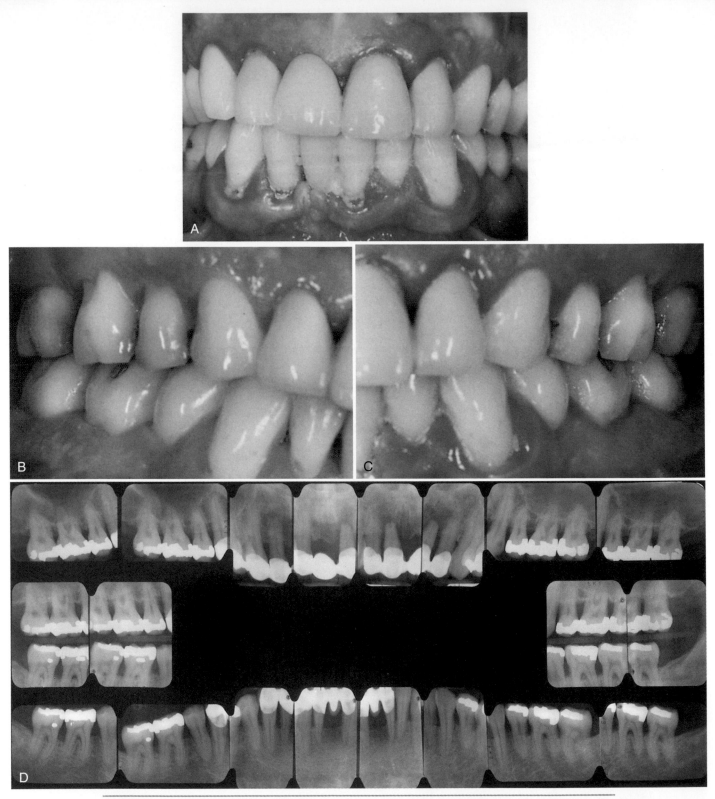

FIGURE 7-10 ■ **Rapidly progressing periodontitis.** This aggressive form of periodontal disease is characterized by rapid loss of bone in young adults. In this 30-year-old man, clinical assessment showed plaque, calculus, signs of inflammation, and recession. The radiographs showed generalized advanced bone loss. **A,** Clinical presentation of the anterior teeth with heavy deposits of plaque and calculus. **B,** Clinical presentation of the right side. **C,** Clinical presentation of the left side. **D,** Full-mouth radiographs of rapidly progressing periodontitis. The amount of bone loss is remarkable. Note that it is not horizontal in nature, but some areas have lost extensive amounts of support. Furcation involvement is seen in all molar regions and external resorption is seen at the apex of the maxillary left central incisor, probably as a result of past trauma. (Courtesy of Dr. Craig Y. Yonemura.)

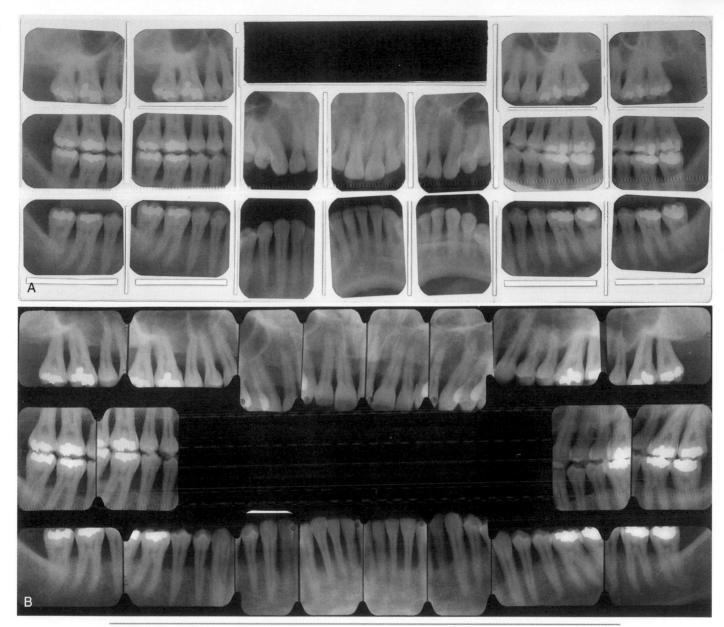

FIGURE 7-11 ■ **Refractory periodontitis.** This form of aggressive periodontitis was unresponsive to periodontal therapy. Bone and attachment loss continued despite good plaque control and all appropriate treatment. **A,** Radiographs of a 35-year-old man with moderate to advanced bone loss on all teeth. **B,** Two years later, the bone loss continued to progress despite excellent plaque control, nonsurgical and surgical periodontal therapy, systemic antibiotics, and 2- to 3-month periodontal maintenance visits. Bone loss has proceeded almost to the apices of the maxillary molars.

TABLE 7-2	Comparison of Major Characteristics of Chronic and Aggressive Periodontal Diseases	
CHARACTERISTIC	**CHRONIC PERIODONTITIS**	**AGGRESSIVE PERIODONTITIS**
Progression	Slow, <1 mm/year	Rapid, >1 mm/year May be extremely rapid
Bone loss	Generalized Primarily horizontal	Generalized May be localized to specific areas
Age	35 years of age or older	Prepubertal—children Juvenile—teens, young adults Rapidly progressive—20s and 30s Refractory—50 years or older
Plaque biofilm	Gram-negative Some microorganisms in a set of pathogens often associated with disease	Gram-negative Specific pathogens present with some forms
Systemic characteristics	Not related	Often related to defects in immune system
Relation to local factors	Severity of disease consistent with amounts of plaque biofilm and calculus present	Amount of plaque biofilm and calculus not always consistent with severity of disease

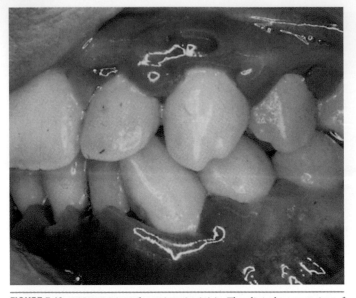

FIGURE 7-12 ■ **Necrotizing ulcerative gingivitis.** The clinical presentation of this form of aggressive periodontitis includes intense inflammation, punched-out interdental papillae, and attachment loss. In this patient, the attachment loss was most obvious on the mesial aspect of the mandibular canine. The condition was extremely painful, and the patient had severe breath odor. (Courtesy of University California, San Francisco, Division of Periodontology.)

change the character of periodontal disease. Although most patients with advanced disease can be classified correctly as having chronic periodontitis or aggressive periodontitis, sometimes the periodontal disease has systemic origins or complicating factors.

Systemic diseases, such as Down syndrome, IDDM, acquired immunodeficiency syndrome (AIDS), and Papillon-Lefèvre syndrome, can increase the severity of periodontal disease. The use of this diagnosis may be beneficial to the dental hygienist and dentist by emphasizing the presence of an underlying systemic problem, altering patient management. For example, diabetes increases both the severity of bone loss and the rate of progression of periodontal disease. As mentioned earlier, chronic periodontal disease is now considered a major complication of diabetes.[12,15]

For all patients, significant periodontal disease beyond what would be expected for the level of plaque and calculus present should suggest a more thorough medical evaluation. Life-threatening diseases, such as uncontrolled diabetes and leukemia, may first be seen as changes in the gingival and periodontal structures. Other systemic diseases, such as hypophosphatasia, alter tooth development and therefore affect periodontal attachment. These oral signs and symptoms of systemic disease mimic those of aggressive periodontal infections. It is important that the physician be included as a member of the oral health care team to collaborate in the evaluation of patients with unusual forms of periodontitis. A number of systemic diseases and treatment considerations for the associated periodontal disease are described in Chapter 9.

ABSCESS OF THE PERIDONTIUM

Periodontal abscess is an acute, localized purulent infection of the periodontium. Although they are discussed in greater detail in Chapter 16, abscesses are presented here because they

represent a separate diagnosis of periodontal disease and conditions in the accepted classification scheme.[1,8]

Periodontal abscesses most often occur in patients with chronic periodontitis, frequently cases that have been untreated. Figure 7-13 shows examples of periodontal abscesses. They may be acute or chronic in nature. The abscess is thought to occur because the periodontal pocket containing pathologic bacterial plaque becomes occluded, allowing the infection to become localized and pus to accumulate in the adjacent tissues. Acute periodontal abscesses are associated with rapid bone loss and should be treated immediately to minimize bone loss and maximize the healing potential of the lesion. Acute periodontal abscesses are commonly thought to occur more frequently after periodontal scaling or prophylaxis[26]; however, other studies dispute this finding.[27]

If the acute abscess is left untreated, the infection will seek a route to drain. It then becomes a chronic periodontal abscess, constantly inflamed, and will result in continued bone loss. Chronic periodontal abscesses are frequently asymptomatic and the patient is unaware of any draining pus. On questioning, patients often recall vague symptoms such as episodes of localized swelling in the area or "funny" feelings in the gingiva around the chronic abscess. These symptoms may be related to episodes of acute infection when the chronic abscess has lost its ability to drain. A clinical case showing a chronic periodontal abscess is presented in Figure 7-14.

Usually, periodontal abscesses occur in deepened pockets, but they may appear only in the gingival tissues, where they are called gingival abscesses (see Chapter 6). A gingival abscess is most often caused by a foreign body being forced into the sulcus. The condition resolves when the material is removed and the area is cleaned.

A unique form of periodontal abscess occurs around partially erupted teeth, usually third molars. This abscess occurs around a flap of tissue partially covering the tooth, called an operculum. This is called a pericoronal abscess, often referred to as pericoronitis (see Chapter 16). The pericoronal abscess may be extremely painful and can spread to the submandibular tissues.

> **CLINICAL NOTE 7-10** Treatment of periodontal abscesses, whether they are chronic, pericoronal, or localized in the gingiva, involves careful debridement of the pocket. It often includes surgical removal of the lining of the periodontal pocket through open or closed curettage. Systemic antibiotics must be administered if there is evidence of fascial cellulitis or if the patient has a fever. Treatment for a pericoronal abscess includes removal of the operculum or extraction of the partially erupted molar.

PERIODONTITIS ASSOCIATED WITH ENDODONTIC LESIONS

Periodontal abscesses must be differentiated from abscesses of endodontic origin, which may also have signs and symptoms in the periodontium. An abscess may be entirely periodontal or entirely endodontic in origin, or it may be a combined lesion. In the case of periodontitis associated with an endodontic lesion, a chronic periodontal pocket may have progressed to join an endodontic lesion, or periodontitis may have infected the pulp of the tooth through the apex or lateral canals in the tooth root. Alternatively, the endodontic lesion could drain

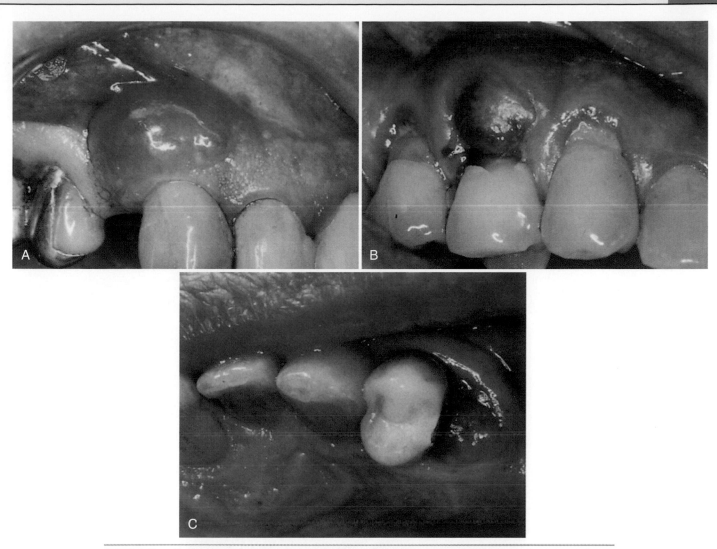

FIGURE 7-13 ■ **Acute periodontal abscess. A,** This large painful abscess arose in the proximity of a 9-mm pocket on the distal surface of the canine. Note the significant color change and fluctuant appearance of the overlying gingiva. **B,** The acute abscess can also arise very close to the marginal gingiva. This abscess is smaller, possibly because it is partially draining through the orifice of the pocket, and associated with a deep pocket on the facial surface of the maxillary first premolar. **C,** Acute abscesses can occur around any surface of the teeth. This abscess arose on the distal of a first premolar. It was very painful to the patient, and the pocketing around the tooth was severe. The tooth was lost after repeated episodes of acute abscess.

through the periodontal ligament, infecting the surrounding tissue. The key to recognizing these lesions is that they usually occur as a single, isolated deep pocket or are present in the furcation of a specific tooth. That specific tooth is frequently also sensitive to percussion.[28] An overview of endodontic lesions and combined lesions is presented in Chapter 16.

> **CLINICAL NOTE 7-11** The treatment of periodontitis associated with endodontic lesions requires endodontic therapy. Combined lesions require both endodontic and periodontal therapy because both conditions are present. It is important to know that scaling and root planing should not be performed on a combined abscess until after the endodontic lesion has healed. This is because scaling and root planing disrupt the attachment of the collagen fibers to the root surfaces. There is a higher likelihood of periodontal reattachment if the draining sinus tract through the periodontal ligament is not disturbed. Leaving the infection undisturbed permits all the cellular elements to remain in place, so the healing potential in the area is preserved.

DEVELOPMENTAL OR ACQUIRED DEFORMITIES AND CONDITIONS

There are a number of acquired or developmental conditions that are seen in the periodontium that may require periodontal treatment. These include **pseudopockets**, recession, and **developmental anomalies**.

Pseudopockets occur when the gingival margin is coronal to the cementoenamel junction and there is often no associated attachment loss. This developmental condition is often seen on the distal surfaces of second or third molars. Pseudopockets make plaque biofilm control difficult and can result in gingivitis and lead to chronic periodontitis.

Gingival recession may also be a developmental condition if it is caused by an underlying osseous defect, or it may represent an acquired defect resulting from trauma from toothbrushing or some other abrasion. Whether developmental or acquired, gingival recession may lead to root sensitivity, root caries, periodontal disease and possibly be an aesthetic problem. Examples

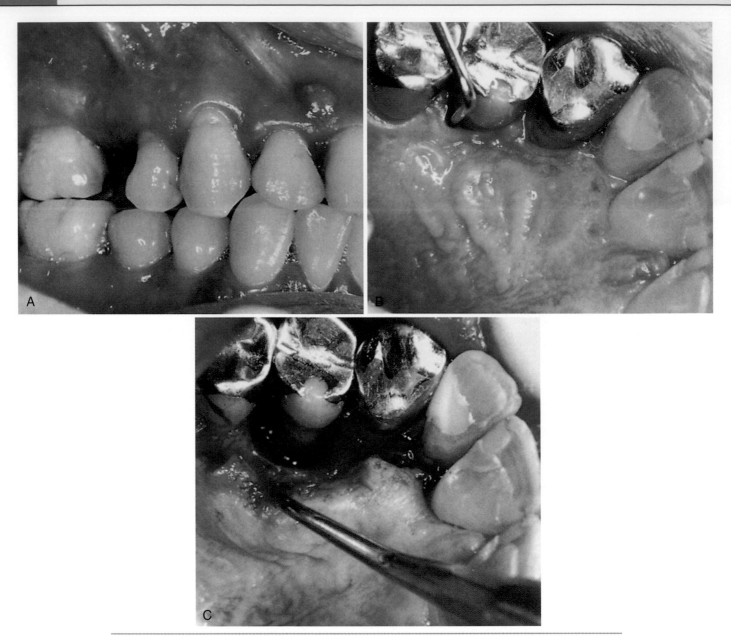

FIGURE 7-14 ■ **Periodontal abscess. A,** This acute periodontal abscess drained through a sinus in the mucosa. The sinus tract in the swelling associated with this lateral incisor is positioned away from the gingiva in the mucosa, mimicking a lesion of endodontic origin. **B,** Chronic periodontal abscesses that drain through the periodontal pocket may exhibit much less swelling, but can be very painful. This abscess was associated with a deep pocket on the lingual aspect of the tooth and drained through the pocket. **C,** Note the extent of the bone loss that could only be seen when a periodontal flap was retracted to expose the root surface and treat the abscess.

of developmental conditions, altered tooth development resulting in a cemental spur, and the periodontal effects of a lateral developmental groove are illustrated in Figure 7-15.

METHODS OF DETECTING PERIODONTAL DISEASE

The most common and accepted method of detecting periodontal disease is careful assessment of the attachment level around all surfaces of all teeth with a graduated periodontal probe. Generally, probing pocket depths of greater than 3 mm indicate attachment loss and evidence of periodontal disease. The location of the gingival margin on a tooth and the degree of bone

loss determines the classification of the disease. The probing pocket depth itself is secondary in diagnostic significance to the clinical attachment level.

The presence of bleeding in response to probing and a visible color change in the gingival tissue are also important factors in the diagnosis of periodontal disease. The relationship between bleeding and progression of disease is not strong, but there is evidence that this information, in conjunction with the probing attachment level and radiographic signs of bone loss, assists in the diagnosis and classification of the disease. Meta-analyses (evaluation of all appropriate clinical studies) have demonstrated that areas are not likely to show progressive bone loss and attachment loss if they do not bleed.[29] Other diagnostic

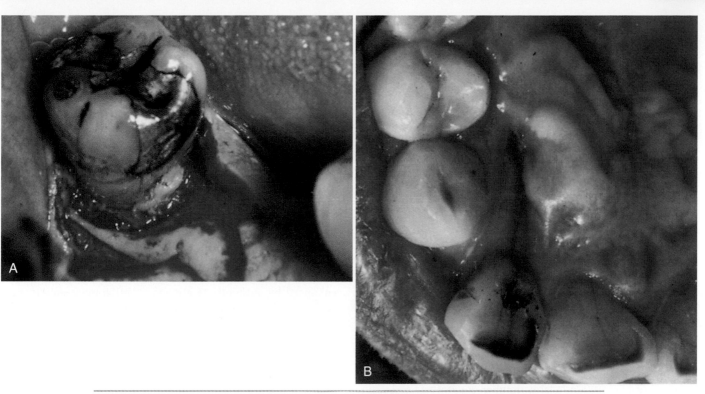

FIGURE 7-15 ■ **Developmental conditions associated with periodontitis. A,** Cementicle. In this case, a cementicle or cemental spur on the mesial aspect of the mandibular molar was located just apical to the cementoenamel junction. This caused plaque retention and resulted in an infrabony defect. Treatment with scaling and root planing was impossible and the spur required surgical removal. Healing was uneventful and the periodontal problem was resolved. **B,** Lingual developmental groove. Maxillary lateral incisors often have lingual grooves extending apically from the cingulum. In this case, the groove extended almost to the apex of the tooth, retaining plaque biofilm and permitting calculus to form in the groove. After repeated instances of periodontal abscess, the tooth required extraction. There was no other periodontal disease present in this patient's mouth. Most developmental grooves are not this extensive and can be treated successfully with surgical removal of bone to the apical extent of the groove and odontoplasty to remove the groove or placement of a tissue-compatible restoration in the groove.

data and tests include mobility and comparison of probing data over time. These are presented in Chapter 8.

ETIOLOGY OF PERIODONTITIS

As in gingivitis, dental plaque biofilm is the principal cause of all forms of periodontitis. Treatment that is directed at elimination or reduction of the amount and quality of plaque biofilm is the most effective. However, the pathogenicity of biofilm bacteria varies widely, as does the susceptibility of each patient. This variability makes the causes of periodontitis less clear-cut than the direct relationship between plaque biofilm and gingivitis. Many other factors are involved. Animal studies in which dental biofilm formation had been arrested or controlled indicated that nutritional deficiencies, hormonal alterations, and trauma from occlusion cannot in themselves cause periodontal pocket formation. However, in the presence of plaque biofilm, these conditions may worsen the progression of periodontitis (see Chapter 4).

Dental calculus is calcified dental plaque biofilm. It does not by itself cause periodontal disease; however, it is covered with and infiltrated by millions of pathogenic bacteria. Because of its large surface area and rough surface, its associated plaque biofilm is difficult to remove and regrows at a rapid rate. The presence of calculus on a root surface indicates that there is always biofilm present, so for this reason scaling, root planing, and periodontal debridement to remove the calculus and associated plaque are the cornerstones of periodontal treatment.

CLINICAL NOTE 7-12 All conditions that retain biofilm or that make dental plaque biofilm difficult to remove by either the patient or the dental hygienist play significant roles in the etiology of periodontal diseases. These include the following:

- Overhanging or poorly contoured dental restorations
- Food retention or impaction areas
- Furcations
- Spaces between teeth
- Missing and drifted teeth
- Alterations in tooth morphologic features (e.g., fluting and grooves)

Deepened periodontal pockets also harbor large amounts of subgingival plaque biofilm that are impossible to control with home care alone. This is the primary rationale for the dental hygienist to debride deep pockets at frequent intervals carefully to arrest and control periodontal disease.

Hormonal changes associated with pregnancy, menopause, and oral contraceptive use have been studied extensively. These hormones change the environment of the gingival sulcus and alter the types of bacteria that grow in the plaque, therefore increasing the likelihood of pathogenic plaque.[30] Hormones definitely increase the flow of gingival fluid by causing proliferation and increased permeability of the microcirculation; however, good plaque biofilm removal appears to control the level of gingival inflammation.

TOBACCO USE

Tobacco use is a known risk factor for periodontal disease that has been clearly associated with increased attachment loss. Young smokers have been demonstrated to have more progression of disease than nonsmokers, even when controlled for the level of plaque present, and smokers are at higher risk for tooth loss than nonsmokers. Tobacco use also has an effect on healing after periodontal therapy. Studies have shown that smokers have less probing depth reduction and less attachment gain than nonsmokers after scaling and root planing.[31]

There are several possible explanations for this increased risk, including both direct and indirect effects of tobacco smoke. Tobacco smoke contains a large number of cytotoxic and vasoactive components, including nicotine. Nicotine ingestion causes vasoconstriction, possibly explaining why smokers have less gingival bleeding than nonsmokers. Smokers also have diminished neutrophil function, possibly explaining why smokers rather than nonsmokers are more likely to have refractory periodontitis.[32] Smoking is also thought to impair fibroblast function and reduce the capacity of the periodontal tissues to heal. Reduced healing characterized by slower turnover in gingival tissues may upset the balance between the disease process and the healing process, resulting in progression of periodontal disease.

The role of other forms of tobacco use (e.g., cigar smoking, smokeless tobacco) is less clear. The particular effects of cigars have been much less studied than cigarettes, although the effects are likely to be quite similar. Localized gingival recession is commonly seen in the oral areas in which smokeless tobacco is held, often between the gingiva and vestibular mucosa.[32]

CLINICAL NOTE 7-13 All patients who smoke or use any form of tobacco should be informed of the effects of tobacco on the disease process. The dental hygienist should have tobacco cessation materials and referrals available and be proactive in encouraging patients to quit. It is also very important for patients to refrain from tobacco use during periodontal therapy to maximize the healing potential.

GENETIC FACTORS PROMOTING PERIODONTITIS

There is increasing evidence that susceptibility to periodontal diseases may be genetically determined because individuals respond to their oral microbiota in unique ways. It has been known for some time that rare periodontal diseases in systemic conditions, such as Papillon-Lefèvre syndrome, Chédiak-Higashi syndrome, and leukocyte adhesion deficiency, are genetically induced. However no specific genes have been

identified for chronic periodontitis, although studies on twins have suggested that susceptibility to chronic periodontitis may also be genetically linked. There is tremendous opportunity for advances in therapy based on our increasing knowledge of the genetics of periodontal disease.[33]

ANTIBIOTICS IN THE TREATMENT OF PERIODONTAL DISEASES

The treatment of periodontal infections involves altering the subgingival bacterial biofilm to remove the cause of infection and allow tissues to heal and inflammation to resolve. Because of the nonspecific anaerobic nature of the infection, this goal is most often accomplished through mechanical procedures, such as scaling and root planing, and possibly periodontal surgery.

Some periodontal diseases, particularly the aggressive and refractory forms, continue to progress, but therapy can be enhanced by antibiotic treatment.[34] Antibiotic treatment may be either systemic (given to the patient orally or by injection) or applied locally to the specific site of infection.

SYSTEMIC ANTIBIOTICS

Antibiotics used for systemic administration in the treatment of periodontal diseases include tetracyclines, metronidazole, penicillins, clindamycin, and cephalosporins. In addition, several of these antibiotics have been used in combination, with varying results. A summary of the uses for these antibiotics follows.

Tetracyclines are a particularly useful group of antibiotics for treating periodontal disease because they are concentrated in the gingival fluid. In other words, when administered orally, a higher concentration of the antibiotic is available in the gingival fluid than in the circulating plasma. *A. actinomycetemcomitans* is usually susceptible to tetracycline. Therefore, this antibiotic is particularly helpful in the treatment of aggressive forms of periodontitis. In addition to their antimicrobial effect, tetracyclines may be helpful in periodontal therapy because they inhibit collagenase activity and thus help control the spread of disease.[34,35]

Metronidazole has been used to treat periodontal diseases because of its ability to inhibit several periodontal pathogens, including spirochetes, *Porphyromonas* species, and *Prevotella* species. Because metronidazole kills anaerobic bacteria, its use in treating rapidly progressing periodontitis seems logical. It is not effective against *A. actinomycetemcomitans*, so it is not as effective for some forms of aggressive periodontitis.[34,35]

Penicillin is less appropriate to use against periodontal infections than other drugs because it does not increase attachment, and many periodontal pathogens may become resistant to it. Resistance occurs when bacteria produce enzymes that break down the antibiotic.[34,35]

Other agents, such as clindamycin and amoxicillin, have been recommended for use in controlling refractory periodontitis and rapidly progressing periodontitis on the basis of limited studies. However, their effectiveness and place in periodontal therapy is still being investigated. A promising supplemental treatment has been to use several of these agents in combination. Although metronidazole and amoxicillin are not effective alone in eliminating *A. actinomycetemcomitans* in aggressive periodontitis and rapidly progressing periodontitis, studies have shown that they may work well when used together.[34]

Systemic antibiotics can be useful when conventional scaling and root planing provide an insufficient therapeutic effect. Rapid identification of the predominant microbial forms in periodontal infections also facilitates the appropriate use of antibiotics in the treatment of periodontal diseases. There are some chairside testing systems in use now. Until the microbiology of periodontitis is better understood and rapid testing is available for all pathogens, antibiotics are prescribed at the discretion of the dentist and periodontist. They are most often used to augment the treatment of aggressive periodontitis and for patients who respond poorly to mechanical therapy.[34]

LOCALLY DELIVERED CONTROLLED-RELEASE ANTIBIOTICS

Locally delivered controlled-release antibiotics are now available to assist in treating periodontal disease. Local delivery has distinct advantages in that it places the drug directly at the site of infection and reduces the risk of allergic side effects from systemic administration.

There are several delivery systems available for a variety of medications. Each places the drug directly into the infected periodontal pockets and has demonstrated some ability to further decrease probing depths and increase clinical attachment further when used in conjunction with scaling and root planing.

Chlorhexidine, a disinfectant, can be placed subgingivally using a biodegradable chip. It degrades in about 10 days and does not require removal by the clinician. The chip has been shown to increase the number of healed sites with 2 mm or more of probing depth reduction and does not stain. Doxycycline (a form of tetracycline) gel has shown improved clinical measures after 3 and 6 months, including improved probing depths, attachment levels, and fewer bleeding sites. Minocycline (another form of tetracycline) gel has also been shown to improve clinical parameters of healing in clinical trials. Metronidazole gel (also an antibiotic) is used outside the United States and has demonstrated the ability to shift the microbiota to those more associated with health. Figure 7-16 shows examples of locally delivered antibiotics used in periodontal therapy.

There are major advantages of locally delivered antimicrobial agents over systemically delivered ones. First, local delivery results in much lower amounts of the drug present in the serum. The drug is still absorbed through the periodontium into the serum, but at a very low rate. The total dose required is also much lower than doses required for systemic administration, which greatly reduces any risk of systemic side effects. Second, the active agent is present in high concentration at the site of infection, rather than having to be diffused through the entire circulatory system.[35]

The agents used for local delivery produce relatively small clinical changes, perhaps less than 0.39-mm improvement in clinical attachment loss and probing depths. However, these small increments can be extremely significant to the retention of the periodontally involved teeth, especially when used to treat deep pockets and hard instrument areas, such as furcations. A thoughtful review by Ciancio and Mariotti has concluded that the decision to use these adjunctive agents should be made when considering clinical findings, medical and dental history, patient preferences, and potential benefits.[36]

ENZYME SUPPRESSION THERAPY (INFLAMMATORY INHIBITORS)

A significant portion of the tissue destruction observed in the pathogenesis of periodontal disease results from the enzymes released by the inflammatory response to bacterial plaque.[36] These enzymes are cytokines that mediate the destruction of collagen and therefore damage gingival and periodontal fibers. They also have effects on the alveolar bone and trigger bone resorption by stimulating osteoclastic activity (see Chapter 2, "Host Response"). This information has led to exploring enzyme suppression therapy. Nonsteroidal anti-inflammatory drugs and other drugs may prove to be beneficial in the development of this avenue of therapy.[34]

◎ DENTAL HYGIENE CONSIDERATIONS

- Periodontitis is defined as inflammation that extends from the gingiva to the supporting tissues of the tooth, periodontal ligament, cementum, and alveolar bone.
- Periodontitis is characterized by the presence of pathologic periodontal pockets and bone loss caused by a virulent gram-negative plaque biofilm and other local factors.
- Periodontal disease progresses in episodic bursts that lead to tooth loss if untreated.
- The classification of periodontal diseases includes chronic periodontitis, aggressive periodontitis, periodontitis as a manifestation of systemic disease, necrotizing ulcerative periodontitis, abscesses, periodontitis associated with endodontic lesions, and periodontitis associated with developmental or acquired deformities and conditions.
- Aggressive periodontitis has prepubertal, juvenile (both localized and generalized), rapidly progressing, and refractory forms.
- Periodontitis is a risk factor for systemic diseases, including cardiovascular disease, bacterial pneumonia, diabetes, and preterm birth.
- Tobacco use is a significant risk factor for periodontal disease.
- A genetic component has been associated with periodontal disease, which may lead to future treatments.
- Both systemic and locally delivered antibiotics are useful in treating periodontal diseases that do not respond to mechanical debridement and plaque biofilm control.
- Enzyme suppression therapy (inflammatory inhibitors) may enhance periodontal treatment.

✳ CASE SCENARIO

Mr. Chacon has come to the office seeking treatment for bleeding gums and teeth that "look longer." He is a 40-year old Hispanic male, who is a high school teacher and supports his family of three. He has not attended dental offices regularly for some years. Mr. Chacon is in excellent health; he has no history of illness or hospitalizations and takes no prescription medications. Your assessments show that Mr. Chacon has generalized bone loss and both maxillary and mandibular furcation involvement visible on radiographic images. His clinical examination reveals 5- to 7-mm probe depths, 1 mm of recession throughout his dentition, and bleeding on probing throughout the dentition. There is moderate subgingival calculus and generalized moderate plaque biofilm accumulation, especially in the interproximal areas.

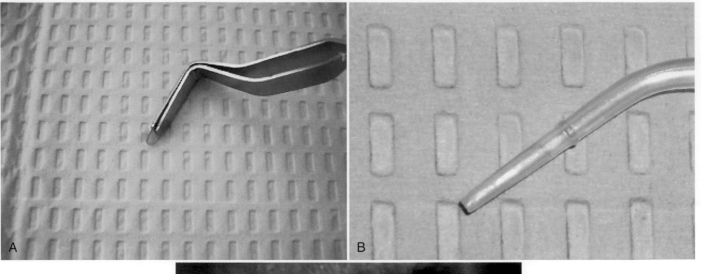

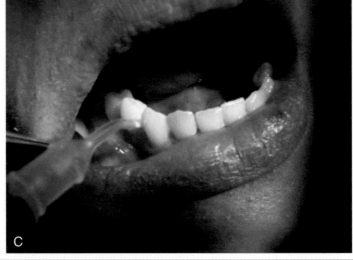

FIGURE 7-16 ■ **Local delivery of antibiotics. A,** An antiseptic chip containing 2.5 mg of chlorhexidine gluconate in a biodegradable gel can be placed in pockets deeper than 5 mm. The chip is placed immediately after scaling and root planing. Antiseptic release peaks after 2 hours and continues for 9 days. Patients should not brush or floss the area for 9 days.[37] **B,** The antibiotic minocycline hydrochloride is available in a bioabsorbable gel system, which is available for syringe application. **C,** Minocycline hydrochloride being delivered to a deep periodontal pocket. This material adheres inside the pocket and does not require any additional packing or adhesive. It maintains a therapeutic drug concentration for up to 10 days. Patients should avoid brushing the area where the antibiotic is placed for 12 hours and refrain from interproximal cleaning for 10 days.[37]

1. How do the periodontal pockets you have been examining extend apically?
   A. Junctional epithelium contracts and shortens, collagen is deposited, and the host response is involved.
   B. Junctional epithelium contracts and shortens, collagen breaks down, and the host response is not involved.
   C. Junctional epithelium elongates and collagen breaks down because of chemotactic substances released by bacteria.
   D. Junctional epithelium elongates and collagen breaks down because of chemotactic substances released by bacteria and reaction of the host immune system.

2. The contents of the deep periodontal pockets you have assessed are predominantly made up of
   A. pus.
   B. gram-positive bacteria.
   C. virulent bacteria and motile forms.
   D. lipopolysaccharides without bacteria.

3. You are unsure about whether Mr. Chacon has an aggressive form of periodontitis because he has not received previous periodontal care and you cannot assess his response to therapy.
   A. Both the statement and the reason are correct and related.
   B. Both the statement and the reason are correct but NOT related.
   C. The statement is correct, but the reason is NOT correct.
   D. The statement is NOT correct, but the reason is correct.
   E. NEITHER the statement NOR the reason is correct.

4. Mr. Chacon has active periodontal disease. You determined this by assessing bleeding.
   A. Both statements are true.
   B. Both statements are false.
   C. The first statement is true, and the second statement is false.
   D. The first statement is false, and the second statement is true.

5. Plaque biofilm control may be challenging for Mr. Chacon because
   A. deep pockets are present.
   B. he has a lot of missing teeth.
   C. deep pockets and furcations are present.
   D. he has not been to the dentist for a long time.

STUDY QUESTIONS

Answers and rationales to these questions can be obtained from your instructor.

MULTIPLE CHOICE

1. What is the principal etiologic agent of periodontitis?
   A. Subgingival calculus
   B. Neutrophil deficiency
   C. Dental plaque biofilm
   D. Antigen-antibody reactions
2. Gingivitis and periodontitis share all the following characteristics EXCEPT one. Which one is the EXCEPTION?
   A. Pocket formation
   B. Alveolar bone loss
   C. Tissue inflammation
   D. Collagen fiber destruction
3. All of the following conditions contribute to the retention of dental plaque biofilm EXCEPT one. Which one is the EXCEPTION?
   A. Deep pockets
   B. Cigarette smoking
   C. Subgingival calculus
   D. Overhanging restoration margins
4. Chronic periodontitis is
   A. a rare disease.
   B. not treatable with antibiotics.
   C. neither localized nor generalized.
   D. usually significant before age 35 years.
5. Localized aggressive periodontitis in its juvenile form is associated with all the following characteristics EXCEPT one. Which one is the EXCEPTION?
   A. Neutrophil defect
   B. Presence of *P. gingivalis*
   C. Patients younger than 20 years
   D. Bone loss around the molars and incisors
6. Which type of bacteria is associated with localized juvenile periodontitis?
   A. *Bacteroides forsythus*
   B. *A. actinomycetemcomitans*
   C. *Prevotella intermedia*
   D. *P. gingivalis*
7. Refractory periodontitis never responds adequately to treatment and the disease essentially continues unabated because of the failure of nonsurgical therapy.
   A. Both the statement and the reason are correct and related.
   B. Both the statement and the reason are correct but NOT related.
   C. The statement is correct, but the reason is NOT correct.
   D. The statement is NOT correct, but the reason is correct.
   E. NEITHER the statement NOR the reason is correct.

8. Cigarette smokers are more likely to have tooth loss and impaired healing than nonsmokers. It is important for patients to refrain from smoking during periodontal therapy.
   A. Both statements are true.
   B. Both statements are false.
   C. The first statement is true, and the second statement is false.
   D. The first statement is false, and the second statement is true.

SHORT ANSWER

9. Why are tetracyclines useful in the treatment of some periodontal infections?
10. What are the roles of the dental hygienist in the treatment of periodontal disease?

Please visit **http://evolve.elsevier.com/Perry/periodontology** for additional practice and study support tools.

REFERENCES

1. Armitage GC. Diagnosis and classification of periodontal diseases. In: Rose LF, Mealey BL, eds. *Periodontics: Medicine, Surgery, and Implants.* St. Louis, MO: Elsevier Mosby; 2004:19–31.
2. Carranza FA, Hogan EL. Gingival enlargement. In: Newman MN, Takei HH, Klokkevold PR, et al, eds. *Carranza's Clinical Periodontology.* 11th ed. St. Louis, MO: Elsevier Saunders; 2012:84–96.
3. Carranza FA, Camargo PM. The periodontal pocket. In: Newman MN, Takei HH, Klokkevold PR, et al, eds. *Carranza's Clinical Periodontology.* 11th ed. St. Louis, MO: Elsevier Saunders; 2012:127–139.
4. Wilkins EM, Towle JH. The older adult patient. In: Wilkins EM, ed. *Clinical Practice of the Dental Hygienist.* 11th ed. Philadelphia, PA: Lippincott Williams & Wilkins; 2013:797–811.
5. Carranza FA, Camargo PM, Takei HH. Bone loss and patterns of destruction. In: Newman MN, Takei HH, Klokkevold PR, et al, eds. *Carranza's Clinical Periodontology.* 11th ed. St. Louis, MO: Elsevier Saunders; 2012:140–150.
6. Listgarten MA. Pathogenesis of periodontitis. *J Clin Periodontol.* 1986;13:418–425.
7. Goodson JM, Tanner ACR, Haffajee AD, et al. Patterns of progression and regression of advanced periodontal disease. *J Clin Periodontol.* 1982;9:472–481.
8. Armitage GC. Development of a classification system for periodontal diseases and conditions. *Ann Periodontol.* 1999;4:1–6.
9. Wilkins EM. Periodontal disease development. In: *Clinical Practice of the Dental Hygienist.* 11th ed. Philadelphia, PA: Lippincott Williams & Wilkins; 2013:244–254.
10. Nield-Gehrig JS, Willmann DE. Biofilms and periodontal infections. In: Nield-Gehrig JS, Willmann DE, eds. *Foundations of Periodontics for the Dental Hygienist.* Philadelphia, PA: Lippincott Williams & Wilkins; 2011:97–114.
11. Teughels W, Quirynen M, Jakuboviks N. Periodontal microbiology. In: Newman MN, Takei HH, Klokkevold PR, et al, eds. *Carranza's Clinical Periodontology.* 11th ed. St. Louis, MO: Elsevier Saunders; 2012:232–270.
12. Mealey BL, Klokkevolde PR. Impact of periodontal infection on systemic health. In: Newman MN, Takei HH, Klokkevold PR, et al, eds. *Carranza's Clinical Periodontology.* 11th ed. St. Louis, MO: Elsevier Saunders; 2012:320–330.
13. Arbes SJ, Slade GD, Beck JD. Association between extent of periodontal attachment loss and self-reported history of heart attack: an analysis of NHANES III data. *J Dent Res.* 1999;78:1777–1782.
14. Mealey BL, Rees TD, Rose LF, et al. Systemic factors impacting the periodontium. In: Rose LF, Mealey BL, eds. *Periodontics: Medicine, Surgery and Implants.* St. Louis, MO: Elsevier Mosby; 2004:790–845.

15. Nield-Gehrig J, Willmann D. Periodontal infections as a risk factor for systemic disease. In: Nield-Gehrig J, Willmann D, eds. *Foundations of Periodontics for the Dental Hygienist*. Philadelphia, PA: Lippincott Williams & Wilkins; 2011:298–320.

16. Grossi SG, Mealey BL, Rose LF. Effect of periodontal infection on systemic health and well-being. In: Rose LF, Mealey BL, eds. *Periodontics: Medicine, Surgery and Implants*. St. Louis, MO: Elsevier Mosby; 2004:846–859.

17. Scannapieco FA, Mylotte JM. Relationships between periodontal disease and bacterial pneumonia. *J Periodontol*. 1996;67:1114–1122.

18. Hobbs HC, Rowe DH, Johnson PW. Periodontal ligament cells from insulin-dependent diabetes exhibit altered alkaline phosphatase activity I response to growth factors. *Periodontol*. 1999;70:736–742.

19. Thomas MV, Mealey BL. Formulating a periodontal diagnosis and prognosis. In: Rose LF, Mealey BL, eds. *Periodontics: Medicine, Surgery and Implants*. St. Louis, MO: Elsevier Mosby; 2004:170–199.

20. Löe H, Anerud A, Boysen H, et al. The natural history of periodontal disease in man: the rate of periodontal destruction before 40 years of age. *J Periodontol*. 1978;49:607–620.

21. Hinrichs JE, Novak MJ. Classification of diseases and conditions affecting the periodontium. In: Newman MG, Takei HH, Klokkevold PR, et al, eds. *Carranza's Clinical Periodontology*. 11th ed. St. Louis, MO: Elsevier Saunders; 2011:34–54.

22. Haffajee AD, Socransky SS. Microbial etiological agents of destructive periodontal diseases. *Periodontol 2000*. 1997;14:12–32.

23. Loomer PM, Armitage GC. Microbiology of periodontal diseases. In: Rose LF, Mealey BL, eds. *Periodontics: Medicine, Surgery and Implants*. St. Louis, MO: Elsevier Mosby; 2004:69–84.

24. Nevins M, Becker W, Kornman K, eds. *World Workshop in Clinical Periodontics*. Chicago, IL: American Academy of Periodontology; 1989:123–131.

25. Genco RJ. Systemic antimicrobials in the management of periodontal diseases. In: *Periodontal Disease Management*. Chicago, IL: American Academy of Periodontology; 1994:237–252.

26. Klokkevold PR. Necrotizing ulcerative periodontitis. In: Newman MB, Takei HH, Klokkevold PR, et al, eds. *Carranza's Clinical Periodontology*. 11th ed. St. Louis, MO: Elsevier Saunders; 2011:165–168.

27. Dello Russo MM. The post-prophylaxis periodontal abscess: etiology and treatment. *Int J Periodont Restor Dent*. 1985;5:29–34.

28. Perry DA, Taggert EJ. Occurrence of periodontal abscess in incompletely treated periodontal disease [abstract]. *J Dent Res*. 1996;76:A568.

29. Rossman LE. Endodontic-periodontal considerations. In: Rose LF, Mealey BL, eds. *Periodontics: Medicine, Surgery and Implants*. St. Louis, MO: Elsevier Mosby; 2004:772–789.

30. Armitage GC. Periodontal disease: diagnosis. *Ann Periodontol*. 1996;1:37–215.

31. Nield-Gehrig J, Willmann D. Systemic factors associated with periodontal disease. In: Nield-Gehrig J, Willmann D, eds. *Foundations of Periodontics for the Dental Hygienist*. Philadelphia, PA: Lippincott Williams & Wilkins; 2011:171–194.

32. Ramseier C, Southard C, Walter C. Smoking and periodontal disease. In Nield-Gehrig J, Willmann D, eds. *Foundations of Periodontics for the Dental Hygienist*. Philadelphia, PA: Lippincott Williams & Wilkins; 2011:195–208.

33. Bento E, Cotter J. That patient who uses tobacco. In: Wilkins EM, ed. *Clinical Practice of the Dental Hygienist*. 11th ed. Philadelphia, PA: Lippincott Williams & Wilkins; 2013:474–495.

34. Diehl SR, Chou C-H, Kuo F, et al. Genetic factors and periodontal disease. In: Newman MG, Takei HH, Klokkevold PR, et al, eds. *Carranza's Clinical Periodontology*. 11th ed. St. Louis, MO: Elsevier Saunders; 2012:271–284.

35. Kinane DF. Systemic chemotherapeutic agents. In: Rose LF, Mealey BL, eds. *Periodontics: Medicine, Surgery and Implants*. St. Louis, MO: Elsevier Mosby; 2004:288–296.

36. Ciancio S, Mariotti A. Antiinfective therapy. In: Newman MG, Takei HH, Klokkevold PR, et al, eds. *Carranza's Clinical Periodontology*. 11th ed. St. Louis, MO: Elsevier Saunders; 2012:482–491.

37. Matsuda SA, Wilkins E. Nonsurgical periodontal therapy: supplemental care procedures. In: Wilkins EM, ed. *Clinical Practice of the Dental Hygienist*. 11th ed. Philadelphia, PA: Lippincott Williams & Wilkins; 2013:639–650.

Assessment of Periodontal Diseases

The first step in dental hygiene care is the evaluation of the patient. Data collected and analyzed permit the hygienist to assess patient concerns, evaluate the disease present, define a treatment plan, and decide upon the need for therapy by other members of the health care team. The following questions are addressed in Part III:

8

Clinical Assessment

Cheryl A. Cameron, Gina D. Evans, and Dorothy A. Perry

LEARNING OUTCOMES

- Describe the connection between patients' overall health and their oral health.
- Define the aspects of clinical assessment in the dental hygiene process of patient care.
- List and describe the indices that measure:
  - Plaque biofilm accumulation
  - Periodontal status
  - Furcation involvement
  - Tooth mobility
  - Dental caries
  - Root caries
  - Tooth wear

- Describe the intrinsic and extrinsic dental stains and their associated causes.
- Compare and contrast normal and abnormal clinical presentation of the periodontium and dentition.
- Identify the radiographic changes seen in periodontal diseases.
- Compare and contrast normal and abnormal clinical and radiographic presentation of the periodontal structures surrounding dental implants.

KEY TERMS

Assessment	Evaluation	Periodontal assessment
Bleeding on probing	Furcation	Probing measurements
Clinical examination	Oral hygiene assessment	Radiographic examination
Dentinal sensitivity	Peri-implant mucositis	Tooth mobility
Documentation	Peri-implantitis	Tooth wear

The **assessment** is the first stage in the dental hygiene process of patient care. It provides the foundation for the subsequent diagnosis, planning, implementation, and **evaluation** of dental and dental hygiene care. It is essential to the overall quality of care provided. **Documentation** of the information gathered is critical to have as a reference tool, a historical record, and a patient educational resource. It also serves an important medicolegal function as a record of your care.

The information and procedures essential to the assessment of a patient's periodontal status include the chief complaint, medical and dental histories, **clinical examination,** and **radiographic examination.**[1] The value of the assessment process is enhanced when data collection follows a comprehensive and systematic protocol. This chapter describes the elements of an assessment protocol for dental hygiene practice. An overview of the assessment process is presented in Box 8-1.

PATIENT HISTORY

MEDICAL HISTORY

The medical history is obtained at the initial appointment and is reviewed or updated at each subsequent visit. Patients need to understand the importance of sharing their medical history so that they do not omit information that they may consider irrelevant to their dental health. The medical history ensures patient safety, health, and well-being by aiding the clinician in the following: (1) evaluating oral manifestations of systemic disease; (2) detecting systemic conditions that may affect the periodontal tissue response; and (3) detecting systemic and infectious conditions that require special precautions and modifications in treatment procedures.

Medical history questionnaires vary in length, content, and format.[2,3] It is important that the medical history survey remains current with evolving connections between overall health issues and dental and periodontal health, and that it gathers information critical to ensuring patient safety, health, and well-being (e.g., bisphosphonate use for conditions such as osteoporosis and associated dental implications).[4] Regardless of which questionnaire is used, it is critical to supplement the information by interviewing the patient.[5] All patient responses should be documented in the patient record and there should be no unanswered questions on the medical history form. Supplementing the medical history through consultation with other treating health care providers may also be necessary to fully address the goal of patient safety, health, and well-being. For example the patient's orthopedic surgeon may need to be contacted regarding the need for premedication in the case of joint replacement.[6]

Patient vital signs must be taken and documented in the medical history. This includes blood pressure, pulse, and respiration. Although the taking of blood pressure may seem time-consuming, the increased understanding of the connection among hypertension, cardiovascular disease, and periodontal disease provides important support for its regular administration.[6] Vital signs should be noted at the initial interview and all subsequent medical history updates. It is also critical that the medical history be dated and signed by both the patient and the dental hygienist to validate the patient's responses.

> **CLINICAL NOTE 8-1** Because of the connection between oral health and general health, it is essential to take and record vital signs.

BOX 8-1 Assessment Protocol

Interview	Dentition Assessment
Medical history	Caries
Dental history	Restorations
Extraoral and Intraoral Assessment	Overhanging Margins
Head and neck examination	Proximal contact relationships
Oral mucosa assessment	Tooth abnormalities
Oral Hygiene Assessment	Parafunctional habits
Plaque biofilm	Tooth wear
Calculus	Sensitivity or hypersensitivity
Stain	**Radiographic Assessment**
Periodontal Assessment	Interdental septa
Probe depth	Bone destruction
Clinical attachment loss	Furcation areas
Bleeding and suppuration	Dental implants
Furcation evaluation	
Tooth mobility	
Tooth migration	
Implant status	

DENTAL HEALTH HISTORY

Patients should be asked to identify their chief complaints or reasons for seeking oral health care. Chief complaints and problems and possible oral health connections are described in Table 8-1. Patients should also describe any pain they may be experiencing. Common sources of oral pain are described in Table 8-2.

Patient reports of dental problems are often very general. It is essential that the dental hygienist assist the patient in providing the necessary details required for the dental diagnosis. The pertinent information may include, but is not limited to, the following:

- Specific location
- Stimulus that elicits pain
- Duration of stimulation
- Frequency of occurrence
- Date of the initial problem
- Changes in the problem since the initial identification

TABLE 8-1 Common Chief Complaints and Their Possible Oral Health Connections

CHIEF COMPLAINT	POSSIBLE ORAL HEALTH CONNECTIONS
Bleeding gums (gingival inflammation)	Pathogenic bacteria, drug-induced bleeding (e.g., aspirin, anticoagulant therapy), drug-induced gingival hyperplasia (e.g., antihypertensive and antiseizure medications), and systemic disease–induced gingival inflammation and hyperplasia (e.g., diabetes, HIV)
Loose teeth (mobility)	Loss of periodontal support, bruxism, traumatic tooth injury, and root fracture
Spreading of the teeth with the appearance of spaces where none existed before (tooth migration)	Loss of periodontal support, missing teeth (e.g., lack of posterior dental support), myofunctional habits (e.g., tongue thrusting), and failure to use or maintain orthodontic retainers
Bad taste in mouth	Fungal infection, periodontal disease, smoking, and xerostomia
Bad breath (halitosis)	Chronic or acute periodontal disease, xerostomia, nasopharyngeal infection (e.g., sinus, tonsil, and throat infections), deep caries, and coated tongue
Food catching between teeth	Restoration defect resulting in a lack of interdental contact, tooth migration (e.g., high bite in dental restoration, bruxism, missing teeth), loss of periodontal support or interdental papilla, and marginal ridge defect
Rough spot on tooth	Supragingival calculus, chipped tooth, restoration defect, dental caries, wear facet, and recession
Dry mouth (xerostomia)	Medications (e.g., tricyclic antidepressants, antipsychotics, antihistamines, antihypertensive medications, diuretics), diseases of the salivary glands (e.g., Sjögren's syndrome), head and neck radiation therapy, dehydration, smoking, and aging
Itchy feeling in gums	Chronic gingival inflammation, open contact, ill-fitting restoration (e.g., overhang)

TABLE 8-2   Common Pain Descriptions and their likely Oral Health Connections

CHIEF PAIN-RELATED COMPLAINTS	POSSIBLE ORAL HEALTH CONNECTIONS
Cannot open mouth wide enough or painful to open, or to brush or floss	Temporomandibular joint (TMJ) dysfunction, muscle fatigue associated with bruxism and clenching, muscle spasm, trauma associated with dental treatment or oral habit (e.g., dental restoration or extraction, chewing hard foods)
Headaches on the side of the head	TMJ, muscle fatigue associated with bruxism and clenching
Hurts to bite hard things	Tooth or root fracture, defective restoration, occlusal attrition or erosion, dental caries, bruised periodontal ligament (PDL) (e.g., high bite or traumatic injury)
Hurts to eat sugar or sweet things	Dental caries, defective restoration, tooth wear condition (i.e., attrition, abrasion, erosion, abfraction), dentin exposure from recession
Hurts to brush teeth at the gum line	Tooth wear condition, dentin exposure from recession, gingival inflammation, traumatic injury to the tooth and/or gingival tissue (e.g., toothbrushing technique, biting on hard foods, consuming acidic foods and beverages), acute manifestations of systemic and periodontal conditions (e.g., lichen planus, acute necrotizing ulcerative gingivitis [ANUG], herpes simplex)
Constant dull gnawing pain or dull pain after eating	Bruised PDL, pulpitis, periodontal disease, open contact with food impaction
Acute throbbing pain	Bruised PDL, pulpitis, food impaction (e.g., popcorn kernel), periodontal or endodontic abscess, deep dental caries, thermal sensitivity (hot or cold), systemic or localized infection (e.g., ANUG, primary herpes simplex, acute mucositis, infected oral piercing)
Sensitivity to hot and cold	Dental caries, pulpitis, recession, tooth wear condition, traumatic injury (e.g., recent restoration, malocclusion, blunt force tooth injury), bruxism, clenching, tooth fracture
Burning sensation in the gums	Fungal infection (e.g., candidiasis), xerostomia, chronic manifestation of systemic conditions (e.g., lichen planus), allergic reactions (e.g., sodium lauryl sulfate, cinnamon, palladium, nickel)

CLINICAL NOTE 8-2   Information about the chief complaint allows you to assess immediate needs and is a critical part of establishing rapport with the patient and developing a treatment plan that meets the patient's personal goals of care.

A dental history should also include information about the patient's previous dental experiences, current oral hygiene practices, and attitudes toward dentistry. Information about the patient's family, social history, and habits (e.g., caffeine consumption, tobacco use, alcohol use, recreational drug use), are important elements of your assessment. Sometimes seemingly healthy lifestyle routines can have untoward effects on the dentition or oral health. For example, physical fitness and competitive sport activities can lead to high consumption of acidic sport drinks. The information gathered in the dental history may affect the plan and delivery of oral health care, as well as patient education. Always be aware that patients may not be willing to disclose health history information fully because they think it is not relevant to dental care or because of a concern for personal privacy.[7]

The interview is important for gathering information that patients may not realize is important to their care plan. An example is the patient who fails to inform the dental hygienist of a recent joint replacement surgery, but later informs the dentist because the surgeon told the patient to tell the dentist. Patients can be unaware of the invasive nature of dental hygiene therapy (e.g., bleeding and bacteremia) and not intuitively make the connection to their general health. The interview is also an

opportunity to supplement the standard medical or dental history on the basis of clinical observations. For example, a patient with no prior history of tooth wear presents with notable tooth wear lesions at a recall appointment. The patient's updated medical and dental history did not note any changes. An interview that inquires about information such as new medications (e.g., bruxism-inducing medications), changes in dietary habits (e.g., consumption of acidic foods and beverages), and changes in lifestyle or habits (e.g., physical fitness routine or drug use) would be warranted.

PATIENT EDUCATION

The prevention and educational strategies for each patient are aimed at the factors identified during the clinical assessment. These are generally focused on plaque biofilm removal, periodontal disease and dental caries prevention, diet modification, and the use of fluorides.

CLINICAL NOTE 8-3   Oral hygiene instruction must be tailored to the clinical assessment of each patient. Visualization is a key instructional strategy for helping patients understand their oral health status and can be achieved in a variety of ways:
- Direct observation using a mirror
- Intraoral photographs to view soft tissue conditions, enamel cracks, dental caries, and oral abnormalities
- Radiographic images to point out bone loss, dental caries, furcations in molars, and hard tissue abnormalities

Recommendations of preventive protocols, such as plaque biofilm control and removal aids and fluoride use should be introduced and demonstrated as part of this assessment. It is also important that the oral hygiene aids that have been prescribed, dispensed, and introduced to the patient be documented in the patient record.

CLINICAL EXAMINATION

Accurate patient evaluation requires a comprehensive clinical examination. This examination should include extraoral, intraoral, oral mucosal, oral hygiene, periodontal, and dentition assessments.

EXTRAORAL AND INTRAORAL ASSESSMENT

The head, neck, and oral cavity should be examined using visual and tactile techniques. This is the time to look for pathologic conditions, physical deviations, or modifications such as oral piercing. In addition, lymph chains and salivary glands should be palpated to identify swelling or masses. Additional visual adjunctive aids, such as autofluorescence and chemiluminescence, have been developed with the goal of early identification and intervention of high-risk oral lesions; however, their benefit to the dental practice has not yet been established.[8,9]

Findings from this assessment support the development of the dental and dental hygiene treatment plan and patient education plans. For example, when oral piercings are observed, the associated risks of gingival recession, tooth fracture, and infection should be discussed.[10,11] The findings of the extraoral and intraoral assessment may also identify a need for dental specialty referral and for medical consultation and/or referral.

ORAL MUCOSA ASSESSMENT

The oral mucosa assessment requires an understanding of the normal clinical features of the intraoral soft tissues. Three types of oral mucosa line the oral cavity: masticatory mucosa, specialized mucosa, and lining mucosa as described in Chapter 2. Figure 8-1 presents the anatomy of the normal gingiva adjacent to a tooth in diagrammatic form.

One clinically significant observation is noting the amount of attached gingiva extending from the free gingival groove to the movable alveolar mucosa. This junction is called the mucogingival junction. It is usually seen as a slightly scalloped line, as seen in Figure 8-2. The attached gingiva on the buccal aspect of the mandible and maxilla extends from the free gingival groove to the mucogingival junction and is continuous with the vestibule. The width of the attached gingiva is determined by subtracting the sulcus or pocket depth from the total width of the keratinized gingiva (from the gingival margin to the mucogingival junction). This measurement is performed by stretching the lip or cheek to demarcate the mucogingival line while the pocket is probed. The amount of attached gingiva is considered insufficient when stretching the lip or cheek induces movement of the free gingival margin. The attached gingiva on the lingual aspect of the mandible also extends from the free gingival groove to the mucogingival junction, but is continuous with the lining of the floor of the mouth. On the palatal aspect of the maxilla, the attached gingiva is continuous with the

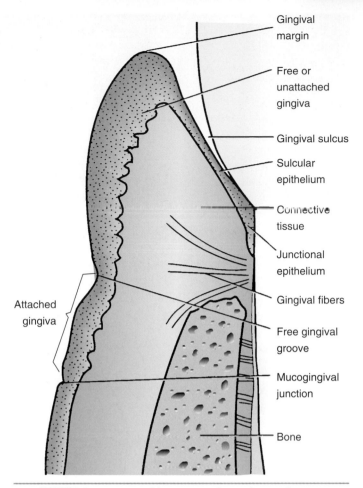

FIGURE 8-1 ■ Diagram of the anatomy of normal gingival tissues.

masticatory palatal mucosa. The amount of attached gingiva can be important for some restorative procedures.

The interdental papilla is the tissue between two adjacent teeth. It consists of a facial or buccal papilla, a lingual papilla, and a col. The col is the valley, or depression, connecting the facial or buccal papilla and the lingual papilla. The col is shown in Figure 8-3. It is usually nonkeratinized and conforms to the interproximal contact area. The col is often absent in areas in which teeth are not in contact.

The health status of the gingiva can be determined by considering four universally accepted descriptive categories: color, contour, consistency, and texture.

Color

The color of a normal marginal and attached gingiva is a pale coral pink, but can vary as a result of individual skin pigmentation, degree of vascularity, and epithelial keratinization. Bright red gingival tissues indicate acute inflammation. Dark red to cyanotic gingival tissues indicate chronic inflammation.

Contour

The contour (also referred to as shape or form) of a healthy marginal gingiva is uniformly scalloped. Healthy interdental papillae appear as pointed knifelike tissues that fill the embrasure spaces between teeth.

Inflamed gingival margins appear swollen, rounded, or shiny and the scalloped appearance may be lost. When the papillae

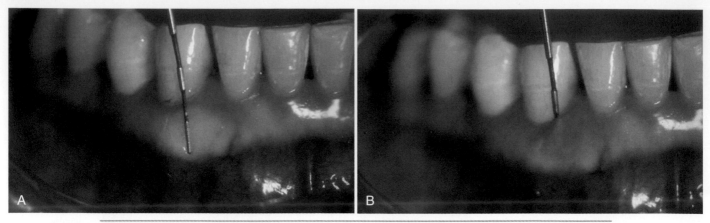

FIGURE 8-2 ■ The width of the attached gingiva is important to assess. **A,** Probe measuring the clinically apparent width of the attached gingiva. **B,** Probe inserted into the pocket penetrates beyond the apparent width of the attached gingiva, indicating epithelial attachment apical to the mucogingival line.

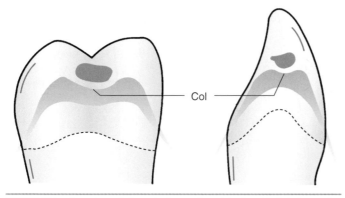

Col

FIGURE 8-3 ■ Location of the col, the nonkeratinized epithelial depression connecting the buccal and lingual papillae of teeth, apical to the contact area *(in gray).*

are inflamed, their appearance may be flattened, blunted, bulbous, cratered, or hyperplastic. Festoons are inner tube–like swellings at the gingival margin. They are thought to be the result of an increase in the number of cells; inflammation may increase the inner tube–like appearance. Clefts, such as a Stillman cleft, appear as slitlike depressions on the facial or lingual gingival margins.

Consistency

The consistency of marginal and interdental gingiva should be firm when palpated with the side of a blunt instrument, such as a periodontal probe. In the presence of inflammation, the gingiva may be soft and spongy, swollen, shiny, and easily deflected away from the tooth with an instrument or a blast of air.

In health, the attached gingiva has a stippled, orange peel–like texture. When inflamed, the gingiva loses its stippled texture and appears rolled, shiny, and smooth. In the case of very fibrotic tissue, the stippling may still be apparent, even in the presence of inflammation.

CLINICAL NOTE 8-4 Gingival descriptive categories provide baseline assessment and comparisons over time. They include color, contour, consistency, and texture.

Assessment of the lining mucosa includes examination of the alveolar mucosa and frenum attachments.

Alveolar Mucosa

Alveolar mucosa is loosely attached, movable tissue that is not keratinized. It is darker than the attached gingiva because the mucosa is thinner and the underlying blood vessels are visible. The alveolar mucosa begins at the mucogingival junction and is continuous with the lining mucosa of the oral cavity.

Frenum Attachments

Frenum attachments are folds of mucosal tissues, often including muscle fibers, that join the movable mucosa to attached or specialized mucosa. Maxillary and mandibular anterior frenum attachments are located at the midlines of the maxillary and mandibular central incisors, as shown in Figure 8-4. The lingual frenum attachment is located on the underside of the tongue. Maxillary and mandibular buccal frenum attachments are located at the canines and premolars.

The assessment of the periodontal health of patients includes the description and documentation of the oral mucosal features. This documentation provides a baseline for planning dental and dental hygiene treatment and assessing the outcome of care. It is essential to describe clinical features, size, location, and severity clearly. Gingival observations may support the identification of underlying systemic, environmental, or behavioral contributing factors that may warrant further evaluation.[12-15] Sample gingival descriptions are shown in Figures 8-5 and 8-6. Routine digital intraoral photographic images with supplemental narrative clinical observations are also useful for documenting and comparing the oral mucosa assessment at baseline and subsequent appointments, and for sharing with other members of the patient's health care team. The electronic record is now commonly used and is a valuable resource to retain and compare images and other documentation over time.

ORAL HYGIENE ASSESSMENT

The **oral hygiene assessment** includes a clinical evaluation of the presence of plaque biofilm, calculus, and stain. The data collected during this assessment help the dental hygienist to draw connections with the clinical periodontal and dentition

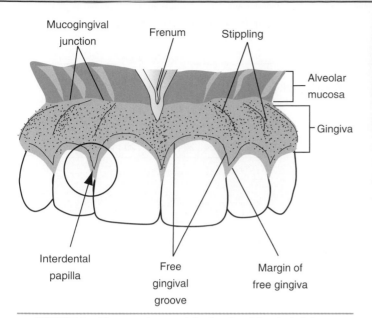

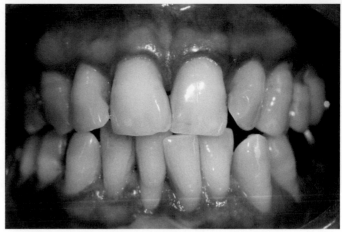

FIGURE 8-6 ■ **Gingival description.** The gingiva appears inflamed, with generalized rolled borders. Papillae do not fill the interdental spaces, and there is some loss of stippling. The marginal gingival tissues appear reddened.

FIGURE 8-4 ■ The normal anatomic landmarks of the gingival tissue.

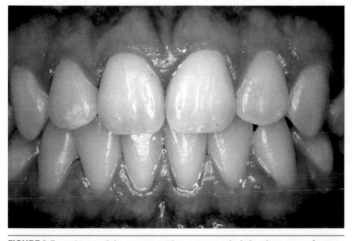

FIGURE 8-5 ■ **Gingival description.** The gingiva is slightly edematous, showing loss of stippling. Papillae are rounded and fill the interdental spaces. There is a localized rolled margin in the lower anterior area. The marginal gingival tissues appear reddened.

assessments, develop a dental hygiene treatment plan, design patient education strategies, and evaluate the outcome of oral hygiene instruction.

Plaque Biofilm

Plaque biofilm is a structured and functioning synergistic community of bacteria that support their combined metabolism and together enhance their overall bacterial virulence. It is described in detail in Chapter 4. Eighty-five percent of all dental treatment is related to the diagnosis, treatment, and prevention of plaque biofilm–related diseases. Periodontal disease and dental caries are the reason for 75% of all extractions.[16]

Identifying and documenting the location of plaque biofilm on the teeth can be used to educate patients on their specific oral hygiene prevention needs and provide a record over time. The plaque biofilm can be stained with a red disclosing solution to help patients see it or it can be shown to the patient when removed with an explorer or other instrument. The O'Leary

Plaque Control Record provides a simple method of recording the presence of plaque biofilm at the gingival third of the buccal, lingual, mesial, and distal surface of each tooth.[17] The plaque biofilm record quantifies the percentage of total tooth surfaces with plaque biofilm (e.g., 20 surfaces with recorded plaque biofilm ÷ 40 total surfaces = 50%). This method is particularly useful in research protocols requiring standardized recording of patient data.

In the clinical practice setting, the amount of plaque biofilm is more easily described as light, moderate, or heavy and the location is noted as generalized or localized, such as anterior, posterior, buccal, lingual, interproximal, and cervical or marginal. This documentation is kept in the patient's permanent record and can be used to compare and evaluate the success of the plaque biofilm prevention program. An example of a plaque biofilm control record is presented in Figure 8-7.

Calculus

The assessment of calculus is very important for developing the dental hygiene treatment plan. The presence of supragingival calculus can be observed directly. Light supragingival calculus deposits are more easily seen when dried with air. Subgingival calculus is detected using an explorer by carefully examining each tooth surface to the level of the periodontal attachment. Figure 8-8 shows the topography evaluated by explorer detection. Gentle blasts of air may be used to deflect the gingiva and permit some visualization of the calculus in the pockets.

Radiographic images may show heavy interproximal calculus deposits, as seen in Figure 8-9. However, calculus is usually present in greater amounts on the teeth than can be seen on the two-dimensional images. Detection methods can be enhanced through the use of fiberoptic endoscopy, spectro-optical scanning, autofluorescence, ultrasound, and combined laser-autofluorescence technologies.[18-20] These technologies are not routinely available in general dental practice so the combination of tactile, radiographic, and visual detection of subgingival calculus remains the general professional standard for the assessment of calculus.

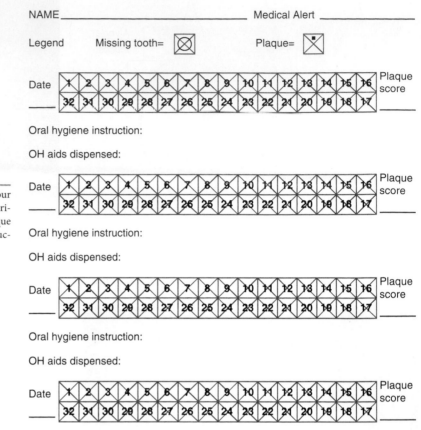

PLAQUE BIOFILM CONTROL RECORD

NAME _____ Medical Alert _____

Legend   Missing tooth= ⊗   Plaque= ⊠

Date ____   Plaque score ____

Oral hygiene instruction:

OH aids dispensed:

Date ____   Plaque score ____

Oral hygiene instruction:

OH aids dispensed:

Date ____   Plaque score ____

Oral hygiene instruction:

OH aids dispensed:

Date ____   Plaque score ____

Oral hygiene instruction:

OH aids dispensed:

FIGURE 8-7 ■ Example of a plaque biofilm control record. Four plaque scores can be recorded to provide the patient with a comparison over time, monitor improvement, and reinforce better plaque control. There is also space to record the oral hygiene (OH) instructions given at each session and to list the aids dispensed.

CLINICAL NOTE 8-5 The documentation of calculus includes description of the type (supragingival and subgingival), location (tooth, surface, generalized, localized, interproximal, or marginal), quantity (heavy, moderate, or light), and nature (white and chalky, spicules, rings, black, and tenacious).

Dental and Oral Tissue Stain

Pigmented deposits on the tooth surface are called extrinsic stains. They are primarily aesthetic problems that result from the pigmentation of ordinarily colorless acquired pellicular and dental plaque biofilm by chromogenic bacteria, foods, and chemicals. These removable stains vary in color, composition, and firmness of adherence to the tooth surface. In contrast, intrinsic stains occur within the tooth structure and cannot be mechanically removed by scaling or polishing. A commonly recognized cause of intrinsic staining is discoloration from pre-eruption and posteruption drug interactions (e.g., tetracycline or minocycline stains).

Extrinsic Stains

Brown Stain. Brown stain is a thin, translucent, acquired, bacteria-free pigmented pellicle. It is frequently associated with poor oral hygiene and not using dentifrice. Brown stain is the most commonly occurring stain. It can be very diffuse and appear at varying intensities throughout the dentition. The

discoloration is usually greater on irregular tooth surfaces and places that tend to concentrate pellicle, such as the gingival margins and interproximal areas. The brown staining is often caused by tannin, which has a denaturing effect on pellicular proteins and is found in coffee, tea, fruits, and red wine.[21]

Tobacco produces tenacious dark brown or black surface deposits and brown discoloration of tooth structures. Staining is not necessarily proportional to the amount of tobacco used, but depends to a considerable degree on preexisting acquired coatings that attach the tobacco products to the tooth surface.

Chlorhexidine was introduced to U.S. dental practice in the 1980s as a general antiseptic with broad antibacterial action against gram-positive and gram-negative bacteria and yeasts. An undesirable side effect of continued use of chlorhexidine solution is that it imparts a yellow-brown to brown color to the tissues of the oral cavity. The staining also appears in the cervical and interproximal regions of the teeth, on restorations, in plaque biofilm, and on the surface of the tongue.[22] Chlorhexidine also has a denaturing effect on proteins that may result in increased staining of the acquired pellicle by metal ions. There may also be increased binding of dietary chromogens after treatment with chlorhexidine.[23] Chlorhexidine staining is shown in Figure 8-10.

The anticaries benefits of stannous fluoride have long been recognized. In addition, stannous fluoride is used for the control

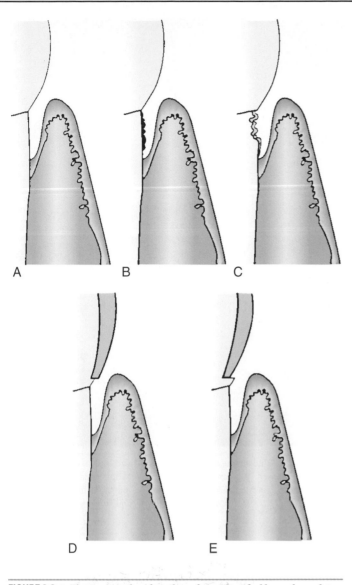

FIGURE 8-8 ■ **The topography of tooth surfaces identified by explorer detection. A,** Pathologically deepened sulcus with normal topography. **B,** Calculus on the root surface. **C,** Caries on the root surface. **D,** Overhanging restoration margin. **E,** Undercontoured restoration margin.

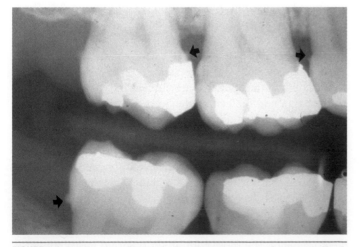

FIGURE 8-9 ■ **Bitewing radiograph showing interproximal subgingival calculus.** Radiographic appearance of spicules (spurs) of calculus is evident between the teeth.

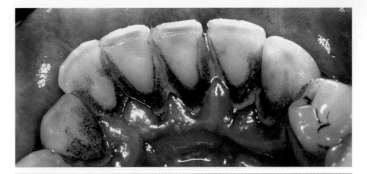

FIGURE 8-10 ■ **Chlorhexidine stain on the lower anterior teeth.** Note the formation of supragingival calculus, which is also stained.

of plaque biofilm formation, gingivitis, and dentinal hypersensitivity. Stannous fluoride imparts a yellow-brown or golden discoloration of the tongue and teeth. It has been suggested that this stain is primarily stannous sulfide.[24]

Black Stain. Black stain usually occurs as thin black lines on the facial and lingual surfaces of the teeth near the gingival margin and also as diffuse patches on proximal surfaces. It is firmly attached, tends to recur after removal, is more common in women, and may occur in mouths with excellent hygiene. The black stain that occurs in children is typically associated with a low incidence of caries. The microflora of black stain is dominated by chromogenic bacteria, which may be the cause of the black pigmentation.[25] Another theory is that the black pigmentation is an insoluble ferric sulfide produced as a result of an interaction of hydrogen sulfide–producing bacteria and iron from the saliva and gingival fluid.[26] Black stain tends to recur, and in some cases a 3- or 4-month recall program is required to respond to the patient's aesthetic concerns.

Green Stain. Green stain is a green-yellow stain, sometimes of considerable thickness. It is most often associated with children. The stain is considered to be stained remnants of the enamel cuticle, but this theory has not been substantiated. The discoloration has been attributed to fluorescent bacteria and fungi, such as *Penicillium* and *Aspergillus*.[27] Green stain usually occurs on the gingival half of the facial surfaces of anterior teeth. It is associated with poor oral hygiene.[28]

Orange Stain. Orange stain is less common than green or brown stain. It may occur on both the facial and lingual surfaces of anterior teeth. Orange stain is often associated with poor oral hygiene and is observed to form on loosely attached debris. *Serratia marcescens* and *Flavobacterium lutescens* have been suggested as the responsible chromogenic organisms.[29]

Preeruption Intrinsic Stains

Fluorosis. The excessive ingestion of fluoride from sources such as toothpaste, fluoride supplements, and water can cause hypomineralization of enamel during development, known as fluorosis. Although the enamel remains decay-resistant, the aesthetic appearance is discolored and mottled. In its mildest form, fluorosis can appear as white flecks primarily on the cusp tips and facial surfaces of permanent dentition. The more severe forms of fluorosis, which result from source fluoride of a higher dosage or longer duration of exposure, may appear as white opaque areas or darkly stained and pitted enamel.[30]

Tetracycline Stains. Tetracycline can also cause tooth discoloration when used during tooth development. The

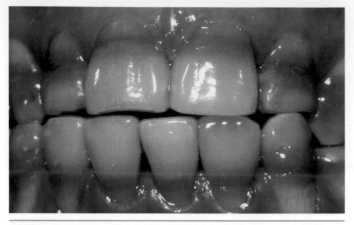

FIGURE 8-11 ■ **Tetracycline stain in the gingival third of the upper and lower teeth.** Also note recession, attrition, and erosion.

appearance may range from yellow to gray-brown in color in teeth simultaneously developing during tetracycline exposure. This staining is extrinsic in the dentin so it cannot be removed. The discoloration takes on a banded appearance in the section of the tooth developing at the time of exposure, as seen in Figure 8-11.[31]

Other Intrinsic Stains. In addition to drug-related intrinsic stains, tooth discoloration may occur as a result of metabolic disorders (e.g., hypothyroidism), inherited disorders (e.g., amelogenesis imperfecta, dentinogenesis imperfecta), systemic disorders (e.g., cystic fibrosis), or environmental factors (e.g., trauma).[32]

Posteruption Intrinsic Staining

Minocycline Stains. Minocycline, a commonly used medication with a broad range of clinical indications (e.g., acne, rosacea, rheumatoid arthritis, periodontal disease), has been shown to cause intrinsic dental and oral tissue discoloration, as seen in Figure 8-12. The onset of discoloration can occur within 1 month or many years after initiation of treatment.[31] The discoloration ranges in color from green-gray to blue-gray.

Other Intrinsic Discoloration. Pink tooth is observed in cases of internal resorption and invasive cervical resorption as a result of inflamed pulp tissue and inflamed periodontal granulation tissue, respectively.[33]

CLINICAL NOTE 8-6 Stains are documented according to color (brown, black, green blue, gray, yellow, or orange), location (tooth, surface, intrinsic or extrinsic), extent (amount of tooth surface or tissue covered, localized or generalized), and intensity (light, moderate, or heavy).

PERIODONTAL ASSESSMENT

Periodontal assessment includes a clinical evaluation of the periodontium, looking for signs of inflammation and damage to periodontal tissues. The clinical detection of inflammatory lesions and damage to periodontal tissues is essential for diagnosis, treatment planning, and monitoring therapeutic effectiveness.[34] The clinical assessments include the following:

- Measuring periodontal probe depths and clinical attachment levels

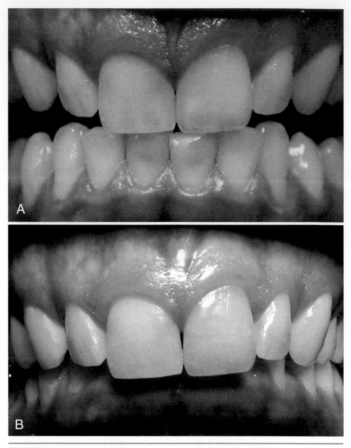

FIGURE 8-12 ■ **Minocycline stain on the dental and oral tissue of a 27-year-old patient with a 10-year history of minocycline treatment for acne. A,** Intrinsic blue-gray dental staining of the upper and lower incisors. **B,** Intrinsic blue-gray oral tissue staining of the upper and lower attached gingival mucosa.

- Assessing gingival bleeding and suppuration
- Identifying and measuring **furcations**
- Testing mobility
- Recognizing pathologic tooth migration[35]

The assessment should follow an established sequence to ensure that it is comprehensive and complete. The diagnoses for periodontal diseases and conditions are defined by the American Academy of Periodontology's Classification System for Periodontal Diseases and Conditions in Box 8-2.[36] These are defined in detail in Chapters 6 and 7.

Probing Measurements

Periodontal probing provides a numeric assessment of the apical extent of the epithelial attachment in relation to the gingival margin and the cementoenamel junction. **Probing measurements** are used to evaluate periodontal disease status, support treatment planning decisions, design individualized prevention plans, and determine the success of treatment. Periodontal probing depths are a critical component of a complete periodontal charting, which also includes assessments of radiographic images, bleeding, clinical attachment loss, furcation involvement, and bone loss.

A periodontal probe is used to obtain two types of probing measurements. The most commonly reported measurement is the distance between the gingival margin and the base of the gingival sulcus. This distance is known as the periodontal

I. Gingival diseases
  A. Dental plaque–induced gingival diseases
    1. Gingivitis associated with dental plaque only
      a. Without other local contributing factors
      b. With local contributing factors
    2. Gingival diseases modified by systemic factors
      a. Associated with the endocrine system
        1) Puberty-associated gingivitis
        2) Menstrual cycle–associated gingivitis
        3) Pregnancy-associated
          a) Gingivitis
          b) Pyogenic granuloma
        4) Diabetes mellitus–associated gingivitis
      b. Associated with blood dyscrasias
        1) Leukemia-associated gingivitis
        2) Other
    3. Gingival diseases modified by medications
      a. Drug-influenced gingival diseases
        1) Drug-influenced gingival enlargements
        2) Drug-influenced gingivitis
          a) Oral contraceptive–associated gingivitis
          b) Other
    4. Gingival diseases modified by malnutrition
      a. Ascorbic acid–deficiency gingivitis
      b. Other
  B. Non–plaque-induced gingival lesions
    1. Gingival diseases of specific bacterial origin
      a. *Neisseria gonorrhoeae*–associated lesions
      b. *Treponema pallidum*–associated lesions
      c. *Streptococcus* species–associated lesions
      d. Other
    2. Gingival diseases of viral origin
      a. Herpesvirus infections
        1) Primary herpetic gingivostomatitis
        2) Recurrent oral herpes
        3) Varicella zoster infections
      b. Other
    3. Gingival diseases of fungal origin
      a. *Candida* species infections
        1) Generalized gingival candidiasis
      b. Linear gingival erythema
      c. Histoplasmosis
      d. Other
    4. Gingival lesions of genetic origin
      a. Hereditary gingival fibromatosis
      b. Other
    5. Gingival manifestations of systemic conditions
      a. Mucocutaneous disorders
        1) Lichen planus
        2) Pemphigoid
        3) Pemphigus vulgaris
        4) Erythema multiforme
        5) Lupus erythematosus
        6) Drug-induced
        7) Other
      b. Allergic reactions
        1) Dental restorative materials
          a) Mercury
          b) Nickel
          c) Acrylic
          d) Other
        2) Reactions attributable to
          a) Toothpastes, dentifrices
          b) Mouth rinses, mouthwashes
          c) Chewing gum additives
          d) Foods and additives
        3) Other
    6. Traumatic lesions (e.g., factitious, iatrogenic, accidental)
      a. Chemical injury
      b. Physical injury
      c. Thermal injury
      7. Foreign body reactions
      8. Not otherwise specified
II. Chronic periodontitis
  A. Localized (≤30% of involved sites)
  B. Generalized (>30% of involved sites)
III. Aggressive periodontitis
  A. Localized
  B. Generalized
IV. Periodontitis as a manifestation of systemic disease
  A. Associated with hematologic disorders
    1. Acquired neutropenia
    2. Leukemias
    3. Other
  B. Associated with genetic disorders
    1. Familial and cyclic neutropenia
    2. Down syndrome
    3. Leukocyte adhesion deficiency syndromes
    4. Papillon-Lefèvre syndrome
    5. Chédiak-Higashi syndrome
    6. Histiocytosis syndromes
    7. Glycogen storage disease
    8. Infantile genetic agranulocytosis
    9. Cohen syndrome
    10. Ehlers-Danlos syndrome (types IV and VIII)
    11. Hypophosphatasia
    12. Other
  C. Not otherwise specified
V. Necrotizing periodontal disease
  A. Necrotizing ulcerative gingivitis (NUG) (described in Chapter 6)
  B. Necrotizing ulcerative periodontitis (NUP)
VI. Abscess of the periodontium
  A. Gingival abscess
  B. Periodontal abscess
  C. Pericoronal abscess
VII. Periodontitis associated with endodontic lesions
  A. Combined periodontal-endodontic lesions
VIII. Developmental or acquired deformities and conditions
  A. Localized tooth-related factors that modify or predispose to plaque-induced gingival diseases or periodontitis
    1. Tooth anatomic factors
    2. Dental restorations, appliances
    3. Root fractures
    4. Cervical root resorption and cemental tears
  B. Mucogingival deformities and conditions around teeth
    1. Gingival, soft tissue recession
      a. Facial or lingual surfaces
      b. Interproximal (papillary)
    2. Lack of keratinized gingiva
    3. Decreased vestibular depth
    4. Aberrant frenum, muscle position
    5. Gingival excess
      a. Pseudopocket
      b. Inconsistent gingival margin
      c. Excessive gingival display
      d. Gingival enlargement
    6. Abnormal color
  C. Mucogingival deformities and conditions on edentulous ridges
    1. Vertical or horizontal ridge deficiency
    2. Lack of gingiva, keratinized tissue
    3. Gingival, soft tissue enlargement
    4. Aberrant frenum muscle position
    5. Decreased vestibular depth
    6. Abnormal color
  D. Occlusal trauma
    1. Primary occlusal trauma
    2. Secondary occlusal trauma

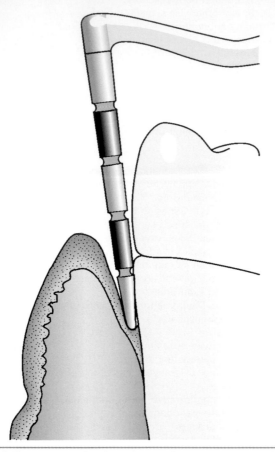

FIGURE 8-13 ■ **Diagram of probing the periodontal pocket depth.** The millimeter measurement indicates the distance from the margin of the gingiva to the base of the pocket, in this example 5 mm.

pocket depth, probing depth or, in the case of periodontal health, gingival sulcus depth. Probing measurements should be taken at six sites on each tooth: distobuccal, buccal, mesiobuccal, distolingual, lingual, and mesiolingual. Probing the periodontal pocket depth is shown in Figure 8-13.

Clinical Attachment Loss. The other important measurement is clinical attachment loss, the distance between the cementoenamel junction and the most apical extent of the epithelial attachment. The significance of clinical attachment loss, along with probing depth, is shown in Figure 8-14.

When the cementoenamel junction is visible, clinical attachment loss is determined by adding the periodontal pocket depth to the gingival recession measurement. Gingival recession is the distance between the cementoenamel junction and the gingival margin.

When the gingival margin is coronal to the cementoenamel junction, the distance between the gingival margin and the cementoenamel junction is subtracted from the periodontal pocket depth to calculate the clinical attachment loss.

Clinical attachment loss provides the most accurate and reliable means of assessing the progression and remission of periodontal disease.[37] In many cases, other factors such as previous periodontal therapy and surgery, orthodontic treatment, occlusal trauma, occlusal attrition, erosion leading to extrusion, and traumatic toothbrushing can contribute to attachment loss. In addition, the observation of clinical attachment loss may support the identification of underlying systemic, environmental, or behavioral contributing factors that may warrant further investigation, such as diabetes, smoking, or head and neck radiation therapy.[38-40] Figures 8-15 and 8-16 explain the difference between clinical attachment loss and periodontal probing depth.

CLINICAL NOTE 8-7 Periodontal probing measurements cannot detect disease activity or predict destruction. Clinical attachment loss is only an indication that destructive disease has occurred. Accurate records are essential to assess changes in the disease process over time.

Probing depths are affected by the clinician's insertion force, the probe's tip size or measurement scale, the insertion point and angulation, and the patient's gingival inflammation status. The probe tip easily penetrates the inflamed epithelial attachment and typically results in measurements that are generally 1 mm deeper than the histologic depth of the pocket, even with the most careful technique.[41]

Bleeding. Bleeding on probing is not an absolute predictor of active disease.[42] However, the presence of persistent bleeding on probing, in patients seen for periodontal maintenance, has been shown to be an indicator of disease progression.[43] Therefore, the presence of bleeding on probing is important but does not necessarily indicate that active disease is present. Increased bleeding on probing is also seen in patients on a drug regimen, such as aspirin or anticoagulant therapy, and during pregnancy.[44,45] It is important to note that the absence of bleeding on probing generally indicates current stability of the periodontium.[46]

CLINICAL NOTE 8-8 Bleeding on probing does not mean that disease is active; however, sites that exhibit bleeding over time are more likely to present with increasing attachment loss.

Reduced bleeding and suppressed clinical signs of gingival inflammation are also observed in smokers due to the effects of nicotine on periodontal tissues and cellular function.[47] The number of years of smoking exposure and the number of daily exposures (dosage) may also increase the smoking-associated risk of periodontal disease. It has been shown that the suppressed inflammatory response is reversible on smoking cessation.[48] In addition, a reduction in smoking may have a beneficial effect on associated periodontal disease in heavy smokers. Patients who reduce or quit smoking with the assistance of nicotine substitutes, such as patches and gum, may continue to exhibit reduced bleeding on probing.[49] In the absence of bleeding in smokers, calculus and increased probing depths can be viewed as signs of suppressed inflammatory response and active periodontal disease.[50]

Areas that bleed when probed should be documented in the patient's periodontal record. Gingival bleeding can be assessed during the probing process. This assessment can be as simple as noting and recording the presence or absence of bleeding, or it can be more detailed and include the amount and quickness of the bleeding response. Gingival bleeding can also be assessed using an interproximal brush. This is a technique that can be used as part of the oral hygiene instruction plan and can

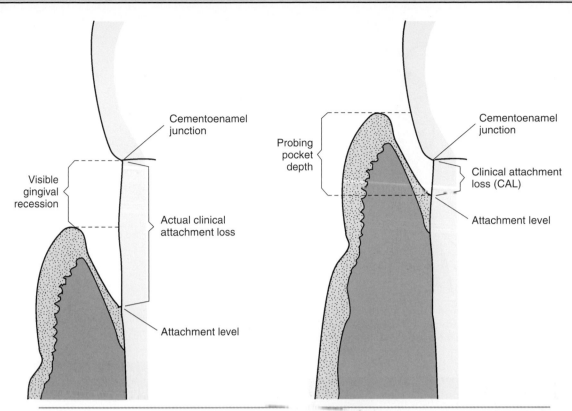

FIGURE 8-14 ■ **The difference between probing pocket depth and clinical attachment loss.** Clinical attachment loss is often the more critical assessment for the long-term health of the tooth and success of treatment. It is important to understand the distinction between clinical attachment loss, gingival recession, and pocket depth. The 3-mm probing depths represented here depict distinctly different levels of clinical attachment loss.

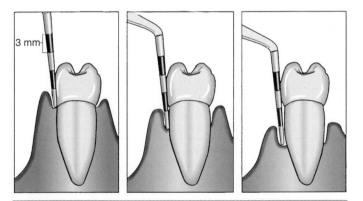

FIGURE 8-15 ■ **Diagram of 3-mm probing pocket depths in relation to different clinical attachment levels.** Greater attachment loss indicates more periodontal destruction.

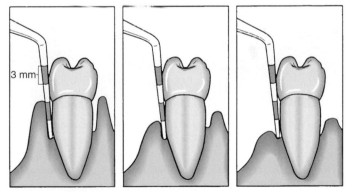

FIGURE 8-16 ■ **Diagram of different probing pocket depths related to the same level of clinical attachment loss.** Deeper probing pocket depths do not necessarily indicate more periodontal destruction.

provide a mechanism for the patient to assess improvement as treatment progresses.[51]

Suppuration. The presence of suppuration, also called purulent exudate or pus, in combination with periodontal pockets and bleeding on probing, can indicate that a site is in an active disease state and attachment loss is increasing.[52] Clinical assessment of pus within a periodontal pocket is performed by gently placing a finger against the marginal gingiva and pressing toward the crown of the tooth, as shown in Figure 8-17. Suppuration is formed on the inner pocket wall, but the external appearance of the pocket may be unchanged. Therefore, visual examination and digital pressure is required.

Suppuration does not occur in all periodontal pockets; however, its absence is not an indicator of periodontal stability. Clinically detectable suppuration should be documented in the patient's periodontal record.

Furcation Identification and Measurement

In the normal dentition, furcations are not clinically visible or detectable. Furcations can be detected and evaluated when attachment loss has occurred. Evaluating the presence, type, location, and extent of involvement of furcations is critical because it dramatically affects the treatment and prognosis of the tooth. A furcation probe, such as the Nabers probe seen

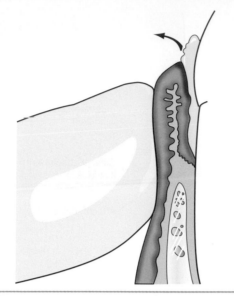

FIGURE 8-17 ■ Suppuration can be expressed from infected periodontal pockets by gentle finger pressure. (Modified from Newman MG, Takei HH, Klokkevold PR, Carranza FA, eds. *Carranza's Clinical Periodontology.* 10th ed. St. Louis, MO: Elsevier Saunders; 2006.)

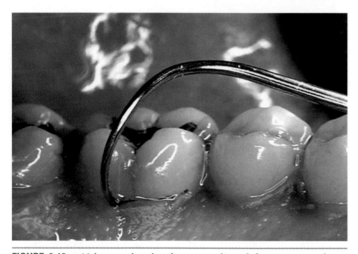

FIGURE 8-18 ■ Nabers probe placed to assess lingual furcation on a lower molar.

penetrating a furcation area in Figure 8-18, and radiographic images (discussed later in the section on radiographic assessment) are the primary furcation diagnostic tools.

Furcations may be visually observed, but they are more commonly manually detected as an indentation during probing or exploration. Once a furcation is identified, its type must be determined. The type of furcation present in a two-rooted tooth is a bifurcation involvement. The type of furcation present in a three-rooted tooth may be either a bifurcation (if it involves two roots) or a trifurcation (if it involves all three roots). Bifurcations in the following locations:

- In two-rooted mandibular molars on the buccal and lingual aspects
- In two-rooted maxillary first premolars on the mesial and distal aspects
- In three-rooted maxillary molars on the buccal, mesiolingual, and distolingual aspects; trifurcation involvement includes all three roots.

Molar furcation areas are shown in Figure 8-19.

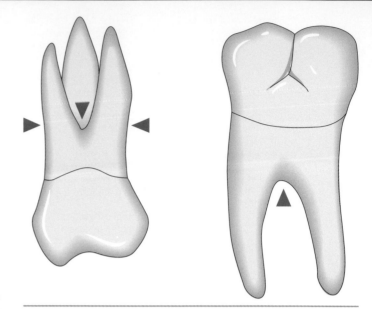

FIGURE 8-19 ■ The locations of furcation areas *(arrows)* on maxillary three-rooted and mandibular two-rooted teeth.

TABLE 8-3	Glickman Index of Furcation Classifications
GRADE	**DESCRIPTION**
Grade I	Early stage furcation involvement with pocket formation into the flute of the furca that may include limited bone loss; without radiographic changes
Grade II	Furcation involvement of one or more furcations of a tooth with bone loss that does not extend beyond the dome of the root; with or without radiographic changes
Grade III	Extension of bone loss beyond the dome of the root that may permit probing through the furcation; with radiolucency in the furcation crotch
Grade IV	Extensive bone loss permitting complete passage throughout the furcation with clinically visible furcation openings

Adapted from Sims T, Takei HH, Ammons WF, Harrington GW. Furcation: involvement and treatment. In: Newman MN, Takei HH, Klokkevold PR, et al, eds. *Carranza's Clinical Periodontology.* 11th ed. St. Louis, MO: Elsevier Saunders; 2012:592.

Estimations of horizontal and vertical bone loss within a bifurcation or trifurcation are used to determine the degree of involvement. The horizontal component is the measurement of bone loss horizontally under the anatomic crown of the tooth. Table 8-3 shows the Glickman Index of horizontal furcation classifications.[53] The vertical component is the measurement of bone loss within the bifurcation or trifurcation vertically from the roof or dome of the furcation (crotch of the tooth) to the current bone level. The vertical component may be difficult to assess if the furcation entrance is covered by soft tissue that obstructs access and vision. Horizontal and vertical bone loss measurements are illustrated in Figure 8-20. The area between the cementoenamel junction and the coronal aspect of the furcation is generally concave or fluted, which makes it particularly susceptible to plaque and calculus accumulation and more difficult for the patient and dental hygienist to access.

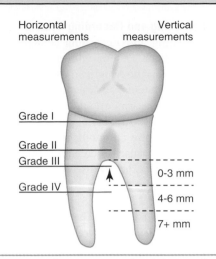

Horizontal   Vertical
measurements   measurements

Grade I

Grade II
Grade III   0-3 mm
Grade IV
                                             4-6 mm

                                             7+ mm

FIGURE 8-20 ■ Assessing furcations using the Glickman Index requires two measurements, a vertical measurement recorded in millimeters from the crotch of the furcation measuring apically to the level of the bone, and a horizontal assessment of the depth of the furcation involvement taken at the level of the bone.

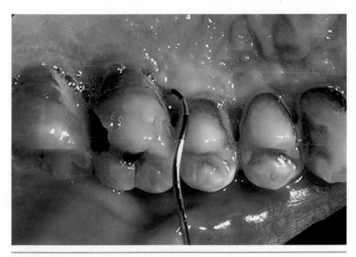

FIGURE 8-21 ■ The curved, calibrated Nabers probe is designed to assess furcations on any tooth surface, including the difficult to assess mesial surface shown.

Probing a furcation area with a traditional periodontal probe can provide an accurate measurement as long as the furcation entrance is visible. A curved, calibrated furcation probe is designed to adapt to furcations universally (Figure 8-21). A furcation should be probed with care. The probe tip can easily penetrate through inflamed epithelial attachment and result in inaccurate measurements. The furcation probe should be guided into the furcation entrance by sliding the probe along the hard surfaces of the tooth to ensure that the probe does not penetrate the attached soft tissues within the furcation.

Once a bifurcation or trifurcation is found during clinical assessment, further investigation should be performed to determine its cause. Radiographic images can be instrumental in this assessment. They help to visualize anatomic abnormalities, defective restorations, or destruction of the periodontium caused by periodontal or endodontic lesions. Teeth with furcation involvement have been shown to be at greater risk for continued bone loss and tooth loss.[43,54]

TABLE 8-4 Tooth Mobility Classification

GRADE	DESCRIPTION
Grade 0	Physiologic mobility only
Grade 1/2	Clinical mobility that is slightly greater than physiologic mobility, but <1 mm buccolingually (can also be assigned as "+")
Grade 1	Slight pathologic mobility, approximately 1 mm buccolingually
Grade 2	Moderate pathologic mobility, approximately 2 mm buccolingually, but no vertical displacement
Grade 3	Sever pathologic mobility, >2 mm buccolingually or mesiodistally, combined with vertical displacement

Tooth Mobility

Tooth mobility can be an indicator of periodontal disease and other pathology. The dental hygienist must be able to distinguish between physiologic mobility and pathologic mobility.

Physiologic Mobility. All teeth have a slight degree of mobility because they are supported by the periodontal ligament. Physiologic mobility may vary in different teeth and at different times of the day.[55]

Pathologic or Abnormal Mobility. Pathologic or abnormal mobility is horizontal or vertical movement of a tooth beyond its physiologic limits. It is caused by factors affecting the periodontal ligament space and loss of alveolar bone. Loss of tooth support can be the result of horizontal or vertical bone loss from periodontal disease or periodontal surgical therapy. The amount of mobility depends on the severity and distribution of the bone loss around each tooth, the length and shape of the roots, and the ratio of the crown-to-root length.[55]

Occlusal Trauma. Occlusal trauma can also cause tooth mobility. Primary occlusal trauma occurs when teeth in a normal periodontium are subjected to excessive occlusal forces that cause pathologic mobility. Abnormal occlusal habits, such as grinding (bruxing) and clenching, are a common cause of tooth mobility. Secondary occlusal trauma occurs when teeth in a compromised periodontium (e.g., teeth exhibiting bone loss from previous episodes of periodontal disease) become mobile because they cannot withstand normal occlusal forces. Occlusal forces are described in Chapter 11.

Inflammatory Changes. Gingival inflammation extending into the periodontal ligament results in changes that can increase tooth mobility, even in the absence of bone loss. Therefore, increased tooth mobility is often seen in patients with gingivitis or periodontal disease. The spread of inflammation from an acute periapical abscess produces a temporary increase in tooth mobility in the absence of periodontal disease. Increased mobility is often seen after traumatic injury to the mouth, surgical periodontal therapy, restoration placement, and endodontic therapy.[55]

Tooth mobility may be associated with any condition that manifests inflammation of the periodontal tissues, including pregnancy or a reaction to an anticonvulsant medication for seizure control. Mobility is graded according to the ease and extent of tooth movement, using the criteria shown in Table 8-4.[56]

Pathologic Migration of Teeth

Pathologic migration is tooth displacement that occurs when the balance among the factors that maintain physiologic tooth position is disturbed. Pathologic migration is commonly associated with periodontal disease. The teeth may move in any direction, and the migration is usually accompanied by mobility and rotation. Pathologic migration in the occlusal or incisal direction is termed *extrusion* or *elongation.*

Pathologic migration may be caused by occlusal forces against weakened periodontal support, primarily bone loss, which renders the teeth unable to maintain normal positions in the arch. The problem arises from lack of periodontal support, not necessarily from abnormal occlusal forces, and is frequently observed in maxillary anterior teeth.[57]

The presence of pathologic migration will also increase with tooth loss. Unreplaced missing teeth may change the occlusal forces, allowing other teeth to drift into the spaces left by their absence. Drifting does not result from destruction of the periodontal tissues, but it creates conditions that can lead to periodontal disease. In the molar region, drifting is primarily in the mesial direction. When the first molar is missing, the premolars may drift distally. With a loss of posterior teeth, most commonly the first molars, the associated posterior bite collapse causes an adverse change in the occlusal forces that may lead to flaring of the anterior teeth.[57]

Pathologic migration leads to spaces between teeth, which are called diastemas or diastemata. The disturbed proximal contact relationships can lead to food impaction, tooth caries, gingival inflammation, and pocket formation, followed by bone loss and tooth mobility. The integrity of proximal contact relationships can also be disturbed by tooth loss, leading to dental caries, difficulty in maintaining oral hygiene, and severe tooth wear. Reduction in periodontal support can lead to further migration of the teeth and occlusal imbalance. Figure 8-22 presents an example of severe pathologic tooth migration.

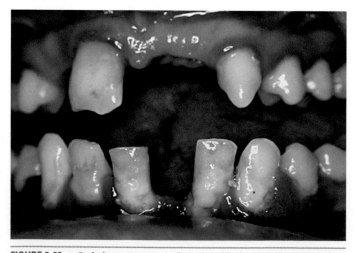

FIGURE 8-22 ■ Pathologic migration of upper and lower incisors accompanied by acute gingival inflammation.

Periodontal Screening and Recording System

Periodontal Screening and Recording (PSR)[58] is a simplified periodontal assessment system endorsed by the American Dental Association and the American Academy of Periodontology. This screening system was designed to promote efficiency in the periodontal assessment and documentation process without compromising the quality of patient care. Although the PSR does not replace the comprehensive periodontal assessment, it is recognized as a useful screening tool that can enhance the identification of periodontal disease.[59]

A specially designed periodontal probe with a ball tip and colored calibrations at 3.5 and 5.5 mm is used to probe the standard six sites on each tooth. The dentition is evaluated by sextants. A PSR code is assigned to each sextant and recorded in the patient record. The code that most accurately describes the most periodontally involved tooth in a sextant is assigned to that sextant. When two or more sextants are scored Code 3, one sextant is scored Code 3 and Code*, or one sextant is scored Code 4, and a comprehensive full mouth periodontal examination and charting should be performed. The PSR system is described in Table 8-5.

Periodontal Considerations of Implants

Dental implants are an increasingly important procedure for the replacement of missing teeth. The dental hygienist plays an integral role in the clinical evaluation of implants and in increasing patients' understanding of their periodontal health. Many

TABLE 8-5	Periodontal Screening and Recording System
CODE	**DESCRIPTION**
Code 0	Colored area of probe remains completely visible in the deepest crevice in the sextant. • No calculus or defective margins are detected. • Gingival tissues are healthy, with no bleeding on probing.
Code 1	Colored area of probe remains completely visible in the deepest probing depth in the sextant. • No calculus or defective margins are detected. • There is bleeding on probing.
Code 2	Colored area of probe remains completely visible in the deepest probing depth in the sextant. • Supragingival or subgingival calculus is detected or defective margins are detected.
Code 3	Colored area of the probe remains partly visible in the deepest probing area in the sextant.
Code 4	Colored area of the probe completely disappears, indicating probing depth > 5.5 mm.
Code *	The symbol * is added to the sextant score whenever findings indicate clinical abnormalities such as the following: • Furcation invasion • Mobility • Mucogingival problems • Recession extending to the colored area of the probe (3.5 mm or greater

Adapted with permission from the American Academy of Periodontology, Chicago, IL, and the American Dental Association, Chicago, IL. Periodontal Screening and Recording and PSR are service marks and trademarks of the American Dental Association.

of the clinical parameters used to assess the periodontium are also used to evaluate dental implants; however, the interpretation differs.

The clinical assessment of implants includes an evaluation of the soft tissue and supporting structures surrounding an implant. An implant is considered to have **peri-implant mucositis** when there is inflammation of the soft tissue surrounding the implant. However, when inflammation progresses to include a loss of the peri-implant bone, it is considered to be **peri-implantitis**. Patients with a history of periodontitis have been reported to be at greater risk of peri-implantitis.[60]

The first step in the implant assessment process is to indicate the presence and location of implants on the dental records. As with the natural dentition, plaque biofilms are the primary causative agents in peri-implant gingival inflammation, and they are associated with implant failure.[61,62] Therefore, the presence and location of plaque biofilm and calculus should also be documented. As with natural teeth, it is important to evaluate gingival color, contour, consistency, and texture. The gingival tissue surrounding the implant may be keratinized or nonkeratinized, depending on the implant recipient tissue. Increased redness and a smoother texture may be associated with healthy nonkeratinized gingival tissues.

Peri-implant probing is an essential step in assessing implant health. Probing should be performed using a standard periodontal probe and applying light pressure. In healthy implants, probing depth will measure the apical extent of the barrier epithelium and the height of the marginal bone can be expected to be approximately 1 mm apical to the location of the probe tip. When the peri-implant tissue is inflamed, the probe will penetrate into the connective tissue.[63]

Successful healthy implants generally have probing depths of approximately 3 to 4 mm; probing depths of 6 mm or greater are an indication of peri-implantitis.[62] The maintenance of baseline probing depths is an indication of peri-implant stability. An increase in peri-implant probing depths is a sign of bone loss. To measure such changes accurately, the assessment of probe depths requires that measurements be taken in relation to a fixed reference point on the implant or prosthesis. Documentation of the fixed reference point is required to permit repeated assessments of attachment level, which is essential for evaluating progressive attachment loss. The anatomic shape of some implants, or the associated restorations, can complicate insertion and angling of the periodontal probe. Although it may not be possible to access all surfaces for proper probing, a minimum of one surface needs to be consistently monitored.[63]

CLINICAL NOTE 8-10 Healthy implants maintain their probing depths after initial healing.

A higher diagnostic value is attached to bleeding on probing of implants than on probing of teeth.[62] Bleeding on probing is an indicator of inflammation in the peri-implant mucosa and a predictor for the loss of implant support. The presence of clinically visible suppuration is also a sign of likely infection and progressive peri-implantitis. The presence of bleeding on probing and suppuration should be routinely assessed and

recorded. Many restorations are cemented on to the implant, and residual cement has been reported to lead to peri-implant disease.[64]

Implants with clinically detectable mobility have a lack of osseointegration and are considered to have failed.[63] Implant mobility is measured with the same technique as prescribed for mobility testing of the natural dentition.[65] Radiographic imaging evaluation of implants is also recommended to monitor bone height, with baseline radiographs taken at the time of restoration and subsequently with signs of peri-implantitis.[63] Also, note that implants placed in the maxilla have been reported to have a slightly higher incidence of failure.[66] Recognized systemic, environmental, or behavioral risk factors, including poor oral hygiene, history of periodontitis, diabetes, history of head and neck radiation treatment, smoking, implant overload, poor-fitting superstructure, and bruxism, can also lead to implant failure.[60,63,66,67]

Documentation of Periodontal Assessment

The patient record provides a continuous historical accounting of the patient's oral health status and the delivery of oral health care services. The format of the patient record will vary with each clinical setting; however, it must be comprehensive and systematic to provide the information necessary for the diagnosis, planning, implementation, and evaluation of dental and dental hygiene care. A paper-based periodontal charting record is shown in Figure 8-23. Computerized charting and electronic patient records are becoming increasingly common. They contain all the elements of the paper-based charts and have the advantage of assisting the dental hygienist in comparing data over time.

CLINICAL NOTE 8-11 All patients require regular comprehensive periodontal assessments to detail their status, provide a historical accounting, and alert the dental hygienist to evidence of disease activity.

DENTITION ASSESSMENT

The dentition assessment includes a clinical evaluation of the teeth for caries, restoration status, presence of implants, proximal contact relationships, anomalies of form, evidence of parafunctional habits, tooth wear conditions, and tooth sensitivity. This assessment should follow an established sequence to ensure that the evaluation is comprehensive. These observations help identify underlying systemic, environmental, or behavioral contributing factors that may be of concern, such as xerostomia or methamphetamine use.[68-70]

Caries

Caries assessment includes visual, tactile, and radiographic image assessments. Locations of carious lesions and visual changes in the dentition, such as white spot lesions, must be noted. Tactile changes in teeth range from actual cavitation of pits and fissures or smooth surfaces to the tacky, sticky, or leathery sensations of root surfaces. Carious lesions appear as radiolucent areas in the tooth structure on images. Transillumination is now sometimes used to identify fractures or other alterations in the surface layers of tooth structure.

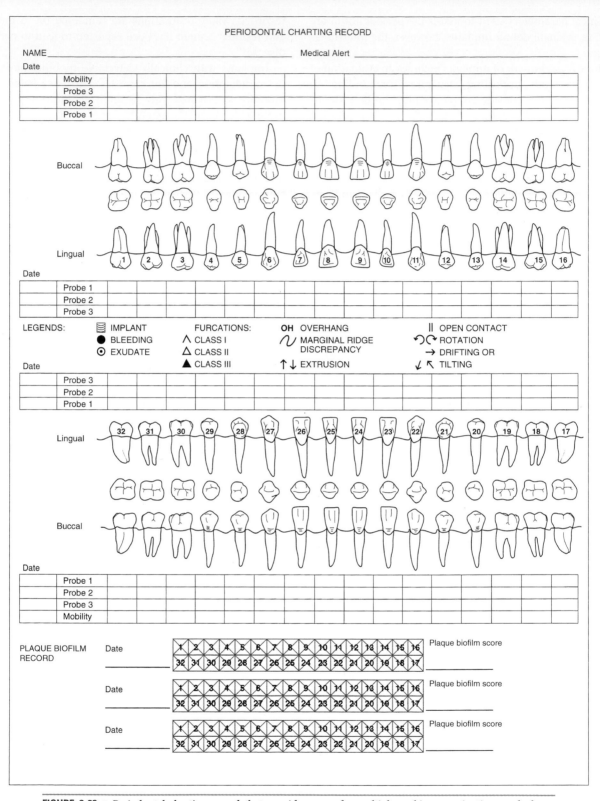

FIGURE 8-23 ■ **Periodontal charting record that provides space for multiple probing examinations and plaque biofilm assessment.** This type of record permits easy comparison of probe depths, recession to compute clinical attachment loss, and plaque biofilm scores over a series of appointments.

Because of their periodontal structural implications, root surface caries are of particular concern in periodontal assessment. These lesions provide a reservoir for bacteria that can contribute to further caries and periodontal inflammation. Root surface caries are usually associated with age and gingival recession.[71] Color changes in the root surface range from yellow to dark brown or black. Incipient lesions may be yellow or light tan, round or oval, and slightly soft, without cavitation or pain. Root surface lesions may rapidly progress and completely encircle the tooth, making restoration difficult. Lesions in remission appear black or dark brown and are more leathery in texture than the surrounding normal cementum. Table 8-6 presents

TABLE 8-6 Black's Cavity Classification

CLASS	DESCRIPTION
Class 1	Pit and fissure cavities • Occlusal surfaces of premolars and molars • Occlusal two thirds of facials and linguals on molars • Lingual surface of maxillary incisors
Class 2	Proximal cavities in premolars and molars
Class 3	Proximal cavities in incisors and canines (does not involve incisal angle)
Class 4	Proximal cavities in incisors and canines (involves incisal angle)
Class 5	Gingival third cavities (does not include pit and fissure cavities)
Class 6	Incisal edge and cusp tip cavities

Used with permission from Black GV. *Operative Dentistry.* 8th ed. Woodstock, IL: Medico-Dental Publishing; 1947-1948.

TABLE 8-7 Severity of Root Caries Index by Newbrun

GRADE	DESCRIPTION
Grade I Incipient	Surface texture is soft, can be penetrated with a dental explorer No surface defect or cavitation Pigmentation from light tan to brown
Grade II Shallow	Surface texture is soft, irregular and rough; can be penetrated by a dental explorer Surface defect < 0.5 mm deep Pigmentation ranges from tan to dark brown
Grade III Cavitation	Surface texture is soft; can be penetrated with a dental explorer Penetrating lesion with cavitation that is >0.5 mm; no pulpal involvement Pigmentation from brown to dark brown
Grade IV Pulpal	Deeply penetrating lesion with pulpal involvement Pigmentation from brown to dark brown

Adapted by permission from Newbrun E. Problems in caries diagnosis. *Int Dent J.* 1993;43:133-142.

Black's cavity classification[72] and Table 8-7 shows the classification for assessing and documenting the severity of root surface caries described by Newbrun.[73]

Restoration Status

Assessment of restoration status should include documentation of existing restorations, poorly contoured restorations, removable prosthetic appliances, and implants. This documentation is essential in the collection of baseline data for comprehensive treatment planning and medicolegal liability protection. The restoration status should be updated periodically to support ongoing treatment planning and to evaluate treatment outcomes.

Overhanging restorations, open contacts with food impaction, undercontoured restorations, and poorly fitting crown margins are of particular concern in periodontal assessment because of their direct effect on periodontal health and therapy.

Several studies have confirmed that overhanging dental restorations contribute to increased gingival inflammation, attachment loss, and bone loss. Despite major advances in restorative material technology, overhangs continue to be created, are not always clinically detected, and are not always removed when obviously evident in radiographs.[74] Patients are often unaware of poor margins and their detrimental effects. The dental hygienist should document these findings and, with the dentist, encourage the patient to undergo treatment for these problems. Restorative considerations are described in detail in Chapter 5.

Proximal Contact Relationships

The dental assessment should include an evaluation of proximal contact relationships. Open contacts permit food impaction that may affect periodontal health. Tight contacts may discourage patient compliance with interproximal plaque biofilm removal. Therefore, the tightness of contacts should be assessed to aid in the development of a plan of care and patient education. Proximal contacts are usually most effectively evaluated with dental floss. Proximal contact relationships can change over time based on physiologic or pathologic tooth migration, marginal ridge defects, or parafunctional habits. The identification and correction of proximal contact deficiencies can prevent periodontal deterioration and dental caries or help resolve periodontal inflammation that has already developed.

Anomalies of Tooth Form

Some developmental anomalies directly affect periodontal health and therapy—for example, the enamel projections shown in Figure 8-24. These anomalies include enamel and dentinal defects and anatomic formations that promote plaque biofilm retention, inhibit plaque biofilm removal, and influence the selection of therapy.

Parafunctional Habits

Parafunctional habits subject the teeth to forces outside the normal scope of functional occlusion. These include tooth to tooth contact, contact between teeth and soft tissue, and contact between teeth and foreign objects. All can result in damage to the periodontal and tooth structures and soft tissues of the oral cavity. Common parafunctional habits are clenching, grinding; biting or chewing of the cheeks, lips, tongue, or fingernails, and using the teeth to hold foreign objects, such as office supplies, personal care products, occupational tools, and food or food containers. These habits can cause traumatic damage to the dentition, such as broken cusps, defective restorations, dental attrition and abrasion, and craze lines and cracks.[75]

Tooth Wear

Tooth wear is the loss of tooth structure caused by chronic destructive processes other than dental caries. These destructive processes include abrasion, abfraction, attrition, and erosion. Determining the cause of tooth wear lesions is critical for the prevention of their progression, but may be complicated by a combination of destructive processes and oral hygiene, demographic, nutritional, health, occupational, and lifestyle factors. In addition to clinical examination, patient interviews may help to identify circumstances that contribute to tooth destruction. Documentation of the presence of tooth wear lesions, the extent

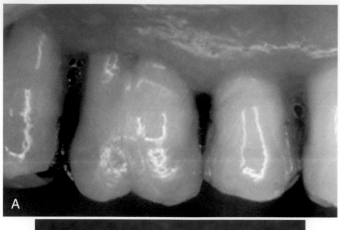

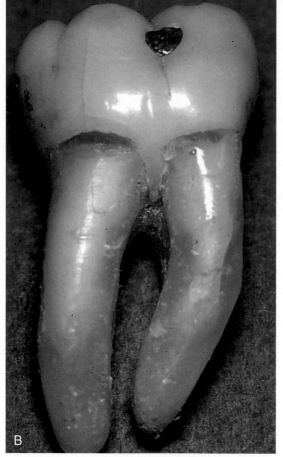

FIGURE 8-24 ■ **A,** Enamel projections. An enamel projection on the buccal surface of an upper first molar predisposes the patient to periodontal disease because there is no epithelial attachment on enamel. **B,** An enamel projection extends into the furcation, interfering with epithelial attachment and furcation health. (Courtesy of Dr. Gary C. Armitage, University of California, San Francisco, School of Dentistry, Division of Periodontology).

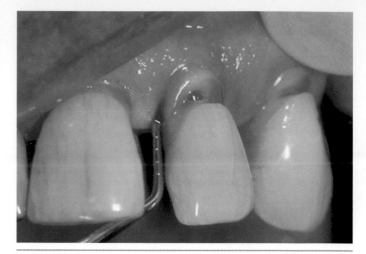

FIGURE 8-25 ■ Abrasion and abfraction (notching) of buccal root surfaces.

- Brushing technique, typically horizontal scrubbing
- Frequency and amount of time spent brushing
- Forces applied during brushing
- Type and hardness of toothbrush bristles
- Acidity of the oral cavity caused by acidic foods and beverages, regurgitation, and acid reflux
- Dentifrice abrasiveness and amount

Figure 8-25 shows abrasion and abfraction. Personal habits, such as fingernail or thread biting and holding foreign objects with the teeth, such as a pipe stem, may cause abrasions.

Abfraction. Abfraction is a term used to describe cervical V- or wedge-shaped lesions that are generally located apical to the cementoenamel junction in incisors and premolars. These lesions can be located on a single tooth or on nonadjacent teeth and are thought to be caused by microfractures in enamel and dentin that are linked to large, eccentric occlusal loads. For example, during bruxism, the changing back and forth direction of the occlusal forces bends the tooth, causing side to side fatigue and small fractures at the most flexed area in the cervical region of the tooth. The etiology of abfraction lesions is also considered multifactorial because these lesions can progress as a result of toothbrush abrasion and other tooth wear conditions.[78,79]

Attrition. Attrition occurs primarily on the occlusal and incisal surfaces of the teeth as wear from tooth to tooth functional contact. However, attrition can occur on any surface exposed to tooth to tooth contact, as on the buccal and lingual surfaces of anterior teeth in a deep overbite relationship, as seen in Figure 8-26. Parafunctional attrition is often related to excessive grinding motions. The tooth wear results in matching wear patterns between the opposing tooth surfaces. Reduced salivary flow may contribute to tooth wear as a result of increased tooth to tooth friction.[79]

Erosion. Erosion is the loss of enamel and dentin, primarily by the chemical action of acids other than those produced by oral bacteria. Dietary and gastric acids are the most common causes of dental erosion. Dietary erosion is most commonly observed as moderate generalized erosion of the cervical, buccal, and lingual surfaces of the maxillary teeth and the occlusal and buccal surfaces of the mandibular teeth, as shown in Figure 8-27. Gastric erosion is commonly observed on the

of destruction, and contributing factors is essential to the development of an appropriate plan of care and prevention.[76]

Abrasion. Abrasion is the wearing away of tooth structures, usually on the buccal, incisal, and occlusal surfaces as a result of excessive abrasive forces by a foreign object. Buccal lesions are most typically attributed to oral hygiene habits, may be more frequent in premolars, and are concavities and notches at or apical to the cementoenamel junction.[77] Factors that may influence toothbrush abrasion include the following:

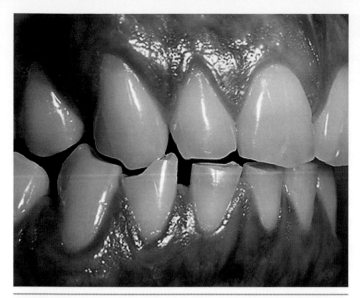

FIGURE 8-26 ■ This patient exhibits extreme tooth wear from tooth to tooth contact. Note that the maxillary teeth fit precisely into the notching on the mandibular teeth.

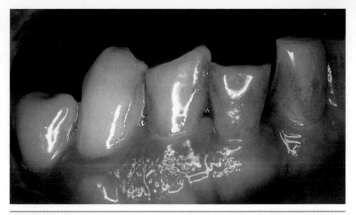

FIGURE 8-27 ■ Severe incisal erosion caused by tooth to tooth contact in the anterior teeth.

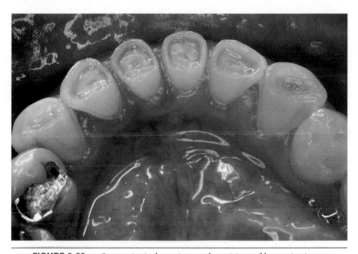

FIGURE 8-28 ■ Severe incisal erosion and attrition of lower incisors.

lingual aspects of the anterior and posterior maxillary teeth, buccal aspects of the mandibular posterior teeth, and occlusal aspects of the mandibular and maxillary posterior teeth, which may initially appear as a cupping of the cusp tips. Dietary analysis of the consumption, frequency, and duration of exposure to acidic foods and beverages may help to identify the cause of erosion. Acidic food and beverage sources include fruit, foods containing vinegar, carbonated drinks containing citric acid, phosphoric acid, or carbonic acid, acidic sports drinks, herbal tea, wine, and acidic foods such as yogurt, which contains high amounts of calcium and phosphate.[80-82]

Patients may be challenging to educate about erosion because they feel that their diet is part of a healthy lifestyle and because regurgitation from vomiting caused by health conditions such as anorexia nervosa, bulimia, gastroesophageal reflux disease, obesity, and other chronic conditions is difficult to treat. Figure 8-28 shows extreme incisal edge erosion. Toothbrushing immediately after eating highly acidic foods will exacerbate erosive tooth wear. Tooth-bleaching products may also contribute to erosion of already exposed dentin.[83]

Medications should not be overlooked as a potential cause of dental erosion. Medications can have the effect of reducing the pH of the oral environment, inducing vomiting, or decreasing salivary flow and its buffering capacity. Drug abuse of substances such as cocaine and amphetamines can also accelerate tooth wear conditions.[84]

Conventional tooth wear conditions are described as ditching, notching, or flattening of the tooth structure. Less common tooth wear conditions include cupping of the incisal or occlusal surfaces, projection of restorations above the tooth surface, and reduction of tooth length that results in a disproportional width-to-length ratio, as described in Table 8-8. Tooth wear conditions and patterns can be documented on the dental chart, described narratively in the record, or recorded with intraoral photographs or study casts. The Basic Erosive Wear Examination (BEWE) was designed as a simple index for use in the dental practice.[85] With the BEWE, the dental provider scores the most severely affected tooth in each sextant. The scoring criteria for the BEWE are presented in Table 8-9. The scores for all sextants are then summed to provide a general index of a patient's tooth wear condition. The risk levels for the BEWE have been described as follows:

- None = cumulative score of 0 to 2
- Low = cumulative score of 3 to 8
- Medium = cumulative score of 9 to 13
- High = cumulative score of more than 14

Tooth wear increases with age. With an aging population that is retaining its dentition for a lifetime, the complications associated with tooth wear will likely increase and benefit from documentation and monitoring.[86]

Dentinal Sensitivity or Hypersensitivity

Patients frequently report pain or sensitivity related to their teeth; this is known as dentinal sensitivity. In order to develop an understanding of the source or origin of the sensitivity, it is critical to gather information from the patient about what causes the pain. The most common stimuli are: thermal, mechanical, and chemical.[87,88] Table 8-10 describes common conditions associated with these stimuli. Sensitive areas with their associated stimuli and dental conditions should be noted in the patient record and considered in the overall treatment plan.

TABLE 8-8 Summary of Tooth Wear Conditions

TOOTH WEAR CONDITION	LOCATION	CLINCIAL DESCRIPTION	PATIENT CHIEF COMPLAINT	ETIOLOGY
Abrasion	Buccal surface at cementoenamel junction Incisal and occlusal surfaces	Wedge-shaped defects, concavities, or notches Ditches, notches, or indentations	Sensitivity to brushing, temperature, sweets and/or tactile pressure Aesthetic concerns	Mechanical process from foreign object, often a toothbrush Commonly related to oral habits with foreign objects
Abfraction	Cervical surfaces (mostly buccal) Usually in incisors and premolars	V- or wedge-shaped lesions with sharp edges that are greater in depth than width Generally supragingival	Hot and cold sensitivity Pain when biting Food trap	Mechanical process from tooth flexure by eccentric occlusal bruxing
Attrition	Incisal or occlusal surfaces Buccal and lingual surfaces	Flattening or well-defined wear facets Wear facets and ledges	Hot and cold sensitivity Sweets Tooth pain on incisal or occlusal edges when biting	Mechanical process involving tooth to tooth contact May be related to deep overbite, crossbite, or other functional contact
Erosion	Cervical and buccal surfaces of maxillary teeth; occlusal and buccal surfaces of mandibular teeth (dietary erosion)	Early lesions: wide, shallow, silky smooth concavities that are greater in width than depth	Temperature and tactile sensitivity, increased staining in the wear lesions	Chemical actions of acids other than those produced by oral bacteria, mostly dietary and gastric acids
	Lingual surfaces of anterior and posterior maxillary teeth, buccal surfaces of mandibular posterior teeth, and occlusal surfaces of mandibular and maxillary posterior teeth (gastric erosion)	Advanced lesions: dentin involvement, restorations rising above adjacent tooth structure, cupping of cusp tips	Temperature and tactile sensitivity, increased staining in the wear lesions	Chemical actions of acids other than those produced by oral bacteria, mostly dietary and gastric acids

TABLE 8-9 Basic Erosive Wear Examination

SCORING CRITERIA FOR GRADING EROSIVE WEAR

0 = No erosive tooth wear
1 = Initial loss of surface texture
2 = Distinct defect, hard tissue loss < 50% of the surface area*
3 = Hard tissue loss > 50% of the surface area*

*In scores 2 and 3, dentin often is involved.
From Bartlett D, Ganss C, Lussi A. Basic Erosive Wear Examination: A new scoring system for scientific and clinical needs. *Clin Oral Invest.* 2008;12:565-568.

RADIOGRAPHIC IMAGING

Radiographic images are an essential adjunct to the clinical examination. They play an integral role in assessing the destruction associated with periodontal disease. Because of the episodic nature of periodontal disease, radiographic images may permit comparison of changes over time in periodontal status, but they are indicators of past, not active, disease.

RADIOGRAPHIC ASSESSMENT
Radiographic Image Surveys of the Periodontium
Radiographic image surveys include horizontal and vertical bitewing radiographs, panoramic radiographs, and periapical images. The bitewing image is particularly valuable because of its ability to represent the bone height of the interdental septa.

TABLE 8-10 Stimuli and Conditions Associated with Dentinal Sensitivity

STIMULUS	CONDITIONS ASSOCIATED WITH DENTINAL SENSITIVITY
Thermal Cold	Recent restoration, defective restoration, dental caries, cracked tooth syndrome, endodontic lesion, tooth wear conditions, recession, periodontal therapy (e.g., scaling, root planing, surgery), occlusal trauma (e.g., high restoration)
Hot	Recent restoration, endodontic lesion
Mechanical (e.g., toothbrush, fingernail, dental instruments, such as explorers, probes, and scalers)	Tooth wear conditions (e.g., toothbrush abrasion), recent periodontal therapy, dental caries, defective restoration, recession (or contact with unexposed root structure)
Chemical (e.g., acidic dietary source, gastric acid, tooth bleaching)	Tooth wear conditions, dental caries, defective restoration, recession

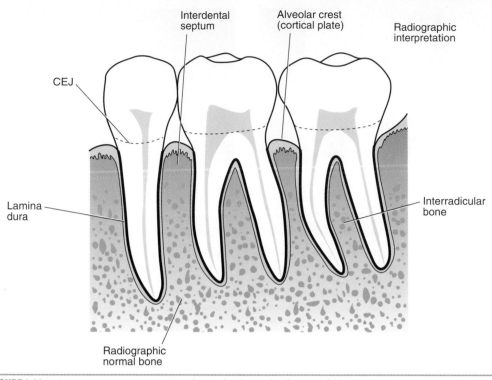

Interdental septum

Alveolar crest (cortical plate)

Radiographic interpretation

CEJ

Lamina dura

Interradicular bone

Radiographic normal bone

FIGURE 8-29 ■ Diagrammatic representation of normal radiographic features of the periodontium. CEJ, Cementoenamel junction.

With proper technique, the x-ray beam is perpendicular to the bone, long axis of the tooth, and film or sensor plane, thus minimizing distortion. When a nonperpendicular beam is used, the result is elongation or foreshortening of the image, causing an inaccurate appearance of an increase or decrease in the bone level. The cusp tips are a good guide; when the buccal and lingual cusp tips are level, the x-ray beam was probably correctly angled.[89] Horizontal bitewings are adequate for the assessment of bone height in patients without periodontal disease; however, vertical bitewings are necessary to capture an image of the existing bone in patients with moderate to advanced periodontal disease. In comparison with periapical radiographs, bitewing radiographs limit the patient's radiation exposure because fewer images are required for the survey.

All radiographic image surveys should be logged in the patient record and be accompanied by a documented interpretation of the patient's radiographically evident periodontal status. The assessment value of radiographic images is enhanced when the exposure, projection technique, and processing of radiographs are standardized.

CLINICAL NOTE 8-12 Radiographic image assessment of bone loss reflects the history of periodontal disease and does not assess disease activity.

Radiographic Appearance of the Periodontium

The radiographic evaluation of bone changes associated with periodontal disease is primarily based on the appearance of the interdental septa. In conventional radiographs, the buccal and lingual alveolar crests are obscured by the relatively dense root structure, limiting their use in assessing the patient's periodontal status on the buccal and lingual surfaces. The interdental septum normally has a thin radiopaque border, adjacent to the

periodontal ligament space, referred to as the lamina dura. This radiopaque image appears continuous with the alveolar crest, which is the shadow of the cortical plate at the crest of the septum. This border appears radiographically as a continuous white line; however, anatomically, it is perforated by numerous small foramina that contain blood vessels, lymphatics, and nerves passing between the periodontal ligament and the bone. It represents the bone lining the tooth socket. The periodontal ligament space appears as a thin radiolucent line between the lamina dura and tooth root. Figure 8-29 illustrates the radiographic features of the periodontium.

The width and shape of the interdental septum and the angle of the alveolar crest normally vary according to the convexity of the proximal tooth surfaces and the level of the cementoenamel junctions of the approximating teeth. The interdental septa between teeth with prominently convex proximal surfaces in the posterior teeth are wider anteroposteriorly than are those between teeth with relatively flat proximal surfaces found in anterior teeth. The buccolingual diameter of the bone is related to the proximal root width. The alveolar crest generally runs parallel to a line between the cementoenamel junctions of the approximating teeth. When there is a difference in the levels of the cementoenamel junctions through variation in the degree or inclination of eruption of adjacent teeth, the alveolar crest is angulated rather than horizontal, as illustrated in Figure 8-30.

Radiographic Changes with Periodontal Disease

Interdental Septa. In periodontal disease, the interdental septa undergo changes that affect the radiodensity of the crestal cortical plate, the size and shape of the medullary spaces, and the height and contour of the bone. When the inflammation process is permitted to progress, fuzziness, loss of radiopacity,

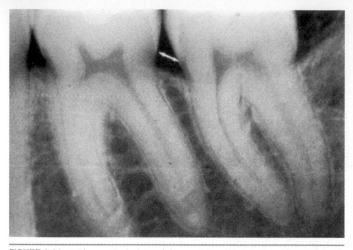

FIGURE 8-30 ■ The cortical plate of the crest usually appears radiographically as a horizontal line running between and slightly apical to the cementoenamel junctions of adjacent teeth. It may appear angled between teeth *(arrow)* and result in deeper probe depths if the cementoenamel junctions of adjacent teeth are not level. This appearance is a variation of normal. The radiograph has been cropped to emphasize the periodontal condition of the teeth. (Used with permission from Carranza F, Newman M. *Glickman's Clinical Periodontology.* 8th ed. Philadelphia, PA: WB Saunders; 1996.)

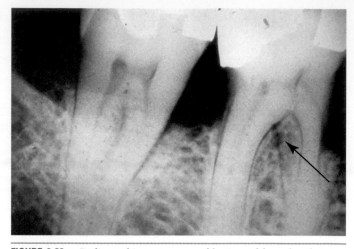

FIGURE 8-32 ■ **Radiographic appearance of horizontal bone loss between two molars.** The crestal cortical plate is absent and some wedge-shaped bone loss is apparent next to the tooth roots. The *arrow* points to an area of furcation involvement. The radiograph has been cropped to emphasize the periodontal condition of the teeth.

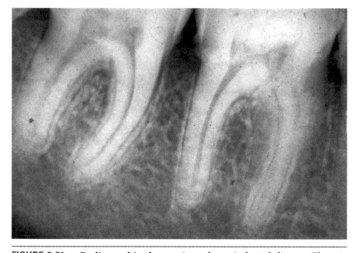

FIGURE 8-31 ■ **Radiographic changes in early periodontal disease.** There is fuzziness in the lamina dura and an indistinct crest of the interdental septa. The radiograph has been cropped to emphasize the periodontal condition of the teeth.

and breaks in the continuity of the crestal plate and the lamina dura at the mesial and distal aspect of the alveolar crest may occur. This is illustrated in Figure 8-31, which demonstrates the early radiographic signs of periodontal disease progression. Subsequent formation of wedge-shaped radiolucent areas at the mesial and distal aspects of the crest of the interdental septum are observed, as seen in Figure 8-32. The apices of these triangulated areas point apically in the direction of the affected roots. These areas are produced by resorption of the bone of the lateral aspect of the interdental septum and an associated widening of the periodontal ligament space. As periodontal disease progresses, the height of the interdental septum is reduced by the extension of inflammation and the resorption of bone.

The measurement between the cementoenamel junction and crestal cortical plate is critical for assessing the extent of bone loss. The measurement of normal crestal bone height ranges from 0.5 to 2 mm from the cementoenamel junction.[90] When the alveolar crest appears to be approximately parallel to the line drawn between the cementoenamel junctions of adjacent teeth, reduction in height of the interdental septum is known as horizontal bone loss. An example is shown in Figure 8-33. Horizontal alveolar bone loss has been shown to be a normal physiologic response to aging. Therefore, even in periodontally healthy patients, small amounts of bone loss may be observed. When the crest no longer appears parallel to the line formed by the adjacent cementoenamel junctions, the reduction in bone height is known as vertical or angular bone loss. The bone loss is observed to progress vertically along the root to form an angular defect. Vertical bone loss is more common in the posterior than in the anterior periodontium.[91] This type of defect is shown in Figure 8-34.

Furcations. Furcation involvement may be detected by radiographic assessment of the interradicular bone, as seen in Figure 8-34. However, furcation involvements that can be detected clinically are often not seen in radiographs. An example of this is presented in Figure 8-35. The anatomic location of the furcation involvement and variations in radiographic technique may obscure the radiographic image of a furcation. It is not uncommon for one film to show significant involvement, whereas another film of the same tooth shows no involvement because of differences in projection and exposure. To assist in the detection of furcation involvement, the following criteria are suggested:

1. The slightest radiographic change of the periodontal ligament space in the furcation area should be investigated clinically for definitive diagnosis.
2. Diminished radiodensity in the furcation area, as shown by visible outlines of bony trabeculae, suggests furcation involvement.
3. Whenever there is marked bone loss in relation to one root of a molar, it may be assumed that the furcation is also involved.

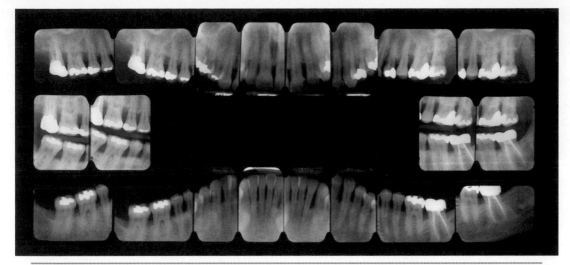

FIGURE 8-33 ■ A full-mouth radiographic survey of a patient with moderate periodontal disease characterized by generalized horizontal bone loss.

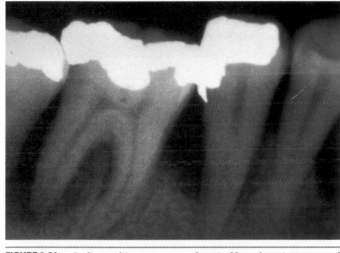

FIGURE 8-34 ■ **Radiographic appearance of vertical bone loss.** A pronounced vertical defect appears between the mandibular second premolar and the first molar. The radiograph has been cropped to emphasize the periodontal condition of the teeth.

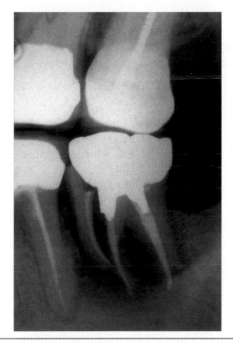

FIGURE 8-36 ■ Endodontically treated second molar with a separated vertical root fracture.

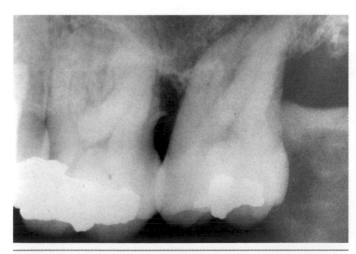

FIGURE 8-35 ■ **Radiographic appearance of maxillary molar furcations.** The absence of bone on the distal surfaces requires a careful assessment of furcation involvement. Buccal furcations are not obvious. The radiograph has been cropped to emphasize the periodontal condition of the teeth.

Root Fractures

Root fractures may be horizontal or vertical in direction and may or may not be detected by radiographic assessment.

Horizontal root fractures appear on images as radiolucent lines running horizontally across the root. Vertical root fractures are commonly associated with endodontically and prosthetically restored posterior teeth.[92] They are often difficult to see on images unless there is separation of the fractured fragments, as seen in Figure 8-36. In the absence of an obvious separation, other radiographic observations may include a periapical and perilateral radiolucency, also called the halo appearance, and a lateral periodontal radiolucency of the root, as seen in Figure 8-37.[93] Without such separation, radiographic

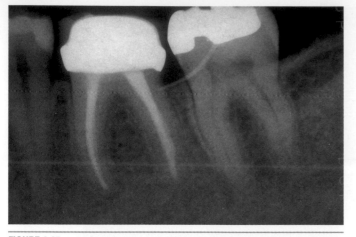

FIGURE 8-37 ■ Radiopaque gutta percha point has been placed in a clinically visible sinus tract exhibiting a small amount of suppuration. The gutta percha points toward the distal root at bone level where a vertical root fracture begins. There is crestal bone loss at the coronal-most point of the vertical root fracture.

signs of bone loss may need to be supplemented by clinical examinations such as probing depth. The probing depth associated with vertical fractures often presents as narrow (1 to 3 mm in width) and deep (8 to 10 mm in length), and may not present with obvious mucosal signs of gingival inflammation.

Root Resorption. Root resorption is a condition that is most often clinically asymptomatic and is discovered during the radiographic assessment. Root resorption can occur after a traumatic injury to the tooth, chronic inflammation of the pulp, or periodontal ligament irritation. It is the result of the stimulation of the osteoclast cells by infection or pressure.[94]

There are two types of periodontal-related root resorption, described in Table 8-11. When root resorption is identified, it is important that an accurate diagnosis be made because the treatment modalities vary depending on the nature of the resorption. To facilitate diagnosis and treatment planning, the radiographic assessment should facilitate the review of the factors outlined in Table 8-12. Figure 8-38 illustrates external and internal root resorption.

TABLE 8-11   Types of Periodontal-Related Root Resorbtion[67]

EXTERNAL RESORPTION	INTERNAL RESORPTION
Direction of the root resorption is from the outside to the inside, generally at the level of the connective tissue attachment.	Direction of the root resorption is from the inside to the outside, beginning at any location within the pulp.
Causes of external resorption include trauma, orthodontic treatment, periodontal disease treatment, dentoalveolar surgery, or other circumstances that impose increased pressure on the periodontal attachment structures.	Causes of internal resorption include pulpal trauma and inflammation resulting from events such as injury to a tooth, orthodontic treatment, and intracoronal bleaching.
Frequently asymptomatic to the patient unless it has extended to invade the pulp canal.	Frequently asymptomatic to the patient depending on the level of inflammation in the pulp or the perforation of the lesion into the periodontal ligament.
Clinically, the resorption lesion will generally exhibit rough asymmetrical margins just below the epithelial attachment. When probing at the site of an undiagnosed lesion, there can be a sudden dropping of the probe tip into the lesion just apical to the crown; what is identified with the increased probe depth is a resorption lesion as opposed to a periodontal pocket. Another form of external resorption is called an invasive cervical resorption, which in many ways will mimic an internal resorption that has perforated the periodontal ligament.	Clinically, the resorption lesion will generally exhibit symmetrical, smooth, well defined margins. Pink tooth is also a possible clinical observation. These lesions occur most frequently in anterior teeth, males, and the middle third of the tooth.

TABLE 8-12   Radiographic Appearance of Periodontal-Related Root Resorption[67]

EXTERNAL RESORPTION (see Figure 8-38A)	INTERNAL RESORPTION (see Figure 8-38B)
Variations in density lead to a moth-eaten appearance. In contrast, an invasive cervical resorptive lesion will radiographically mimic an internal resorptive lesion by presenting with a uniform radiolucency and smooth regular outline.	Will present with a uniform radiolucency.
The nerve canal is unaltered, which may be evidenced by the ability to see the pulp canal through the resorptive defect. Lesions that progress untreated can lead to an eventual invasion of the pulp canal, in which case it becomes increasingly difficult to distinguish between external and internal resorption.	The nerve canal will increase in size as the resorptive lesion progresses due to chronic inflammation.
The relationship of the pulp canal to the resorptive lesion will shift as the x-ray beam is reangled. Therefore, an additional periapical radiograph may be particularly useful in diagnosis of the type of root resorption a patient presents.	An internal resorptive lesion is within the pulp canal; therefore, additional periapical radiographs will show an unaltered relationship of the canal to the defect.

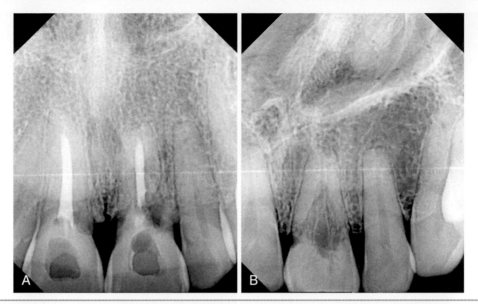

FIGURE 8-38 ■ **External and internal root resorption.** Root resorption is often severe by the time it is seen on radiographic images. **A,** External resorption appears as a moth-eaten, or extremely thin root surface with ragged edges. It is often visible only on one side of the tooth in the image and surrounding teeth may appear unaffected. **B,** Internal resorption appears on images as a hollowed out area of the root.

Limitations of Radiographic Assessment of Periodontal Disease

Even slight changes observed in radiographic images mean that periodontal disease has progressed beyond the earliest stages.[95] This is because images are two-dimensional representations of three-dimensional structures, so they do not reflect the complete extent of bone loss, especially on the buccal and lingual surfaces of teeth. Importantly, images do not show the internal morphologic features of bone or the depth of the crater-like interdental defects that appear as angular or vertical defects. It is possible to have deep bony craters between the buccal and lingual plates without any indication of their presence on images.

Radiographic Assessment of Dental Implants

The radiographic assessment of dental implants includes examination of the presence of peri-implant radiolucencies and the height of the marginal bone. The accuracy of this assessment depends on the diagnostic quality of the images. Diagnostic quality is enhanced with the use of the paralleling technique, in which the x-ray beam is perpendicular to the film or sensor plane and implant. As with the natural dentition, only proximal bone levels can be distinguished because of the superimposition of the buccal and lingual cortical plates and the implant. The bony destruction associated with peri-implantitis appears as saucer-shaped defects on images because the lesion extends the full circumference of the implant. These defects must be verified by periodontal probing of the implant.[96]

Marginal bone height is the measurement between the marginal bone and an established reference point on the implant (e.g., the implant abutment junction, the top of the abutment, or the implant threads). Bone loss of 0.5 to 1.5 mm may be observed in the first year after connection of the abutment to the implant. An annual loss of 0.05 to 0.2 mm may be observed in subsequent years. The intervals for radiographic assessment of implants should be based on the clinical assessment.[97] Figure 8-39 presents a radiographic survey of a single implant over an 11-year period.

Advancements in Imaging Assessment of Periodontal Disease

Advances in imaging techniques have been pursued to respond to the recognized deficiencies of conventional radiography. Of particular note for the diagnosis of periodontal disease is digital subtraction radiography (DSR).[98] DSR measures changes in bone density over time and therefore requires two standardized images with similar projection geometry and exposure parameters. Structures that have not changed in the time between the two radiographs are subtracted from the image. The remaining visible structure is the bone loss or gain appearing on a neutral background. DSR can reduce the delay between the destruction of bone and its detection on images by more efficiently using captured information. It may also be used to assess regeneration of bone in response to periodontal therapy.

TECHNOLOGIC ADVANCES IN ASSESSMENTS

Scientists and clinicians are working toward the development of cost-effective, efficient technologic advancements to aid in the assessment and diagnosis of periodontal disease and other dental diseases. Of particular interest are methods that will enhance the accuracy of the diagnosis of active periodontal disease, such as controlled-force probes for measuring clinical attachment loss, automated tooth mobility equipment for measuring mobility of teeth and implants, risk calculators, microbiologic testing, and genetic analysis.[99,100] These and other advances will soon be practical for use in daily dental hygiene practice.

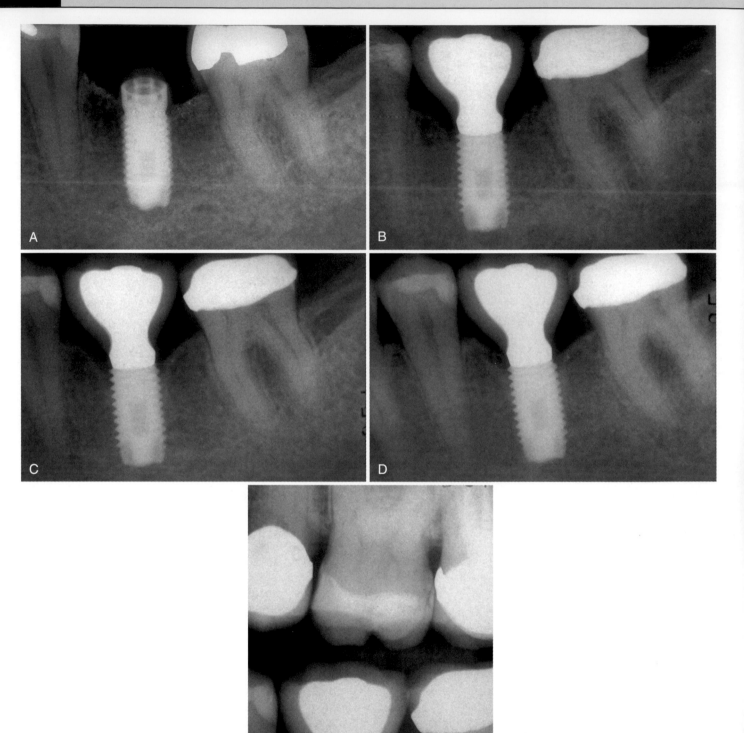

FIGURE 8-39 ■ **Radiographic assessment of a single titanium implant taken over an 11-year period after placement.** **A,** Baseline image of the implant at the time of initial restoration 8 months after surgical placement. **B,** One year post-prosthesis placement. **C,** Two years postprosthesis placement with an observable level of normal bone loss. **D,** Seven years postprosthesis placement with healthy osseous integration. **E,** Eleven years postprosthesis placement with expected bone loss surrounding the implant.

◎ DENTAL HYGIENE CONSIDERATIONS

- The assessment process begins with the very first observation of the patient in the waiting room and continues throughout the course of each appointment.
- The assessment protocol is intended to reflect the entire patient, not just the periodontal structures.
- Patients may not understand the interconnections between their oral health and their general health. The dental hygienist is uniquely positioned to help make these connections, which can lead to improved oral health, increased awareness of overall health, and even life-saving interventions.
- The medical history helps ensure patient safety, health, and well-being by aiding the clinician in the following:
  - Evaluating the oral manifestations of systemic disease
  - Detecting systemic conditions that may affect the periodontal tissue response
  - Identifying systemic conditions that require special precautions and modifications in treatment procedures
- A dental history should include information about the patient's chief complaint, previous dental experiences, current oral hygiene practices, and attitudes toward dentistry in order to design a care plan that meets the needs of the patient fully.
- Oral hygiene instruction needs to be individualized and based on the findings of the clinical assessment.
- The extraoral and intraoral assessments may identify a need for dental specialty or medical consultation and/or referral.
- Descriptions of oral mucosal features that are universally recognized, including clinical features (color, contour, consistency, and texture), location, and severity are important for assessment and evaluation.
- Gingival observations and clinical attachment loss may support the identification of underlying systemic, environmental, or behavioral contributing factors.
- Clinical evaluation of the presence of plaque biofilm, calculus, and stain are essential for a comprehensive assessment of a patient's oral hygiene status.

- It is important to evaluate oral tissue and dental stains and assess their local and systemic causes because patients are overwhelmingly aware of and concerned about tooth color and stains.
- Recorded probe depths in conjunction with current radiographic images provide detailed information on pocket depths and bleeding, clinical attachment loss, furcation involvement, and bone loss.
- The absence of bleeding on probing generally indicates current stability of the periodontium.
- The clinical signs of periodontal disease are suppressed in active smokers, and the effects of smoking are dose-dependent.
- Clinical and radiographic image assessments of furcations are important because patients with furcation involvement have an increased risk for continued bone loss and tooth loss.
- Tooth mobility beyond slight physiologic movement is considered pathologic.
- Pathologic migration is tooth displacement that occurs when the balance among the factors that maintain physiologic tooth position is disturbed.
- Peri-implant mucositis is an inflammation of the soft tissue surrounding an implant. When the inflammation extends to a loss of peri-implant bone, the condition is called peri-implantitis.
- Root caries are associated with age and gingival recession and can contribute to periodontal inflammation.
- Overhanging, poorly contoured, or defective restorations can have a detrimental effect on periodontal health.
- Attrition, abrasion, abrasion, and erosion are tooth wear conditions that are common and of significance in periodontal health.
- Dentinal sensitivity is a common patient complaint that can often be alleviated.
- Radiographic images provide valuable adjuncts to the clinical examination and historical documentation of the health and course of destruction of the periodontium.

★ CASE SCENARIO

You are seeing Mr. George, a 44-year-old Asian American for the first time. Mr. George is in good general health except for, as he reports, "a long history of dental problems, missing teeth, and gum disease." He was evaluated last week by Dr. Morrison who instructed you to complete full-mouth radiographs and record assessments. Mr. George has two single-tooth implants replacing his congenitally missing maxillary lateral incisors. Your assessments reveal generalized 5- to 7-mm probing pocket depths around all teeth and the implants. There is also 1 to 2 mm of recession around all teeth, missing first molars in all quadrants, no visible plaque biofilm, and light accumulation of supragingival calculus on the lower anterior teeth. All the teeth are mobile beyond what would be expected from physiologic movement.

1. How much clinical attachment loss does Mr. George have around tooth #6, the maxillary right canine, based on your measurement of 5-mm probing depths on all aspects and 2 mm of recession around that tooth?
   A. 2 mm
   B. 5 mm
   C. 7 mm
   D. Impossible to determine

2. You should be concerned about furcation involvement in the posterior sextants because Mr. George has deep pockets around all remaining teeth.
   A. Both the statement and the reason are correct and related.
   B. Both the statement and the reason are correct but NOT related.
   C. The statement is correct, but the reason is NOT correct.
   D. The statement is NOT correct, but the reason is correct.
   E. NEITHER the statement NOR the reason is correct.

3. The best way to evaluate the extent of Mr. George's furcation involvement is to
   A. use an explorer to evaluate vertical and horizontal dimensions of the furcations.
   B. use a curved probe to evaluate vertical and horizontal dimensions of the furcations.
   C. rely on the most recent radiographic images to measure the furcation involvement.
   D. use the periodontal probe to evaluate vertical and horizontal dimensions of the furcations.

4. What has caused Mr. George's tooth mobility?
   A. Loss of alveolar bone.
   B. Loss of periodontal ligament.
   C. Loss of both periodontal ligament and alveolar bone.
   D. Mr. George does not have mobility beyond what you would expect to find.

5. You are concerned about Mr. George's implants because they have deeper probe depths than you would expect to find with healthy implants.
   A. Both the statement and the reason are correct and related.
   B. Both the statement and the reason are correct but NOT related.
   C. The statement is correct, but the reason is NOT correct.
   D. The statement is NOT correct, but the reason is correct.
   E. NEITHER the statement NOR the reason is correct.

STUDY QUESTIONS

Answers and rationales to these questions can be obtained from your instructor.

MULTIPLE CHOICE

1. The first step in the dental hygiene process of patient care is
   A. planning.
   B. diagnosis.
   C. assessment.
   D. implementation.
2. A type of stain that occurs as a thin black line on the facial and lingual surfaces of the teeth of individuals who have excellent oral hygiene is called
   A. black stain.
   B. orange stain.
   C. tobacco stain.
   D. chlorhexidine stain.
3. What is the most important parameter for assessment of the failure of an implant?
   A. Attachment loss
   B. Mobility
   C. Probing
   D. Radiographs
4. The health status of the gingiva should be described with all of the universal descriptive categories listed below EXCEPT one. Which one is the EXCEPTION?
   A. Color
   B. Consistency
   C. Contour
   D. Stimuli
   E. Texture
5. The causes of pathologic mobility include all of the following EXCEPT one. Which one is the EXCEPTION?
   A. Bone loss
   B. Acidic diet
   C. Missing teeth
   D. Occlusal forces
   E. Parafunctional habits
6. The most significant measure that the periodontal probe provides is
   A. bleeding.
   B. mobility.
   C. pocket depth.
   D. clinical attachment loss.

7. The radiograph image assessment shows evidence of all of the following EXCEPT one. Which one is the EXCEPTION?
   A. Interdental craters
   B. Vertical bone loss
   C. Horizontal bone loss
   D. Furcation involvement
8. Bleeding on probing indicates
   A. disease activity.
   B. presence of inflammation.
   C. presence of subgingival calculus.
   D. presence of supragingival calculus.

SHORT ANSWER

9. How does assessment of the medical history help the clinician to ensure the safety and health of the patient?
10. Where are the furcations located on the tooth?

Please visit **http://evolve.elsevier.com/Perry/periodontology** for additional practice and study support tools.

REFERENCES

1. American Academy of Periodontology. Parameters on comprehensive periodontal examination. *J Periodontol.* 2000;71:847–848.
2. Minden NJ, Fast TB. Evaluation of health history forms used in U.S. dental schools. *Oral Med Oral Pathol.* 1994;77:105–109.
3. Jacobsen PL, Fredekind R, Budenz AW, et al. An updated multiple language health history for dental practice. *J Calif Dent Assoc.* 2000;28:492–502.
4. Dao V, Kraut R. Bisphosphonate use and health history questionnaire. *N Y State Dent J.* 2008;74:20–22.
5. Carey B. An audit comparing the discrepancies between a verbal enquiry, a written history, and an electronic medical history questionnaire: a suggested medical history/social history form for clinical practice. *J Ir Dent Assoc.* 2011;57:54–59.
6. Friedewald VE, Kornman KS, Beck JD, et al. The American Journal of Cardiology and Journal of Periodontology editors' consensus: periodontitis and atherosclerotic cardiovascular disease. *J Periodontol.* 2009;80:1021–1032.
7. McDaniel TF, Miller D, Jones R, et al. Assessing patient willingness to reveal health history information. *J Am Dent Assoc.* 1995;126:375–379.
8. Patton LL, Epstein JB, Kerr AR. Adjunctive techniques for oral cancer examination and lesion diagnosis. *J Am Dent Assoc.* 2008;139:896–905.
9. Awan KH, Morgan PR, Warnakulasuriya S. Utility of chemiluminescence (ViziLite) in the detection of oral potentially malignant disorders and benign keratoses. *J Oral Pathol Med.* 2011;40:541–544.
10. Vilchez-Perez MA, Fuster-Torres MA, Figueiredo R, et al. Periodontal health and lateral low lip piercings: a split-mouth cross-sectional study. *J Clin Periodontol.* 2009;36:558–563.
11. Hennequin-Hoenderdos NL, Slot DE, Van der Weijden GA. Complications of oral and peri-oral piercings: a summary of case reports. *Int J Dent Hygiene.* 2011;9:101–109.
12. Seymour RA, Preshaw PM, Thomason JM, et al. Cardiovascular diseases and periodontology. *J Clin Periodontol.* 2003;30:279–292.
13. Klokkevold PR, Mealey BL. Influence of systemic conditions on the periodontium. In: Newman MN, Takei HH, Klokkevold PR, et al, eds. *Carranza's Clinical Periodontology.* 11th ed. St. Louis, MO: Elsevier Saunders; 2012:304–319.
14. Novak MJ, Novak KF, Preshaw PM. Smoking and periodontal disease. In: Newman MN, Takei HH, Klokkevold PR, et al, eds. *Carranza's Clinical Periodontology.* 11th ed. St. Louis, MO: Elsevier Saunders; 2012:294–300.

15. Lambert R, Sauvaget C, de Camargo Cancela M, et al. Epidemiology of cancer from the oral cavity and oropharynx. *Eur J Gastroenterol Hepatol.* 2011;23:633–641.

16. Flemmig TF, Beikler T. Control of oral biofilms. *Periodontol 2000.* 2011;55:9–15.

17. O'Leary TJ, Drake RB, Naylor JE. The plaque control record. *J Periodontol.* 1972;43:38.

18. Krause F, Braun A, Frentzen M. The possibility of detecting subgingival calculus by laser-fluorescence in vitro. *Lasers Med Sci.* 2003;18:32–35.

19. Buchalla W, Lennon AM, Attin T. Fluorescence spectroscopy of dental calculus. *J Periodontal Res.* 2004;39:327–332.

20. Stambaugh RV, Myers G, Ebling W, et al. Endoscopic visualization of the submarginal gingival dental sulcus and tooth root surfaces. *J Periodontol.* 2002;73:374 382.

21. Eriksen HM, Nordbo H. Extrinsic discoloration of teeth. *J Clin Periodontol.* 1978;5:229–236.

22. Nordbo H. Discoloration of human teeth by a combination of chlorhexidine and aldehydes or ketones in vitro. *Scand J Dent Res.* 1971;79:356–361.

23. Eriksen HM, Nordbo H, Kantanen H, et al. Chemical plaque control and extrinsic tooth discoloration: a review of possible mechanisms. *J Clin Periodontol.* 1985;12:345–350.

24. Rolla G, Ellingsen JE. Clinical effects and possible mechanisms of action of stannous fluoride. *Int Dent J.* 1994;44:99–105.

25. Slots J. The microflora of black stain on human primary teeth. *Scand J Dent Res.* 1974;82:484–490.

26. Reid JS, Beeley JA, MacDonald DG. Investigations into black extrinsic tooth stain. *J Dent Res.* 1977;56:895–899.

27. Badanes BB. The role of fungi in deposits upon the teeth. *Dent Cosmos.* 1933;75:1154.

28. Leung SW. Naturally occurring stains on the teeth of children. *J Am Dent Assoc.* 1950;41:191–194.

29. Bartel HA. A note on chromogenic microorganisms from an organic colored deposit on the teeth. *Int J Orthod.* 1939;25:795–799.

30. Den Besten PK. Mechanism and timing of fluoride effects on developing enamel. *J Public Health Dent.* 1999;59:247 251.

31. Tredwin CJ, Scully C, Bagan-Sebastian JV. Drug induced disorders of teeth. *J Dent Res.* 2005;84:596–602.

32. Watts A, Addy M. Tooth discolouration and a review of the literature. *Brit Dent J.* 2001;190:309–316.

33. Caliskan MK, Türkün M. Prognosis of permanent teeth with internal resorption: a clinical review. *Endod Dent Traumatol.* 1997;13:75–81.

34. Armitage GC, Robertson PB. The biology, prevention, diagnosis and treatment of periodontal diseases: scientific advances in the United States. *J Am Dent Assoc.* 2009;140:36S–43S.

35. Highfield J. Diagnosis and classification of periodontal disease. *Aust Dent J.* 2009;54:S11–S26.

36. Armitage GC. Development of a classification system for periodontal diseases and conditions. *Ann Periodontol.* 1999;4:1–6.

37. Savage A, Eaton KA, Moles DR, et al. A systematic review of definitions of periodontitis and methods that have been used to identify this disease. *J Clin Periodontol.* 2009;39:458–467.

38. Heitz-Mayfield LJA. Disease progression: identification of high-risk groups and individuals for periodontitis. *J Clin Periodontol.* 2005;32(suppl 6):196–209.

39. Borrell LN, Papapanou PN. Analytical epidemiology of periodontitis. *J Clin Periodontol.* 2005;32(suppl 6):132–158.

40. Douglass CW. Risk assessment and management of periodontal disease. *J Am Dent Assoc.* 2006;137:27S–32S.

41. Armitage GC, Svanberg GK, Löe H. Microscopic evaluation of clinical measurements of connective tissue attachment levels. *J Clin Periodontol.* 1977;4:173–190.

42. Haffajee AD, Socransky SS, Lindhe J, et al. Clinical risk indicators for periodontal attachment loss. *J Clin Periodontol.* 1991;18:117–125.

43. Lang NP, Tonetti MS. Periodontal diagnosis in treated periodontitis: why, when and how to use clinical parameters. *J Clin Periodontol.* 1996;23:240–250.

44. Royzman D, Recio L, Badovinac RL, et al. The effect of aspirin intake on bleeding on probing in patients with gingivitis. *J Periodontol.* 2004;75:679–684.

45. Gürsoy M, Pajukanta R, Sorsa T, et al. Clinical changes in periodontium during pregnancy and post-partum. *J Clin Periodontol.* 2008;35:576–583.

46. Lang NP, Adler R, Joss A, et al. Absence of bleeding on probing. *J Clin Periodontol.* 1990;17:714–721.

47. Goncalves RB, Coletta RD, Silvério KG, et al. Impact of smoking on inflammation: overview of molecular mechanisms. *Inflamm Res.* 2011;60:409–424.

48. Nair P, Sutherland G, Palmer RM, et al. Gingival bleeding on probing increases after quitting smoking. *J Clin Periodontol.* 2003;30:435–437.

49. Rosa EF, Corraini P, de Carvalho VF, et al. Prospective 12-month study of the effect of smoking cessation on periodontal clinical parameters. *J Clin Periodontol.* 2011;38:562–571.

50. Dietrich T, Bernimoulin JP, Glynn RJ. The effect of cigarette smoking on gingival bleeding. *J Periodontol.* 2004;75:16–22.

51. Hofer D, Sahrmann P, Attin T, et al. Comparison of marginal bleeding using a periodontal probe or an interdental brush as indicators of gingivitis. *Int J Dent Hyg.* 2011;9:211–215.

52. Baderstein A, Nilveus R, Egelberg J. Scores of plaque, bleeding, suppuration and probing depth to predict probing attachment loss. 5 years of observation following nonsurgical periodontal therapy. *J Clin Periodontol.* 1990;17:102.

53. Sims T, Takei HH, Ammons WF, et al. Furcation: involvement and treatment. In: Newman MN, Takei HH, Klokkevold PR, et al, eds. *Carranza's Clinical Periodontology.* 11th ed. St. Louis, MO: Elsevier Saunders; 2012:589–594.

54. Huynh-Ba G, Kuonen P, Hofer D, et al. The effect of periodontal therapy on the survival rate and incidence of complications of multirooted teeth with furcation involvement after an observation period of at least 5 years: a systematic review. *J Clin Periodontol.* 2009;36:164–176.

55. O'Leary TJ. Tooth mobility. *Dent Clin North Am.* 1969;13:567–579.

56. Miller SC. *Textbook of Periodontia.* 3rd ed. Philadelphia, PA: Blakiston; 1950:125.

57. Brunsvold MA. Pathologic tooth migration. *J Periodontol.* 2005;76:859–866.

58. American Dental Association and American Academy of Periodontology. *Periodontal Screening and Recording.* Chicago, IL: American Dental Association and American Academy of Periodontology; 1992.

59. Khocht A, Zohn H, Deasy M, et al. Assessment of periodontal status with PSR and traditional clinical periodontal examination. *J Am Dent Assoc.* 1995;126:1658–1665.

60. Levin L, Ofec R, Grossman Y, et al. Periodontal disease as a risk for dental implant failure over time: a long-term historical cohort study. *J Clin Periodontol.* 2011;38:732–737.

61. Mombelli A, Décaillet F. The characteristics of biofilms in peri-implant disease. *J Clin Periodontol.* 2011;38:203–213.

62. Lang NP, Bosshardt DD, Lulic M. Do mucositis lesions around implants differ from gingivitis lesions around teeth? *J Clin Periodontol.* 2011;38:182–187.

63. Lindhe J, Meyle J; Group D of European Workshop on Periodontology. Peri-implant diseases: consensus report of the Sixth European Workshop on Periodontology. *J Clin Periodontol.* 2008;35(suppl):282–285.

64. Wilson TG. The positive relationship between excess cement and peri-implant disease: a prospective clinical endoscopic study. *J Periodontol.* 2009;80:1388–1392.

65. Chavez H, Ortman LF, DeFranco RL, et al. Assessment of oral implant mobility. *J Prosthetic Dent.* 1993;70:421–426.

66. Moy PK, Medina D, Shetty V, et al. Dental implant failure rates and associated risk factors. *Int J Oral Maxillofac Implants.* 2005;20:569–577.

67. Koldsland OC, Scheie AA, Aass AM. The association between selected risk indicators and severity of peri-implantitis using mixed model analyses. *J Clin Periodontol.* 2011;38:285–292.

68. Shetty V, Mooney LJ, Zigler CM, et al. The relationship between methamphetamine use and increased dental disease. *J Am Dent Assoc.* 2010;141:307–318.

69. Bachanek T, Pawlowicz A, Tarczydlo B, et al. Evaluation of dental health in mill workers. Part I. The state of dentition. *Ann Agric Environ Med.* 2001;8:103–105.

70. Bachanek T, Chalas R, Pawlowicz A, et al. Exposure to flour dust and the level of abrasion of hard tooth tissues among the workers of flour mills. *Ann Agric Environ Med.* 1999; 6:147–149.

71. Banting DW. The diagnosis of root caries. *J Dent Educ.* 2001;65: 991–996.

72. Black GV. *Operative Dentistry.* 8th ed. Woodstock, IL: Medico-Dental Publishing Co.; 1947-48.

73. Newbrun E. Problems in caries diagnosis. *Int Dent J.* 1993;43:133–142.

74. Brunsvold MS, Lane JJ. The prevalence of overhanging dental restorations and their relationship to periodontal disease. *J Clin Periodontol.* 1999;17: 67–72.

75. Pettengill CA. Interaction of dental erosion and bruxism: the amplification of tooth wear. *J Calif Dent Assoc.* 2011;39:251–256.

76. Lussi A, Jaeggi T. Erosion—diagnosis and risk factors. *Clin Oral Invest.* 2008;12:S5–S13.

77. Pikdöken L, Akca E, Gürbüzer B, et al. Cervical wear and occlusal wear from a periodontal perspective. *J Oral Rehabil.* 2011;38:95–100.

78. Imfeld T. Dental erosion. Definition, classification and links. *Eur J Oral Sci.* 1996;104:151–155.

79. Rees JS, Jagger DC. Abfraction lesions: myth or reality? *J Esthet Restor Dent.* 2003;15:263–271.

80. Lussi A. Dental erosion. Clinical diagnosis and case history taking. *Eur J Oral Sci.* 1996;104:191–198.

81. Brand HS, Tjoe Fat GM, Veerman ECI. The effects of saliva on the erosive potential of three different wines. *Aust Dent J.* 2009;54:228–232.

82. Noble WH. Sports drinks and dental erosion. *J Calif Dent Assoc.* 2011;39:233–238.

83. Engle K, Hara AT, Matis B, et al. Erosion and abrasion of enamel and dentin associated with at-home bleaching: an in vitro study. *J Am Dent Assoc.* 2010;141:546–551.

84. McGrath C, Chan B. Drug abuse. *Brit Dent J.* 2005;198:159–162.

85. Bartlett D, Ganss C, Lussi A. Basic Erosive Wear Examination (BEWE): a new scoring system for scientific and clinical needs. *Clin Oral Invest.* 2008;12:S65–S68.

86. Steele JG, Walls AWG. Using partial recording to assess tooth wear in older adults. *Community Dent Oral Epidemiol.* 2000;28:18–25.

87. Orchardson R, Gillam DG. Managing dentin hypersensitivity. *J Am Dent Assoc.* 2006;137:990–998.

88. Porto ICCM, Andrade AKM, Montes MAJR. Diagnosis and treatment of dentinal hypersensitivity. *J Oral Sci.* 2009;51:323–332.

89. Jeffcoat MK, Wang IC, Reddy MS. Radiographic diagnosis in periodontics. *Periodontol 2000.* 1995;7:54–68.

90. Miles DA, Thomas MV. Radiography for the periodontal examination. In: Rose LF, Mealey BL, eds. *Periodontics: Medicine, Surgery, and Implants.* St. Louis, MO: Elsevier Mosby; 2004:146.

91. Vrotsos JA, Parashis AO, Theofanatos GD. Prevalence and distribution of bone defects in moderate and advanced adult periodontitis. *J Clin Periodontol.* 1999;26:44–48.

92. Tang W, Wu Y, Smales RJ. Identifying and reducing risks for potential fractures in endodontically treated teeth. *J Endod.* 2010;36:609–617.

93. Tsesis I, Rosen E, Tamse A, et al. Diagnosis of vertical root fractures in endodontically treated teeth based on clinical and radiographic indices: a systematic review. *J Endod.* 2010;36:1455–1458.

94. Claiskan MK, Türkün M. Prognosis of permanent teeth with internal resorption: a clinical review. *Endod Dent Traumotol.* 1997;13:75–81.

95. Bender IB, Seltzer S. Roentgenographic and direct observation of experimental lesions in bone. *J Am Dent Assoc.* 1961;62:152–155.

96. Klinge B, Hultin M, Berglundh T. Peri-implantitis. *Dent Clin N Am.* 2005;49:661.

97. Lang NP, Berglundh T, Heitz-Mayfield LJ, et al. Consensus statements and recommended clinical procedures regarding implant survival and complications. *Int J Oral Maxillofac Implants.* 2004;19:150–154.

98. Gröndahl HG, Gröf Cndahl K. Subtraction radiography for the diagnosis of periodontal bone lesions. *Oral Surg.* 1993;55:208–213.

99. Ryan ME. Clinical attachment level change as an outcome measure for therapies that slow the progression of periodontal disease. *J Int Acad Periodontol.* 2005;7(suppl):162–174.

100. Tenenbaum HC, Tenenbaum H, Zohar R. Future treatment and diagnostic strategies for periodontal diseases. *Dent Clin N Am.* 2005;49:677–694.

Systemic Factors Influencing Periodontal Diseases

Gary C. Armitage

LEARNING OUTCOMES

- Understand systemic factors that influence dental hygiene care.
- Describe conditions that require consultation with a patient's physician.

- Describe changes in oral tissues observed with systemic diseases and conditions.
- List modifications needed for optimal treatment of patients with systemic conditions.

KEY TERMS

Blood dyscrasias
Cardiovascular diseases
Dermatologic diseases

Endocrine disturbances and
abnormalities
Infectious diseases
Joint diseases and disorders

Neurologic disorders
Oral cancer
Tobacco use

Systemic factors can have a profound effect on the diagnosis, pathogenesis, and treatment of periodontal infections. Some systemic diseases have signs and symptoms that mimic those of plaque-induced gingivitis or periodontitis, thereby increasing the likelihood of a misdiagnosis. Systemic problems in some patients can result in the following:

- Increase susceptibility to infection.
- Interfere with wound healing.
- Require modification of standard approaches to treatment.
- Complicate factors associated with patient cooperation.

In many cases, medical treatment of systemic diseases affects the clinical presentation and course of periodontal infections. People are now living longer than ever before. As a result, the patient population in a typical dental practice includes an increasing number of individuals with complex systemic problems, many of which are being treated with a wide variety of medications. The knowledgeable clinician must understand how the patient's systemic problems influence the selection of periodontal treatment and the anticipated response to therapy. This chapter provides an introduction to this subject and reviews some common systemic conditions encountered in dental hygiene and dental practice.

CARDIOVASCULAR DISEASES

In the United States, more than 40 million people have some form of cardiovascular disease. In this group of diseases, the most common conditions include hypertension (high blood pressure), coronary artery disease, heart valve disease, cardiac arrhythmias, and congestive heart failure. Because **cardiovascular diseases** are so prevalent in the population, many patients who seek dental care will have these conditions. In general, dental and periodontal treatment is not contraindicated in most patients with cardiovascular disease. In many cases, it is advisable to obtain a written medical consultation from the patient's physician before treatment is initiated. It is important to include a summary of which type of dental or periodontal treatment is planned. This information is useful to the physician in deciding whether any special precautions are required for the anticipated dental treatment. When dentists or dental hygienists request medical consultations, it is their responsibility to have a reasonable idea of which pretreatment precautions might be necessary.

HYPERTENSION (HIGH BLOOD PRESSURE)

High blood pressure is a major risk factor for cardiovascular disease, stroke, and kidney failure. Tens of millions of people in the United States have high blood pressure or are taking antihypertensive medications.[1] Hypertension has been called the "silent killer" because it is frequently asymptomatic and more than half of patients with hypertension are unaware that they have it. The prevalence of the disease increases dramatically with age,[2] and variations also occur by gender and race.[3] Blood pressure is the force of the blood pushing against the walls of arteries. It is highest when the heart beats (systolic pressure) and lowest when the heart is resting (diastolic pressure). Blood

TABLE 9-1   Classification of Adult Blood Pressure and Dental Treatment Modifications

CATEGORY	SYSTOLIC PRESSURE (mm Hg)	DIASTOLIC PRESSURE (mm Hg)	DENTAL TREATMENT
Normal	<120	<80	No modification of dental care
Prehypertension	120-139	80-89	No modification of dental care
Hypertension			
Stage I	140-159	90-99	No modification of dental care, medical referral, inform patient
Stage II	160-179	100-109	Selective dental care,* medical referral
Stage III	180-209	110-119	Emergency nonstressful procedures,† immediate medical referral/consultation
Stage IV	≥210	≥120	Emergency nonstressful procedures,† immediate medical referral

*Selective dental care may include, but is not limited to, dental prophylaxis, nonsurgical periodontal therapy, restorative procedures, and nonsurgical endodontic therapy.

†Emergency nonstressful procedures may include, but are not limited to, dental procedures that may help alleviate pain, infection, or masticatory dysfunction. These procedures should have limited physiologic and psychological effects. An example of an emergency nonstressful procedure might be a simple incision and drainage of an intraoral fluctuant dental abscess. The medical benefits achieved by performing emergency nonstressful procedures in stages III and IV hypertensive patients should outweigh the risk of complications caused by the patient's hypertensive state.

Used with permission. Modified from Muzyka BC, Glick M. The hypertensive dental patient. *J Am Dent Assoc.* 1997;128:1109–1120.[6] Copyright 1997, American Dental Association.)

See: http://www.nhlbi.nih.gov/.

pressure is recorded as two numbers, the systolic over the diastolic pressure (e.g., 110/70 mm Hg).[4] In general, patients with readings greater than 140/90 mm Hg are considered to be hypertensive.[5,6] Patients with a systolic pressure from 120 to 139 mm Hg and a diastolic pressure from 80 to 89 mm Hg are considered to have prehypertension.[4] Table 9-1 shows a classification of hypertension from the Joint National Committee on the Detection, Evaluation, and Treatment of High Blood Pressure.[5]

Dental hygienists play an important role in detecting previously undiagnosed and asymptomatic cases of hypertension. Adult dental patients should have their blood pressure measured at each visit. When elevated blood pressure is detected, patients should be advised to see their physician. In individuals with uncontrolled hypertension, elective dental treatment should be deferred because stress associated with dental procedures can further elevate blood pressure and thereby increase the risk of stroke and assorted cardiovascular or renal problems. However, patients with medically well-controlled hypertension can safely receive nearly all forms of dental and periodontal therapy.

CLINICAL NOTE 9-1   The dental hygienist must routinely take blood pressure readings on adult patients.

The use of epinephrine-containing local anesthetics is not contraindicated in patients with well-controlled hypertension. However, it is advisable to use minimal amounts of epinephrine, such as 0.04 mg per dental visit (approximately two cartridges containing 1:1000,000 parts epinephrine). If pain is anticipated in association with the planned dental or periodontal treatment, very good local anesthesia is desirable to minimize the release of endogenous epinephrine.[7,8]

Physicians prescribe many types of medications for hypertensive patients, including diuretics (e.g., thiazides), sympatholytics (e.g., beta-adrenergic blockers such as propranolol), vasodilators (e.g., hydralazine HCl), and angiotensin-converting enzyme inhibitors (e.g., enalapril). As with all patients who are taking medication, it is important for the dental hygienist to review the list of drugs taken by the patient and become familiar with their mode of action and potential side effects. Some of the side effects of these medications are drowsiness, mental depression, confusion, and xerostomia (dry mouth).

Coronary Artery (Ischemic Heart) Disease

Atherosclerosis is the deposition of cholesterol-containing material in the walls of arteries that results in a narrowing of the affected blood vessels. This can eventually lead to the complete blocking of blood flow. Ischemia is the insufficient supply of blood to an organ or tissue. Atherosclerotic changes in the coronary arteries that feed the heart can lead to ischemic heart disease, the leading cause of sudden death in the United States. The two most common clinical manifestations of ischemic heart disease are angina pectoris and myocardial infarction, commonly referred to as a heart attack.

Angina pectoris is a severe recurring chest pain that frequently radiates into the left shoulder and arm. It is an intense crushing pain that can also move across the chest and down each arm. Sometimes the pain involves the neck, lower jaw, and face. It is caused by the deprivation of oxygen to the cardiac muscle as a result of reduced blood flow, frequently as a consequence of atherosclerotic narrowing of the coronary arteries. However, it also can be caused by specific situations in which the oxygen demands of the heart muscle are not met, such as strenuous physical exertion or extreme psychological stress.

A condition in which anginal pain is predictable and controlled by medication is called stable angina.[9] Patients with stable angina frequently control their anginal pain by taking one or more of the following types of drugs: nitrates (e.g., nitroglycerin), beta-adrenergic blockers, and calcium channel blockers (e.g., nifedipine). Gingival enlargement is one of the common side effects of nifedipine (Procardia) and some other calcium channel blockers.[10-14] The gingival enlargement can

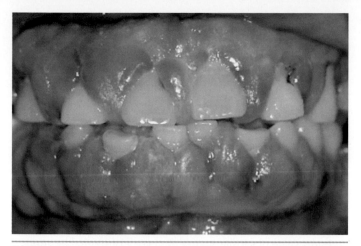

FIGURE 9-1 ■ Drug-influenced gingival enlargement in a 53-year-old male who was taking verapamil for a cardiac arrhythmia, nifedipine to control anginal pain, and cyclosporine for its immunosuppressive effect to combat rejection of a transplanted kidney. A reported side effect of all three drugs is gingival enlargement. (Courtesy of Dr. V. Godfrey.)

make oral hygiene difficult and thereby increase the risk of plaque-induced diseases, such as dental caries and periodontal disease, (Figure 9-1).

Patients with stable angina can safely receive routine dental care, but it is advisable to minimize stress by scheduling relatively short morning appointments so that the patient is well rested. As with hypertensive patients, local anesthesia should be used for potentially painful procedures to minimize the release of endogenous epinephrine.[7,8] If an anginal attack occurs during the delivery of dental care, treatment should be discontinued, the patient should be placed in a semisupine position, and standard emergency procedures should be performed.

Myocardial infarction, or heart attack, is caused by sudden occlusion or blocking of the blood supply to a portion of the heart. Heart attacks are frequently caused by occlusion of a coronary artery by atherosclerotic deposits or a blood clot (thrombus). Patients who are recovering from a recent heart attack should not receive elective dental treatment until their condition is medically stabilized, usually for 6 months or until treatment is approved by their physician.

CLINICAL NOTE 9-2 Patients with stable angina or those with a history of ischemic heart disease whose condition is medically stable can receive almost any routine dental treatment.

DISEASES OF HEART VALVES

Any dental or periodontal procedure that introduces bacteria into the bloodstream of patients with heart valve disease can increase their risk of a potentially fatal heart infection called infective endocarditis. In general, damaged heart valves are more susceptible to colonization by bacteria. In addition, the stasis of blood, frequently associated with defective heart valves, increases the likelihood that bacteria will be able to attach successfully to fibrin deposits that can form on the heart at sites at which blood flow is impaired. In the past, some patients with heart valve problems were prescribed antibiotics before undergoing any procedures in which gingival bleeding might be induced, including periodontal examination and scaling of the teeth. It was believed that the antibiotics lowered

the risk of developing infective endocarditis. However, this is no longer routinely recommended because the risks of taking antibiotics often outweigh the risk of developing infective endocarditis.[15]

It is important for dental hygienists to have a basic understanding of the general types of diseases that affect heart valves so they can more effectively consult physicians about any pretreatment precautions that should be taken for high-risk patients.

The primary function of heart valves is to allow the unidirectional forward flow of blood through the heart. Diseases of the heart valves can be either acquired or congenital. Acquired diseases are far more common. Approximately half of all acquired heart valve lesions occur as isolated stenosis, or narrowing, of the orifice of the aortic or mitral valve. Stenosis leads to the failure of a valve to open completely, thereby retarding the forward flow of blood through the heart. Heart valve insufficiency is the failure of a valve to close completely, thereby leading to regurgitation, or flow of blood in a reverse direction. Stenosis and insufficiency often affect the same valve.

Many methods are used by physicians to detect heart disease. One of them is to listen to heart sounds with a stethoscope to detect, among other things, the presence or absence of a heart murmur. Murmurs are simply the sounds that are produced by the turbulent flow of blood through the heart. Heart valve disease is only one of many possible causes of a heart murmur. Some murmurs are caused by abnormalities of the heart (organic murmurs); others are termed *innocent* or *functional* murmurs. When patients report that they have a heart murmur, it is usually advisable to consult their physician to determine whether any precautions are necessary before dental procedures are performed. Patients with heart murmurs rarely require preoperative coverage with antibiotics, although this was common in the past.

Acquired heart valve disease is often found in patients with a history of rheumatic fever[16] and several other systemic diseases.[17-19] Rheumatic fever is an acute systemic inflammatory disease that sometimes follows throat infections with group A streptococci. Antistreptococcal antibodies that form in response to these infections can react with heart valve tissues and cause inflammation and damage to the valves. This damage may lead to rheumatic heart disease in which there is scarring of the heart valves. In the past, a history of rheumatic heart disease was one of the conditions for which antibiotics were routinely prescribed in an attempt to reduce the risk of infective endocarditis. Other conditions for which preoperative antibiotics are no longer recommended include mitral valve prolapse, bicuspid valve disease, calcified aortic stenosis, and some congenital heart conditions such as ventricular or atrial septal defects.[15] The American Heart Association (AHA) has published guidelines on when antibiotic prophylaxis for dental procedures are recommended (Table 9-2).[15] However, before performing dental procedures (including oral examinations with periodontal probing or exploring) in a patient with a history of heart valve problems, the clinician should consult the patient's physician to determine whether preoperative coverage with antibiotics is necessary.

CLINICAL NOTE 9-3 Most patients with heart murmurs can be safely treated without antibiotic premedication.

TABLE 9-2 AHA Recommendations of Prophylactic Antibiotic Coverage for Dental Procedures in Patients at High and Moderate Risk for Infective Endocarditis

SITUATION	AGENT	REGIMEN*
Standard general prophylaxis	Amoxicillin	Adults: 2.0 g; children: 50 mg/kg orally 1 hr before procedure
Unable to take oral medications	Ampicillin	Adults: 2.0 g IM or IV; children: 50 mg/kg IM or IV within 30 min before procedure
Allergic to penicillin	Clindamycin OR Cephalexin[†] or cefadroxil[†] OR Azithromycin or clarithromycin	Adults: 600 mg; children: 20 mg/kg orally 1 hr before procedure Adults: 2.0 g; children: 50 mg/kg orally 1 hr before procedure Adults: 500 mg; children: 15 mg/kg orally 1 hr before procedure
Allergic to penicillin and unable to take oral medications	Clindamycin OR Cefazolin[†]	Adults: 600 mg; children: 20 mg/kg IV within 30 min before procedure Adults: 1.0 g; children: 25 mg/kg IM or IV within 30 min before procedure

*Total children's dose should not exceed adult dose.
[†]Cephalosporins should not be used in individuals with immediate-type hypersensitivity reaction (urticaria, angioedema, or anaphylaxis) to penicillins.
Used with permission from Dajani AS, Taubert KA, Wilson W, et al. Prevention of bacterial endocarditis: recommendations by the American Heart Association. *J Am Dent Assoc.* 1997;128(28):1142–1151.[20]; and Hancock EW. Coronary artery disease: epidemiology and prevention. In: Rubenstein E, Federman DD, eds. *Scientific American Medicine.* New York, NY: Scientific American; 1991:1(section VIII):1–10. Copyright American Dental Association. Excerpted by JADA with permission of *The Journal of the American Medical Association. JAMA.* 1997;277(22):1794–1801; Copyright 1997 American Medical Association. Adapted 2006 with permission of the American Dental Association.)
IM, Intramuscularly; *IV,* intravenously.

CARDIAC ARRHYTHMIAS

Irregular heartbeat can be associated with a variety of systemic conditions, such as high fevers from certain infectious diseases, ischemic heart disease, congestive heart failure, mitral valve prolapse, rheumatic heart disease, myocardial infarction, hypertension, certain allergic reactions (anaphylaxis), and hyperthyroidism. There are many forms of cardiac arrhythmia, some of which can be controlled by medications. Others require the insertion of electronic devices (e.g., pacemakers and defibrillators).

Dental procedures can be safely performed in most patients who are under medical treatment for cardiac arrhythmias. However, patients who are taking antiarrhythmic drugs can experience a variety of side effects that may complicate or worsen their dental and periodontal problems. For example, some antiarrhythmic drugs, such as disopyramide (Norpace), mexiletine (Mexitil), verapamil (Calan), and diltiazem (Cardizem), may lead to xerostomia, which can facilitate plaque retention and increase the patient's susceptibility to dental caries

and periodontal disease. Drugs such as phenytoin (Dilantin), verapamil, and diltiazem may lead to severe gingival enlargement, which makes plaque control difficult (see Figure 9-1). In some patients, mexiletine and quinidine (Cardioquin) may cause neutropenia (a decrease in circulating neutrophils), which can increase their susceptibility to periodontal and other infections.

CLINICAL NOTE 9-4 The dental hygienist must be familiar with the actions and side effects of the medications that patients are taking in order to determine whether the drugs might adversely influence or complicate periodontal therapy.

Some cases of cardiac arrhythmia are best treated by surgical insertion of a battery-operated electronic device (pacemaker) under the skin of the upper chest wall. Wire leads connect the pacemaker to an electrode that is placed in contact with heart tissue. The pacemaker sends periodic electrical impulses to the heart, thereby regulating its rate of contraction. The AHA guidelines do not recommend that patients with pacemakers be given antibiotics before dental procedures.[15] However, for certain patients, the physician or cardiologist might recommend antibiotic coverage.

In one type of arrhythmia, portions of the heart undergo rapid irregular twitching, referred to as fibrillation. Defibrillators are designed to send electrical impulses to the heart to shock it into a normal pattern of contraction. Defibrillators can be implanted subcutaneously in the abdomen with electrodes connected to the heart. The devices detect the onset of fibrillation and automatically send small electrical shocks to the heart to correct the situation. As with pacemakers, prophylactic antibiotic coverage is not usually required before dental procedures.[15]

CONGESTIVE HEART FAILURE

Elective dental procedures should not be performed in patients with congestive heart failure unless their condition has been stabilized by medical treatment. In cases of congestive heart failure, the heart is unable to supply the body with sufficient oxygenated blood. As a result, the patient has difficulty breathing after minimal exertion.

Patients whose condition is under good medical control can safely receive routine dental treatment. However, appointments should be kept short to minimize stress. When these patients are treated, the dental chair should be kept in an erect or partially reclining position. If these patients are placed in a fully reclining position, gravity promotes the return of peripheral blood to the central circulation, thereby placing an extra burden on the heart. For these patients, it is a good idea to have supplemental oxygen on hand in case they encounter any difficulty in breathing.

PATIENTS WHO ARE TAKING ANTICOAGULANTS

Many patients with a history of cardiovascular disease often take anticoagulants (blood thinners). These reduce the risk of the development of blood clots that can block the circulation to vital organs such as the brain, heart, and lungs. Patients who have prosthetic heart valves or have had a recent heart attack or stroke (blockage of blood flow to the brain) frequently receive anticoagulant therapy. The medications that are usually administered for these conditions are heparin or warfarin (Coumadin) derivatives. Warfarin is the agent that is most often used on an outpatient basis. Subgingival instrumentation associated with routine dental hygiene procedures in anticoagulated patients can result in more gingival bleeding than is ordinarily encountered. However, the bleeding is usually easily controlled by applying pressure with a gauze sponge. When treating these patients, it is important to minimize the soft tissue trauma associated with subgingival instrumentation.

Many patients with a history of cardiovascular disease take small daily doses (80 to 325 mg) of aspirin, which retards the formation of blood clots by inhibiting platelet aggregation. At these doses, aspirin does not significantly alter the bleeding time,[20] and postoperative bleeding from dental hygiene procedures is usually not a problem.

> **CLINICAL NOTE 9-5** Anticoagulants and aspirin may cause more bleeding than expected during subgingival instrumentation.

JOINT DISEASES AND DISORDERS

Joint diseases and disorders that are frequently seen in dental patients and can complicate or modify the approach to dental or periodontal treatment include arthritis and artificial or prosthetic joints.

ARTHRITIS

Arthritis is a general term that means inflammation of a joint. It is a common condition that affects, in one form or another, as many as 85% of adults older than 45 years. It is associated with many systemic diseases, including rheumatoid arthritis (rheumatism), osteoarthritis, systemic lupus erythematosus, scleroderma, and gout. The primary dental problem that arthritis causes in some patients is difficulty in performing oral hygiene procedures. This problem is particularly common in patients with rheumatoid arthritis and osteoarthritis involving the hands. Arthritic involvement of the hands can result in the inability to grasp such items as a toothbrush and to manipulate dental floss or other interproximal cleaning devices. This inability may stem from actual loss of joint flexibility or from intense pain associated with inflamed joints of the hands and fingers. Dental hygienists must recognize this potential problem and determine whether special plaque control devices, such as a powered toothbrush, are needed. In addition, as with all patients who have difficulty cleaning their teeth, it is advisable to schedule more frequent professional care.

Patients with severe arthritis often take antiinflammatory medications to reduce local inflammation and decrease the amount of joint pain. In some cases, relatively high doses of aspirin are prescribed by the patient's physician. Aspirin can retard the formation of blood clots, so some increased bleeding may occur during routine scaling and root planing procedures. In most patients, this problem is not significant, and any localized gingival bleeding resulting from subgingival instrumentation can be controlled by pressure with a gauze sponge.

> **CLINICAL NOTE 9-6** During periodontal treatment, increased bleeding may be encountered in patients who take aspirin for their arthritis, similar to the increased bleeding found in patients taking blood thinners. Applying pressure usually controls the bleeding.

It is important to remember that arthritis can be the result of many systemic diseases and that it is only one of several medical problems that may have dental implications. For example, patients with progressive systemic sclerosis (PSS), or scleroderma, experience multiple dental and periodontal problems that are directly attributable to their systemic disease.[21] PSS is a chronic connective tissue disease of unknown cause in which abnormal amounts of collagen are continuously deposited in a variety of organ systems, including the skin, lungs, and kidneys. PSS can cause death due to kidney or respiratory failure. As the disease progresses, the skin loses much of its elasticity and becomes almost leather-like. Severe arthritis and stiffening of the hands are common (Figure 9-2). It is difficult for these patients to hold or manipulate plaque control devices, and their firm inflexible skin often prevents them from opening their mouths wide enough to allow the dentist or dental hygienist access to perform routine procedures. As a result, patients with PSS tend to experience high rates of dental caries and periodontal disease. Significant gingival recession is a common feature (Figure 9-3). An unusual oral finding in some patients with PSS is the uniform widening of the periodontal ligament space seen in radiographs (Figure 9-4).[22] Although PSS is not a common disease, it is a dramatic example of a systemic disease that can present challenges to the dentist and dental hygienist in providing adequate oral health care.

ARTIFICIAL JOINTS

In some patients with arthritis, the destruction of joint tissues can result in severe pain and loss of function. In such cases, it is often necessary to replace the affected joint with an artificial or prosthetic device. Through modern orthopedic surgery, it is possible to replace joints of the hip, knee, elbow, wrist, and shoulder. Complete replacement of the hip joint is the most common procedure. Insertion of an artificial knee joint is often performed. Because more than 450,000 joint prostheses are placed annually in the United States, most dental practices will encounter patients with these devices.[23]

Infection, in one form or another, occurs in approximately 1% of joint prostheses and is a major cause of their failure.[24] The sources of infections of joint prostheses (infections that occur more than 3 months after joint placement) are not known, but bacteremias originating from acute dental, respiratory tract, dermatologic, or urinary tract infections are prime suspects.[24-28] It appears that the highest risk of late infections of joint prostheses is up to 2 years after joint replacement.[29]

All patients with total joint replacements, orthopedic pins, and plates do not routinely require antibiotic prophylaxis before dental treatment.[23] However, some patients may be at increased risk of hematogenous joint infection and should be considered as candidates for antibiotic coverage before extensive bacteremia-producing dental procedures. Guidelines for antibiotic regimens for these patients are currently being revised. Because there are no universally approved antibiotic

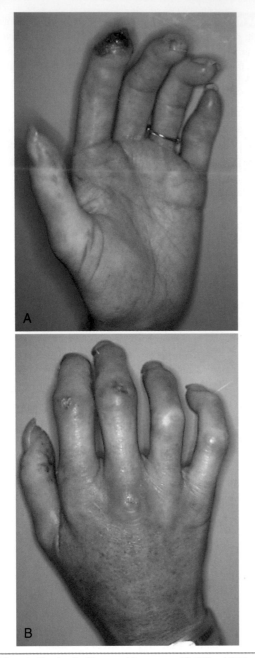

FIGURE 9-2 ■ **A,** Hands of a 50-year-old woman with PSS exhibiting arthritic enlargement of the finger joints. **B,** Sores on the hands and tips of the fingers (Raynaud's disease) are secondary to inadequate circulation from blood vessel involvement. In addition to these changes, loss of skin flexibility made it impossible for the patient to grasp a toothbrush.

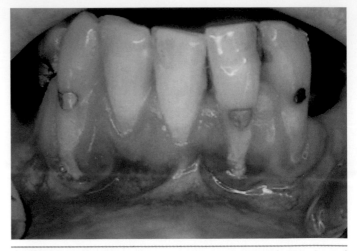

FIGURE 9-3 ■ **Marked gingival recession in a patient with PSS.** Gingival recession is a common feature in patients with long-standing PSS. Same patient as shown in Figure 9-2.

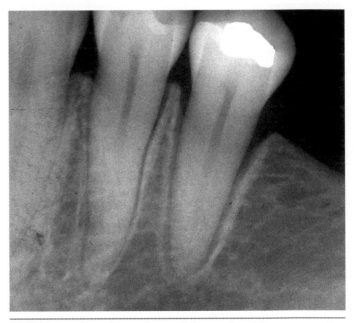

FIGURE 9-4 ■ The uniform widening of the periodontal ligament space in a 38-year-old woman with PSS. The tooth was not mobile.

prophylaxis guidelines, it is recommended that the patient's physician be consulted prior to performing dental hygiene procedures in an individual with artificial joints.

> **CLINICAL NOTE 9-7** All patients with artificial joints are candidates for antibiotic prophylaxis prior to dental procedures. Consultation with the patient's physician is necessary.

ENDOCRINE DISTURBANCES AND ABNORMALITIES

DIABETES MELLITUS

It is estimated that more than 16 million people in the United States have diabetes mellitus (DM), but only half of them have

been diagnosed.[30] Due to the obesity epidemic, the number of people with the disease is increasing. DM is a group of disorders that share the common feature of an elevated glucose level in the blood. The underlying problem in DM is an insufficient supply or impaired availability of insulin, a pancreatic hormone that is necessary for the regulation of carbohydrate metabolism. Based on the newest method of classification there are two main types of DM, type 1 and type 2.[31] Although different groups of genes have been linked to the risk of developing of each of these two forms of diabetes, both forms have a genetic component.

Approximately 10% to 20% of all cases of diabetes mellitus are of the type 1 variety. In this form of the disease, there is a severe deficiency of insulin as a result of the destruction of pancreatic beta cells. Destruction occurs because of autoimmune reactions to beta cells that develop in response to environmental injury from some viruses.[32] In other cases, destruction of beta cells may be caused by tumors, surgery, and toxic reactions to drugs or chemicals.[32] Onset of the disease is usually rapid and occurs around the time of puberty. Medical control of type 1 DM requires periodic self-injection with one or more prescribed insulin preparations.

Patients with type 2 DM account for 80% to 90% of all cases of diabetes mellitus. In the early stages, the pancreatic beta cells are intact and capable of producing insulin. There are, however, two general metabolic defects associated with the development of type 2 DM, impaired secretion of insulin and insulin resistance.[33] Although the precise reasons for these abnormalities are unknown, defective cell receptors for insulin are believed to play a role in insulin resistance.[31] The onset of the disease is slow and it usually affects overweight individuals older than 30 years.[32] The incidence of the disease increases with age. Medical control of early forms of type 2 DM can frequently be achieved by dietary modifications. If problems persist, oral hypoglycemic agents are used that stimulate insulin release from the pancreas and enhance insulin uptake by the tissues. In many patients with long-standing type 2 DM, loss of pancreatic beta cells eventually occurs, and periodic insulin injections are required to achieve medical control of the disease.

Patients with either form of diabetes suffer a wide variety of cardiovascular, kidney, eye, and neurologic problems.[32] In addition, patients with uncontrolled or poorly controlled DM appear to be more susceptible to infections, including periodontal disease.[33,34] The precise reasons for this increased susceptibility are unknown, but certain antibacterial functions of neutrophils appear to be abnormal.[35-38] Other common oral problems associated with diabetes include asymptomatic parotid gland enlargement[39] and dry mouth resulting from decreased salivary flow.[40]

> **CLINICAL NOTE 9-8** Patients with poorly controlled diabetes mellitus have an increased susceptibility to periodontal infections.

There is a long-standing clinical impression that control of gingival inflammation through periodontal therapy and good daily oral hygiene reduces insulin requirements in patients with diabetes.[41] In other words, satisfactory metabolic control of diabetes is made easier if periodontal infections are arrested. There is a growing body of scientific evidence supporting this clinical impression.[42-45]

> **CLINICAL NOTE 9-9** In many patients, metabolic control of diabetes is enhanced by periodontal treatment. Decreased gingival inflammation is linked to improved diabetic control.

Treatment Considerations

Patients with diabetes mellitus tolerate most routine dental procedures well, and no special precautions are usually necessary. However, because they are at greater risk for periodontal disease, it is advisable to schedule preventive dental care at more frequent intervals. Before dental visits, patients with diabetes should be instructed to continue their medication schedule as prescribed by their physician. For morning appointments, they should eat a normal breakfast to reduce the chances of becoming hypoglycemic during the visit.

Occasionally, before a dental visit, diabetic patients do not eat their normal diet and self-administer too much insulin. This practice can precipitate a dangerous emergency called insulin shock, in which the patient becomes severely hypoglycemic. The condition frequently develops rapidly and with little warning. The initial signs and symptoms of insulin shock include mental confusion, slurred speech, rapid heartbeat, nausea, and cold clammy skin. If the condition is not promptly treated, the patient's blood pressure may drop precipitously. As a result, the patient may lose consciousness and have seizures. Death can occur if emergency measures are not taken. Fortunately, insulin shock is relatively easy to recognize, and the initial management of the emergency is simple. Because the underlying problem in cases of insulin shock is dangerously low levels of blood sugar (glucose), initial emergency care involves the prompt administration of a sugar-containing beverage, such as orange juice. Any easily administered sugar source will suffice (e.g., candy, honey, soft drinks). In addition, many patients will know what is happening and why they are being asked to consume a sugar-containing substance. Once the patient has consumed the sugar, recovery usually begins within a few minutes. If the patient does not respond, a medical emergency response team should be called.

PREGNANCY

Increased gingival inflammation (gingivitis) is frequently associated with pregnancy.[46-50] The gingivitis can be severe, with the tissues becoming swollen and red (Figure 9-5). Patients often report bleeding gums because the tissues bleed on the slightest provocation. The gingivitis is most severe during the first and second trimesters. It decreases somewhat around the eighth month and after parturition.[47,48] If left untreated, the severe gingivitis associated with pregnancy may lead to the development of periodontitis, with the loss of alveolar bone and even teeth.[46,50]

It is not known precisely why gingival inflammation intensifies during pregnancy, but it has been clearly established that the inflammation is caused by plaque.[47,48] However, vascular

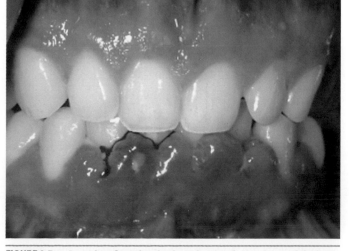

FIGURE 9-5 ■ Severely inflamed and enlarged gingival tissues around the lower anterior teeth of a 28-year-old woman who was in the fifth month of an uncomplicated pregnancy. The patient's chief dental complaint was bleeding gums.

alterations associated with the hormonal changes of pregnancy (i.e., elevated serum levels of estrogen and progesterone) make the gingiva more susceptible to plaque-induced inflammation.[50] Increased estrogen and progesterone can promote the growth of certain suspected periodontal pathogens such as *Prevotella intermedia*.[51,52] In addition, changes in the immune system associated with pregnancy alter the host defenses against some infections.[49]

CLINICAL NOTE 9-10 Hormonal and immunologic changes associated with pregnancy can affect the composition of the subgingival microbiota, thereby promoting the development of gingivitis and, in some cases, even periodontitis.

Treatment Considerations

Because pregnant women may be more susceptible to periodontal disease, they should receive closely supervised oral health care and intensified preventive services during pregnancy. Pregnant patients should be informed that they are at increased risk for periodontal disease. They should then be shown how to perform thorough oral hygiene procedures. In addition, when a patient becomes pregnant, it is usually advisable to schedule professional teeth cleaning at more frequent intervals. For example, a patient who was being followed at 6-month intervals before her pregnancy might be seen at 3-month intervals during her pregnancy.

CLINICAL NOTE 9-11 Preventive oral health services should be a routine part of prenatal care.

FLUCTUATIONS IN FEMALE SEX HORMONE LEVELS

Increased gingival inflammation associated with physiologic fluctuations in the levels of female sex hormones is observed during puberty[53] and the menstrual cycle.[54] Acquired fluctuations occur in some patients who are taking oral contraceptives.[55-60] The mechanisms responsible for this increased susceptibility to plaque-induced gingival inflammation are probably the same as those in pregnancy. In addition, the clinical features of the gingival changes that occur during puberty or the menstrual cycle and in patients who are taking oral contraceptives sometimes resemble those seen in pregnant women. When oral contraceptives were introduced, relatively high doses of hormones were used and the gingival effects were significant.[61,62] Gingival changes associated with modern low-dose contraceptives are not as severe.[60]

CLINICAL NOTE 9-12 The gingival inflammation in patients with physiologic or acquired fluctuations in female sex hormone levels is caused by plaque. Therefore, the oral hygiene practices in these patients must be carefully monitored to reduce the likelihood of periodontal disease.

PSYCHOLOGICAL STRESS

Many patients are under psychological stress because of pressures associated with daily life. The effect of stress on the general systemic well-being of patients is a complex and often

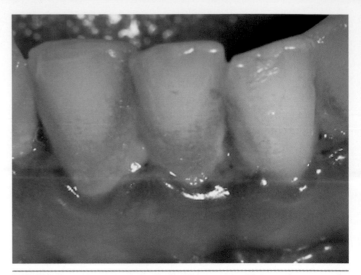

FIGURE 9-6 ■ NUG in a medically healthy 21-year-old man who was under severe emotional stress. Note the interproximal necrosis and ulceration.

controversial subject. However, there is a long-standing clinical impression that patients who are under emotional tension have an increased susceptibility to certain periodontal infections.[63,64] It has been firmly established that in some patients, stressful life events can partially suppress certain components of the immune system.[65-69]

The clinical impression that stress is an important factor in the pathogenesis of certain periodontal diseases is strongest in the case of necrotizing ulcerative gingivitis (NUG).[70-72] This periodontal infection, also known as trench mouth or Vincent's infection, is characterized by the rapid onset of gingival pain and the presence of interproximal necrosis and ulceration (Figure 9-6). Most patients with NUG exhibit one or more of the following predisposing factors: recent emotional stress, heavy cigarette smoking, lack of sleep, and poor dietary habits.[73]

CLINICAL NOTE 9-13 Emotional stress and associated partial suppression of the immune system are associated with an increased risk for periodontitis.

Treatment Considerations

A growing body of evidence is emerging that certain psychosocial factors, including emotional stress, are associated with an increased risk of developing periodontitis.[69] Nevertheless, when patients with certain periodontal diseases (especially aggressive ones such as NUG) state that they have recently been under considerable stress, it is possible that their emotional state may be contributing to their disease. Depending on a variety of circumstances, it may be advisable to inform some patients of the possible relationship between stress and periodontal infections. For some patients, merely knowing that stress might negatively affect the course of their periodontal disease encourages them to modify their lifestyle or to seek psychological counseling. However, even in patients who make no effort to change their stress level, local treatment of the periodontal infection through plaque control instruction and scaling and root planing is the most significant step toward arresting the disease. At best, stress may be a modifying factor, not the cause of the periodontal infection.

INFECTIOUS DISEASES

The presence of certain **infectious diseases** in patients is a source of concern to oral health care providers. Some infections may have one or more of the following effects:

1. Modify or increase the patient's susceptibility to oral diseases
2. Create diagnostic challenges because of their oral manifestations
3. Cause infection control problems that increase the risk of transmitting the disease to other patients and health care workers

VIRAL HEPATITIS

The liver is a multifunctional vital organ that plays a major role in metabolizing lipids and carbohydrates, producing serum proteins, and detoxifying drugs (e.g., alcohol). Hepatitis, or inflammation of the liver, can be caused by a variety of factors. The two most common factors are certain viral infections and ingestion of drugs or toxic chemicals. Viral hepatitis is a general term that refers to a group of liver infections caused by at least five distinct deoxyribonucleic acid (DNA)–containing viruses designated as types A, B, C (non-A, non-B), D, and E (non-A, non-B). Hepatitis A virus (HAV) is primarily transmitted in food that has been contaminated with sewage. The liver disease caused by HAV is sometimes called infectious hepatitis. The hepatitis E virus (HEV) is an enteric form of non-A, non-B hepatitis that is primarily found in the water supply after catastrophic seasonal flooding in third-world countries throughout Central and South America, Asia, India, and Africa. All of the other hepatitis viruses (B, C, and D) are primarily transmitted by the inadvertent introduction of infected blood or blood products into the circulation. Liver infections caused by this group of viruses are often collectively referred to as serum hepatitis. Infection with the hepatitis B virus (HBV) is the most common cause of this form of hepatitis.

Serum hepatitis (types B, C, and D) is of particular concern to oral health care workers because they are at increased risk for the disease if they come in contact with saliva or blood from infected patients. In addition, hepatitis viruses survive on inadequately sterilized dental instruments and therefore can be transmitted to other patients. Approximately 90% of all patients infected with HBV completely recover from the infection, and 60% to 70% never have any symptoms (i.e., subclinical infection). However, the disease is fatal 0.2% to 0.5% of the time.[74] Once infected with HBV, approximately 2% to 10% of patients remain chronically infected and become carriers of the virus.[74] Chronic infection with the virus often leads to further liver damage, and in many patients, a fatal liver malignancy (hepatocellular carcinoma) develops. Therefore, all health care providers who are exposed to the blood and saliva of potential carriers of HBV must be immunized against the disease, and appropriate infection control procedures must be used at all times. It is not possible to determine from a self-reported medical history whether a patient is a carrier of HBV because many infected patients are asymptomatic. Therefore, it is necessary to assume that all patients are potential carriers of HBV. For this reason, rigorous infection control procedures must be followed for every patient.

ACQUIRED IMMUNODEFICIENCY SYNDROME

Acquired immunodeficiency syndrome (AIDS) is caused by infection with the human immunodeficiency virus (HIV), which is a ribonucleic acid–containing retrovirus. It is transmitted primarily through sexual activities that result in the transfer of certain body fluids, such as blood or semen, from one individual to another. Other major routes of transmission include the sharing of contaminated needles by intravenous drug users (parenteral route) and transmission from infected mothers to their newborns. In comparison to many other viruses, HIV is relatively difficult to transmit. It is not passed from person to person through food, clothing, sneezing, shaking hands, or casual contact.[75-77]

HIV infects and eventually kills a wide range of cells, but it has a particular predilection for subpopulations of CD4-positive helper T cells (thymus-derived lymphocytes that promote certain immunologic reactions and carry a cell surface receptor designated as CD4). The depletion of CD4-positive helper T cells can result in severe immunosuppression that makes the patient susceptible to many life-threatening fungal, bacterial, and viral infections. Infection with one or more of these opportunistic pathogens is the major cause of AIDS-related deaths.[75] Some other common cellular targets of the virus are monocytes, endothelial cells, and certain cells of the central nervous system. HIV infection of the brain can result in severe neurologic dysfunction, including paralysis and dementia.[75]

Depending on the population examined and the diagnostic criteria used, epidemiologic surveys indicate that 15% to 74% of HIV-infected individuals have oral manifestations of the disease.[75] The most frequently reported oral lesion in patients with AIDS is a fungal infection called candidiasis.[78-82] This infection is caused by the overgrowth of *Candida albicans*, a yeast commonly found in the normal oral microbiota. Approximately half of patients with AIDS have oral candidiasis.[78-82] Lesions can develop on virtually any mucosal surface in the mouth and perioral tissues. The clinical features of candidiasis are variable. However, in one common form (thrush, or acute pseudomembranous candidiasis), the palate and buccal mucosa are covered with white patches that can be wiped off, leaving a reddened, ulcerated, and tender mucosal surface (Figure 9-7). Treatment usually involves the administration of topical or systemic antifungal agents. Because the condition is frequently uncomfortable, elective dental and periodontal procedures should be delayed until the infection is controlled. Candidiasis can also occur in HIV-negative patients. This infection usually occurs in patients who take an antibiotic, such as tetracycline, which suppresses the oral microbiota and allows *Candida* to overgrow. It also can occur under ill-fitting artificial dentures and partial dentures in older patients who are not infected with HIV.

HIV-infected patients, especially those who already have AIDS or are on the verge of manifesting it, often contract several viral infections of the oral cavity. According to most epidemiologic reports, the most common of these is caused by a herpesvirus called the Epstein-Barr virus (EBV).[82] Before the era of AIDS, EBV was primarily associated with two types of malignancies, Burkitt's lymphoma (a neoplasm of B lymphocytes) and certain nasopharyngeal carcinomas. In HIV-positive patients, EBV has been strongly linked to a generally

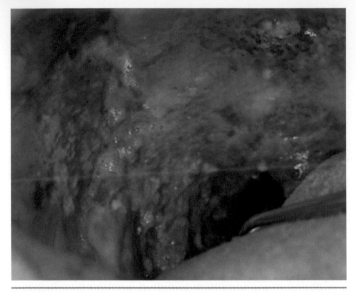

FIGURE 9-7 ■ Acute pseudomembranous candidiasis of the soft palate and buccal mucosa in a 43-year-old man with AIDS.

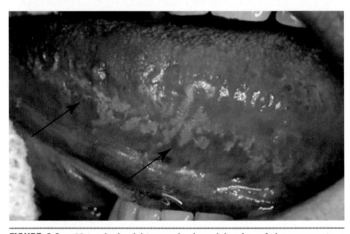

FIGURE 9-8 ■ Hairy leukoplakia on the lateral border of the tongue in a 36-year-old man with AIDS.

asymptomatic oral lesion called hairy leukoplakia.[75] This corrugated white lesion usually occurs on the lateral border of the tongue (Figure 9-8). In some patients, hairy leukoplakia is the first sign of HIV infection. Many HIV-positive individuals with the lesion have full-blown AIDS within 36 months of its appearance.[83] In addition to EBV, other DNA-containing viruses cause oral lesions at a higher rate in HIV-positive patients compared with HIV-negative patients. These include human papilloma viruses, which cause oral warts, herpes simplex, which is the cause of herpetic ulcerations, and herpes zoster, which causes chickenpox and shingles.

Some HIV-positive patients also have severe forms of periodontal disease, such as NUG or necrotizing ulcerative periodontitis (NUP) and rapidly progressing periodontitis.[84-86] The amount and rapidity of tissue destruction in patients with NUP can be particularly striking (Figure 9-9). These diseases of bacterial origin are not unique to immunosuppressed HIV-positive individuals, but most studies show that they occur with some regularity in this population of patients.[83-86] The types of bacteria that have been associated with severe cases of periodontitis appear to be similar in both HIV-positive and HIV-negative

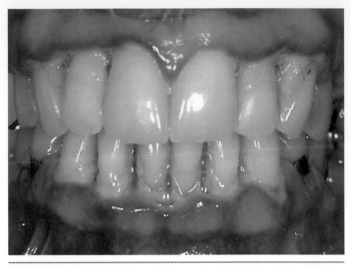

FIGURE 9-9 ■ NUP in a 42-year-old man with AIDS. The periodontal tissues were sore and tender. Other oral manifestations of HIV infection in this patient included candidiasis and hairy leukoplakia. (Courtesy of Dr. R. Fujitaki.)

patients.[87,88] These bacteria include, but are not limited to, *Actinobacillus actinomycetemcomitans*, *Porphyromonas gingivalis*, *Campylobacter rectus*, *P. intermedia*, *Micromonas (Peptostreptococcus) micros*, *Eikenella corrodens*, and various *Treponema* species (spirochetes).

Treatment Considerations

The initial treatment of NUG, NUP, and severe periodontitis in all patients, regardless of their HIV serostatus, involves oral hygiene instructions and thorough scaling and root planing. In immunosuppressed patients, it is particularly advisable to recommend the use of an antimicrobial mouth rinse containing chlorhexidine to assist in the reduction of the plaque bacteria.[89] Because patients with NUG or NUP frequently have tender gingival tissues, multiple visits and local anesthesia are usually required.

The risk to a dentist or dental hygienist of contracting HIV from an infected patient during dental and periodontal procedures is low.[75] The primary danger to health care providers is through the accidental introduction of the patient's blood into the care provider's bloodstream (i.e., parenteral exposure). In a dental setting in which proper infection control procedures are used, practically the only way that this type of accident can occur is through needle sticks or cuts from sharp instruments. Even if this type of accident occurs, the risk of becoming infected with HIV is still small. For example, in one study of 860 medical personnel who had parenteral exposure to HIV-infected blood, only 4 (0.5%) seroconverted.[90]

> **CLINICAL NOTE 9-14** The risk of contracting HIV from the accidental puncture of the skin with an HIV-contaminated needle is very low.

HERPES SIMPLEX INFECTIONS

Herpesviruses are a group of DNA-containing viruses. One member of this group, known as herpes simplex virus-1 (HSV-1), primarily binds to nerve terminals within the epithelial tissues of the mouth and skin.[91] A second virus, herpes simplex-2

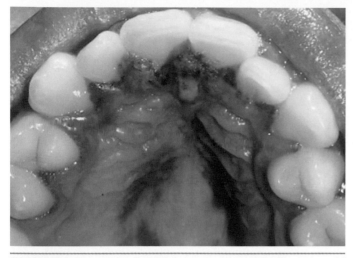

FIGURE 9-10 ■ Herpetic gingival infection in an otherwise healthy 18-year-old male. Note the interproximal lesions. As is the case with ANUG, the disease is of sudden onset and painful. However, unlike ANUG, there is no cratering of the interproximal papillae (compare with Figure 9-6).

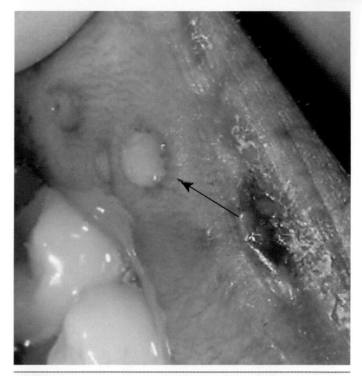

FIGURE 9-11 ■ Herpetic ulcerations of the buccal mucosa of the same patient shown in Figure 9-10.

(HSV-2), primarily affects the genitals. In a few cases, HSV-1 affects the genitals and HSV-2 can affect the oral tissues. Previous exposure and infection with HSV-1 is common, with approximately 90% of the population demonstrating antibody to the virus.[92] Most of the time, infection with HSV-1 occurs during childhood. Patients usually have some symptoms of the common cold, such as a low-grade fever and a runny nose. HSV-1 has an unusual natural cycle. After initial infection of an epithelial surface, the virus migrates along branches of the main sensory nerve of the face, the trigeminal nerve, to the trigeminal ganglion, where it becomes latent, or inactive. Later in life, the virus can be reactivated by a variety of stimuli, migrate to the original site of infection, and cause mucosal or dermal ulcerations.[91] This condition is called secondary, or recurrent, HSV infection. It occurs in approximately 40% of the population at some point.[92]

Intraoral herpetic ulcerations may appear on the tongue, buccal mucosa, and gingiva (Figures 9-10 and 9-11). The lesions are of rapid onset and painful. The patient usually has a fever and does not feel well. Herpetic gingival lesions are sometimes confused with gingival changes associated with NUG because both diseases have a rapid onset and are painful. It is important to distinguish clinically between the two diseases because bacterial infections, such as NUG, can be treated by removal and control of dental plaque, whereas viral infections do not respond to such treatment. It is usually easy to eliminate NUG as the problem because patients with this bacterial infection rarely have ulcerations of the buccal mucosa or tongue. In addition, the gingival lesions of NUG are usually confined to interproximal gingival tissues that have a cratered, or punched-out, appearance (see Figure 9-6). In medically healthy individuals, herpetic lesions are usually self-limiting and resolve without therapy within 10 to 14 days (Figure 9-12). Supportive measures, such as adequate bed rest and ingestion of fluids, are usually all that is necessary. However, it is sometimes advisable to have patients see their physician to determine whether there is a serious underlying medical problem that has precipitated the recurrent herpetic infection.

HUMAN PAPILLOMAVIRUS INFECTIONS

DNA-containing human papillomaviruses (HPVs) target epithelial cells. Certain subtypes of HPV cause the widely familiar skin (cutaneous) wart. There are more than 65 known subtypes of HPV, of which at least 11 affect the oral epithelium.[93] The HPV subtypes that cause cutaneous warts are usually different from those that cause oral lesions, but there are some exceptions. The most common oral lesion associated with HPV is a benign epithelial tumor called an oral squamous cell papilloma. As many as 80% of these lesions are caused by HPV subtypes 6 and 11.[93] They can appear on any soft tissue surface in the mouth, but have a predilection for the soft palate. Gingival lesions occasionally occur (Figures 9-13 and 9-14). They have a characteristic cauliflower-like appearance and a white or pink exterior. They can usually be successfully treated by surgical removal. Transmission is believed to occur by direct contact with a lesion that is actively shedding virus particles.

Some HPV (primarily subtype 16), in conjunction with other risk factors, such as tobacco and alcohol use, are believed to have an association with a type of **oral cancer** called squamous cell carcinoma.[94,95] However, most papilloma-like lesions do not lead to oral cancer. As with all soft tissue lesions or abnormalities, their presence should be pointed out to the patient and the dentist should be notified so that the lesions can be appropriately treated.

DERMATOLOGIC DISEASES

Many diseases that involve the skin can also affect the soft tissues of the mouth. This observation is not surprising because the skin and oral mucous membranes share many histologic characteristics. The list of diseases with skin involvement that may have an oral counterpart is long, but a few of the more

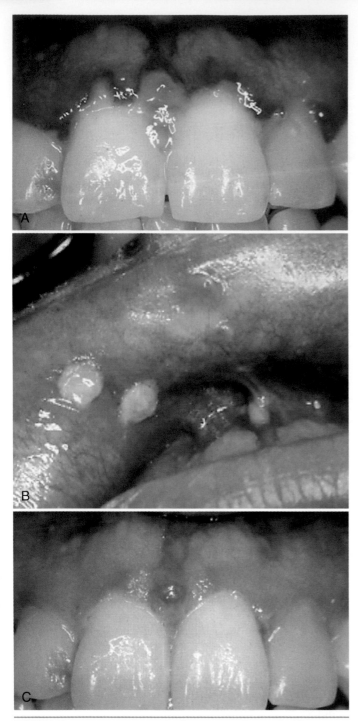

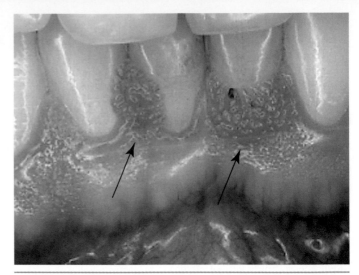

FIGURE 9-13 ■ Multiple gingival papillomas *(arrow)* in the lower anterior area of a medically healthy 32-year-old male. The lesions had been present for 3 years.

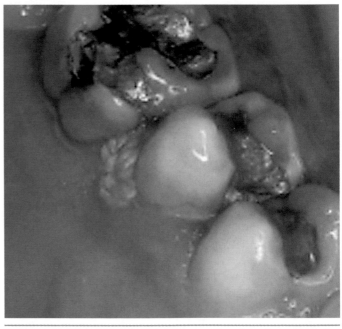

FIGURE 9-14 ■ Solitary gingival papilloma with a hyperkeratotic surface between an upper first molar and a second premolar in a medically healthy 15-year-old female. The patient was unaware of the lesion.

FIGURE 9-12 ■ **A,** Herpetic gingival infection in an otherwise healthy 25-year-old male. **B,** Ulcerations of the adjacent oral mucosa of the upper lip were also present. **C,** The same patient 11 days later. There has been spontaneous resolution of the gingival lesions. No periodontal therapy was administered because herpetic lesions are usually self-limiting and run their course in 10 to 14 days. (Courtesy of Dr. R. E. Robinson.)

notable diseases are malignant melanoma, squamous cell carcinoma, Kaposi's sarcoma, candidiasis, HPV infection, psoriasis, and vesiculobullous diseases, such as erythema multiforme, pemphigus vulgaris, pemphigoid, and lichen planus.

The dental hygienist is sometimes the first member of the oral health care team to detect soft tissue lesions of the mouth. If such a lesion is observed, it may be impossible to determine immediately whether the lesion is an infection, an innocent oral manifestation of a skin condition, or a potentially lethal oral cancer. Dental hygienists should be able to distinguish between normal and abnormal hard and soft oral tissues. The dental hygienist is expected to detect oral lesions, not to diagnose them. The importance of detecting abnormalities cannot be overemphasized. For example, prompt detection of a white lesion of the oral mucosa, which is later found to be an early squamous cell carcinoma, can be lifesaving. Detection of oral cancers at an early stage in their growth, when they are small and easy to treat, is the single most important factor in the successful treatment or cure of oral cancer.

In addition to their role in the detection of abnormalities, dental hygienists frequently treat patients who have painful oral lesions associated with certain **dermatologic diseases.**

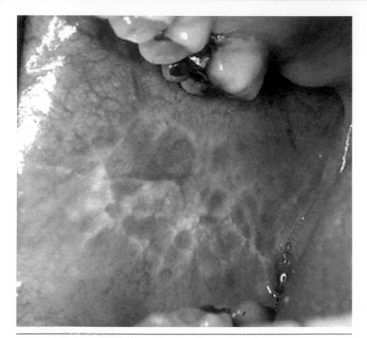

FIGURE 9-15 ■ Reticular form of lichen planus on the right buccal mucosa of a 48-year-old female. The lacelike white lesions (striae of Wickham) are characteristic of lichen planus.

Uncomfortable oral lesions can complicate routine approaches to periodontal therapy by preventing the patient from performing adequate oral hygiene procedures or by making subgingival instrumentation more difficult. There are many examples of systemic conditions in which this problem occurs, but lichen planus is probably the most common dermatologic disease that may cause painful oral lesions.

LICHEN PLANUS

Lichen planus is a chronic inflammatory skin and mucosal disease that affects approximately 1% of the general population.[96] Although the causes of lichen planus are unknown, cell-mediated autoimmune reactions against basal epithelial cells are involved. Lesions of the oral mucosa appear in approximately 75% of patients with lichen planus and 30% have only oral lesions.[96] It affects men and women more or less equally.

The most common type of lichen planus is the reticular form, which is characterized by the presence of lacelike white lesions on the buccal mucosa (Figure 9-15). The tongue and gingiva are also frequently involved.[97] The lesions usually produce no symptoms, but in one prospective study of 181 patients with reticular lichen planus, 55% reported some oral discomfort because of the lesions.[97] Two other, less common types of lichen planus are the atrophic and erosive forms. Both types frequently cause painful gingival lesions. Gingival lesions in the atrophic form usually consist of fiery red tissues that are sore and tender (Figure 9-16). Erosive forms of lichen planus are also uncomfortable because of the development of mucosal ulcerations. Approximately 85% of patients with the atrophic or erosive forms of lichen planus report pain and soreness.[97]

The pain associated with oral lichen planus lesions can often be reduced by the topical or systemic administration of steroids.[98] Some success has also been reported in reducing the gingival discomfort by instituting a professionally supervised

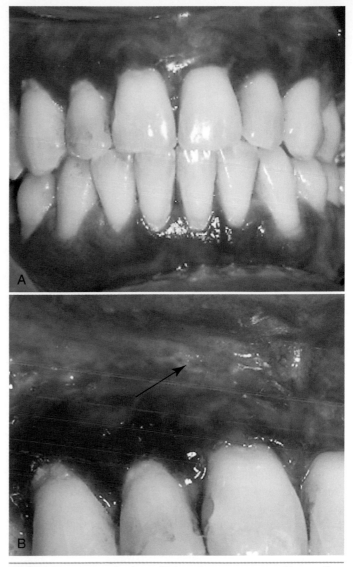

FIGURE 9-16 ■ **A,** Atrophic form of lichen planus in a 52-year-old man affecting gingival tissues around the upper and lower teeth. In this form of lichen planus, the gingival tissues are usually bright red and tender. The tenderness interfered with the patient's ability to perform plaque control procedures. **B,** Lacelike white lesions of the alveolar mucosa, apical to the mucogingival junction of the upper right lateral and central incisors (*arrow*).

intensive program of oral hygiene instruction in which an antimicrobial mouth rinse (0.2% chlorhexidine) is used.[99] Even though dental plaque is not the cause of lichen planus, it appears that plaque-induced inflammation superimposed on sites affected by lichen planus can contribute to the patient's discomfort.[99]

ORAL CANCER

Cancer is a general term for a large group of potentially fatal diseases in which there is an uncontrolled growth of genetically altered abnormal cells. Such cells are generally referred to as malignant because, if not eliminated, they can lead to death. Death is usually the result of the destruction or replacement of tissues of one or more vital organs by cancer cells. Certain cancers are sometimes referred to as malignant neoplasms (new growths) or malignant tumors (swellings). Some neoplasms and

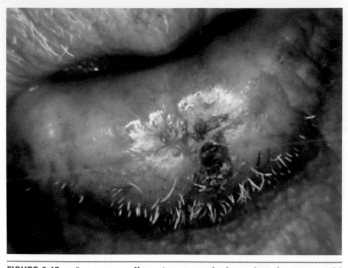

FIGURE 9-17 ■ **Squamous cell carcinoma on the lower lip of a 68-year-old man.** The patient had noticed the lesion for 18 months and wanted to know, "Why hasn't the sore healed?" Long-standing unhealed sores can be a sign of cancer.

tumors are composed of morphologically and genetically normal cells. Such growths are usually not life-threatening and are called benign neoplasms or tumors.

There are many causes of cancer. Frequently, more than one factor leads to the formation of cancer cells. Important risk factors that predispose people to the development of oral cancer include smoking or other tobacco use, excessive alcohol intake, exposure to ionizing radiation, ingestion of environmental toxins and chemicals, and infection with certain viruses. Cancers can affect essentially all organ systems and types of tissues. An oral cancer is any malignant growth that originates from tissues of the mouth. There are two basic ways in which cancer cells can spread:

- By local invasion of adjacent tissues
- By metastasis

Metastasis is the process whereby malignant cells are carried away from the site of origin to another part of the body. It occurs when malignant cells are shed by the tumor, enter the bloodstream or lymphatic system, and are carried to other tissues.

Oral cancers can cause a variety of signs and symptoms. For example, white or red lesions of the oral mucosa could be cancerous. Long-standing ulcerations or unhealed sores of the mouth or lips should be particularly suspected of being cancerous (Figure 9-17). Unexplained lumps or swellings of the mouth or face could be the first sign of certain cancers. In rare cases, even common signs of periodontitis, such as loose teeth and radiographically visible bone loss, can be signs of a malignant lesion (Figure 9-18).

The most frequent type of oral cancer is squamous cell carcinoma, a malignancy that develops from epithelial cells. In the United States, approximately 30,000 new cases of oral squamous cell carcinoma are diagnosed each year. The development of oral squamous cell carcinoma is strongly linked to pipe and cigarette smoking.[100] Heavy smokers frequently have visible changes in their palatal tissues (Figure 9-19). The chronic use of smokeless tobacco (snuff) has also been linked to the development of this type of oral cancer.[101] Most snuff users habitually

place the tobacco between the gingiva and cheek and leave it there for prolonged periods. In almost all cases, the oral mucosa has dramatic and clinically obvious changes (Figure 9-20).

Treatment of cancer usually involves a combination of approaches, all of which are aimed at eradicating the malignancy. Basic cancer therapy techniques involve the following:

- Surgical excision of the lesion
- Administration of anticancer drugs (chemotherapy)
- Irradiation of the malignancy

TREATMENT CONSIDERATIONS

Oral health care practitioners are frequently called on to provide important dental and periodontal services before or during cancer treatment. In some forms of cancer therapy, such as bone marrow transplantation and chemotherapy, patients may become susceptible to infections because of the severe immunosuppression induced by the cancer treatment. In such cases, it is important to eliminate all ongoing oral infections before the cancer treatment.

Most chemotherapeutic approaches to the treatment of cancer use toxic drugs that are capable of killing malignant cells. Unfortunately, when such drugs are systemically administered, they also kill normal cells, thereby creating a variety of severe side effects. Some cancer-fighting drugs cause painful oral ulcerations that make routine plaque control procedures impossible (Figures 9-21 and 9-22). Therefore, it is important to bring the patient's oral disease(s) under control before toxic anticancer drugs are administered.

Radiation therapy is sometimes used to treat some cancers of the head and neck. Although during modern radiation therapy, attempts are made to shield nondiseased tissues from the lethal doses of radiation, some damage to the salivary glands can occur. In such cases, the patient may experience a temporary, but sometimes permanent, reduction in salivary flow. The resulting xerostomia (dry mouth) can promote plaque retention and increase the patient's risk of severe dental caries. Another possible side effect of radiation treatment of head and neck tumors is temporary damage to the oral mucosa. In such cases, mucosal tissues lining the oral cavity receive radiation burns. These burns make the mouth tender. This condition is sometimes called radiation-induced mucositis. Because routine oral hygiene procedures are difficult in these situations, it is often advisable to see patients at frequent intervals for prophylaxis during the course of the radiation treatment. Frequent treatment may minimize the chances of plaque-induced diseases.

CLINICAL NOTE 9-15 Dental hygienists play an important role in preventing radiation-induced mucositis by helping affected patients improve their oral hygiene practices.

BLOOD DYSCRASIAS

The term **blood dyscrasias** refers to a large group of disorders that affect cellular elements of the blood (i.e., red or white blood cells). Patients with blood dyscrasias are occasionally encountered in most dental practices. In some of these disorders, there is impaired function of infection-fighting white blood cells, such as polymorphonuclear neutrophilic leukocytes

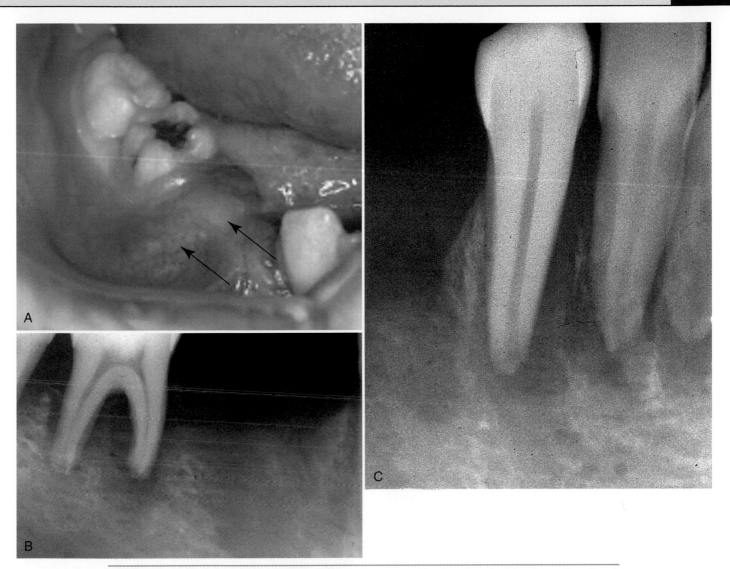

FIGURE 9-18 ■ A, Painless swelling in the lower right jaw of a 19-year-old male with Burkitt's lymphoma. Several teeth in the quadrant were loose. B and C, Radiographs of the lower right quadrant. The diffuse radiolucencies around the teeth and in the surrounding alveolar bone show sites where the malignancy has destroyed bone.

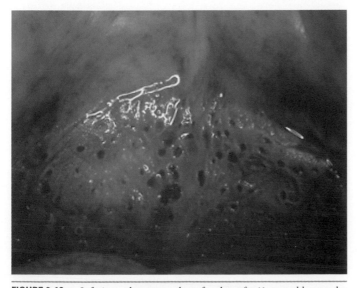

FIGURE 9-19 ■ Soft tissue changes on the soft palate of a 41-year-old man who was a heavy drinker and cigarette smoker (three packs/day). The lesions were not yet malignant, but extensive use of alcohol and tobacco products increases the risk of oral cancer (squamous cell carcinoma).

(PMNs, or neutrophils). As a result, periodontal disease and other oral infections can worsen in patients who have either impaired PMN function or a significant decrease in normal numbers of PMNs (i.e., leukopenia). Commonly encountered blood disorders that affect white blood cell populations include aplastic anemia, agranulocytosis, cyclic neutropenia, and several forms of leukemia.

APLASTIC ANEMIA, AGRANULOCYTOSIS, AND CYCLIC NEUTROPENIA

The term *aplastic anemia* refers to a dramatic reduction in the ability of bone marrow to produce most of the cellular components of blood. It can be caused by a variety of factors, but environmental exposure to toxic chemicals (e.g., benzene) or certain drugs (e.g., chloramphenicol) has been implicated as the cause in some patients. In some cases, no cause can be identified (known as idiopathic aplastic anemia). Patients with this disease experience a rapidly progressing form of periodontitis (Figure 9-23), probably because of the significant decline in the numbers of neutrophils, which are necessary to fight infection.[102,103]

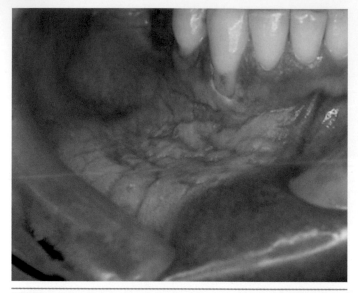

FIGURE 9-20 ■ Changes in the oral mucosa associated with the use of smokeless tobacco (snuff) in a 42-year-old male. For 20 years (approximately 10 times/day), the patient had placed snuff between the buccal mucosa and gingiva. Use of smokeless tobacco can lead to the development of squamous cell carcinomas. Note the gingival recession on the facial surface of the lower canine. Such recession is a common finding at sites where the snuff is placed.

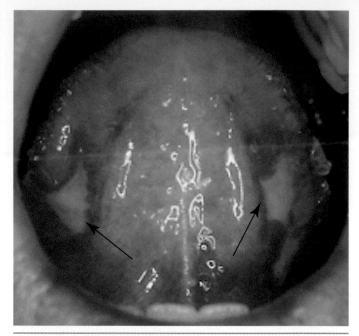

FIGURE 9-22 ■ Severe ulcerations on the ventral surface of the tongue in a 20-year-old male who was being treated for testicular cancer (choriocarcinoma) with a toxic anticancer drug (dactinomycin).

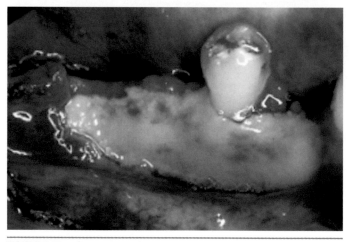

FIGURE 9-21 ■ Severe gingival ulcerations in a 27-year-old woman who was treated for cancer (lymphosarcoma) with a systemically administered toxic anticancer drug (methotrexate). Oral ulcerations can be a side effect of some drugs used for cancer treatment (see Figure 9-22).

Agranulocytosis is the depletion of the granulocyte precursors in the bone marrow. Because PMNs are one type of granulocyte, severe periodontal infections are frequently a feature of this disease.[104,105] In addition, oral ulcerations occur with some regularity. As with aplastic anemia, this disorder can be caused by a reaction to certain medications (e.g., chloramphenicol, methimazole).

Cyclic neutropenia is a blood dyscrasia of unknown etiology in which there are periodic reductions in neutrophil populations in the blood and bone marrow. As might be expected, patients with this disease experience flare-ups of any existing periodontal infection during the period of PMN depletion.[106]

Treatment Considerations

Periodontal diseases in affected patients are all caused by dental plaque. Therefore, because these patients are at increased risk

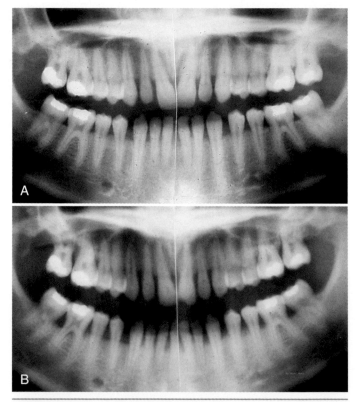

FIGURE 9-23 ■ **A,** Rapidly progressing periodontitis in a 19-year-old male with aplastic anemia. **B,** Radiograph of the same patient taken 12 months after the one shown in A. Note the marked loss of alveolar bone that had occurred in this young patient in only 1 year. Patients with aplastic anemia and some other blood dyscrasias are highly susceptible to periodontal infections.

for periodontal infection, they should be given a rigorous program designed to prevent gingivitis and periodontitis. Even in these high-risk patients, periodontal damage will not occur if dental plaque is adequately controlled.

CLINICAL NOTE 9-16 Dental hygienists play an important role in the management of the oral problems experienced by patients with blood dyscrasias.

LEUKEMIAS

Leukemias are a group of cell malignancies of the bone marrow. Although the precise causes of leukemia are unknown, some forms have been strongly linked to certain viruses or exposure to ionizing radiation.[107] In these diseases, abnormal white blood cells replace and actively suppress the differentiation of normal bone marrow tissue. As the normal marrow is replaced, a significant depletion of infection-fighting normal white blood cells occurs. In addition, there is a drastic reduction in the production of platelets, which are necessary for the normal clotting of blood. As a result, patients with leukemia (particularly those with acute forms) are at increased risk for infections and bleeding problems. Overwhelming infection and uncontrollable bleeding are the two primary causes of death in patients with leukemia.

There are several forms of leukemia. The major types are acute lymphoblastic leukemia, acute myeloblastic leukemia, chronic myeloid leukemia, and chronic lymphocytic leukemia.[107] The acute forms have a sudden onset and lead to death within a few months unless treated. Chronic forms develop slowly and usually have a relatively long clinical course. In general, 80% of patients with acute lymphoblastic leukemia are younger than 15 years, whereas most patients with acute myeloblastic leukemia are between the ages of 15 and 39 years. The chronic forms of leukemia usually affect adults. In all types of leukemia, increased susceptibility to infection (including periodontal disease) can be a problem because of the immunosuppression associated with the disease or its treatment. Of all patients with leukemia, those with the chronic forms are most likely to be seen in a dental practice because they are often being medically managed on an outpatient basis.

CLINICAL NOTE 9-17 Because of their increased susceptibility to periodontal infections, patients with chronic leukemia should have their teeth professionally cleaned at frequent intervals and should be given a rigorous plaque control program.

In some forms of leukemia (particularly acute myeloblastic leukemia), gingival enlargement occurs as a result of the accumulation of leukemic cells in the gingival tissues and swelling caused by plaque-induced inflammation.[108] This oral manifestation of leukemia is relatively rare and is usually seen only in very sick, hospitalized patients.

Some patients with acute leukemia are treated with bone marrow transplantation. This treatment involves the intentional destruction of the abnormal marrow before the insertion of normal marrow cells. Because severe immunosuppression occurs with this treatment, it is advisable to eliminate all sources of oral infection before the patient's malignant bone marrow is

destroyed.[108] This step is important because uncontrolled oral infections can be fatal in severely immunosuppressed patients. For this reason, dentists and dental hygienists are an important part of the medical team that performs bone marrow transplantation procedures.

NEUROLOGIC DISORDERS

Patients with a variety of neurologic disorders are frequently encountered in dental practices. Many diseases affect the nervous system, and an equally large number of conditions have neurologic manifestations.[109] Patients with diseases of the nervous and neuromuscular systems present three basic problems:

1. Physical inability to perform adequate oral hygiene procedures because of difficulties associated with hand and movement coordination
2. Mental or physical inability to cooperate with the practitioner
3. Changes in oral tissues that increase the risk for dental diseases

The first two present an obvious set of patient management difficulties. Because these patients often have low levels of cooperation and poorly executed personal oral hygiene procedures, they should be seen regularly for professionally administered oral care.

CLINICAL NOTE 9-18 Dental hygienists can play a very important role in teaching the patient's daily caregiver how to perform oral hygiene procedures for the patient.

PHENYTOIN-INFLUENCED GINGIVAL ENLARGEMENT

Gingival enlargement associated with the administration of anticonvulsant drugs, such as phenytoin, is probably the most common change in the oral tissues of patients with neurologic problems. Phenytoin is often prescribed by neurologists to control cerebral seizures (epilepsy), which are disorders in which the brain undergoes an involuntary burst of chaotic electrical activity. Most patients with cerebral seizures are of normal intelligence and can lead productive lives if their seizures are controlled. A troublesome side effect of phenytoin is the development of gingival enlargement, which can cause aesthetic and plaque control problems for the patient (Figure 9-24). Approximately 50% of patients who take phenytoin for a long period experience this side effect, although its reported incidence varies from 0% to 84.5%, depending on the criteria used for enlargement.[110] Plaque control problems associated with gingival enlargement can lead to periodontitis and tooth loss. In cases of severe enlargement, surgical excision of the gingival tissue is required.

Treatment Considerations

Although the mechanisms associated with phenytoin-influenced gingival enlargement are not completely understood, evidence shows that plaque-induced inflammation plays an important role in the process.[110,111] Therefore, patients who have this side effect should be urged to practice meticulous oral hygiene procedures. In addition, frequent visits for

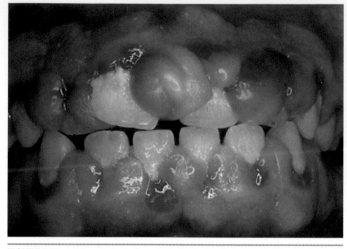

FIGURE 9-24 ■ **Phenytoin-influenced gingival enlargement.** This 23-year-old male was taking phenytoin to help control cerebral seizures. He had been taking the drug for 5 years.

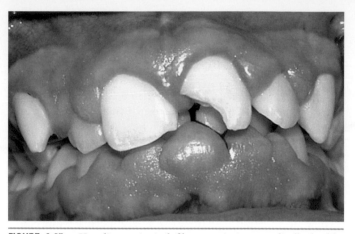

FIGURE 9-25 ■ **Hereditary gingival fibromatosis in a medically healthy 15-year-old male.** Although the gingival enlargement resembles that associated with the ingestion of phenytoin (see Figure 9-24), the patient was not taking any medications. The chipped front tooth was caused by a sports accident.

professionally administered cleaning of the teeth is advisable. Patients who have undergone periodontal surgery to remove the enlarged gingiva are likely to experience a recurrence unless rigorous daily plaque control procedures are practiced.[111] Recurrence is also likely for patients who experience drug-influenced gingival enlargement as a side effect of certain immunosuppressive drugs (e.g., cyclosporine) that are used to combat rejection of transplanted organs or some medications (e.g., verapamil, nifedipine) that are used to treat cardiovascular problems.

Gingival enlargement also occurs in some patients who are not taking any medications. Such patients have a rare condition known as hereditary gingival fibromatosis (Figure 9-25).[112,113] The disease is transmitted as an autosomal dominant trait that is not fully expressed in every case.[114]

CLINICAL NOTE 9-19 Meticulous oral hygiene and frequent visits for professional tooth cleaning help minimize recurrence of drug-influenced and hereditary forms of gingival enlargement.

TOBACCO USE AND PERIODONTAL DISEASE

In addition to the catastrophic consequences of cigarette smoking, such as emphysema, lung cancer, heart disease, and oral cancer, there is strong evidence that tobacco use is an important risk factor for periodontal disease.[115-117] The mechanisms where by smoking increases susceptibility to periodontal infections are not completely known, but it is likely that smoking suppresses certain components of the immune system.[118,119] Impaired neutrophil function induced by products of tobacco smoke appears to be particularly important.[120-123]

Dental hygienists can play an important role in smoking cessation programs. However, understanding and tact are needed. Patients with periodontitis frequently ask the dentist or dental hygienist, "Does cigarette smoking play a role in my gum disease?" When such questions are asked, it is advisable to inform the patient that periodontal diseases are infections and that smoking reduces the resistance to infections. However, even in smokers, it is possible to treat periodontitis if the plaque

bacteria are well controlled. Because smokers are addicted to their habit, it is not wise to tell them that their gum disease will worsen unless they stop smoking. This statement only discourages the patient. Addictions are difficult to break, and patients should be given hope that their periodontal disease can be controlled without cessation of smoking. However, controlling periodontal disease is more difficult if the patient continues to smoke.

◎ DENTAL HYGIENE CONSIDERATIONS

- Systemic conditions are often encountered in typical dental practices. As a key member of the oral health care team, the dental hygienist will be called on to treat patients with medical problems.
- It is necessary to consider the entire patient in order to provide optimal prevention and treatment of dental and periodontal diseases.
- The dental hygienist must realize how a patient's systemic condition influences the development and progression of dental and periodontal diseases.
- Plaque-induced oral diseases in most patients with medical problems can be safely and effectively treated in a dental setting.
- Even in very ill patients, treatment of plaque-induced infections is important because a comfortable, disease-free mouth can greatly improve the patient's quality of life.
- Treatment of dental diseases in patients with medical problems is helpful and causes no harm as long as appropriate precautions and modifications in therapeutic approaches are taken, as dictated by the medical history and condition of the patient.

✳ CASE SCENARIO

Mrs. Henry is a 52-year-old African American female whom you are seeing for the first time. She is a new patient in the practice and the dentist has interviewed her and has now asked you to review her medical history and assess her oral condition. Mrs. Henry completed the medical history form and has stated that she is in excellent health, with no history of illness, and that she is taking no medications. Her dental history indicates that she has regular dental check-ups and cleanings. You take her vital signs, which are respirations 20, pulse 82, and blood pressure 189/94. You take her vital signs a second time after having her relax in the chair for 10 minutes and the reading is unchanged. You inform Mrs. Henry of these results and tell her that before any treatment can be done she needs to have her blood pressure evaluated by her physician. She becomes very angry and accuses you of practicing medicine without a license.

1. According to the American Dental Association guidelines regarding hypertension, Mrs. Henry may have
   A. prehypertension.
   B. stage 1 hypertension.
   C. stage 2 hypertension.
   D. stage 3 hypertension.

2. Patients with this level of blood pressure can be treated
   A. for selective dental procedures.
   B. for nonemergent procedures only.
   C. for emergent dental procedures and then provided with immediate medical referral.
   D. for emergent dental procedures but not provided with immediate medical referral.

3. You are quite distressed by Mrs. Henry's reaction to your concern for her health. The most appropriate response is to
   A. call the dentist in to speak to her.
   B. explain to her the significance of hypertension.
   C. offer to assist her in getting an appointment with her physician for an evaluation.
   D. all of the above.

STUDY QUESTIONS

Answers and rationales to these questions can be obtained from your instructor.

MULTIPLE-CHOICE

1. High blood pressure is a major risk factor for all of the following EXCEPT one. Which one is the EXCEPTION?
   A. Stroke
   B. Liver disease
   C. Kidney failure
   D. Cardiovascular disease

2. Patients are considered to have prehypertension if their blood pressure is routinely found to be which of the following?
   A. 110/75 mm Hg
   B. 119/79 mm Hg
   C. 132/84 mm Hg
   D. 142/91 mm Hg
   E. 155/90 mm Hg

3. Gingival tissue enlargement is a common side effect of
   A. nitroglycerin.
   B. corticosteroids.
   C. local anesthetics.
   D. endogenous epinephrine.
   E. calcium channel blockers.

4. The deposition of cholesterol-containing material in the walls of arteries is called angina pectoris. Severe recurring chest pain from angina pectoris often radiates into the kidneys and lower back.
   A. Both statements are true.
   B. Both statements are false.
   C. The first statement is true, and the second statement is false.
   D. The first statement is false, and the second statement is true.

5. Antibiotic coverage (prophylaxis) prior to periodontal scaling and root planing is usually recommended for patients who have a
   A. cardiac pacemaker.
   B. cardiac defibrillator.
   C. functional heart murmur.
   D. history of atherosclerosis.
   E. history of infective endocarditis.

6. Rheumatic fever is an acute systemic inflammatory disease that sometimes follows throat infections with
   A. group A streptococci.
   B. *P. intermedia.*
   C. *Streptococcus mutans.*
   D. *P. gingivalis.*
   E. *A. actinomycetemcomitans.*

7. Soon after sitting down in a dental chair, a patient with type 1 DM rapidly develops the following signs and symptoms: mental confusion, slurred speech, rapid heartbeat, nausea, and cold clammy skin. These signs and symptoms are characteristic of
   A. insulin shock.
   B. hyperglycemia.
   C. angina pectoris.
   D. myocardial infarction.
   E. fear of having dental work done.

8. HIV can be transmitted by all of the following EXCEPT one. Which one is the EXCEPTION?
   A. Aerosols from sneezing
   B. Unprotected sexual contact
   C. Sharing of contaminated needles
   D. Nonsterilized dental instruments
   E. Blood from infected mothers to newborns

SHORT ANSWER

9. A patient tells you that smoking has nothing to do with his periodontal disease and does not see why he should stop. What would you tell him?

10. When providing routine dental care to patients with a history of congestive heart failure, how should the dental chair should be placed?

Please visit **http://evolve.elsevier.com/Perry/periodontology** for additional practice and study support tools.

REFERENCES

1. Council on Community Health, Hospital, Institutional and Medical Affairs. Hypertension update: a survey of the literature of interest to dentists. *J Am Dent Assoc.* 1989;118:645–646.
2. Council on Dental Health and Health Planning, Bureau of Health Education and Audiovisual Services. Breaking the silence on hypertension: a dental perspective. *J Am Dent Assoc.* 1985;110:781–782.
3. Fay JT, O'Neal R. Dental responsibility for the medically compromised patient. *J Oral Med.* 1984;39:148–156.
4. National Heart, Lung, and Blood Institute. What is high blood pressure? 2012 (http://www.nhlbi.nih.gov/health/health-topics/topics/hbp).
5. Chobanian AV, Bakris GL, Black HR, et al; Joint National Committee on Detection, Evaluation and Treatment of High Blood Pressure. Seventh report of the Joint National Committee on Detection, Evaluation and Treatment of High Blood Pressure. *Hypertension.* 2003;42:1206–1252.
6. Muzyka BC, Glick M. The hypertensive dental patient. *J Am Dent Assoc.* 1997;128:1109–1120.
7. Hasse AL, Heng MK, Garrett NR. Blood pressure and electrocardiographic response to dental treatment with use of local anesthesia. *J Am Dent Assoc.* 1986;113:639–642.
8. Abraham-Inpijn L, Borgmeijer-Hoelen A, Gortzak RAT. Changes in blood pressure, heart rate, and electrocardiogram during dental treatment with use of local anesthesia. *J Am Dent Assoc.* 1988;116:531–536.
9. Farkas JA, Goebel WM. Assessing the risk of angina for dental therapy. *Oral Surg Oral Med Oral Pathol.* 1984;58:253–256.
10. Miranda J, Brunet L, Roset P, et al. Prevalence and risk of gingival enlargement in patients treated with nifedipine. *J Periodontol.* 2001;72:605–611.
11. Nery EB, Edson RG, Lee KK, et al. Prevalence of nifedipine-induced gingival hyperplasia. *J Periodontol.* 1995;66:572–578.
12. Katz J, Givol N, Chaushu G, et al. Vigabatrin-induced gingival overgrowth. *J Clin Periodontol.* 1997;24:180–182.
13. Jorgensen MG. Prevalence of amlodipine-related gingival hyperplasia. *J Periodontol.* 1997;68:676–678.
14. Bullon P, Machuca G, Martinez-Sahuquillo A, et al. Clinical assessment of gingival size among patients treated with diltiazem. *Oral Surg Oral Med Oral Pathol.* 1995;79:300–304.
15. Wilson W, Taubert KA, Gewitz M, et al. Prevention of infective endocarditis. Guidelines from the American Heart Association. *Circulation.* 2007;116:1736–1754.
16. Little JW, Falace DA. Rheumatic fever, rheumatic heart disease, and murmurs. In: *Dental Management of the Medically Compromised Patient.* 3rd ed. St. Louis, MO: CV Mosby; 1988:100–110.
17. Zysset MK, Montgomery MT, Redding SW, et al. Systemic lupus erythematosus: a consideration for antimicrobial prophylaxis. *Oral Surg Oral Med Oral Pathol.* 1987;64:30–34.
18. Perloff JK. Evolving concepts of mitral-valve prolapse. *N Engl J Med.* 1982;307:369–370.
19. Devereux RB, Kramer-Fox R, Kligfield P. Mitral valve prolapse: causes, clinical manifestations, and management. *Ann Intern Med.* 1989;111:305–317.
20. Hancock EW. Coronary artery disease: epidemiology and prevention. In: Rubenstein E, Federman DD, eds. *Scientific American Medicine.* New York, NY: Scientific American; 1991;1(section VIII):1–10.
21. Nagy G, Kovács J, Zeher M, et al. Analysis of the oral manifestations of systemic sclerosis. *Oral Surg Oral Med Oral Pathol.* 1994;77:141–146.
22. Alexandridis C, White SC. Periodontal ligament changes in patients with progressive systemic sclerosis. *Oral Surg Oral Med Oral Pathol.* 1984;58:113–118.
23. Fitzgerald RH Jr, Jacobson JJ, Luck JV Jr, Nelson CL, Osmon DR, et al. Advisory statement: Antibiotic prophylaxis for dental patients with total hip joint replacements. *J Am Dent Assoc.* 1997;128:1004–1008.
24. Little JW. The need for antibiotic coverage for dental treatment of patients with joint replacements. *Oral Surg Oral Med Oral Pathol.* 1983;55:20–23.
25. Ahlberg A, Carlsson AS, Lindberg L. Hematogenous infection in total joint replacement. *Clin Orthop Rel Res.* 1978;137:69–75.
26. Thyne GM, Ferguson JW. Antibiotic prophylaxis during dental treatment in patients with prosthetic joints. *J Bone Joint Surg.* 1991;73B:191–194.
27. Ching DWT, Gould IM, Rennie JAN, et al. Prevention of late haematogenous infection in major prosthetic joints. *J Antimicrob Chemother.* 1989;23:676–680.
28. Bartzokas CA, Johnson R, Jane M, et al. Relation between mouth and haematogenous infection in total joint replacements. *Br Med J.* 1994;309:506 508.
29. Hanssen AD, Osmon DR, Nelson CL. Prevention of deep periprosthetic joint infection. *J Bone Joint Surg[Am].* 1996;78-A:458–471.
30. Mokdad AH, Ford ES, Bowman BA, et al. Diabetes trends in the United States, 1990-98. *Diabetes Care.* 2000;23:1278–1283.
31. American Diabetes Association. Report of the expert committee on the diagnosis and classification of diabetes mellitus. *Diabetes Care.* 2001;24(suppl 1):S5–S20.
32. Mealey BL, Moritz AJ. Hormonal influences: effects of diabetes mellitus and endogenous female sex steroid hormones on the periodontium. *Periodontol 2000.* 2003;32:59–81.
33. Taylor GW. Bidirectional interrelationships between diabetes and periodontal diseases: an epidemiologic perspective. *Ann Periodontol.* 2001;6:99–112.
34. Soskolne WA, Klinger A. The relationship between periodontal diseases and diabetes: an overview. *Ann Periodontol.* 2001;6:91–98.
35. Kjersem H, Hilsted J, Madsbad S, et al. Polymorphonuclear leucocyte dysfunction during short term metabolic changes from normo- to hyperglycemia in type 1 (insulin dependent) diabetic patients. *Infection.* 1988;16:215–221.
36. Wilson RM, Reeves WG. Neutrophil phagocytosis and killing in insulin-dependent diabetes. *Clin Exp Immunol.* 1986;63:478–484.
37. Marhoffer W, Stein M, Maeser E, et al. Impairment of polymorphonuclear leukocyte function and metabolic control of diabetes. *Diabetes Care.* 1992;15:256–260.
38. McMullen JA, Van Dyke TE, Horosweicz HU, et al. Neutrophil chemotaxis in individuals with advanced periodontal disease and a genetic predisposition to diabetes mellitus. *J Periodontol.* 1981;52:167–173.
39. Russotto SB. Asymptomatic parotid gland enlargement in diabetes mellitus. *Oral Surg Oral Med Oral Pathol.* 1981;52:594–598.
40. Conner S, Iranpour B, Mills J. Alteration in parotid salivary flow in diabetes mellitus. *Oral Surg Oral Med Oral Pathol.* 1970;30:55–59.
41. Williams RC, Mahan CJ. Periodontal disease and diabetes in young adults. *JAMA.* 1960;172:776–778.
42. Katagiri S, Nitta H, Nagasawa T, et al. Multi-center intervention study on glycohemoglobin (HbA1c) and serum, high sensivity CRP (ha-CRP) after local anti-infectious periodontal treatment in type 2 diabetic patients with periodontal disease. *Diabetes Res Clin Pract.* 2009;83:308–315.
43. Sun W-L, Chen L-L, Zhang S-Z, et al. Inflammatory cytokines, adiponectin, insulin resistance and metabolic control after periodontal intervention in patients with type 2 diabetes and chronic periodontitis. *Intern Med.* 2011;50:1569–1574.
44. Engebretson SP, Hey-Hadavi J. Sub-antimicrobial doxycycline for periodontitis reduces hemoglobin A1c in subjects with type 2 diabetes: a pilot study. *Pharmacol Res.* 2011;64:624–629.
45. Preshaw PM, Alba AL, Herrera D, et al. Periodontitis and diabetes: a two-way relationship. *Diabetologia.* 2012;55:21–31.
46. Maier AW, Orban B. Gingivitis and pregnancy. *Oral Surg Oral Med Oral Pathol.* 1949;2:334–373.
47. Löe H, Silness J. Periodontal disease in pregnancy: I. Prevalence and severity. *Acta Odontol Scand.* 1963;21:533–551.
48. Silness J, Löe H. Periodontal disease in pregnancy: II. Correlation between oral hygiene and periodontal condition. *Acta Odontol Scand.* 1964;22:121–135.
49. Poole JA, Claman HN. Immunology of pregnancy. Implications for the mother. *Clin Rev Allergy Immunol.* 2004: 26: 161–170.
50. Sooriyamoorthy M, Gower DB. Hormonal influences on gingival tissue: relationship to periodontal disease. *J Clin Periodontol.* 1989;16:201–208.
51. Kornman KS, Loesche WJ. The subgingival microbial flora during pregnancy. *J Periodontal Res.* 1980;15:111–122.
52. Kornman KS, Loesche WJ. Direct interaction between estradiol and progesterone with *Bacteroides asaccharolyticus* and *Bacteroides melaninogenicus. Infect Immun.* 1982;35:256–263.
53. Sutcliffe P. A longitudinal study of gingivitis and puberty. *J Periodontal Res.* 1972;7:52–58.

54. Holm-Pedersen P, Löe H. Flow of gingival exudate as related to menstruation and pregnancy. *J Periodontal Res.* 1967;2:13–20.

55. Lindhe J, Björn A-L. Influence of hormonal contraceptives on the gingiva of women. *J Periodontal Res.* 1967;2:1–6.

56. El-Ashiry GM, El-Kafrawy AH, Nasr MF, et al. Comparative study of the influence of pregnancy and oral contraceptives on the gingivae. *Oral Surg Oral Med Oral Pathol.* 1970;30:472–475.

57. Knight GM, Wade AB. The effects of hormonal contraceptives on the human periodontium. *J Periodontal Res.* 1974;9:18–22.

58. Kalkwarf KL. Effect of oral contraceptive therapy on gingival inflammation in humans. *J Periodontol.* 1978;49:560–563.

59. Pankhurst CL, Waite IM, Hicks KA, et al. The influence of oral contraceptive therapy on the periodontium: duration of drug therapy. *J Periodontol.* 1981;52:617–620.

60. Perry DA. Oral contraceptives and periodontal health. *J West Soc Periodontol.* 1981;29:72–80.

61. Lynn BD. "The pill" as an etiologic agent in hypertrophic gingivitis. *Oral Surg Oral Med Oral Pathol.* 1967;24:333–334.

62. Kaufman AY. An oral contraceptive as an etiologic factor in producing hyperplastic gingivitis and a neoplasm of the pregnancy tumor type. *Oral Surg Oral Med Oral Pathol.* 1969;28:666–670.

63. Burstone MS. The psychosomatic aspects of dental problems. *J Am Dent Assoc.* 1946;33:862–871.

64. Moulton R, Ewen S, Thieman W. Emotional factors in periodontal disease. *Oral Surg Oral Med Oral Pathol.* 1952;5:833–860.

65. Kardachi BJR, Clarke NG. Aetiology of acute necrotizing ulcerative gingivitis: a hypothetical explanation. *J Periodontol.* 1974;45:830–832.

66. Roberts A, Matthews JB, Socransky SS, et al. Stress and the periodontal diseases: effects of catecholamines on the growth of periodontal bacteria in vitro. *Oral Microbiol Immunol.* 2002;17:296–303.

67 Ader R, Cohen N, Felten D. Psychoneuroimmunology: conditioning and stress. *Lancet.* 1995;345:99–103.

68. Kiecolt-Glaser JK, Dura JR, Speicher CE, et al. Spousal caregivers of dementia victims: longitudinal changes in immunity and health. *Psychosom Med.* 1991;53:345–362.

69. LeResche L, Dworkin SF. The role of stress in inflammatory disease, including periodontal disease: review of concepts and current findings. *Periodontol 2000.* 2002;30:91–103.

70. Shannon IL, Kilgore WG, O'Leary TJ. Stress as a predisposing factor in necrotizing ulcerative gingivitis. *J Periodontol Periodontics.* 1969;40: 240–242.

71. Formicola AJ, Witte ET, Curran PM. A study of personality traits and acute necrotizing ulcerative gingivitis. *J Periodontol.* 1970;41:36–38.

72. Shields WD. Acute necrotizing ulcerative gingivitis: a study of some of the contributing factors and their validity in an Army population. *J Periodontol.* 1977;48:346–349.

73. Armitage GC. *Biologic Basis of Periodontal Maintenance Therapy.* Berkeley, CA: Praxis; 1980:146–154.

74. Hollinger FB. Hepatitis B virus. In: Fields BN, Knipe DM, eds. *Fields Virology.* 2nd ed. New York, NY: Raven Press; 1990:2171–2236.

75. Greenspan D, Schiødt M, Greenspan JS, Pindborg JJ. *AIDS and the Mouth.* Copenhagen, Denmark: Munksgaard; 1990:15–198.

76. Ward JW, Drotman DP. Epidemiology of HIV and AIDS. In: Wormser GP, ed. *AIDS and Other Manifestations of HIV Infection.* 2nd ed. New York, NY: Raven Press; 1992:1–15.

77. Tindall B, Cooper DA, Donovan B, et al. Primary human immunodeficiency virus infection: clinical and serologic aspects. In: Sande MA, Volberding PA, eds. *The Medical Management of AIDS.* Philadelphia, PA: WB Saunders; 1988:75–89.

78. Silverman S, Migliorati CA, Lozada-Nur F, et al. Oral findings in people with or at risk for AIDS: a study of 375 homosexual males. *J Am Dent Assoc.* 1986;112:187–192.

79. Patton LL, McKaig R, Strauss R, et al. Changing prevalence of oral manifestations of human immunodeficiency virus in the era of protease inhibitor therapy. *Oral Surg Oral Med Oral Pathol Oral Radiol Endod.* 2000;89:299–304.

80. Meiller TF, Jabra-Rizk MA, Baqui AAMA, et al. Oral *Candida dubliniensis* as a clinically important species in HIV-seropositive patients in the United States. *Oral Surg Oral Med Oral Pathol Oral Radiol Endod.* 1999;88:573–580.

81. Ceballos-Salobreña A, Gaitaín-Cepeda L, Ceballos-García L, et al. The effect of antiretroviral therapy on the prevalence of HIV-associated oral candidiasis in a Spanish cohort. *Oral Surg Oral Med Oral Pathol Oral Radiol Endod.* 2004;97:345–350.

82. Chattopadhyay A, Journ D, Caplan DJ, et al. Incidence of oral candidiasis and oral hairy leukoplakia in HIV-infected adults in North Carolina. *Oral Surg Oral Med Oral Pathol Oral Radiol Endod.* 2005;99:39–47.

83. Greenspan D, Greenspan JS, Hearst NG, et al. Relation of oral hairy leukoplakia to infection with the human immunodeficiency virus and the risk of developing AIDS. *J Infect Dis.* 1987;155:475–481.

84. Shulten EAJM, ten Kate RW, van der Waal I. Oral manifestations of HIV infection in 75 Dutch patients. *J Oral Pathol Med.* 1989;18:42–46.

85. Porter SR, Luker J, Scully C, et al. Orofacial manifestations of a group of British patients infected with HIV-1. *J Oral Pathol Med.* 1989;18: 47–48.

86. Winkler JR, Robertson PB. Periodontal disease associated with HIV infection. *Oral Surg Oral Med Oral Pathol.* 1992;73:145–150.

87. Moore LVH, Moore WEC, Riley C, et al. Periodontal microflora of HIV positive subjects with gingivitis or adult periodontitis. *J Periodontol.* 1993;64:48–56.

88. Paster BJ, Russell MK, Alpagot T, et al. Bacterial diversity in necrotizing ulcerative periodontitis in HIV-positive subjects. *Ann Periodontol.* 2002;7:8–16.

89. Winkler JR, Murray PA, Grassi M, et al. Diagnosis and management of HIV-associated periodontal lesions. *J Am Dent Assoc.* 1989;119(suppl): 25S–34S.

90. Marcus R. Surveillance of health care workers exposed to blood from patients infected with human immunodeficiency virus. *N Engl J Med.* 1988;319:1118–1123.

91. Scully C. Orofacial herpes simplex virus infections: current concepts in the epidemiology, pathogenesis, and treatment, and disorders in which the virus may be implicated. *Oral Surg Oral Med Oral Pathol.* 1989;68: 701–710.

92. Regezi JA, Sciubba J, Jordan RCK. Vesiculo-bullous diseases. In: *Oral Pathology: Clinical Pathological Correlations.* 4th ed. Philadelphia, PA: WB Saunders; 2003:1–21.

93. Chang F, Syrjanen S, Kellokoski J, et al. Human papillomavirus (HPV) infections and their associations with oral disease. *J Oral Pathol Med.* 1991;20:305–317.

94. Woods KV, Shillitoe EJ, Spitz MR, et al. Analysis of human papillomavirus DNA in oral squamous cell carcinomas. *J Oral Pathol Med.* 1993;22: 101–108.

95. Ostwald C, Müller P, Barten M, et al. Human papillomavirus DNA in oral squamous cell carcinomas and normal mucosa. *J Oral Pathol Med.* 1994; 23:220–225.

96. Plemons JM, Gonzales TS, Burkhart NW. Vesiculobullous diseases of the oral cavity. *Periodontol 2000.* 1999;21:158–175.

97. Silverman S, Gorsky M, Lozada-Nur F. A prospective follow-up study of 570 patients with oral lichen planus: persistence, remission, and malignant association. *Oral Surg Oral Med Oral Pathol.* 1985;60:30–34.

98. Vincent SD, Fotos PG, Baker KA, et al. Oral lichen planus: the clinical, historical, and therapeutic features of 100 cases. *Oral Surg Oral Med Oral Pathol.* 1990;70:165–171.

99. Holmstrup P, Schiøtz A, Westergaard J. Effect of dental plaque control on gingival lichen planus. *Oral Surg Oral Med Oral Pathol.* 1990;69: 585–590.

100. Silverman S, Gorsky M. Epidemiologic and demographic update in oral cancer: California and national data—1973 to 1985. *J Am Dent Assoc.* 1990;120:495–499.

101. Winn DM, Blot WJ, Shy CM, et al. Snuff dipping and oral cancer among women in the southern United States. *N Engl J Med.* 1981;304: 745–749.

102. Opinya GN, Kaimenyi JT, Meme JS. Oral findings in Franconi's anemia: a case report. *J Periodontol.* 1988;59:461–463.

103. Stamps JT. The role of oral hygiene in a patient with idiopathic aplastic anemia. *J Am Dent Assoc.* 1974;88:1025–1027.

104. Awbrey JJ, Hibbard ED. Congenital agranulocytosis. *Oral Surg Oral Med Oral Pathol.* 1973;35:526–530.

105. Hou G-L, Tsai C-C. Oral manifestations of agranulocytosis associated with methimazole therapy. *J Periodontol.* 1988;59:244–248.

106. Smith JF. Cyclic neutropenia. *Oral Surg Oral Med Oral Pathol*. 1964;18: 312–320.

107. Scheinberg DA, Golde DW. The leukemias. In: Isselbacher KJ, Braunwald E, Wilson JD, et al, eds. *Harrison's Principles of Internal Medicine*. 13th ed. New York, NY: McGraw-Hill; 1994:1764–1771.

108. Barrett AP. Gingival lesions in leukemia: a classification. *J Periodontol*. 1984;55:585–588.

109. Haerer AF. *DeJong's The Neurologic Examination*. 5th ed. Philadelphia, PA: JB Lippincott; 1992:1–844.

110. Angelopoulos AP, Goaz PW. Incidence of diphenylhydantoin gingival hyperplasia. *Oral Surg Oral Med Oral Pathol*. 1972;34:898–906.

111. Donnenfeld OW, Stanley HR, Bagdonoff L. A nine-month clinical and histological study of patients on diphenylhydantoin following gingivectomy. *J Periodontol*. 1974;45:547–557.

112. Becker W, Collings CK, Zimmerman ER, et al. Hereditary gingival fibromatosis. *Oral Surg Oral Med Oral Pathol*. 1967;24:313–318.

113. Kilpinen E, Raeste A-M, Collan Y. Hereditary gingival hyperplasia and physical maturation. *Scand J Dent Res*. 1978;86:118–123.

114. Jorgenson RJ, Cocker ME. Variation in the inheritance and expression of gingival fibromatosis. *J Periodontol*. 1974;45:472–477.

115. Rivera-Hidalgo F. Smoking and periodontal disease. *Periodontol 2000*. 2003;32:50–58.

116. Labriola A, Needleman I, Moles DR. Systematic review of the effect of smoking on nonsurgical periodontal therapy. *Periodontol 2000*. 2005;37:124–137.

117. Grossi SG, Zambon JJ, Ho AW, et al. Assessment of risk for periodontal disease: I. Risk indicators for attachment loss. *J Periodontol*. 1994;65: 260–267.

118. Bergström J, Preber H. Tobacco use as a risk factor. *J Periodontol*. 1994;65:545–550.

119. Bennet KR, Read PC. Salivary immunoglobulin A levels in normal subjects, tobacco smokers, and patients with minor aphthous ulcerations. *Oral Surg Oral Med Oral Pathol*. 1982;53:461–465.

120. Costabel U, Bross KJ, Reuter C, et al. Alterations in immunoregulatory T-cell subsets in cigarette smokers: a phenotypic analysis of broncho-alveolar and blood lymphocytes. *Chest*. 1986;90:39–44.

121. Kenney EB, Kraal JH, Saxe SR, et al. The effect of cigarette smoke on human oral polymorphonuclear leukocytes. *J Periodontal Res*. 1977; 12:227–234.

122. Lannan S, McLean A, Drost E, et al. Changes in neutrophil morphology and morphometry following exposure to cigarette smoke. *Int J Exp Pathol*. 1992;73:183–191.

123. Selby C, Drost E, Brown D, et al. Inhibition of neutrophil adherence and movement by acute cigarette smoke exposure. *Exp Lung Res*. 1992;18: 813–827.

CHAPTER 10

Treatment Planning for the Periodontal Patient

Phyllis L. Beemsterboer

LEARNING OUTCOMES

- Describe the goals and rationale for periodontal treatment planning.
- Define the role of the dental hygienist in determining the dental hygiene care plan.
- Classify the phases of dental treatment included in the comprehensive care plan.
- List the major classifications of periodontal disease.
- Identify the considerations for sequencing dental hygiene treatment with periodontal diseases.
- Identify the patient factors to be considered when establishing the treatment plan sequence.
- Discuss informed consent and its importance to the process of patient care.

KEY TERMS

1 month evaluation
Assessment
Dental hygiene care plan
Dental hygiene process of care
Dental hygiene treatment plan
Diagnosis
Informed consent

Informed refusal
Periodontal maintenance
Phase I treatment
Phase II treatment
Phase III treatment
Phase IV treatment
Preliminary phase

Progress notes
Prognosis
Reevaluation
Tissue check
Treatment sequence

D efining a treatment plan for the periodontal patient is a process that requires the **assessment**, preventive, therapeutic, and evaluative skills of the dental hygienist and the dentist. The treatment plan is the blueprint for management of the dental case and is an essential aspect of successful therapy.[1] This plan includes all procedures performed to attain and maintain the long-term oral health of the patient and should involve all members of the health care team and the patient. This chapter describes current strategies and classifications for planning the treatment of the periodontal patient. No treatment should be provided to a patient until a treatment plan has been established and agreed on. The only exception to this would be emergency care to relieve a patient of pain due to injury or acute disease.

GOALS OF TREATMENT

The total treatment plan is the sequential outline of the essential services and procedures to be provided to eliminate disease and restore the oral cavity to health and function. The **dental hygiene treatment plan** consists of services that are performed by the dental hygienist within the total treatment plan.[2] Treatment planning occurs after the assessment of all clinical data and reflects the **diagnosis** and **prognosis** of the patient. The treatment plan defines the methods and sequence of delivering appropriate treatment.[1,3,4]

The goals of the treatment plan are to eliminate and control etiologic and predisposing factors of disease, maintain health, and prevent recurrence of disease.[1,4] These goals are the same, regardless of the sequence of treatment or the individual who is delivering the dental care. Treatment planning provides an opportunity to explain problems and treatment goals to the patient in understandable terms.[4-6] Listening to the patient's concerns is a crucial element in the treatment planning process so that the plan can address the patient's perceived needs along with the disease identified by the clinician. The dental hygienist must also use the visual and verbal feedback from the patient to judge the patient's level of understanding. A true partnership between the patient and the dental team working toward mutual treatment goals has the greatest opportunity for success.

> **CLINICAL NOTE 10-1** All treatment plans must be understood by the patient and reflect the patient's wishes and preferences.

For coordination of the total treatment of the patient, the treatment plan can be divided into various segments or phases. An individualized, well thought-out treatment plan must be established before the beginning of treatment, and it must be carefully monitored. The role of the dental hygienist may vary depending on the type of case, experience of the hygienist, requirements of the state dental practice act, practice setting, and philosophy of the periodontist or general dentist.

PHASES OF TREATMENT

Carranza and collaborators divided the treatment plan into four main phases. Each phase suggested a particular group of procedures and included evaluation of the patient's response. The treatment sequence begins with a preliminary phase (incorporating immediate treatment needs), followed by Phase I (etiologic treatment), Phase II (surgical treatment), Phase III (restorative treatment), and Phase IV (maintenance treatment). The phases of therapeutic periodontal procedures, along with the sequence of other needed dental procedures, are presented in Box 10-1.

The purpose of the preliminary phase of treatment is to bring all emergency and other critical situations under control. Dental and periodontal abscesses should be treated. Hopeless

---

BOX 10-1   Sequence of Periodontal Procedures

Preliminary Phase
- Treatment of emergencies
  - Dental or periapical
  - Periodontal
- Extraction of hopeless teeth and provisional replacement if needed (may be postponed to a more convenient time)

Phase I Therapy (Nonsurgical Phase)
- Plaque biofilm control
- Diet control (for patients at high caries risk)
- Scaling and root planing to remove bacterial plaque biofilm and calculus
- Correction of contributing restorative and prosthetic factors
- Removal of caries and restoration of teeth (temporary or final, depending on whether a definitive prognosis for the tooth has been arrived at and on the location of the caries)
- Antimicrobial therapy (local or systemic)
- Occlusal therapy
- Minor orthodontic movement
- Provisional splinting
- Evaluation of response to Phase I (occurs 1 month or longer after completion)
  - Reassess gingival condition and pocket depth
  - Rechecking for plaque, calculus, and caries

Phase II Therapy (Surgical Phase)
- Periodontal surgery, including placement of implants
- Endodontic therapy

Phase III Therapy (Restorative Phase)
- Final restorations
- Fixed and removable prosthodontics
- Evaluation of response to restorative phase
  - Periodontal examination

Phase IV Therapy (Maintenance Phase)
- Plaque biofilm and calculus removal
- Monitoring
  - Periodontal condition (pockets, inflammation)
  - Occlusion and tooth mobility
  - Other pathologic changes

(Reprinted and adapted by permission from Newman MG, Takei HH, Klokkevold PR, et al, eds. *Carranza's Clinical Periodontology.* 11th ed. St. Louis, MO: Elsevier Saunders; 2012.)

---

teeth should be removed and provisional restorations, such as temporary partial dentures, should be fabricated. Endodontic therapy can be performed to relieve pain, even if its completion carries over to other phases of treatment, and oral lesions of any type should be evaluated and treated or referred.

Phase I therapy describes the procedures that are designed to control or eliminate the etiologic factors of the disease process. Patient education and plaque control instruction occur at the beginning of this phase. Scaling, root debridement and planing are performed. Antimicrobial agents are used or recommended for home use. This stage has also been referred to as initial therapy, nonsurgical therapy, cause-related therapy, or the hygienic phase of treatment.[7,8]

Phase II therapy is the surgical phase of treatment. During this phase, procedures are undertaken to reduce the effects of disease. Regenerative techniques are performed to help restore periodontal tissues that have been lost due to disease.

Phase III therapy usually involves restorations and replacement of missing teeth. Procedures in this phase included restorative dentistry, extensive orthodontics, and any needed occlusal therapy.

Phase IV therapy is the maintenance phase. Patients remain in this phase for a lifetime. Although this phase is often referred to as "recall," the accepted terms are periodontal maintenance or periodontal recall because the patient's periodontal health must be continuously monitored from this point. The maintenance phase begins after Phase I, but not necessarily before all phases of treatment have been completed. Patients with extensive surgical and restorative needs often have treatment extend over many months, even years. Periodontal maintenance occurs while the other phases of treatment are ongoing because the completion of the entire treatment plan can take months or years, and decline in the status of periodontal patients has been observed much earlier, after as little as 90 days. In their classic studies, Ramfjord and Ash demonstrated that 3-month maintenance intervals were responsible for the long-term success of periodontal treatment.[7]

The interval between periodontal maintenance appointments is determined by the periodontal condition and the plaque control that the patient is able to attain and maintain. Most patients who have been treated for moderate to advanced periodontal disease require maintenance visits every 3 months.[9-12]

ROLE OF THE DENTAL HYGIENIST

The dental hygienist is often responsible for treatment of the periodontal patient in the nonsurgical, or Phase I, and maintenance, or Phase IV, stages of periodontal treatment. Because of the complexity of the periodontal treatment required to meet planned goals, a series of appointments is often required. The sequence of treatment depends on a number of factors, including the periodontal diagnosis and prognosis, the patient's systemic and periodontal condition, and the patient's preferences. Figures 10-1 to 10-4 are examples of successful therapeutic results achieved by a dental hygienist providing Phase I therapy.

Disease classifications are useful for diagnosis, prognosis, and treatment planning because they help define the extent of disease and facilitate communication among members of the

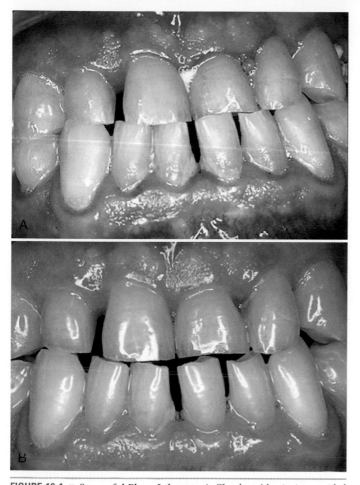

FIGURE 10-1 ■ **Successful Phase I therapy. A,** The dental hygienist provided four quadrants of scaling and root planing with the use of local anesthetics, plus home care instruction and reinforcement, for this 60-year old man. The patient had 4- to 6-mm probe depths, slight CAL, and heavy deposits of plaque biofilm and subgingival calculus. **B,** One month after the last treatment appointment, the pocket depths have resolved by 2 mm and the patient's home care has improved dramatically. Note the tissue changes from red and edematous to a uniform coral pink.

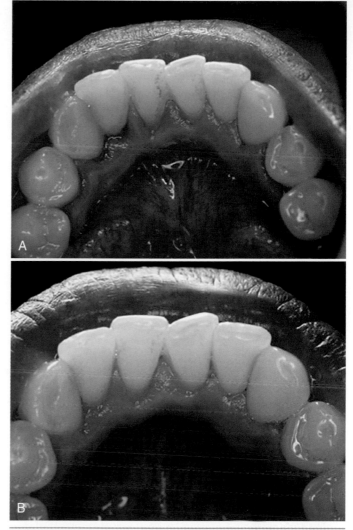

FIGURE 10-2 ■ **Dental hygiene care. A,** This 27-year-old woman had relatively shallow pocket depths, 2 to 4 mm throughout, but moderate subgingival calculus accumulated on the lingual and interproximal surfaces of the mandibular teeth. The patient sought treatment because she was concerned about breath odor and stains on the teeth. The dental hygiene care plan included oral hygiene instruction, scaling and root planing half of the mouth at each visit, polishing to remove extrinsic stains, and a follow-up assessment. **B,** One month after the second treatment visit, the tissue had improved significantly. Probing depths were 2 to 3 mm, the tissue was firm and pink, and the patient's home care habits had improved greatly. The patient was very pleased because the stains were gone from her teeth and she thought that her breath odor was gone. The patient was initially placed on a 4-month recall to help reinforce her good oral hygiene habits and is now maintained (Phase IV) with therapy at 6-month intervals.

treatment team. Various periodontal classification systems have been used over the years and have been modified to reflect advances in knowledge and research.[1] A classification system is simply a method for comparing treatment approaches and likely results. Using a system that is understood and used by a large number of dental professionals greatly facilitates communication regarding cases.

In 1999, an international group of periodontal experts approved the classification system currently in use. This system is based on the clinical manifestations of disease and conditions. The overall approach of this classification system separates gingival disease from periodontal disease and conditions affecting the periodontium. This system was adopted by the American Academy of Periodontology (AAP) and is widely accepted by the dental community as the preferred classification system.[13] The classifications are outlined in Box 10-2.

Many clinicians may still use an earlier version of an AAP-designed system that has a case type structure containing five descriptive groups. The dental hygienist will still find many references to this system in patient charts and journal articles.[1,2] The case type classification system is presented for reference,

but it is important to note that the more recent system better reflects current evidence and understanding of disease processes. The case types are:

- Case Type I Gingivitis
- Case Type II Slight Chronic Periodontitis
- Case Type III Moderate Chronic or Aggressive Periodontitis
- Case Type IV Advanced Chronic or Aggressive Periodontitis
- Case Type V Refractory Chronic or Aggressive Periodontitis

For treatment planning purposes, identifying the extent and severity of periodontal disease is helpful in determining the

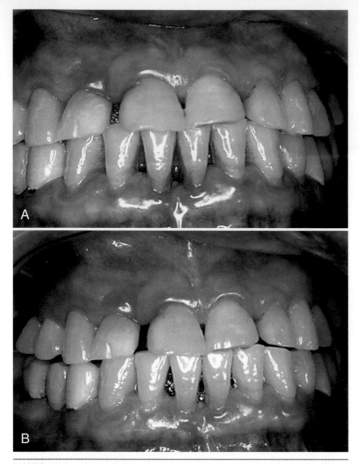

FIGURE 10-3 ■ **Phase I therapy. A,** This 36-year-old woman was concerned about bleeding gingivae. She had heavy subgingival calculus and 5 to 6 mm of CAL in most areas of her mouth. Probing depths were 4 to 6 mm throughout the mouth, with class II furcations involvement in the molar teeth. **B,** The patient was treated with quadrant scaling and root planing requiring local anesthesia, oral hygiene instruction, and reinforcement. She required periodontal surgery to reduce the remaining pockets and permit cleaning of the furcation areas. Note the improved tissue color and tone in the anterior areas. The patient was maintained on a 3-month recall regimen that began after Phase I therapy was completed. She had the periodontal surgery performed while on the maintenance regimen, and the dental hygienist was able to maintain the successfully treated areas of the mouth and modify recommended oral hygiene procedures to assist her in cleaning the furcation areas.

appropriate treatment time and sequence. Severity of disease is appropriately described in terms of clinical attachment loss (CAL) and generally defined as follows:

- Slight periodontal disease is characterized by 1 to 2 mm CAL
- Moderate periodontal disease is characterized by 3 to 4 mm CAL.
- Severe periodontal disease is characterized by 5 mm or more of CAL.

Disease is also characterized as generalized or localized depending on the extent of the dentition that is affected. The severity of disease, the extent of disease, the amount of calculus, and the patient education process will influence the number of visits required to treat the patient's periodontal needs appropriately and comprehensively.

Patient education to attain plaque biofilm control is a critical element of treatment. It is often the responsibility of the dental hygienist and includes oral hygiene instruction and prevention

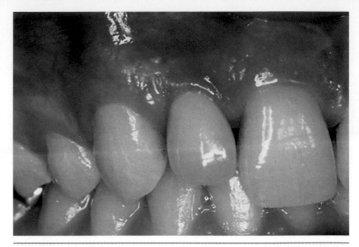

FIGURE 10-4 ■ **The significance of reassessment after Phase I therapy.** This 41-year-old male patient had completed Phase I therapy consisting of quadrant scaling and root planing and oral hygiene instructions. The maxillary right area did not respond well around tooth #7. The dental hygienist noted the redness and swelling that remained in the tissue and reinstrumented the area. Substantial amounts of calculus remained on the tooth. After this second treatment, the pocket depth resolved to 2 to 3 mm, and tissue color and texture then appeared similar to the other areas of the mouth—pink and firm. Note the residual calculus on the mesial surface of tooth #9, at the right edge of the figure. Calculus at this location adheres to the root surface right at the cementoenamel junction and is very difficult to remove.

BOX 10-2	Classification of Periodontal Disease and Conditions

Gingival Disease
- Dental plaque–induced gingival disease
- Non–plaque-induced gingival lesions

Chronic Periodontitis
- Localized
- Generalized

Aggressive Periodontitis
- Localized
- Generalized

Periodontitis as a Manifestation of Systemic Disease

Necrotizing Periodontal Disease
- Necrotizing ulcerative gingivitis
- Necrotizing ulcerative periodontitis

Abscesses of the Periodontium
- Gingival abscess
- Periodontal abscess
- Pericoronal abscess

Periodontitis Associated with Endodontic Lesions
- Combined periodontal-endodontic lesion

Developmental or Acquired Deformities and Conditions
- Localized tooth-related factors that predispose to plaque-induced gingival disease or periodontitis
- Mucogingival deformities and conditions around teeth
- Mucogingival deformities and conditions on edentulous ridges
- Occlusal trauma

From Armitage GC. Development of a classification system for periodontal diseases and conditions. *Ann Periodontol.* 1999;4:1-6.

education. Effective behavioral change is difficult to achieve if the patient does not understand the relationship between his or her oral condition and plaque biofilm control procedures. Time spent providing the patient with plaque control and prevention instruction makes a significant difference in the overall success of periodontal treatment. The patient education process continues throughout the treatment sessions and during all phases of care. The most successful approach to patient education and ultimate behavioral change is to involve the patient as a partner in the journey and provide repeated positive reinforcement.

Patient education for plaque biofilm control must be initiated after the assessment and classifications are established. This component of dental hygiene care is often postponed or even ignored. The appropriate time to begin discussing the cause of periodontal disease, and its control by the patient, is as early as possible in the sequence of care, beginning during Phase I rather than waiting for Phase IV. The patient must understand that the cause of gingivitis and periodontitis is the accumulation of bacterial plaque biofilm in and around the tissues of the periodontium. Any time devoted to this activity is time well spent and will positively influence the outcome of treatment.

CLINICAL NOTE 10-2 Patient education to attain plaque biofilm control is a critical element of treatment.

Decisions about the number of appointments needed to provide appropriate dental hygiene care, the sequence of treatments, and the required adjunctive techniques, such as the use of local anesthetics, are based on the complexity of the case. There are many factors to consider in making these decisions and they determine the degree of difficulty involved in providing periodontal debridement. Factors to be considered in determining each patient's specific treatment plan are presented in Box 10-3.

TREATMENT PLANNING FOR PERIODONTAL DISEASE

Treatment plans can be estimated for periodontal patients based on the classification and extent of disease. These plans should be considered estimates, not templates for dental hygiene care. Every case must be considered individually and treatment visits must be varied according to the degree of difficulty involved in treating the conditions present. A suggested outline of treatment plans by case severity is shown in Box 10-4.

BOX 10-3 Considerations for Determining the Dental Hygiene Care Plan

Patient general health and tolerance of treatment
Number of teeth present
Amount of supragingival calculus
Amount of subgingival calculus
Probing pocket depths (amount of attachment loss is less significant during treatment planning than when assessing the case or considering the prognosis)
Furcations
Alignment of teeth
Margins of restorations
Caries
Developmental anomalies
Physical barriers to access (e.g., gagging or limited opening)
Patient cooperation
Patient prevention education needs
Patient sensitivity (requiring use of anesthesia or analgesia)

The systemic and periodontal conditions of the patient dictate how the dental hygienist sequences either a single session or a series of nonsurgical treatment sessions. The normal procedures for clinical assessment completed at every treatment session for every patient include a review of the medical history, monitoring of vital signs, extraoral and intraoral examination, and review or reexamination of dental and periodontal charting.

The patient may have systemic conditions that alter the number and length of treatment appointments. For example, patients with chronic illnesses may tolerate shorter treatment appointments very well but may be exhausted after longer ones.

BOX 10-4 Suggested Dental Hygiene Treatment Plans for Gingival and Periodontal Disease

Gingival Disease (no CAL)
Often completed in one treatment visit
1. Assessments
2. Patient education and plaque biofilm control instruction
3. Scaling and periodontal debridement
4. Establish appropriate maintenance interval
5. Reevaluation at subsequent appointment or first maintenance visit

Slight Periodontitis (1-2 mm CAL)
Often requires more than one treatment visit
1. Assessments
2. Patient education and plaque biofilm control instruction; probably more complex, requiring augmentation and reinforcement at subsequent visits
3. Scaling, root planing, and periodontal debridement, probably requiring anesthesia and analgesia
4. Establish appropriate maintenance interval
5. Reevaluation by dental hygienist and dentist

Moderate Periodontitis (3-4 mm CAL)
Often treated by quadrants, requires several treatment visits
1. Assessments, consider referral to periodontist
2. Patient education and plaque biofilm control instruction, probably more complex, requiring augmentation and reinforcement at subsequent visits
3. Scaling, root planing, and periodontal debridement by quadrant, often requiring anesthetic use
4. Establish appropriate maintenance interval
5. Reevaluation by dental hygienist and dentist

Severe Periodontitis (≥5 mm CAL)
Often treated by quadrants, but may require therapy by sextants, requires several visits
1. Assessments, strongly consider referral to periodontist
2. Patient education and plaque biofilm control instruction, probably more complex, requiring augmentation and reinforcement at subsequent visits
3. Scaling, root planing, and periodontal debridement by quadrant or sextant
4. Establish appropriate maintenance interval

Aggressive Periodontitis
Presents with a variety of signs and symptoms; may be treated in single or multiple treatment visits
1. Assessments will require referral to periodontist
2. Patient education and plaque biofilm control instruction
3. Scaling, root planing, and periodontal debridement
4. More frequent recalls often required
5. Courses of antibiotics and microbiologic diagnostic monitoring may be required
6. Establish appropriate maintenance interval.
7. Reevaluation by dental hygienist and periodontist

Various medications can also complicate treatment and they should be carefully noted and monitored. Patients with physical or mental disabilities can also present challenges that require modification of treatment plans.[14]

A common practice that is now considered outdated is referred to as gross scaling. Gross scaling was an approach to removing calculus by removing large deposits at the beginning of the periodontal treatment. Successive appointments then allowed the clinician to fine-scale and remove the remaining deposits. This two-stage approach was developed when calculus was considered a mechanical irritant, before it was understood that periodontal disease is a bacterial infection. It was thought that partial debridement encouraged localized healing around a tooth, possibly trapping bacteria at the base of the pocket, leaving unresolved infection, and masking deeper infection in the periodontal pockets.[15] The currently accepted technique is to scale a sextant, quadrant, or more teeth completely at a session. This practice often requires the use of local anesthesia so that treatment can be completed painlessly. Effective anesthesia allows the clinician to gain better access to the periodontal pockets for thorough instrumentation. The immediate goal for each session of instrumentation is complete removal of all adherent bacterial plaque biofilm and calculus deposits. The dental hygienist judges the smoothness of the root surfaces as the indicator for effective and complete calculus and plaque removal. The long-term goal—restored oral health—is the true measure of successful therapy. This goal is evaluated through examination of the tissue response to debridement and maintenance of clinical attachment.

A treatment planning option has been proposed that includes one or two appointments on consecutive days for debridement. The treatment is provided in conjunction with the aggressive use of antimicrobial agents for full-mouth disinfection and has been tested on patients with aggressive and severe forms of periodontal diseases. Complete scaling and root planing were performed within 24 hours in two separate 4-hour appointments, chlorhexidine solution was applied to all periodontal defects where pathogens would likely remain after the thorough scaling, twice-daily chlorhexidine rinses were added to the oral hygiene routine, and the tonsils were sprayed daily with chlorhexidine. The disinfectant rinses and spray continued daily for 2 months. Results showed greater probe depth reductions in deeper pockets after 8 months compared to treatment provided by quadrant at 2-week intervals with no additional use of disinfectant, essentially treatment that relied on traditional mechanical debridement.[16] In addition to probe depth improvements in the disinfection group, periodontal pathogens were reduced or eliminated in greater proportion when compared to the mechanical therapy group.[17] These data suggest that as our understanding and use of antimicrobial agents in periodontal therapy increases, treatment plans will evolve to maximize therapeutic results. More information and application of evidence-based research will help us refine how we evaluate and treat periodontal diseases in the future.

CLINICAL NOTE 10-3 The currently accepted technique is to scale a quadrant, sextant, or more teeth completely at a session, often with anesthesia.

BOX 10-5   Elements of Informed Consent

Reason for the procedure
Description of the procedure
Benefits from the procedure
Risks that could result from the procedure
Prognosis with recommended procedures
Prognosis if recommended procedures not performed
Presentation of other available options or alternatives

INFORMED CONSENT

Informed consent is the permission granted by the patient for the health care provider to proceed with treatment. All treatment plans must be understood by the patient and reflect the patient's wishes and preferences. Patients must be fully aware of the extent of the disease and the treatment options that are being considered and understand all the aspects available to them in their dental health care.

Informed consent can be verbal or written. Verbal consent is often called implied consent and is used in routine clinical situations in which there is little or no apparent risk. Written or express consent is common practice with most periodontal therapy in which invasive and surgical care are rendered and the risks are greater. The elements of informed consent are presented in Box 10-5.

Every state has laws that address the issue of informed consent. The patient should always be informed of the disease process present in the mouth, the treatment proposed, and the alternatives to that treatment.[18] This discussion should also include the consequences of providing no treatment or partial treatment, usually termed informed refusal. Patients have the right to refuse any treatment even if it is not in their best interest or can contribute further to health-related problems.

Typically, informed consent is a written or electronic document on which the treatment plan is listed and the signatures of all concerned parties are recorded. It is the basis of the legal relationship between the health care provider and the patient.[4] Communication is very important in the informed consent process. The patient must have the opportunity to ask questions and understand the answers before signing any document or proceeding with any treatment option. The dental hygienist should always be careful not to promise a particular result or outcome. Patients need to understand their treatment options, and this process takes time. Specific statements that clearly describe the dental problems greatly help patients and the dental care team.

Sometimes patients are confused when faced with various treatment options. The written agreement clarifies the treatment plan for all parties. A written treatment plan is truly the blueprint for care.

DOCUMENTATION

Documentation is essential in all aspects of dental hygiene and periodontal care. After the patient fully understands the risks, benefits, and alternatives to treatment, has agreed to treatment, and has signed a consent document, the dental hygienist must be equally careful in documenting treatment at every visit. These records are referred to as the chart notes or progress notes, and they reflect all aspects of treatment

BOX 10-6 Elements of Acceptable Progress Notes

Progress notes should do the following:

Be accurate and concise

Be chronologic in sequence

Include descriptions of service, teeth or area, anesthetic, and any noteworthy clinical occurrences

Include dates of changed and canceled appointments

Include summaries of telephone calls related to treatment or problems

Include notes of prescriptions, drugs, or materials dispensed

Include referrals and requests for radiographs and results

Include the recall plan

Be dated and electronically signed by the clinician

---

performed at a particular time. As an example, notes for a typical treatment visit would include review of health, oral examination, oral hygiene instruction, premedication(s) taken, scaling and root planing, anesthetic used, patient response to treatment, postoperative instructions, and any other activities. Accurate documentation of progress notes at all visits is essential and must become as much a part of treatment as infection control practices. To ensure accuracy, written entries should be made soon after treatment; postponing entries until the end of the day can lead to information being left out of the records. All entries in the patient's clinical chart should meet a high standard for completeness and clarity. In a written record, if an error is made while entering information, a line should be drawn through the incorrect statements (so they are still legible) and the correct information should be entered next to it. Electronic notes entered after the original date should reflect the actual date entered and the reason for the correction. Standards for chart documentation have been defined by Schoen[19] and are presented in Box 10-6.

CLINICAL NOTE 10-4 Accurate documentation of progress notes at all visits is essential and must become as much a part of treatment as infection control practices.

Confidential handling of patient records is also important because patients expect that their health information will be protected and kept private. Unauthorized disclosure to other patients or providers is considered negligence.[20] Careful documentation is the foundation of sound risk management practice.

The dentist is ultimately responsible for the actions of the dental hygienist; however, a dental hygienist can still be found negligent in legal proceedings if malpractice or negligence has been established and proven. The two universally accepted strategies for minimizing the risks associated with providing dental and dental hygiene services are the following:

- Good documentation
- Careful communication with the patient

TREATMENT PLANNING IN DENTAL HYGIENE

The dental hygiene treatment plan is an individualized approach to treatment for a specific patient that details the care to be provided by the dental hygienist. It is a portion of the total treatment plan detailing comprehensive care for the dental patient and is sometimes called the **dental hygiene care plan**. The plan is adapted to the needs of the patient and presented in an orderly sequence to allow for thoroughness in completing each procedure.[2] The time required for each treatment session depends on the oral condition and extent of care to be provided. Generally, 1-hour appointments are recommended for each treatment visit, but this time frame is used only as a guideline. The philosophy and customs of the practice and the preferences of the dental hygienist and patient will influence this aspect of treatment planning.

Determination of a debridement or tissue conditioning[2] treatment sequence is influenced by a number of factors, including the location and extent of infection, the presence of pain, and medical or physical limitations of the patient. All aspects of the patient's condition must be considered in choosing where to begin treatment, length of appointment, and home care recommendations.

The periodontal patient requires a follow-up visit to evaluate the response of the tissues to the scaling and debridement procedures. This appointment is often called the **reevaluation**, or **1-month evaluation**, and sometimes simply a **tissue check**. Tissue healing and the patient's progress toward effective plaque control should be observed and evaluated about 4 weeks after the debridement sequence is completed to allow for healing of the connective tissues. The scaled pockets will reepithelialize in about a week, but the evaluation of connective tissue healing will not be accurately assessed until it is healed sufficiently to keep the periodontal probe from penetrating right through newly forming collagen apical to the junctional epithelium.

At the reevaluation appointment, the dental hygienist will assess and determine the appropriate interval for periodontal maintenance. In many practices, the reevaluation visit is also the logical and convenient time for the periodontist or dentist to examine the patient and initiate the next step in the total treatment plan.

Treatment planning is considered part of the **dental hygiene process of care**,[2,14] which is defined as an organized systematic group of dental hygiene activities that provides the framework for delivering quality dental hygiene care. The components of dental hygiene care are divided into five categories: assessment, diagnosis, planning, implementation, and evaluation. Treatment planning incorporates both assessment and diagnosis in defining a set of procedures to restore the patient to a state of health.

The treatment plan is individualized for each patient based on the knowledge, clinical judgment, and evidence from research that the dental hygienist assimilates and applies to each case. The decision making process that takes place in periodontal therapy comprises treatment options, cost considerations, and patient preferences. Making thoughtful treatment decisions is a process that is receiving increased attention from the dental research community because of the need and desire to ensure high-quality dental care. The treatment plan is the guideline for the management of comprehensive care and is an essential part of successful therapy for every dental patient.

A series of sample treatment plans are presented in Figures 10-5 and 10-6 to assist the dental hygienist in applying the variety of treatment options to specific case examples.

Sample Dental Hygiene Treatment Plan:
Phase I Therapy in Periodontal Practice

Mrs. Garcia is a 36-year-old female Hispanic who presents with elevated blood pressure and concerns about her teeth and gums. Assessment and charting have been completed by the periodontist and scheduled with the dental hygienist. The patient presents with generalized 3- to 5-mm probing, localized recession on teeth #6 and #11 of 2 mm, moderate subgingival calculus throughout, moderate supragingival calculus on the mandibular anterior teeth, and moderate amounts of gingival and interproximal plaque biofilm on all teeth. The patient is worried about getting "cavities," is eager to preserve her teeth, and wants to improve her dental health.

Treatment 1	Treatment 2	Treatment 3 (1-month evaluation)
Review assessment findings and diagnosis from periodontist.	Review assessment findings and diagnosis, and take vital signs.	Review assessment findings and diagnosis and take vital signs.
Take vital signs and baseline indices.	Evaluate previous scaling and root debridement results.	Evaluate previous scaling and periodontal debridement results.
Begin plaque biofilm control instruction and fluoride recommendations.	Reinforce plaque biofilm control and record comparative indices.	Retreat areas that did not respond to debridement.
Review treatment plan and treatment goals.	Scale and perform periodontal debridement of maxillary and mandibular left quadrants with anesthesia, and retreat any areas on the right side with residual calculus.	Reinforce plaque biofilm control instruction and record comparative indices.
Scale and perform periodontal debridement of maxillary and mandibular right quadrants with anesthesia.		Perform selective polishing.
		Review treatment goals with patient.
		Schedule with periodontist for re-evaluation.
		Establish recall interval.

FIGURE 10-5 ■ Sample dental hygiene treatment plan for Phase I therapy in periodontal practice.

Sample Dental Hygiene Treatment Plan:
Phase IV Therapy in General Dental Practice

Mr. Park is a healthy 50-year-old male with a history of rheumatic fever and periodontal disease. The dental hygienist is the first person to see and treat the patient. He has received periodontal maintenance care at regular intervals but it has been about 9 months since his last visit. The patient presents with 3- to 4-mm probe depths, 2 to 3 mm of CAL throughout, light subgingival calculus, moderate supragingival calculus limited to the mandibular anterior teeth, and slight bleeding on probing. Plaque biofilm accumulation is apparent on the proximal surfaces of the posterior teeth. The patient is very cooperative and wishes to establish a more regular maintenance routine in your office, and has brought radiographs from his previous dentist.

Treatment 1	Treatment 2	Treatment 3 (1-month evaluation)
Take medical and dental history.	Review medical and dental history.	Review medical history.
Evaluate need for premedication and consult with MD.	Confirm antibiotic medication.	Confirm antibiotic premedication.
Reappoint for care.	Review radiographs from previous dentist.	Evaluate previous scaling and periodontal debridement results.
Discuss possibility of referral to periodontist with general dentist.	Take vital signs and baseline indices.	Reinforce home care.
	Assess plaque biofilm control status and fluoride needs.	Consider referral to a periodontist.
	Determine treatment plan and goals.	Establish recall interval.
	Provide appropriate home care instructions and education.	
	Scale and perform periodontal debridement of the full mouth in order to minimize the number of appointments requiring antibiotic premedication.	
	Schedule with dentist for examination and evaluation.	

FIGURE 10-6 ■ Sample dental hygiene treatment plan for Phase IV therapy in general dental practice.

DENTAL HYGIENE CONSIDERATIONS

- Treatment planning is a comprehensive plan to restore the patient's oral health that includes a preliminary phase followed by Phases I, II, III, and IV.
- The dental hygienist is primarily involved in Phase I and Phase IV therapy.
- The goals of treatment are to eliminate and control etiologic and predisposing factors of disease, maintain health, and prevent disease recurrence.
- Extent and severity of disease, along with many individual factors, are considered in developing the treatment plan.
- Informed consent is a process that permits full understanding of the disease process, treatment options, and probable outcomes.
- Accurate documentation is a critical element in the dental hygiene process of care.
- Follow-up or reevaluation visits are important for accurate assessment of the success of treatment, reinforcing oral hygiene habits, re-treating areas that have not healed as expected, and planning maintenance intervals.

CASE SCENARIOS

Mrs. Johnson is a 34-year-old Hispanic woman with a history of slightly elevated blood pressure who is new to the periodontal practice and has undergone a complete dental assessment. She is not taking any medications, nor is she allergic to anything except pollen. Her family history is unremarkable and she states that her periodontal condition is of great concern to her because she is a backup singer for a movie studio. She is also concerned about getting cavities. Mrs. Johnson has been diagnosed as having chronic periodontitis with moderate amounts of calculus in all quadrants. The tissue in the lower right sextant is of concern to the periodontist and the patient because it is particularly red and inflamed. You have been asked to create a treatment plan and to manage care before returning the patient to the periodontist for further evaluation. The patient asks how many appointments this treatment will take to complete.

1. What phase of treatment will you be providing for Mrs. Johnson?
   A. Preliminary phase
   B. Phase I therapy
   C. Phase II therapy
   D. Phase III therapy
   E. Phase IV therapy
2. What are the most critical factors to be considered in scheduling Mrs. Johnson?
   A. Periodontal status and amount of calculus
   B. The severity of disease and amount of calculus
   C. Periodontal status and need for patient education
   D. The amount of calculus and length of appointment sessions
3. Effective behavioral change for Mrs. Johnson's oral hygiene will be dependent on
   A. the cost of the treatment.
   B. the level of informed consent.
   C. the number of appointments required.
   D. an understanding of the periodontal disease classifications.
   E. an understanding of the relationship between her gum problems and plaque control.

4. After entering the treatment rendered in Mrs. Johnson's chart, you discover that you wrote down the wrong blood pressure reading. The best course of action is to
   A. erase the wrong numbers and enter the correct ones.
   B. cross out the wrong numbers so they are illegible and enter the correct ones.
   C. use a correction fluid to cover up the wrong numbers and enter the correct ones.
   D. draw a line through the wrong numbers so they are still legible and enter the correct ones next to the last entry.

STUDY QUESTIONS

Answers and rationales to these questions can be obtained from your instructor.

MULTIPLE CHOICE

1. Which phase of treatment describes the periodontal procedures designed to control or eliminate the causative factors of disease?
   A. Preliminary phase
   B. Phase I therapy
   C. Phase II therapy
   D. Phase III therapy
   E. Phase IV therapy
2. The term for when a patient refuses any further recommended periodontal treatment is
   A. negligence.
   B. implied consent.
   C. informed refusal.
   D. informed consent.
3. The goals of treatment planning are to eliminate and control factors of disease and to prevent recurrence of disease. The dental hygienist can use treatment planning as an opportunity to explain problems to patients in understandable terms.
   A. Both statements are TRUE.
   B. Both statements are FALSE.
   C. The first statement is TRUE, and the second statement is FALSE.
   D. The first statement is FALSE, and the second statement is TRUE.
4. All of the following factors influence the number and length of visits for dental hygiene care EXCEPT one. Which one is the EXCEPTION?
   A. Amount of calculus
   B. Severity of periodontal pockets
   C. Height of patient
   D. Amount of dental caries
   E. Willingness of patient to cooperate
5. The treatment plan is a guideline for the management of comprehensive periodontal and restorative care. The treatment plan is essential for every periodontal patient.
   A. Both statements are TRUE.
   B. Both statements are FALSE.
   C. The first statement is TRUE, and the second statement is FALSE.
   D. The first statement is FALSE, and the second statement is TRUE.

6. Severity of periodontal disease is characterized as slight, moderate, or severe because these characterizations are helpful in determining the appropriate treatment time and sequence.
   A. Both the statement and reason are correct and related.
   B. Both the statement and reason are correct but NOT related.
   C. The statement is correct, but the reason is NOT correct.
   D. The statement is NOT correct, but the reason is correct.
   E. NEITHER the statement NOR the reason is correct.

7. The dental hygienist is most often responsible for treating the periodontal patient in
   A. Phase I and Phase II.
   B. Phase I and Phase III.
   C. Phase II and Phase III.
   D. Phase I and Phase IV.
   E. Phase II and Phase IV.

8. The elements of informed consent include all of the following EXCEPT one. Which one is the EXCEPTION?
   A. Implied consent
   B. Risks and benefits
   C. Prognosis if treatment is performed
   D. Prognosis if treatment is not performed

SHORT ANSWER

9. List the elements necessary for informed consent when establishing a treatment plan.
10. Define what is meant by the dental hygiene care plan.

Please visit **http://evolve.elsevier.com/Perry/periodontology** for additional practice and study support tools.

REFERENCES

1. Carranza FA, Takei HH. The treatment plan. In: Newman MG, Takei HH, Klokkevold PR, et al, eds. *Carranza's Clinical Periodontology*. 11th ed. St. Louis, MO: Elsevier Saunders; 2012:284–286.

2. Wyche CJ. Planning for dental hygiene care. In: Wilkins EM, ed. *Clinical Practice of the Dental Hygienist*. 11th ed. Philadelphia, PA: Lippincott Williams & Wilkins; 2013:340–350.

3. American Academy of Periodontology. Parameters of care. *J Periodontol*. 2000;71(suppl):7–14.

4. Stefanac SJ, Nesbit SP. *Treatment Planning in Dentistry*. 2nd ed. St Louis, MO: Mosby; 2006.

5. American Academy of Periodontology. In: *Proceedings of the World Workshop in Clinical Periodontics*. Chicago, IL: American Academy of Periodontology; 1989.

6. Woodall IR, Wiles C. Formulating a treatment plan, case presentation and appointment plan. In: *Comprehensive Dental Hygiene Care*. 4th ed. St. Louis, MO: Mosby; 1993:371–390.

7. Ramfjord SP, Ash MM. *Periodontology and Periodontics: Modern Theory and Practice*. St. Louis, MO: Ishiyaku EuroAmerica; 1989.

8. Schluger S, Yuodelis R, Page R, et al. *Periodontal Disease*. 2nd ed. Philadelphia, PA: Lea & Febiger; 1990.

9. Fedi Jr P. *The Periodontic Syllabus*. 2nd ed. Philadelphia, PA: Lea & Febiger; 1989.

10. Knowles JW, Burgett FG, Nissle RR, et al. Results of periodontal treatment related to pocket depth and attachment level: eight years. *J Periodontol*. 1979;50:225–233.

11. DeVore CH, Beck FM, Horton JE. Plaque score changes based primarily on patient performance at specific time intervals. *J Periodontol*. 1990;61:343–346.

12. Supportive periodontal therapy (SPT). *J Periodontol*. 1998;69:502–506.

13. Armitage GC. Development of a classification system for periodontal diseases and conditions. *Ann Periodontol*. 1999;4:1.

14. Wyche C. Dental hygiene care plan. In: Wilkins EM, ed. *Clinical Practice of the Dental Hygienist*. 11th ed. Philadelphia, PA: Lippincott Williams & Wilkins; 2013:351–360.

15. O'Hehir TE. Gross scaling: an antiquated concept. *Dent Hyg News*. 1993;7:19–20.

16. Mongardini C, van Steenberghe D, Dekeyser C, et al. One stage full- versus partial-mouth disinfection in the treatment of chronic adult or generalized early-onset periodontitis. I. Long-term clinical observations. *J Periodontol*. 1999;70:632–645.

17. Quirymen M, Mongardini C, Pauwels M, et al. One stage full- versus partial-mouth disinfection in the treatment of chronic adult or generalized early-onset periodontitis. II. Long-term impact on microbial load. *J Periodontol*. 1999;70:646–656.

18. Graskemper J. *Professional Responsibility in Dentistry: A Practical Guide to Law and Ethics*. West Sussex, England: Wiley-Blackwell; 2011.

19. Schoen MA. A quality assessment system: the search for validity. *J Dent Edu*. 1989;53:658–661.

20. Beemsterboer, PL. *Ethics and Law in Dental Hygiene*. 2nd ed. St. Louis, MO: Saunders Elsevier; 2010:153–165.

CHAPTER

11

Occlusion and Temporomandibular Disorders

Phyllis L. Beemsterboer

LEARNING OUTCOMES

- Define the role of the dental hygienist in the detection of occlusal abnormalities and jaw dysfunction.
- Describe the biologic basis of occlusal function and the adaptive capability of the oral system.
- Compare and contrast the classification of primary and secondary traumatic occlusion in periodontal diagnosis and treatment.

- List the common signs and symptoms of temporomandibular disorders.
- Describe the procedures for clinically assessing jaw function and occlusion in a screening examination.
- Identify the various modalities used to treat temporomandibular disorders.

KEY TERMS

Biteguard
Bruxism
Clenching
Clinical jaw function
Crepitus
Dysfunction
Fremitus
Hyperfunction

Masticatory system
Myalgia
Nightguard
Occlusal function
Orthofunction
Parafunctional activity
Physiologic mobility
Physiologic occlusion

Primary traumatic occlusion
Secondary traumatic occlusion
Splint
Supracontact
Temporomandibular disorders (TMDs)
TMD screening examination
Traumatic occlusion
Trismus

The dental hygienist has an important role in the detection of occlusal abnormalities and jaw dysfunction. The application of true prevention principles includes attention to the form and function of all aspects of the head and neck. Form is the morphology of the teeth, bones, and temporomandibular joint (TMJ), whereas function includes the jaw muscles and neuromuscular system. Form and function are also important in the masticatory system, a complex apparatus that has an amazing adaptive capacity to function. However, when the masticatory system's adaptive capacity is exceeded, dysfunction can range from discomfort to debilitating pain. Good oral health requires the functional harmony of the teeth, muscles, and TMJ.

Bacterial plaque biofilm is the causative factor in periodontal diseases. However, numerous local and systemic factors can affect the response of the body to inflammatory periodontal diseases. This chapter describes the relationship of normal and abnormal form and function to provide a better understanding of occlusal function and dysfunction in periodontal treatment. In addition, it describes a method of screening for temporomandibular disorders (TMDs). The classification and treatment of these disorders are also discussed. The role of the dental hygienist is to *recognize* the signs and symptoms of pain and dysfunction, *record* the parameters of these signs and symptoms, and *refer* the patient for diagnosis and treatment.

CLINICAL NOTE 11-1 The role of the dental hygienist is to recognize the signs and symptoms of pain and dysfunction, record the parameters of these signs and symptoms, and refer the patient for diagnosis and treatment.

BIOLOGIC BASIS OF OCCLUSAL FUNCTION

The oral cavity in occlusal function—during talking, chewing, and swallowing—is in a dynamic rather than a static state. Orthofunction is a state of morphofunctional harmony in which the forces developed during function are within an adaptive physiologic range. In orthofunction, which means health and comfort for the patient, there are no pathologic changes in the oral tissues. Another term used to describe a range of morphologic variability is physiologic occlusion.[1,2] This term indicates psychologic and physical comfort for the patient, a normal adaptive situation. An occlusal relationship that functions for the patient is considered optimum and does not follow a particular occlusal configuration. For example, a malocclusion, although not ideal, can still be in orthofunction.

Dysfunction is a state of morphofunctional disharmony in which the forces developed during function cause pathologic changes in the tissues. These changes result in abnormal function or pain. The degree of dysfunction can be slight, with no great disturbance to the patient, or significant, making daily activity difficult or impossible.

The range of morphofunctional harmony to disharmony is dependent on the adaptive capability of the oral system.[1,3-6] At one end of the spectrum is the normal range, orthofunction. When the forces directed through the teeth and periodontal attachment in function and parafunction exceed what an individual system can handle, dysfunction may result. This trauma occurs where the greatest force is exerted against a weakened periodontal apparatus. Axial forces directed along the tooth and periodontium usually meet the demands necessary for normal function. **Parafunctional activity**, such as grinding or **clenching**, can stress this system. Antiaxial forces directed along the tooth and periodontium can cause resorption or a hypertrophic response. For this reason, some areas in the oral cavity will break down as a result of these forces, whereas other areas will not show any injury.[7]

Certain factors affect the response of the teeth and periodontal structures to normal and abnormal function. These factors include the size and shape of the roots, the quantity and quality of the alveolar bone, and the presence of microbial plaque biofilm. Oral habits and other occlusal situations, such as missing or shifting teeth, can increase the frequency and force on the teeth. When periodontal disease has weakened the periodontium, these forces may exceed the individual's adaptive capability, causing injury. At this point, a treatment intervention can correct an existing problem and prevent further damage. An occlusal contact relationship that is harmonious does not produce a painful response in the masticatory system.

When the condyles of the TMJ rest in the normal closed superoanterior position and the mandible has a well-distributed, even contact with the maxilla, the maxillary system is in a stable relationship. This situation allows the TMJ system to tolerate such activities as **hyperfunction** and possibly some trauma. The structures of the masticatory system can tolerate a certain amount of functional change. When functional changes exceed a certain level, alteration to the tissues may begin. This structural breakdown will vary depending on the individual and on systemic and local factors.[5]

The area of occlusion and study of occlusal harmony have been surrounded with controversy and confusion. Therefore, it is important to recognize that each component of the masticatory system must be understood within its functional relationship, not as a separate element.[2,4]

TRAUMA FROM OCCLUSION

A **traumatic occlusion** is an occlusion that has caused injury to the teeth, muscles, or TMJ.[2,5,6] A classification of **primary traumatic occlusion** is made when heavy occlusal forces exceed the adaptive range in a normal periodontium, causing injury to tissues and bone. A classification of **secondary traumatic occlusion** is made when normal occlusal forces exceed the capability of a periodontium that is already affected by periodontal disease. Trauma from occlusion does not initiate gingivitis and periodontal disease. When inflammation is present, occlusal trauma can increase tissue attachment loss and supporting bone destruction. Therefore, occlusal trauma is of interest in the diagnosis and treatment of periodontal disease.

Traumatic occlusion does not refer to a malocclusion, as described by Angle's three classifications. Angle's Class I, II, and III occlusion classify and describe the skeletal relationship of the maxillary to the mandibular teeth. Because malocclusion of the teeth may interfere with the removal of bacterial plaque, it is a factor in the attainment of good oral hygiene. Common terms used to describe mandibular function and dysfunction are listed in Box 11-1.

The occlusal relationship of the teeth is not a predictor of pain or problems in the TMJ. Common occlusal features, such as intercuspal position or midline discrepancies, do not provide the dominant factors in defining populations with TMDs.[8,9]

BOX 11-1 Terms Used to Describe Mandibular Function and Dysfunction

Arthralgia Pain in a joint structure.
Arthrocentesis Puncture of a joint space with a needle and removal of fluid.
Bruxism Grinding or gnashing of the teeth, usually during sleep; an oral habit that can cause periodontal injury and pain and discomfort in the jaw.
Clenching Clamping and forcing the teeth together without grinding.
Clicking Cracking or snapping noise in the temporomandibular joint because of disk and condyle incoordination; can occur in one or both joints.
Crepitus Grating noise in the temporomandibular joint because of damage to the disk and articulating joint surfaces.
Dyskinesia Abnormal movement; can describe masticatory muscle incoordination or spasm.
Excursive movement Mandible in movement from side to side and forward; movement away from the intercuspal position.
Fremitus Vibration or movement of a tooth when in function; can be observed or felt by placing a finger over the tooth.
Hypertrophy Enlargement.
Intercuspal position The maximum intercuspation of the mandibular and maxillary teeth; also called centric occlusion and habitual occlusion.
Interference Tooth contact that does not allow the teeth to achieve stable interdigitation; also called supracontact.
Laterotrusion Mandibular movement away from the midline; the laterotrusive side moves away from the midline in function.
Mediotrusion Mandibular movement toward the midline; the mediotrusive side moves toward the midline in function.
Morphofunction Relationship of form and function.
Myalgia Pain in a muscle.
Myositis Inflammation in a muscle.
Occlusal therapy Treatment that alters the occlusal contacts or mandibular position of the jaw.
Occlusal trauma Pathologic changes in the oral cavity as a result of occlusal forces; an occlusion-producing injury.
Orthofunction A state of morphofunctional harmony in which the forces developed during function are within an adaptive physiologic range.
Parafunction Movement of the mandible outside the range of function.
Physiologic occlusion An occlusion that is free of disease and dysfunction and has adapted to some physiologic changes.
Retruded contact position The mandible in the end point of the terminal hinge closure; also called centric relation position.
Spasm Involuntary contraction of a muscle or muscles, usually painful and interfering with function.
Trismus Spasm in the masticatory muscles associated with a disturbance in the trigeminal nerve.

Controversy regarding the clinical significance of trauma from occlusion has existed for some time. It is now widely accepted that in the absence of marginal gingival irritation, trauma from occlusion does not produce gingival inflammation. Trauma associated with orthodontic movement of teeth is self-limiting. Self-limited mobility is greater than normal, but is based on the adaptive capacity of the periodontium. Thus, the increased mobility of the teeth is handled through periodontal adaptation to the excessive forces without causing trauma from occlusion.[1] Dentists may use this rationale when selectively grinding (adjusting) the occlusal surfaces of the teeth after periodontal therapy to create a dentition that does not produce injury. The goal is to establish an occlusal relationship that will foster a favorable periodontal response. True trauma from occlusion (trauma that exceeds the adaptive capacity of the periodontium) increases bone loss and pocket depth formation. This situation may occur with bruxism in a periodontal patient.

Certain tooth relationships can also be detrimental to the attainment of good periodontal health. Open contacts or faulty contacts between teeth can cause areas of food impaction. Food impaction is the forceful wedging of food into the periodontium by occlusal forces. The self-cleansing aspects of the dentition do not exist in these situations, and food impaction can be a contributing factor in periodontal disease.

The dental hygienist must carefully complete the clinical assessment of the patient, noting all of the gingival conditions and determining the reason for the condition, if possible. In the past, certain gingival conditions, such as recession, clefting, or thickening of the gingival margin, were thought to be caused by trauma from occlusion. These causative relationships have not been supported by research.[4]

Understanding the multifactorial origin of jaw dysfunction and how it relates to the treatment of the periodontal patient is important. When an individual can attain and maintain good oral hygiene, malocclusion is of no periodontal significance.[1,5] However, most patients have difficulty with plaque removal, making malocclusion a factor to be considered in the progression of periodontal disease.

TEMPOROMANDIBULAR DISORDERS

TMDs are a grouping of musculoskeletal conditions that produce pain or dysfunction in the masticatory system. When the disorder involves the muscles and not the joint, it is referred to as extracapsular. A problem occurring within the TMJ is known as intracapsular. The percentage of people who have signs or symptoms of a functional disorder can be as low as 5% or as high as 60%, making the prevalence of TMDs significant.[5,10-14] However, it is generally agreed that only 5% to 7% of these patients are in need of TMD intervention therapy.[2,5]

Historically, TMDs have been described with a number of labels, such as temporomandibular joint syndrome and myofascial pain dysfunction syndrome. Most orofacial clinicians and researchers agree that the term *TMD* accurately reflects the scope and complexity of the conditions.[3,8] A diagnosis of a subcondition, such as myofascial pain or arthritis, further describes the problem. It is important for the dental hygienist to remember that there are many orofacial pain problems in addition to TMDs.

> **BOX 11-2** Diagnostic Categories for Temporomandibular Disorders
>
> Muscle and fascial disorders of the masticatory system
> Disorders of the temporomandibular joint
> Disorders of mandibular mobility
> Disorders of maxillomandibular growth

CAUSE

The etiology of TMDs is multifactorial. Because of the many causes, TMDs are frequently difficult to diagnosis and treat. Stress is often a factor in TMDs and patients with TMDs may have a history of other diseases, such as arthritis and psychological problems. In determining the causes of TMDs, a history of macrotrauma or microtrauma may be discovered by the clinician. A macrotrauma is usually a single event that may have caused damage to the masticatory system. Such an event could be a sports-related injury, a whiplash accident, or a fall. The patient may not relate such an event to later occlusal or TMJ pain and discomfort. Microtrauma is a number of minor habits or events that cause damage to the masticatory structures. Examples of microtrauma include bruxism and postural and oral habits.

CATEGORIES OF TEMPOROMANDIBULAR DISORDERS

There are four main diagnostic categories for TMD, which are listed in Box 11-2. These categories are based on criteria derived from the signs and symptoms gathered in the comprehensive TMD evaluation.[3,5,11] The first category is muscle and fascial disorders of the masticatory system. This group includes myalgia (pain in the masticatory muscles), trismus (spasm in the masticatory muscles), dyskinesia (incoordination of the jaw), bruxism (clenching or grinding), and other muscle disorders. Disorders of the TMJ, the second category, include internal derangements that impair mechanical function of the TMJ, such as arthritis. The third category includes disorders of mandibular mobility, such as ankylosis, muscular fibrosis, internal derangement, and adhesions in the joint. The fourth category, disorders of maxillomandibular growth, is less common. These disorders include neoplastic and nonneoplastic conditions.

Oral Habits

Oral habits can contribute to periodontal and dental damage in the oral cavity. Oral habits are repetitive masticatory activities outside the normal range of function. These parafunctional activities can involve tooth to tooth contact or contact with foreign objects. The amount of damage is related to the intensity and duration of the habit. Oral habits can lead to tooth damage, muscular hypertrophy, muscular pain and tenderness, and periodontal tissue injury. Bruxism is the most frequently described oral habit.

> **CLINICAL NOTE 11-2** Oral habits are repetitive masticatory activities outside the normal range of function.

Bruxism

Bruxism is clenching or grinding of the teeth, not including chewing or swallowing. Bruxism can occur as rhythmic side to side movements or as a sustained clench. Clenching is continuous or intermittent closure of the jaws under vertical pressure.[6] Grinding and clenching are parafunctional habits that are involuntary and may be destructive. Bruxism is further categorized into nocturnal (nighttime) and diurnal (daytime) types. Bruxism can be identified by the presence of wear facets that are not caused by masticatory function. The results of bruxism may be tooth wear, tooth fracture, restoration fracture, myalgia, hypertrophy of the masticatory muscles, and headache. Bruxism or periodontal disease can cause mobility in the teeth. Researchers have found that bruxism does not cause damage to the periodontium and that periodontal disease and bruxism seldom occur in the same individual.[12]

The prevalence of bruxism is difficult to estimate because most patients are unaware that they grind their teeth. Stress may contribute etiologically to bruxism. Other causes may be neurologic or occupational. Bruxism is common in children between the ages of 3 and 12 years and disappears as they age.

There is no absolute cure for bruxism. A variety of treatment approaches have been reported, with varying levels of success. Often, awareness of the problem and its consequences helps the patient control the habit. Other treatments include occlusal splints, pharmacologic therapy, physical therapy, and behavioral modification therapy.[5,13] Bruxism can be a significant problem for patients who have advanced loss of support in the periodontal mechanism, as seen in Figures 11-1 and 11-2.

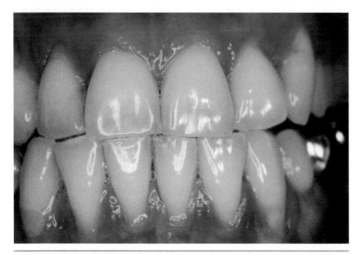

FIGURE 11-1 ■ Bruxism caused mild tooth wear in a 56-year-old woman.

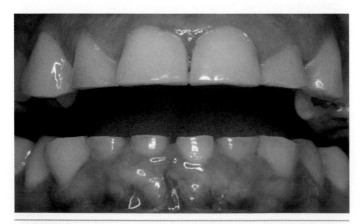

FIGURE 11-2 ■ Bruxism caused severe tooth wear in a 32-year-old man.

SIGNS AND SYMPTOMS OF TEMPOROMANDIBULAR DISORDERS

Four primary symptoms are commonly reported in patients with TMDs. These symptoms are as follows:

- Pain and tenderness in the muscles of mastication
- Pain and tenderness in the TMJ
- Painful clicking of the joint during function
- Limitation of mandibular motion

In addition to these primary symptoms, a number of other symptoms are found in patients with TMDs. An uncomfortable bite, incoordination of the jaw (dyskinesia), ringing in the ears, and muscle swelling may be described by these patients. In the dentition, signs include tooth wear, tooth mobility, and pulpitis. The presence of one or more of these symptoms does not indicate a positive diagnosis of TMD. A diagnosis can be made only after the patient undergoes a complete clinical examination for the signs of TMD and after a careful differential diagnosis is completed.

Pain in the masticatory muscles (myalgia) is the most common symptom reported by patients with a muscle disorder. This pain is usually dull, aching, and continuous or recurrent. Muscle pain may be a normal protective response or may be the result of changes in the muscle tissue caused by hyperactivity or trauma. Stress can cause an increase in the tonicity of the head and neck muscles. Muscle pain is also associated with a reduction in mandibular function, usually the inability to open the mouth widely. Muscle soreness over a long period may be myofascial pain, an acute pain disorder that can occur in any muscle in the body.

Tenderness or pain in the TMJ (arthralgia) is another common finding in TMDs. The pain in this region arises from the soft tissues surrounding the joint because the articular surfaces of the joint are not innervated. This pain is sharp, sudden, and associated with the jaw in function.

The dysfunction that is most common within the TMJ is usually observed as a joint sound. This sound is caused by a disruption of the normal movement of the condyle and articular disk in the joint. This dysfunction is known as a click or a pop if it is a single sound and **crepitus** if it is a grating sound. Within the joint, problems can be caused by incoordination of the disk-condyle complex, restricted translation of the condyle, or dislocation of the condyle.[2,5] Another set of problems results from inflammatory joint disorders, such as osteoarthritis and polyarthritis. For these patients, pain in the TMJ is dull, aching, and constant and increases during function.

The signs and symptoms of TMDs are observed frequently in the dentition. Mobility or movement of the teeth can result from periodontal disease or excessive occlusal forces. Tooth wear or breakdown of the enamel or dentin is a common sign. The functional or parafunctional origin of the wear is determined by locating the position of the worn surfaces on the teeth.

SCREENING FOR TEMPOROMANDIBULAR DISORDERS

The **TMD screening examination** is an important part of the dental hygiene examination. This screening should be completed for each patient. It is simple to accomplish and does not involve a great deal of additional chair time. Once the clinician is comfortable with performing the screening, it should take approximately 5 minutes. The screening examination will lead to one of three conclusions:

1. The jaw system is in orthofunction; there are no contraindications to proceeding with dental hygiene treatment.
2. Problems exist in the jaw system; dental hygiene and dental treatment should proceed with caution and the patient should be informed.
3. The patient should be referred for a comprehensive evaluation before any dental hygiene or dental treatment is administered.

Patients who have signs or symptoms of pain or jaw dysfunction should be referred to the dentist for a comprehensive examination. The dental hygienist is in an excellent position to identify patients with the signs and symptoms of jaw dysfunction and to refer them for treatment. Initial scaling therapy and subsequent maintenance and periodontal recall appointments allow the dental hygienist to screen for TMDs and to gather subjective information that can aid the dentist in diagnosis and treatment.

The screening examination has subjective and objective components. The subjective component is a series of questions the patient is asked during the medical history or examination of the oral cavity. The objective portion is performed by the clinician and is divided into the assessment of clinical jaw function and the assessment of occlusion.

SUBJECTIVE QUESTIONNAIRE

The questions posed in the subjective questionnaire are designed to screen for patient-reported signs and symptoms of TMDs.[1,5,11,15] A positive response to several of these questions does not necessarily indicate a dysfunctional situation. A comprehensive history and complete clinical examination are needed to identify dysfunction. The patient should be asked the following questions:

1. Do you have difficulty opening your mouth?
2. Do you hear noises from the jaw joints?
3. Does your jaw "stick," "lock," or "go out?"
4. Do you have pain in or around the ears, temples, or cheeks?
5. Do you have pain when you chew or yawn?
6. Does your bite feel uncomfortable or unusual?
7. Do you have frequent headaches?
8. Have you had a recent injury to your head or neck?
9. Do you have arthritis?
10. Do you have problems chewing, talking, or using your jaw?
11. Do you clench or grind your teeth? Do others hear you grind?
12. Have you previously been treated for a TMJ problem?
13. Have you experienced previous jaw problems after dental appointments?

ASSESSMENT OF CLINICAL JAW FUNCTION

The techniques in the clinical objective examination are designed to identify certain signs and symptoms of TMDs and can be added to dental hygiene assessment and documentation procedures. Several positive findings do not necessarily indicate a dysfunctional situation. Dysfunction can be assessed only by a comprehensive history and a complete clinical examination. The techniques include muscle palpation and assessment of mandibular movement, joint function, and joint sounds.

Muscle Palpation

Normal muscles are equal in length and contract and relax without discomfort or pain. Muscles that have been overworked or injured are painful and do not contract properly.[7,11] In the clinical objective examination, the temporalis and masseter muscles are examined bilaterally by palpating the origin, body, and insertion of the muscle. Gentle finger pressure lasting 2 seconds along the muscle may elicit a response from the patient. The patient should be instructed to differentiate pressure from pain. Painful reactions should be recorded. This part of the examination is illustrated in Figures 11-3 and 11-4.

Mandibular Movement

The normal opening and closing of the jaw should be smooth and symmetric, and the patient should be able to achieve a minimum of 40 mm of opening distance. The interincisal

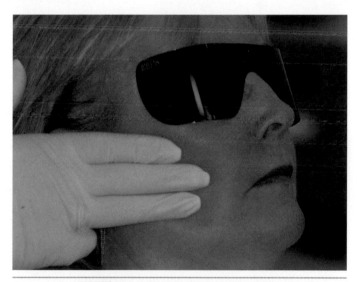

FIGURE 11-3 ■ Palpating the masseter muscle.

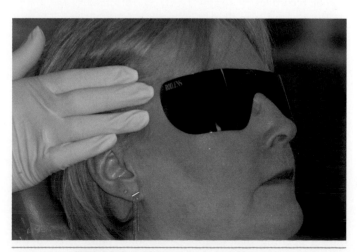

FIGURE 11-4 ■ Palpating the temporalis muscle.

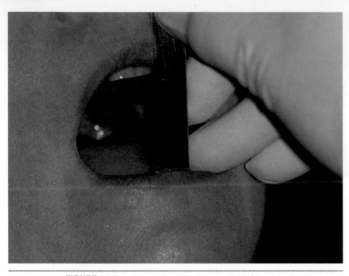

FIGURE 11-5 ■ Measuring the interincisal distance.

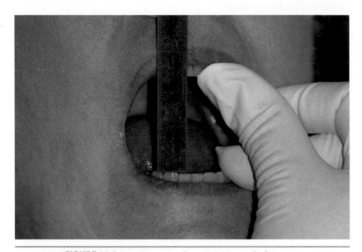

FIGURE 11-6 ■ Measuring the passive stretch distance.

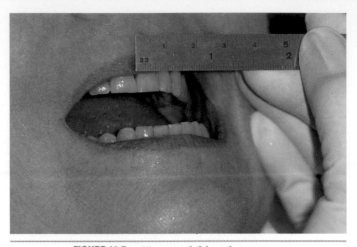

FIGURE 11-7 ■ Measuring left lateral movement.

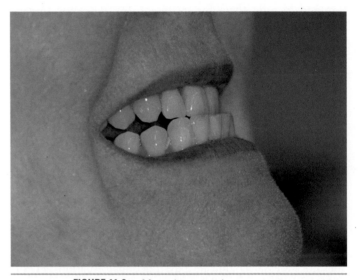

FIGURE 11-8 ■ Measuring protrusive movement.

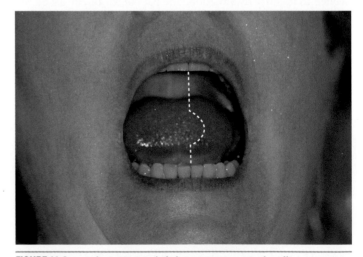

FIGURE 11-9 ■ A deviation is a shift that returns to normal midline at opening.

opening (incisal edge to incisal edge) is measured after the patient opens the mouth as wide as possible, as illustrated in Figures 11-5 and 11-6. Any report of pain should be recorded. If the clinician can passively increase the interincisal distance for a patient (using the thumb and finger to open wider), there may be a muscular problem. The passive stretch distance should also be recorded.

The normal mandibular movement from side to side and forward of the teeth not in contact should be approximately 8 mm. This distance is recorded by measuring the patient's ability to move the mandible laterally and protrusively (forward) from the midline. The left lateral movement, right lateral movement, and protrusive movement are measured and recorded as seen in Figures 11-7 and 11-8.

Joint Function

In function, both TMJs together have the ability to rotate, translate, and move excursively forward and side to side. The normal maximum opening of the jaw should be smooth and straight. The pathway during opening and closing is observed for any alteration from the midline. A deviation is a shift in the midline during opening that disappears at some point later in the opening movement. A deflection is a shift in the midline that becomes greater as the opening movement continues. A deviation may be caused by interference in the disk of the joint, whereas a deflection is caused by a restriction in one joint. These movements are seen in Figures 11-9 and 11-10. Any type of alteration should be recorded.

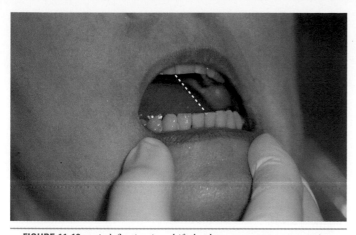

FIGURE 11-10 ■ A deflection is a shift that becomes greater on opening.

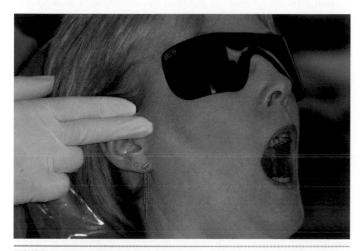

FIGURE 11-11 ■ **Palpating the TMJ.** Light palpation is an excellent way to detect substantial clicks and crepitus.

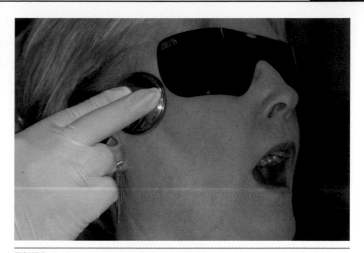

FIGURE 11-12 ■ **Listening for joint sounds.** A stethoscope is helpful, but not necessary, to determine clicking or crepitus.

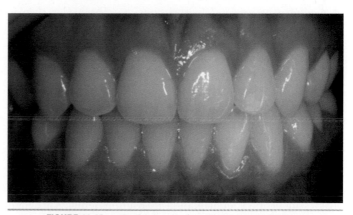

FIGURE 11-13 ■ Teeth in normal maximum intercuspation.

Joint Sounds

On opening, the condyle and disk of the TMJ move forward (anteriorly) to the articular eminence. The normal joint functions smoothly, without noise, irregularities, or pain. Pain or restrictions in the joint can be detected by palpation. The fingers are placed over the condyles and slight pressure is applied. The patient is then asked to open and close the mouth slowly. A sound elicited by the joint in function is either a click or crepitus. The click is a short sound, whereas crepitus is a grating sound. A sound that occurs on opening and closing is called a reciprocal click. Any irregularity, pain, or sound is noted in the chart. This examination is seen in Figures 11-11 and 11-12.

ASSESSMENT OF OCCLUSION
Intercuspal Position

The normal position of the teeth in maximum intercuspation is called centric occlusion. It should be stable, with a firm, well-distributed pattern of occlusal contact. The patient should be able to open and close the mouth several times without searching for a comfortable bite. The dental hygienist should ask the patient to open and close normally while observing the closure pattern. Any difficulty finding a comfortable bite should be noted in the chart.

The posterior teeth should have firm, even contact when together in maximum intercuspation. The anterior teeth may

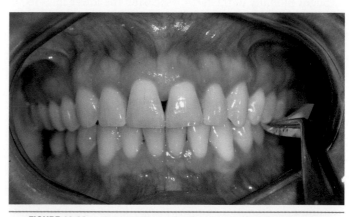

FIGURE 11-14 ■ Determining occlusal contact in the left molar area.

have only light or no contact. To evaluate this contact, polyester film occlusal indicator paper, or Mylar paper, is placed between the teeth at small intervals. The Mylar paper is held with hemostat forceps. The patient is asked to close the mouth and hold on to the Mylar strip with the teeth while the dental hygienist tugs slightly outward. If the Mylar strip holds, there is contact. If the Mylar strip slips through the teeth, there is no contact. The presence or absence of intercuspation contact (Figures 11-13 and 11-14) should be noted for the incisors, canines, premolars, and molars on the right and left sides of the mouth.

Protrusive, Lateral, and Medial Excursive Movements

Normal movement of the jaw with the teeth in contact should be smooth, symmetric, and able to achieve about 8 mm of magnitude. Starting in intercuspation, the patient is asked to protrude the jaw as far as possible. Movement that is limited or deviates on protrusion is recorded.

A **supracontact** (high spot) is an area on a tooth that may prevent well-distributed stable contact between the maxillary and mandibular teeth. Occlusal interferences are supracontacts that are capable of injuring the periodontal tissues or complicating mandibular movement.[2,10]

Lateral movement is examined starting from the intercuspal position. The patient is asked to move the jaw toward the right shoulder. The movement toward the right lateral side is observed and any limitations are recorded. The test is repeated on the left side.

Medial movement is also examined starting from the intercuspal position. Mylar film is used to determine the presence of mediotrusive or laterotrusive contacts. The Mylar strip is placed between the molars on the right side. The patient is asked to move the jaw 2 mm toward the opposite side. If the Mylar film does not hold, no contact exists. If it holds, a mediotrusive contact exists. This contact may prevent proper movement of the jaw in function. The test, as illustrated in Figures 11-15 and 11-16, is repeated on the left side. Supracontacts are noted in the chart.

Tooth Mobility and Wear

The assessment of occlusion also includes an evaluation of tooth mobility, tooth wear, and full-mouth radiographs. These aspects of assessment and documentation are routine elements of dental hygiene care. The results of the related dental hygiene assessment should be included in the TMD screening.

Slight mobility of the teeth, especially the lower incisors, is normal. This is called **physiologic mobility** and occurs because the conical roots of single rooted teeth are suspended in the periodontal ligament, which allows them to move very slightly.

This movement is usually charted to monitor any increases over time. Greater mobility can occur when occlusal forces exceed the adaptive capability of the periodontium. Mobility is evaluated along with the presence of disease in the periodontium. A classification of primary traumatic occlusion is made when heavy occlusal forces exceed the adaptive range in a normal periodontium. A classification of secondary traumatic occlusion is made when normal occlusal forces exceed the capability of a periodontium that is affected by periodontal disease.

The visible and palpable movement of a tooth during function or parafunction is called **fremitus.** Fremitus can be observed or felt. To feel the movement, the dental hygienist places a finger over the tooth root on the attached gingiva (Figure 11-17).

Wear caused by tooth to tooth contact is called attrition. A certain amount of wear is normal, but accelerated wear is the result of parafunctional activity, such as bruxism. Excessive wear may result in a flat tooth surface, a cupped-out occlusal surface, or obliteration of the cusps. A facet is a tooth surface worn by attrition from functional or parafunctional causes. A facet is smooth and shiny because it is the result of the enamel rods becoming fractured and polished. A facet that is shiny is

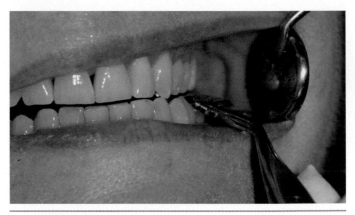

FIGURE 11-16 ■ Determining lateral movement with a Mylar strip.

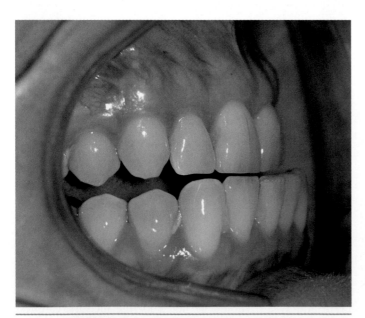

FIGURE 11-15 ■ Determining protrusive movement.

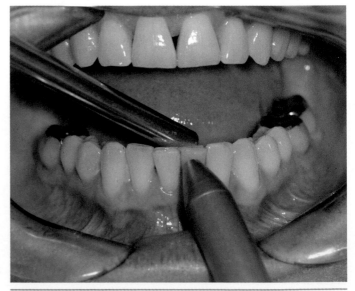

FIGURE 11-17 ■ Determining mobility. The handles of two instruments rather than fingertips should be used to make accurate assessments.

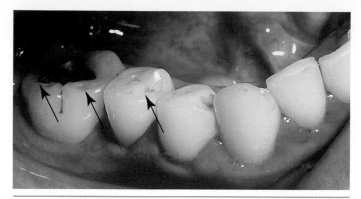

FIGURE 11-18 ■ Wear facets *(arrows)* on premolars and molars.

known as an active facet, whereas a nonshiny or velvet-like facet is termed passive. When the facet is angular, the occlusal forces are directed laterally and increase the risk of periodontal injury.[10] To determine whether wear is from functional or parafunctional use, the patient should be asked to close the mouth and the dental hygienist should observe the position of the mandible. If an occlusal pattern for the wear cannot be established, other factors must be considered. Oral habits, such as nail biting or foreign substance abrasion, can also cause tooth wear, as seen in Figure 11-18.

Radiographic Evaluation

Excessive occlusal forces can cause changes in the teeth and periodontium. These changes can be observed in periapical radiographs. The radiographs should be examined for widening of the periodontal ligament, increased density of the surrounding bone (osteosclerosis), or increased cementum at the apical areas of the root (hypercementosis). The widening of the periodontal ligament is caused by resorption of bony support from the excessive occlusal forces. Osteosclerosis and hypercementosis are hypertrophic responses to the occlusal forces. Examples of these conditions are seen in Figures 11-19 and 11-20.

A temporomandibular screening form for use by the dental hygienist is provided in Figure 11-21. This form can be modified to suit the needs of a particular clinician or dental health care setting.

THE COMPREHENSIVE EXAMINATION

A comprehensive examination for TMDs completed by the dentist or TMD specialist involves an extensive history and physical examination. The physical examination for this expanded evaluation includes examining mandibular motion in all planes, palpating the TMJ, palpating the masticatory muscles, examining and listening to joint sounds, palpating the cervical musculature, and determining the stability of the dentition and skeleton. Additional diagnostic tests and radiographs are used when necessary to aid in the diagnosis and prognosis of TMDs.

CLINICAL NOTE 11-3 Dysfunction of the clinical jaw system can be assessed only by a comprehensive history and a complete clinical examination.

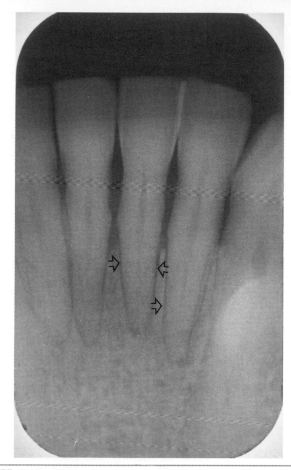

FIGURE 11-19 ■ Widened periodontal ligament *(arrows)*. (Courtesy of Dr. Richard Nagy.)

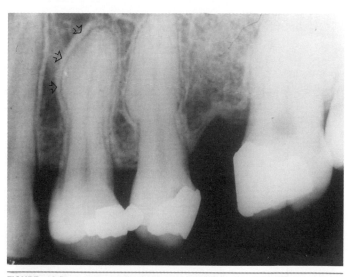

FIGURE 11-20 ■ **Hypercementosis.** Arrows indicate widened cementum. (Courtesy of Dr. Stewart White.)

TREATMENT OF TEMPOROMANDIBULAR DISORDERS

A number of modalities are used to treat TMDs. The goal of treatment is to reduce pain and improve jaw system functionality. The method of treatment should be based on a clear understanding of the problem and should address the cause as well

Temporomandibular Disorders Screening Form

Assessment of Clinical Jaw Function

A. Muscle Palpation

	Pressure (slight discomfort)	Pain (hurts)
Masseter		
Temporalis		

B. Mandibular Movement

	Measurement in millimeters (mm)
Interincisal opening	
Passive stretch	
Lateral movement (left and right)	
Protrusive movement	

C. Joint Function

Opening Pathway	Normal	Deviation (returns to midline)	Deflection (becomes greater)

Palpation of the joint	No discomfort	Pain
Lateral aspect		
Posterior aspect		

D. Joint Sounds

Sounds of the joint	No sounds	Click	Crepitus
Left joint			
Right joint			

Assessment of Occlusion

E. Intercuspal Position

	Easy and repeatable	Difficult and searching
ICP closure pattern		

ICP contact	Right (y/n)	Left (y/n)
Incisors		
Canines		
Premolars		
Molars		

F. Excursive Movements

Protrusive	Forward (mm)	Deviates on movement (y/n)

	Right (mm)	Left (mm)	Supracontact (y/n)
Lateral movement			
Medial movement			

G. Tooth Evaluation

	Anterior teeth (y/n)	Posterior teeth (y/n)
Tooth mobility		
Tooth wear		
Radiographic signs		

Clinical action from screening exam and assessment:

No contraindication to dental hygiene treatment _____
Treat with caution and informed consent for dental hygiene treatment _____
Refer for consult and dental treatment _____

FIGURE 11-21 ■ TMD screening form.

as the symptoms. Clark[10] established three criteria to be used as guidelines for selecting TMD treatments. These criteria state that treatments should be as follows:

- Based on correct differential diagnoses
- Selected with reason and purpose
- Directed toward eliminating or neutralizing the cause of the symptoms

The approach to TMD treatment suggested by most orofacial clinicians and researchers is conservative and reversible.[1,3-5,8] This conservative approach uses simple noninvasive methods rather than irreversible methods, such as open joint surgery. The most frequently recommended approach uses a physical medicine model with a strong behavioral-educational component.[13-17] Usually, this approach requires a combination of dental office therapy and home treatments. The first step in the treatment of a patient with a TMD is to recommend initial therapy. In this model, initial therapy consists of suggesting a soft diet, limited movement of the jaw, application of moist heat to the affected area, and a non-narcotic analgesic. The patient also receives a careful explanation of the disorder and the usual outcome of treatment. Patients frequently improve after 2 to 3 weeks of initial therapy. Often, simply understanding the possible reasons for the symptoms leads to improvement.

Initial therapy is a set of simple noninvasive steps that can provide immediate comfort and relief of symptoms. The first step is to instruct the patient to eat only soft foods. Avoiding foods such as apples and hard rolls allows the overworked jaw muscles to rest. Limited jaw movement is an important part of the treatment. Moist heat provides relief from muscle pain by increasing circulation. A hand towel folded in thirds and moistened with warm water can be placed under the chin and around the neck. Icing of the muscles can also reduce pain. Ice is rubbed against the area until it is numb, approximately 5 minutes. The skin is allowed to warm between applications.

The use of non-narcotic analgesics is often valuable in relieving jaw pain. Common over-the-counter drugs, such as aspirin and ibuprofen, can effectively reduce musculoskeletal discomfort. The dentist may prescribe stronger drugs when symptoms do not respond to non-narcotic analgesics. Medications for TMDs should be prescribed for a limited time.

TREATMENT METHODS

The American Association for Dental Research has endorsed a policy that treatment of TMD patients should initially be based on the use of conservative, reversible, and evidence-based therapeutic modalities, unless there are specific and justifiable indications for therapies to the contrary.[8]

Home Therapy

Home therapy includes initial therapy (soft diet, heat or ice packs, non-narcotic analgesics), rest, and some jaw movement exercises. The jaw movement exercises are demonstrated to the patient and a daily program is recommended. The exercises both relax and stretch the sore muscles so that they can regain their original function.

Physical Therapy

Physical therapy treatments include ultrasound, massage, electrical stimulation of the muscles, soft tissue manipulation, and exercise programs. The goal of home treatment and office treatment programs is the same—to help the patient relieve pain and change any habits that contribute to the problem.

Occlusal Appliances

Occlusal appliances are made of hard acrylic resin and fit over the occlusal and incisal surfaces of the maxillary or mandibular teeth. They are usually called **splints**, **nightguards**, or **biteguards**. A splint is used to protect the teeth and to provide a stable position for them. The goal of a therapeutic splint is to reduce symptoms and encourage normal muscle function. The success or failure of a splint depends on its selection, fabrication, and adjustment.[5,7] The occlusal splint is not a mouthguard.

A mouthguard is used by athletes to protect their teeth, head, and neck during contact sports.

In the past, occlusal adjustment was a common form of treatment for TMDs. Research has shown that this modality is not as effective as more conservative methods; however, limited occlusal adjustment may be appropriate in some situations, but it is rarely considered as a primary TMD treatment.[8]

Behavioral Therapy

Behavioral therapy methods include counseling for stress or anxiety, depression, and psychiatric issues. Pain management clinics and programs, usually offered by universities or hospitals, can provide traditional and nontraditional therapies from multidisciplinary practitioners.

Pharmacologic Therapy

The groups of medications prescribed as part of pharmacologic treatment of TMDs include analgesics, antianxiety drugs, anti-inflammatory agents, muscle relaxants, and local anesthetics. These agents are administered by mouth or by injection.

Pharmacologic therapy can also be used to relieve trigger point pain. A trigger point is a painful hypersensitive band of muscle tissue. A trigger point can refer pain to another area, triggering pain. The use of local anesthetics, such as Carbocaine, can aid in the diagnosis and treatment of this myofascial pain.

Surgical Therapy

Arthroscopic and arthrocentesis surgeries can help patients with acute TMJ derangement–induced hypermobility gain full range of jaw motion. A condylectomy (removal of the condyle), which is more extensive than a condylotomy (partial removal), may be indicated for severe TMJ growth disturbances or tumors. Any surgical procedure should be completed only after a careful diagnosis and the consideration of a second or third opinion.

Irreversible Treatments

Irreversible treatments for TMDs, such as surgery to the joint or disk, are permanent alterations. Surgical treatments are indicated only in a small percentage of patients. Occlusal adjustments are irreversible and there is no evidence that they are effective.[4,8]

> **CLINICAL NOTE 11-4** The patient with TMD requires a series of short appointments, rather than one long appointment, to minimize trauma to the masticatory muscles and joint.

DENTAL HYGIENE APPOINTMENT

Dental hygienists will treat patients who have symptoms of or are in treatment for jaw pain and dysfunction.[18] They must adapt the dental hygiene treatment plan to accommodate these patients. Suggestions to make these appointments more comfortable for the patient are presented in Box 11-3. Patients with TMDs require a series of short appointments, rather than one long one, to minimize trauma to the masticatory muscles and joint. The use of a bite-block to maintain the oral opening is one option for a patient with a history of jaw pain and fatigue. The use of a toothbrush with a small head or other interdental cleaning device can simplify daily oral hygiene care for patients with limited opening or malpositioned teeth. Occasionally, dental hygiene treatment must be postponed until initial TMD therapy is completed and the patient can open the mouth to a greater degree and tolerate a lengthier appointment. Initial therapy, such as a soft diet and moist heat, may be helpful to a dental hygiene patient after a long scaling appointment.

◎ DENTAL HYGIENE CONSIDERATIONS

- Good oral health requires the functional harmony of the teeth, muscles, and TMJ.
- Orthofunction is a state of morphofunctional harmony in which the forces developed during function are within an adaptive physiologic range.
- Dysfunction is a state of morphofunctional disharmony in which the forces developed during function cause pathologic changes in the tissues.
- A classification of primary traumatic occlusion is made when heavy occlusal forces exceed the adaptive range in a normal periodontium, causing injury to tissues and bone.
- Grinding and clenching of the teeth are parafunctional habits that are involuntary and may be destructive.
- The four primary symptoms commonly reported in patients with TMDs are pain and tenderness in the muscles of mastication, pain and tenderness in the TMJ, painful clicking of the joint during function, and limitation of mandibular motion.
- The dental hygienist plays an important role in the detection of occlusal abnormalities and jaw dysfunction by recognizing the signs and symptoms of pain and dysfunction, recording the parameters of these signs and symptoms, and referring the patient for diagnosis and treatment.

✳ CASE SCENARIO

A 34-year-old female patient, Ms. Carrow, presents for dental hygiene treatment with light to moderate subgingival plaque and calculus and states that she is very concerned about the wear on her teeth, especially the lower front incisors. Numerous shiny wear facets are present, there is generalized inflammation around the posterior teeth, and slight bone loss is evident on the radiographs. On reviewing the medical and dental history, you see that Ms. Carrow has also complained of headaches and a sore jaw in the mornings.

1. The most likely cause of Ms. Carrow's chief complaint is
   A. gingivitis.
   B. crepitus.
   C. bruxism.
   D. trismus.

2. Ms. Carrow's symptoms would lead you to consider a condition of
   A. primary occlusal trauma.
   B. secondary occlusal trauma.
   C. malocclusion.
   D. hyperfunction.

3. The bone loss noted on Ms. Carrow's radiographs is probably related to her oral condition of
   A. occlusal trauma.
   B. periodontal disease.
   C. myalgia.
   D. trismus.

4. Ms. Carrow's sore jaw involves only the muscles of mastication and not the TMJ. This type of pain is termed
   A. extracapsular.
   B. intracapsular.
   C. arthralgia.
   D. spasm.

5. After completing Ms. Carrow's initial history and examination, you should
   A. proceed with dental hygiene treatment.
   B. proceed with caution and inform her of potential problems.
   C. refer her for a comprehensive evaluation before any dental hygiene or dental treatment.

STUDY QUESTIONS

Answers and rationales to these questions can be obtained from your instructor.

MULTIPLE CHOICE

1. The term that best describes heavy occlusal forces that have caused injury to tissues and bone in a normal periodontium is
   A. physiologic occlusion.
   B. dysfunctional occlusion.
   C. primary traumatic occlusion.
   D. secondary traumatic occlusion.

2. The etiology of TMDs is described as
   A. behavioral.
   B. neurologic.
   C. psychological.
   D. multifactorial.

3. An oral habit such as bruxism can result in all of the following EXCEPT one. Which one is the EXCEPTION?
   A. Change in microbiota
   B. Muscular hypertrophy
   C. Periodontal tissue injury
   D. Muscular pain and tenderness

4. What are the four primary symptoms of TMDs?
   A. Muscle pain, muscle swelling, jaw pain, and dyskinesia
   B. Muscle pain, clicking, headache, and uncomfortable bite
   C. Muscle pain, jaw pain, clicking, and limitation of motion
   D. Muscle pain, jaw pain, dyskinesia, and limitation of motion

5. Myalgia is best described as
   A. pain in the muscles.
   B. clicking in the joint.
   C. crepitus in the joint.
   D. incoordination of the jaw.
6. The normal jaw should achieve an opening distance of at least 40 mm, Any finding of less than 40 mm should be considered a symptom of a TMD and referred for treatment.
   A. Both statements are true.
   B. Both statements are false.
   C. The first statement is true, and the second statement is false.
   D. The first statement is false, and the second statement is true.
7. A deviation of the mandible to the right on opening would suggest that the patient may have?
   A. Crepitus
   B. Clicking
   C. Restriction of the left condyle
   D. Restriction of the right condyle
8. The most frequently recommended approach for the treatment of TMDs is physical medicine therapy because it is conservative and reversible.
   A. Both the statement and the reason are correct and related.
   B. Both the statement and the reason are correct but NOT related.
   C. The statement is correct, but the reason is NOT correct.
   D. The statement is NOT correct, but the reason is correct.
   E. NEITHER the statement NOR the reason is correct.

SHORT ANSWER

9. Describe the eight aspects of the assessment of clinical jaw function and occlusion.
10. List the three words that summarize the role of the dental hygienist in occlusion and TMD.

Please visit **http://evolve.elsevier.com/Perry/periodontology** for additional practice and study support tools.

REFERENCES

1. Ramfjord SP, Ash MM. *Occlusion.* 4th ed. Philadelphia, PA: WB Saunders; 1995.
2. McDevitt MJ. Occlusal evaluation and therapy. In: Newman MG, Takei HH, Klokkevold PR, et al, eds. *Carranza's Clinical Periodontology.* 11th ed. St. Louis, MO: Elsevier Saunders; 2012:502–504.
3. Griffiths RH. The president's conference of the examination, diagnosis and management of temporomandibular disorders. *J Am Dent Assoc.* 1983;106:75–77.
4. Laskin DM, Greene CS, Hylander WL, eds. *Temporomandibular Disorders: An Evidence-Based Approach to Diagnosis and Treatment.* Chicago, IL: Quintessence; 2006:193–202.
5. Okeson JP: *Management of Temporomandibular Joint Disorders and Occlusion.* 7th ed. St Louis, MO: Elsevier Mosby; 2013.
6. Carranza, FA Periodontal response to external forces. In: Newman MG, Takei HH, Klokkevold PR, et al, eds. *Carranza's Clinical Periodontology.* 11th ed. St. Louis, MO: Elsevier; 2012:151–159.
7. Solberg WK, Clark GT. *Abnormal Jaw Mechanics.* Chicago, IL: Quintessence; 1981.
8. Greene, C. Managing the care of patients with temporomandibular disorders. *J Am Dent Assoc.* 2010;141:1086–1087.
9. Pullinger AG, Seligman DA, Gornbein JA. A multiple logistic regression analysis of the risk and relative odds of temporomandibular disorders as a function of common occlusal features. *J Dent Res.* 1993;72:968–979.
10. Clark GT, Seligman DA, Solberg WK, et al. Guidelines for the examination and diagnosis of temporomandibular disorders. *J Craniomandib Disord.* 1989;3:7–14.
11. Dawson PE. *Evaluation, Diagnosis and Treatment of Occlusal Problems.* St. Louis, MO: CV Mosby; 1989.
12. Lavigne GJ, Khoury S, Abe S, et al. Bruxism physiology and pathology: an overview for clinicians. *J Oral Rehabil.* 2008;35:476–494.
13. Clark GT, Adachi NY, Dornan MR. A review of physical medicine procedures for temporomandibular disorders. *J Am Dent Assoc.* 1990;121:151–162.
14. Clark GT, Beemsterboer PL, Rugh JD. Nocturnal masseter muscle activity and the symptoms of masticatory dysfunction. *J Oral Rehabil.* 1981;8:279–286.
15. Clark GT, Lanham F, Flack VF. Treatment outcome for consecutive TMJ clinic patients. *J Craniomandib Disord.* 1988;2:87–95.
16. Green CS, Laskin DM. Long-term evaluation of treatment for myofascial pain-dysfunction syndrome: a comparative analysis. *J Am Dent Assoc.* 1983;107:235–238.
17. Rugh JD. Behavioral therapy. In: Mohl ND, Zarb GA, Carlsson GE, et al, eds. *A Textbook of Occlusion.* Chicago, IL: Quintessence; 1988;329–338.
18. Forga B. Dental hygienists: first line of defense for TMD patients? *Access.* 2010;November:8–12.

PART IV

Treatment for Periodontal Diseases

Part IV provides the reader with the basis of dental hygiene clinical practice as it particularly relates to treating patients with gingival and periodontal diseases. This information places dental hygiene care in the context of periodontal therapy and expands on basic preventive measures and treatment concepts of the normal dentition. The following questions are addressed in Part IV:

Plaque Biofilm and Disease Control for the Periodontal Patient

Gwen Essex
Based on the original work by Dorothy A. Perry and Phyllis L. Beemsterboer

LEARNING OUTCOMES

- List the goals for plaque biofilm control for the periodontal patient.
- Recognize the role of plaque biofilm removal as an essential element in dental hygiene treatment for patients with periodontal disease.
- Describe why plaque biofilm control is more complex for periodontal patients than for those without clinical attachment loss.
- Evaluate interproximal plaque biofilm removal techniques that permit access to root surface concavities and furcations.

- Differentiate the methods for toothbrushing and interproximal plaque biofilm removal for patients with periodontal disease.
- Compare the effectiveness and uses of supragingival and subgingival irrigation.
- Identify effective chemical plaque biofilm control agents and their indications for use.
- Describe the role of motivation in gaining compliance of patients for plaque biofilm control programs.

KEY TERMS

Anticalculus agents
Bacterial plaque biofilm
Bass toothbrushing method
Charters toothbrushing method
Dental floss
Dr. Charles C. Bass
Interdental brushes

Patient motivation
Permeability
Plaque biofilm control
Powered toothbrushing
Roll toothbrushing method
Rubber tip stimulators
Scrub toothbrushing method

Stillman toothbrushing method
Subgingival irrigation
Substantivity
Supragingival irrigation
Toothpicks
Toxicity

The fundamental role of the dental hygienist that has the most lasting effects in periodontal therapy is that of patient educator. Success in this role permits patients to become knowledgeable about their disease and make lifestyle changes that will help them lead healthier lives. It is essential to incorporate individualized **plaque biofilm control** education into periodontal therapy because dental plaque biofilm is the causative agent of gingival and periodontal diseases. Conscientious, daily plaque biofilm removal inhibits the formation of subgingival plaque and the progression of these diseases and helps the periodontal tissues to heal. In combination with regular calculus removal, adequate plaque control removes a source of infection from the body and facilitates the lifelong maintenance of the natural teeth.

PLAQUE AS A BIOFILM AND AN ETIOLOGIC AGENT

A number of classic studies provide evidence of the importance of supragingival plaque control. Löe and colleagues[1] showed the cause-and-effect relationship between the accumulation of **bacterial plaque biofilm** and the development of gingivitis in

adults within 21 days. The gingivitis was reversible within 7 days when proper plaque control was initiated. Supragingival plaque becomes dominated by gram-negative microbial species as it ages. These gram-negative bacteria are responsible for the development of a subgingival biota associated with periodontal disease.[2] Thorough toothbrushing to remove supragingival plaque has been shown to limit subgingival plaque growth in monkeys.[3] Further more, adequate supragingival plaque control incorporated into periodontal maintenance programs was found to limit periodontal attachment loss in adults.[4] Figure 12-1 shows the effects of plaque accumulation related to gingival inflammation.

Current understanding of plaque as a biofilm (see Chapter 4) highlights the importance of good daily mechanical plaque biofilm control. Mature plaque biofilm is a heterogeneous mass with open, fluid-filled channels used for the movement of nutrients and waste products. The colonies of bacteria making up the plaque mass facilitate each others' growth and the host provides an essential source of nutrients. Plaque bacteria are a complex group of species that are interdependent and adhere to tooth surfaces in such a way as to limit the diffusion of

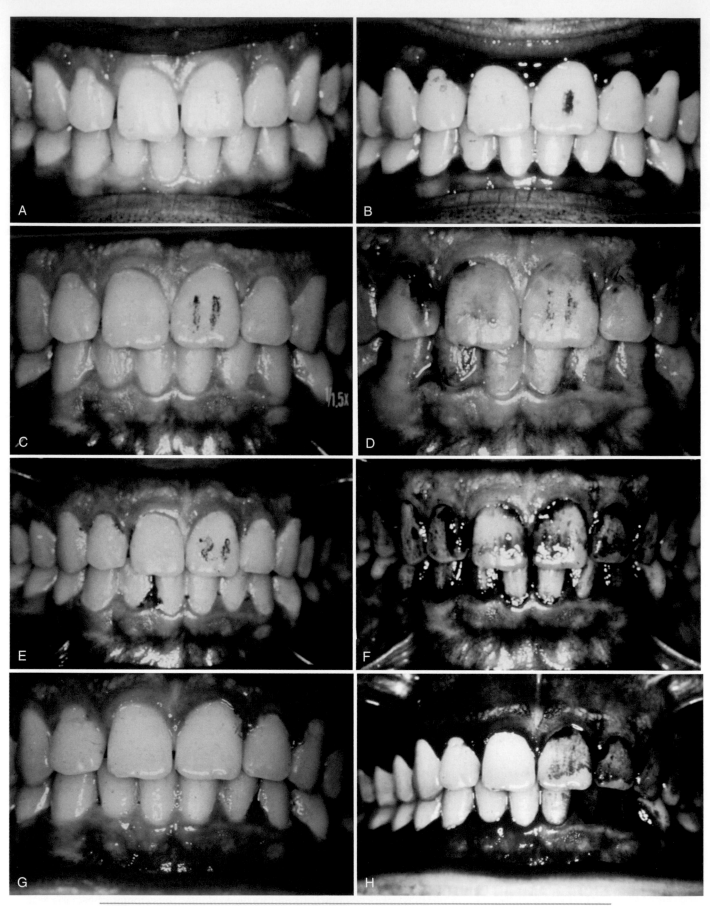

FIGURE 12-1 ■ **Experimental gingivitis in humans. A,** Day 1: A healthy gingiva with pink tissue that conforms to the architecture of the teeth. **B,** Day 1: A healthy gingiva disclosed to show good plaque control (day numbers are marked on central incisor). **C,** Day 11: Gingiva after 11 days with no plaque biofilm control. Note the rolled margins of the free gingiva and reddened marginal gingiva. **D,** Day 11: Disclosed to show biofilm accumulation. **E,** Day 21: Heavy plaque biofilm deposits and gingival swelling; the tissue bleeds on gentle probing. **F,** Day 21: Disclosed plaque biofilm deposits. **G,** Day 28: One week after plaque biofilm control was instituted on the right side of the mouth. Note the improved tissue health, decreased gingival redness, and conformity to the architecture of the teeth on the patient's right side. **H,** Day 28: Disclosed dentition showing mature plaque biofilm remaining on the left side of the mouth.

antimicrobial substances.[5] In light of this understanding, mechanical disruption of the bacterial mass is essential for the treatment of gingival and periodontal diseases.

GOALS OF PLAQUE BIOFILM CONTROL FOR THE PERIODONTAL PATIENT

The goals of plaque biofilm control are numerous. The dental hygienist must understand each goal to develop a successful plaque control program for every periodontal patient. The goals include patient motivation, patient responsibility, management of a complex plaque control routine, caries control, and maintenance of gingival and periodontal health.

PATIENT MOTIVATION

Perhaps the most challenging aspect of plaque control for the periodontal patient is motivation to initiate and continue a lifelong process of improved daily plaque biofilm removal. Most periodontal patients have poor plaque control, which has contributed to the disease process. The habits of a lifetime are hard to change and new oral hygiene procedures will likely require a greater investment in time, from 15 to 30 minutes per day. Research on the topic of compliance and adherence to plaque control procedures indicates that engagement activities such as diaries, logs, quizzes, discussions, positive reinforcement, or other behavioral techniques are more successful than brushing and flossing instructions alone.[6] The dental hygienist should use this knowledge to educate, motivate, and encourage each patient to adopt the recommended procedures and then reinforce the behavioral changes over time. Often, the development of a professional trust and partnership with the patient includes several treatments and recall maintenance visits to facilitate patient adoption of difficult behavioral changes.

PATIENT RESPONSIBILITY

Plaque biofilm control programs help to place responsibility for long-term maintenance of the teeth and periodontium in the hands of the patient. The dental hygienist and dentist play integral roles in therapy and maintenance, but without patient participation, no amount of treatment will succeed. The dental hygienist has the opportunity to individualize the plaque control program, modify it over time, and present it as a way for the patient to assist in the long-term outcome of therapy.

> **CLINICAL NOTE 12-1** Only the patient can perform the necessary daily plaque biofilm control procedures. The dental hygienist provides the critical elements of education, reinforcement, and periodontal maintenance that result in the best treatment outcomes for the periodontal patient.

COMPLEXITY OF PLAQUE BIOFILM CONTROL FOR THE PERIODONTAL PATIENT

Plaque control for periodontal patients usually involves more than toothbrushing and dental flossing, as illustrated by Figure 12-2. Significant areas of attachment loss are often associated with disease and can occur as a result of surgery to reduce periodontal pocket depths. Attachment loss results in

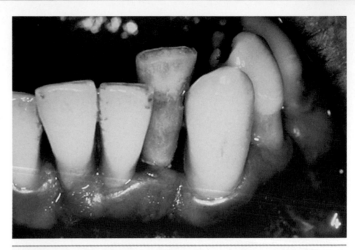

FIGURE 12-2 ■ The complexity of the architecture of the gingiva and tooth anatomy requires more complex cleaning procedures than needed for teeth with no attachment loss. Brushing and flossing alone are not sufficient to clean these exposed root surfaces or periodontal pockets.

exposure of tortuous root anatomy that patients must learn to clean mechanically. This situation is often complicated by deep probing depths.

Periodontal plaque control requires the dental hygienist to apply both knowledge and imagination to find the appropriate plaque control aids for each patient. Describing a favorite brushing technique and encouraging the use of floss will not suffice. The range of aids must be explored, including chemotherapeutic agents, to find a workable combination for the patient.

Often, some trial and error is required to address the periodontal patient's specific cleaning problems. Some aids work better for some people than others, some require more dexterity, and some require more patience. The dental hygienist may ask the patient to try a variety of devices and agents before agreement is reached on the best ones to adopt. For some patients, multiple sessions are needed to master the cleaning techniques for their unique periodontal architecture. If an aid works well for a patient, even if it is not the aid the dental hygienist would prefer to be used, it can be included in the regimen and can help the patient achieve the goals of therapy.

The importance of developing an effective plaque control program is a primary responsibility of the dental hygienist. Dental hygiene treatment, however challenging technically, is not complete without it. The dental hygienist is a teacher and transfers a significant portion of oral health care knowledge and responsibility to the periodontal patient.

> **CLINICAL NOTE 12-2** The aid or technique that the periodontal patient will actually use consistently is the best tool or device to emphasize in your educational discussions.

CARIES CONTROL

A good plaque control program provides all aspects of prevention and maintenance. Proper oral hygiene to control gingival inflammation is important, but the prevention of dental caries is also significant for the periodontal patient. Root caries, as seen in Figure 12-3, is a great threat to the survival of the teeth

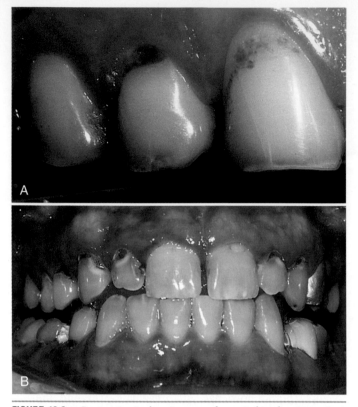

FIGURE 12-3 ■ Root caries is also a concern for periodontal patients. **A,** A single lesion in an area of recession on the maxillary first premolar. The area on the canine is stained but not soft. **B,** Extensive root caries lesions. (Courtesy of Dr. W. Stephen Eakle, University of California, San Francisco, School of Dentistry.)

when attachment loss and recession expose the roots to the oral environment. Teeth that could be maintained for years by treating the periodontal disease can be lost in weeks or months as a result of caries on the root surfaces or in furcation areas. An understanding of caries risk factors and methods for controlling caries make up an essential component of the educational information that dental hygienists must provide for periodontal patients. For a discussion of root caries and its management, see Chapter 17.

MAINTENANCE OF GINGIVAL AND PERIODONTAL HEALTH

Gingival and periodontal health, once restored through therapeutic efforts, however complex, cannot be maintained without the active participation and cooperation of the patient in performing daily supragingival plaque removal. An oral environment that is free of inflammation because of good plaque control rarely becomes reinfected, and further more, satisfactory treatment outcomes are more likely when patients adopt adequate personal plaque control regimens.[7]

MECHANICAL PLAQUE REMOVAL

The most widely accepted prevention methods in periodontology involve both personal and professional mechanical oral hygiene measures. Over the centuries, the rationale for cleaning the teeth has changed from cosmetic intent to disease prevention. However, patients' concerns about maintaining a pleasing appearance should not be underestimated as a motivating factor. In today's health-conscious society, the cosmetic appeal of white teeth and fresh breath are powerful influences on individual behavior. There is ample evidence of this appeal in the quantity of cosmetic dental advertising seen.

Mechanical plaque removal incorporates chemotherapeutic agents as adjuncts to the physical removal of plaque. However, chemical agents alone are not sufficient to remove plaque and control disease. Toothbrushes are still used as standard tools and are augmented by a variety of devices that permit access to interproximal and other areas that are not accessible to toothbrushing techniques. The following section describes toothbrushing and other mechanical techniques for removing plaque.

TOOTHBRUSHING

The toothbrush is the most widely accepted and adopted tool for cleaning the teeth. It is the modern version of the African twig or chew stick, a frayed branch used for mechanical cleansing. There is evidence of toothbrushes in China as early as 1000 BC, but the device did not receive wide distribution until the late eighteenth century. The first brushes were made of hog bristle, often with bone or ivory handles. The Victorians created elaborate handles, including many made of silver. Consequently, early toothbrushes were expensive and were often shared by the entire family. Examples of toothbrushes from the late nineteenth and twentieth centuries are shown in Figure 12-4.

In the 1930s, when nylon-bristled brushes were introduced, toothbrushes became affordable for everyone. Until the 1960s, most brushes sold were stiff-bristled (a legacy of the Victorian era), like the old hog-bristled brushes. Stiff-bristled brushes removed plaque but were associated with trauma to the tooth structure and gingiva.[8] Because of the work of pioneers such as Arnim, Barclay, and Dr. Charles C. Bass, soft-bristled toothbrushes used with a controlled plaque biofilm removal technique have become the standard.

Bass[9] proposed the optimum characteristics of toothbrushes. He studied bristle stiffness, scratching of the gingiva in humans and animals, gingival puncturing, bristle trim, and the presentation of bristles on the brush head. His recommendations are summarized in Box 12-1.

A review of toothbrushing behavior suggests that most Americans brush once daily, with the frequency increasing to twice daily as people get older. Generally, people brush because they believe they are reducing the incidence of decay and are not necessarily aware of the beneficial gingival health effects of plaque biofilm removal by the toothbrush. Interestingly, most people spend less than 1 minute brushing, concentrate on the upper teeth and buccal surfaces, and brush less on the lingual surfaces and lower teeth. Also, effective brushers were most often taught brushing techniques in a dental office.[10] Awareness of the association between good plaque biofilm control and better gingival health may be increasing because of the extensive media advertising about gingivitis. However, the rationale for teaching good brushing techniques and emphasizing the importance of doing the job well is that it improves oral health.

Since Bass's time, many toothbrushes have been marketed to the public. Very complex bristle designs, many with handle modifications, are available. Manufacturers claim superiority in one aspect of cleaning or another, but these claims

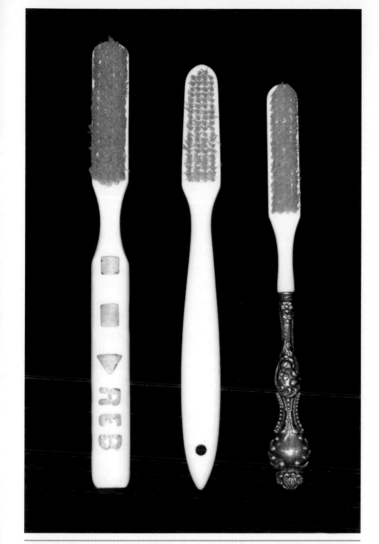

FIGURE 12-4 ■ These ivory-handled toothbrushes are from the nineteenth century. Dental students used them to brush; the handles were also useful for practicing cavity preparations. The shapes and letters on the brush at the left are amalgam-filled "preps." (From Newman MG, Takei HH, Klokkevold PR, et al, eds. *Carranza's Clinical Periodontology.* 11th ed. St. Louis, MO: Elsevier Saunders; 2012.)

BOX 12-1	Characteristics of the Ideal Toothbrush[12]
Handle	Straight, 6 inches long, $\frac{7}{16}$ inches wide
Head	Three evenly spaced rows with six tufts each
Bristles	80 nylon bristles per tuft, 0.007 inches in diameter, $\frac{13}{32}$ inches long
Trim	Rounded finish

are generally related to plaque removal alone, rather than improvements in gingival health. Minor variations in plaque biofilm removal as a result of brush design have not been shown to lead to clinically significant differences in gingival health. One toothbrush may work better than another in the hands of a particular patient, but there is no evidence demonstrating that one toothbrush design is superior to another.[11] An example of an unusual toothbrush design with two brush heads is presented in Figure 12-5.

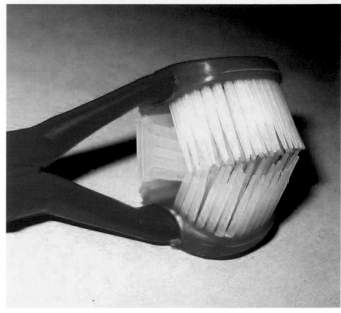

FIGURE 12-5 ■ This unusual toothbrush was designed to clean all surfaces in one motion. (Courtesy of Dr. Sheppard M. Levine.)

TOOTHBRUSHING METHODS

There are several specific toothbrushing techniques that have been proposed and recommended, including the following:

- The Scrub toothbrushing method
- The Roll toothbrushing method
- The Charters toothbrushing method
- The Stillman toothbrushing method
- The Bass toothbrushing method
- Powered toothbrushing

The popularity of various techniques has waxed and waned over the last 50 years. The scrub toothbrushing method is probably the oldest. It merely applies a name to the typical uninstructed action of brushers. The Charters and Stillman methods, which emphasized gingival massage, were popular in the mid-twentieth century, and the roll technique was most commonly recommended in the 1960s and 1970s. Bass's method, which he described in 1948, is probably the most popular method taught today.

CLINICAL NOTE 12-3 The Bass technique is widely taught because it provides mechanical plaque biofilm removal at the gingival margin and minimizes gingival trauma.

No one method of brushing has been found to be superior to the others.[12] The Charters and Stillman methods emphasizing gingival massage are primarily of historical interest because gingival massage has not been shown to improve healing. The best method is the one that suits the individual's needs and abilities, and it is the responsibility of the dental hygienist to work with the patient to develop the most effective technique and to help the patient perform the task thoroughly.

Scrub

The scrub method is the simplest brushing technique, consisting of placing the bristles on the teeth and moving them back and forth, or scrubbing. Nearly everyone, including children, can become adept at this technique. The scrub method does not focus cleaning at the gingival margin, and people who vigorously brush this way believe they have done a thorough job, even if many areas of plaque biofilm have been missed. Extremely vigorous scrubbing, especially with a stiff-bristled brush, can lead to gingival trauma and recession.

CLINICAL NOTE 12-4 Gingival recession is often associated with the scrub method of toothbrushing. The dental hygienist should evaluate the brushing technique of patients who exhibit recession to ensure that they are cleaning using atraumatic techniques.

Roll

The roll technique involves brushing the teeth the way they grow, down on the upper teeth and up on the lower teeth. Bristles are placed on the gingiva, and then the handle of the toothbrush is turned to stroke the bristles along the sides of the teeth. This action is repeated several times in each location, moving around the arches, until all the teeth are brushed. The technique requires a fair amount of concentration to apply the brush to each area and sufficient dexterity to "roll" the brush on the buccal and lingual surfaces. In addition, the rolling strokes must be performed slowly so that the gingival one third of the teeth will be adequately cleaned.[12]

Charters

The Charters technique requires placement of the brush at a 45-degree angle to the tooth surface, with the bristle ends pointing away from the gingiva but toward the interproximal surfaces of the teeth. The bristles rest on the gingiva, and pressure is applied to force the bristles between the teeth using a slight rotary motion. Then the brush is lifted from the gingiva and replaced in the same spot, repeating the massage three or four times. Essentially, the bristles are repeatedly pressed against the gingival margin and then lifted away to massage the tissue and increase blood flow. The bristles are also pressed into the occlusal surfaces with a slight rotary motion so that they fit into the pits and fissures. Charters also recommended the use of metal or wooden toothpicks for interproximal stimulation. Dental floss was to be used only to remove fibrous food caught between faulty contacts.[13]

Although the rationale for massage may be unproven, the effectiveness of the Charters method for plaque removal has been validated by at least one clinical study. The study subjects were instructed to use the technique and its effectiveness in removing all plaque was verified by a dental hygienist every day over the 6-week study period. In this case, the subjects used wooden interdental sticks, rather than metal picks, to ensure interdental cleaning.[14]

CLINICAL NOTE 12-5 The Charters method can be especially useful for patients in orthodontic treatment, because the orientation of the bristles in this technique effectively removes debris trapped by orthodontic brackets and wires.

Stillman

Stillman also advocated toothbrush massage by describing a technique reputed to fill the gingival blood vessels with oxygenated blood. His technique required placement of the bristles pointing apically, but not at right angles to the gingiva, to minimize puncture. Pressure is placed on the bristles, causing them to flex and the tissue to blanch. Then the pressure is released. The procedure is repeated for all teeth in all areas of the mouth and the brush is rinsed several times with a salt water and sodium bicarbonate solution.[15] This technique may result in plaque removal, although its effectiveness around the gingival margin is questionable.

Bass

Bass described his technique in relation to plaque removal as the goal of toothbrushing. He designed a method aimed at gingival and crevicular cleaning and described it as "applying the ends of the bristles to the areas with firm pressure and moving the brush back and forth ('vibratory motion') with short strokes, thereby dislodging soft material by the digging action of the ends of the bristles wherever they can be applied."[16] This technique requires the bristles of a soft, multitufted toothbrush to be placed at a 45-degree angle to the long axis of the teeth. The vibratory motion is used to force the bristles into the sulci and between the teeth as effectively as possible, as illustrated in Figure 12-6. The lingual surfaces of the anterior teeth can be brushed with the heel of the toothbrush for better access and all other areas with the length of the brush head. The occlusal surfaces are brushed with controlled back and forth motions. The Bass technique has been described as modified by the addition of the rolling stroke. This modified stroke is supposed to lift debris away from the gingiva. In practice, clinicians and patients often start with the vibratory motion described by Bass but then modify it in unique ways, such as bigger or circular strokes.

Powered Toothbrushing

Powered, or electric, toothbrushes are popular and useful devices. Many people prefer a powered toothbrush, or find it

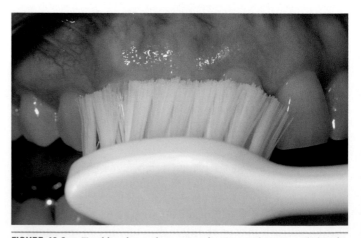

FIGURE 12-6 ■ Toothbrush in place using the Bass technique with bristles placed at a 45-degree angle to the gingival margin, concentrating on the gingival third of the tooth. (From Newman MG, Takei HH, Klokkevold PR, et al, eds. *Carranza's Clinical Periodontology.* 11th ed. St. Louis, MO: Elsevier Saunders; 2012.)

easier to use, particularly if they have dexterity problems. Powered toothbrushes are as effective as manual brushing for reducing plaque, gingivitis, and bleeding.[17]

Powered toothbrushes have different types of actions. The head portion of the brush can be vibrating, oscillating, rotary, or counter-rotary, or it can have a sonic vibration feature. All of these features have been shown to be effective when used correctly. Many studies comparing powered toothbrushes with manual ones have been published over the years. Studies of relatively short duration have demonstrated greater reductions in inflammation and plaque for the powered brushes.[18] The Cochrane Collaboration (http://www.cochrane.org), an international volunteer organization that provides peer-reviewed assessments of published data in scientific literature, has presented a review of studies comparing manual with powered toothbrushes. The group identified 354 studies, of which 29 met the inclusion criteria for their analysis. Their results indicated that rotating-oscillating powered toothbrushes provided a modest clinical benefit to patients in reducing both plaque and gingivitis, whereas the other types of powered brushes performed as well as manual toothbrushes. These small differences in bleeding and plaque scores do not necessarily mean that patients will have less periodontal disease; further studies of the quality required by the Cochrane Collaboration are needed to answer this question.[17] These data demonstrated some plaque biofilm removal advantages for some powered toothbrushes but are not sufficient evidence to recommend that everyone use a powered toothbrush. However, it is clear that powered toothbrushes have a place in the armamentarium of the dental hygienist.

> **CLINICAL NOTE 12-6**   Many powered toothbrushes include features that can support patient home care, such as timers and alerts that assist patients in brushing long enough and in each area of the mouth.

Powered toothbrushes with sonic components cause hydrodynamic shearing forces of water that increase penetration of plaque removal onto the proximal surfaces. Studies have shown that these brushes offer, at best, modest improvements in interproximal cleaning and that they are not substitutes for other interproximal cleaning devices.[7] Figure 12-7 illustrates the placement of the powered toothbrush head on the tooth surface.

Rotary powered toothbrushes designed specifically for access to proximal areas have shaped tips and can readily be applied to both the interproximal surfaces, when there is sufficient space, and the gingival margin. These brush tips have been shown to be as effective in plaque removal and gingivitis reduction as conventional toothbrushing, flossing, and toothpick use.

RECOMMENDATIONS

Regular toothbrushing, whether with a manual or powered brush, is essential. The Bass technique is probably the technique most accepted by the dental profession today, whether for periodontal patients or for patients who have no periodontal disease. The vibratory, back and forth motion of the bristles into the sulcus is simple to perform and seems to have the

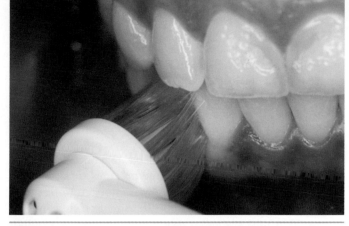

FIGURE 12-7 ■ The brush head of the powered toothbrush must be placed so that the bristles clean the gingival third of the tooth and penetrate proximally as far as possible.

greatest cleaning potential at the gingival margin of the teeth. The technique is adaptable enough that it will remove plaque biofilm from even the complex architecture of severely periodontally damaged dentitions. In addition, patients can be taught to maneuver the brush around the proximal surfaces of teeth with severe attachment loss, including abutment teeth, where long root surfaces and heavy plaque accumulation are common.

Strict adherence to one brushing procedure for all patients is not recommended. The best brushing technique for each patient must be recommended with the knowledge of what works in ideal situations and what difficulties the individual patient faces. An individualized plaque biofilm control program often starts with a simple brushing method, such as the Bass method. Then the technique should be modified by the dental hygienist to permit cleaning of all accessible areas of the teeth.

Powered toothbrushes are useful and good tools for patients who have difficulty brushing or those who simply prefer powered toothbrushes. There is evidence to indicate that periodontal patients significantly decreased their plaque scores over a 3-year period when their manual toothbrushes were replaced with powered toothbrushes.[19] The Cochrane analysis also suggested there are modest benefits in plaque and gingivitis reductions with oscillating-rotating powered brushes. Powered toothbrushes should be considered for plaque control in periodontal patients and adopted if appropriate for the individualized plaque biofilm control program.

INTERPROXIMAL CLEANING WITH MECHANICAL AIDS

Toothbrushes do not adequately clean interproximal surfaces in most cases. For this reason, interdental cleaning with at least one additional device is necessary for thorough plaque removal. Interdental plaque biofilm control may be accomplished with several different aids, including the following:

- Dental floss
- Interdental brushes
- Toothpicks

Several studies have documented that the addition of daily flossing to the toothbrushing regimen leads to reductions in inflammation, plaque biofilm, and calculus deposits.[20-22] Floss is only one of many interproximal cleaning devices available to patients. Some provide better access than others to the long-exposed root surfaces typically found in periodontal patients. The dental hygienist should be knowledgeable about which types of devices are available and recommend appropriate ones for use in individualized plaque biofilm control programs.

Dental Floss

Dental floss is available in a variety of sizes and thicknesses. Waxed, unwaxed, round, flat, thick, thin, tape, red, green, shred-resistant, and fuzzy versions are available, to name a few. When properly used, floss will clean the interproximal surfaces of the teeth, extending under the gingival margin, often to the junctional epithelium, where a toothbrush cannot reach. However, it is likely to miss plaque in root surface grooves and cannot adequately clean furcations.

Bass evaluated dental floss and attempted to define an optimum set of characteristics, although Black suggested that thread would do.[23] Bass believed that floss should be made of nylon (because of the uniformity and strength of fibers), unwaxed (to prevent waxy buildup on tooth surfaces), thin, and multifilamented with few twists per inch.[23] Subsequent research has shown that there is little, if any, difference in cleaning ability among the myriad types of floss.[17] Waxed floss can deposit wax on tooth surfaces in vitro, as first demonstrated by Bass, but in a study of wax deposition on teeth scheduled for extraction, no wax residue could be found on the teeth of human subjects.[24] These data suggest that dental hygienists and patients should select a particular floss on the basis of personal preference and ease of use.

> **CLINICAL NOTE 12-7** Patients may present with individual issues that complicate flossing, such as rotated teeth and tight contacts. It is important to help the patient select the most appropriate type of floss to minimize patient frustration and encourage regular use.

Proper flossing technique requires a piece of floss about 18 inches long to be grasped firmly with both hands. For greater control, a small portion of floss, approximately 1 inch, is held between the thumbs and forefingers. The floss is inserted into the proximal space by working it back and forth, slipped under the papilla by wrapping it around the tooth, and used with up and down strokes to clean the surface, as illustrated in Figure 12-8. Then the floss must be wrapped around the adjacent tooth and the cleaning procedure repeated. After one or two interproximal surfaces are cleaned, the floss often becomes dirty or frayed. The patient must move along the floss, grasping it in a different place, so that a fresh length of the strand can be used to clean the next surface. Dental floss absorbs saliva and bacteria so it is not reusable. After all the tooth surfaces are cleaned, the floss strand must be thrown away.

Floss Threaders. Dental floss can be used to clean under the pontics of fixed partial dentures (bridges) and around abutment teeth when it is threaded under the soldered joints of fixed restorations. Threading is accomplished with a needle-like device called a floss threader or bridge threader. The floss is threaded through the eye of the device and then inserted

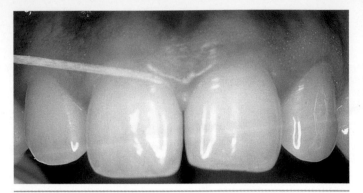

FIGURE 12-8 ■ Dental floss must be wrapped around the tooth and slipped subgingivally for interproximal access. It cleans thoroughly between the teeth when no attachment loss is present.

under the contact area of the bridge. The teeth are cleaned using up and down or back and forth motions, making sure to access the root portions of the abutment teeth, and the floss is pulled out to the side. This task can be difficult for patients to master. There are floss products available that incorporate a stiffer end that acts as a floss threader, thus eliminating the need for a separate device; sometimes this convenience can help a patient establish or maintain the habit of flossing.

Floss Tools or Aids. Many patients have a difficult time learning to floss correctly and give up. They have difficulty holding the floss properly, accessing the proximal surfaces, and then cleaning these surfaces, particularly when the patients are looking at a reversed image of themselves in the mirror. In many cases, the hardest part is holding and manipulating the floss. Floss tools can help with this problem. There are two types of tools, those that are reusable and require the patient to wrap the floss around the device and single-use disposable tools with prestrung floss.

Reusable floss tools have C- or U-shaped working ends. The floss is stretched across the device and the plastic handle is inserted in the mouth; the handle, instead of the fingers, manipulates the floss. The C-shaped ends often work better in the anterior areas and the U-shaped ends work better in the posterior areas. Once the floss tool is threaded, it is inserted interproximally by moving the floss back and forth between the contact areas of the teeth. The cleaning procedure is the same as for finger flossing, wrapping the floss around the tooth and moving it up and down to clean the tooth surfaces.

The advantage of floss tools is that they can make it possible for patients to floss. However, there are some drawbacks. It can be difficult to wind the floss tautly onto the handle because this requires threading around the buttons and grooves on the device. Sometimes, setting up the floss tool is as difficult as learning to floss with the fingers. In addition, floss strung on a tool is harder to move along to obtain a fresh piece when it becomes frayed or dirty. The patient must unwind and then rewind floss more than once, perhaps many times, to floss all the teeth. Also, the floss tool will not substitute for using a bridge threader for access under a fixed partial denture, so another device is required to clean these areas. These disadvantages make the floss tool less attractive than it first appears. Its proper use is usually more time-consuming than finger flossing.

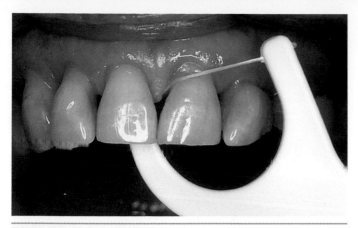

FIGURE 12-9 ■ Disposable floss tools are convenient for some periodontal patients and make flossing possible for those with limited dexterity.

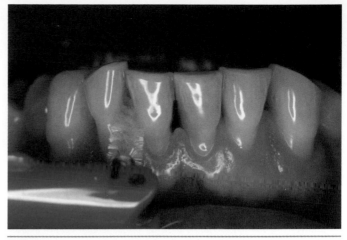

FIGURE 12-10 ■ The interdental brush thoroughly cleans large interdental spaces and complex, exposed interproximal root surfaces.

Disposable floss tools eliminate the problems of threading and winding floss onto a handle. The floss is stretched on the working end of the tool in the manufacturing process. However, the handles are small and may be hard to grasp, and it often takes more than one tool to floss all the teeth. These tools work as well as finger flossing,[25] but they cannot clean under fixed partial dentures either. They are convenient when traveling and for use by children. The use of a floss tool is shown in Figure 12-9.

Other Flossing Materials. Other materials in addition to commercial dental floss can be used for flossing. Using thread as Black recommended, "passing a thread between the teeth,"[10] is inexpensive but not sturdy. However, thicker materials, such as yarn or gauze, can be very useful. These materials can be used like dental floss to clean large interproximal spaces and around abutment teeth. They are thicker than floss, so they may clean large spaces faster and be easier to grasp. In addition, their texture may permit better access into developmental grooves.

A number of automatic flossing devices are now available to simplify the task of flossing and improve compliance. These have prestrung floss that vibrates or a wand of flossing material that penetrates between the teeth and vibrates or spins to remove plaque. There is little evidence to suggest that mechanical flossing is better than using fingers or other tools, but at least one study suggested that patient compliance with flossing is enhanced when the task is made easier through the use of an automatic device.[26]

Interdental Brushes

Interdental brushes facilitate the mechanical cleaning of proximal root surfaces and provide improved access into developmental grooves and furcations. They are useful for periodontal patients who have attachment loss, long-exposed root surfaces, and complex root architecture.

Interdental brush systems usually include a reusable handle and a disposable brush tip. The tip is inserted in the end of the handle, secured at a 90-degree angle to the handle, and used to brush interproximally in spaces that are large enough to permit access. An in and out brushing stroke is used and the interproximal space should be cleaned from both the buccal and lingual aspects. Furcation areas may also be large and accessible enough to permit brushing with this device. The brush can be rinsed and reused, but only by the same patient, and brush tips tend to wear out quickly. Often, periodontal patients must replace the brush tips at least once per week with regular use, and some patients complain about the cost. Figure 12-10 shows the adaptation of an interproximal brush to a large embrasure space. Patients sometimes prefer interproximal brushes to floss,[27] and it is not necessary to floss in areas that are accessible and thoroughly cleaned with an interproximal brush.

In addition to the reusable handle system, there are disposable interproximal brushes. The technique is the same and these tools are discarded when the brush tips wear out. These disposable brushes add to the patient's cost but are convenient for patients who like to carry around cleaning devices, for travel, and for use by children.

Toothpicks

Toothpicks are a very popular interdental cleaning aid. Many people use them to remove large food particles wedged between the teeth, even if their use is sporadic. They are a fixture in society and are available in many public areas, especially restaurants. To take advantage of the popularity of this device, dental hygienists must educate patients to use toothpicks for plaque removal in an organized way, not just sporadic picking. Toothpicks are generally less effective than floss for interproximal cleaning, possibly because of difficult access on lingual surfaces.

Toothpick handles permit the mounting of one or two toothpick tips, several millimeters long, onto a handle. Some handles have curved or bent necks intended to improve access to the posterior teeth. The toothpick end is affixed on the handle and the tip is placed at the gingival margin and used to trace around the necks of the teeth. The handle also permits the tip to slip into proximal spaces, furcation areas, subgingival root surfaces, and developmental grooves to rub biofilm off. In addition, it can be directed subgingivally into periodontal pockets, where plaque biofilm can be dispersed. This plaque biofilm removal technique is shown in Figure 12-11. Some practitioners recommend soaking the tip before use to soften it so that it frays slightly and covers more surface area.

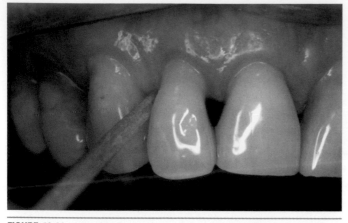

FIGURE 12-11 ■ Toothpicks can be used for plaque biofilm control and are useful in accessing complex root architecture and subgingival areas. They require some dexterity and practice on the part of the patient.

There are also specially designed triangular toothpicks made of soft wood, such as balsa. These can be placed with the base of the triangle on the gingiva and pushed in and out of large proximal spaces. They provide good plaque removal on the buccal surfaces but are difficult to apply to the lingual surfaces and the more posterior teeth. These devices cannot be used with handles and are of less use to periodontal patients because of their access limitations. However, some patients like these devices and carry them around for use during the day, so triangular wooden tips can also be an asset to the individualized plaque biofilm control program.

Plastic Picks. A variety of plastic toothpick-like devices are also available. These devices provide some combination of positive features, depending on the design. Instruction on their use should be predicated on educating the patient about plaque removal. Plastic picks are used like toothpicks and may be convenient for patients to carry in a pocket or purse. They can be rinsed and reused rather than thrown away like wooden picks. This feature is attractive to some individuals.

Rubber Tip Stimulators

Interdental stimulation, commonly called gingival massage, performed by **rubber tip stimulators** was a popular concept in plaque control until the 1970s. Massage was thought to increase keratinization, clean the surface of the gingiva, stimulate blood flow, and squeeze fluid from the gingival sulcus. Manipulation of the interdental tissues with tools such as rubber tip stimulators or toothpicks increases keratinization of the epithelium in treated areas. However, the use of these instruments also results in plaque removal from the surfaces of the teeth. The current concept of mechanical plaque control has evolved to emphasize plaque biofilm removal rather than tissue effects, and it is understood that inflammation starts in the sulcus, not on the keratinized surface of the gingiva. This suggests that tools used to stimulate the interproximal tissue are more likely useful because of their plaque-removing effects.

Rubber tip stimulators are convenient inexpensive devices that can be useful to periodontal patients. The tip is a conical piece of firm rubber or plastic that is several millimeters long. The tip is placed proximally, resting the side of the cone on the gingiva, and worked in a small circular motion.

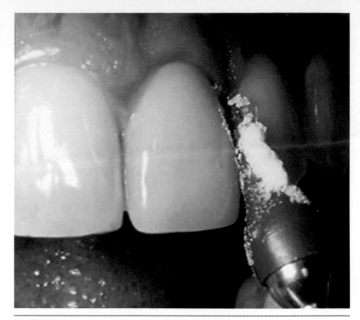

FIGURE 12-12 ■ The rubber tip stimulator can be used for interproximal plaque biofilm removal and for applying chemical agents.

All interdental spaces should be cleaned from both the buccal and lingual surfaces with several revolutions of the cleaning motion. In addition to this technique, the rubber tip may be adapted and applied to the gingival margins of the teeth, traced along the gum line like a toothpick in a holder, as described earlier. Application of the rubber tip stimulator is illustrated in Figure 12-12.

Recommendations

Periodontal patients must understand that plaque biofilm is the etiologic agent in periodontal disease and that daily biofilm control permits them to manage the disease and improve oral health. Plaque control programs consist of identifying tools and mastering techniques to clean around all surfaces of all the teeth at least once daily.

The dental hygienist often begins with toothbrushing, which is a daily habit for most patients. Instruction may involve teaching a new technique or modifying an existing one to ensure maximal cleaning efficiency.

Interproximal cleaning must be emphasized from the beginning, but some experimentation may be required to find the best tool or combination of tools. In addition, the dental hygienist often teaches interproximal plaque control to periodontal patients before surgical treatment. When periodontal surgery is performed, the architecture is changed, sometimes dramatically, resulting in different cleaning needs. Teaching plaque control to periodontal patients is a dynamic process that may require more than one tool and more than one instructional session, and patient needs may change over time.

For patients who have never flossed, refuse to floss, or are beginning interproximal cleaning for the first time, the rubber tip stimulator can be useful. It is easy to use and inexpensive—a real attraction for some patients. The rubber tip stimulator can be a good tool to begin educating patients on cleaning proximal surfaces.

Dental floss is a good tool for periodontal patients, but is rarely the only interproximal aid needed. Even in cases of mild attachment loss, the exposed proximal root anatomy has developmental grooves that the floss glides over, leaving masses of attached plaque biofilm. The situation is more complicated with the maxillary molars, where furcations are present on the mesial and distal surfaces. Regular dental flossing is also a difficult habit to acquire. Studies indicate that although approximately 40% of Americans report using floss, only 10% floss daily and another 10% floss once or twice a week.[10] Although floss is an important oral hygiene tool, it is not the only tool, nor is it always the best tool for the periodontal patient.

Interproximal brushes in various sizes and configurations have the distinct advantage of cleaning the complex architecture on root surfaces. They can clean around abutment teeth and under fixed partial dentures. The brushes must be replaced often, so patients must be committed to the expenditure. It is also difficult for some patients to load the brush onto the handle because it requires threading a thin wire into a small hole and securing it. Any physical impairment, such as arthritic finger joints or poor eyesight, makes this process difficult. Disposable interproximal brushes provide an alternative in these cases.

Individualizing recommendations to meet the needs and abilities of each periodontal patient are very important in mechanical plaque control. A rote presentation of the dental hygienist's favorite toothbrushing technique and interproximal aid will not address the variety of needs and periodontal conditions seen in clinical practice. Individualization, finding the right tools that are easy to use, and reinforcement are the keys to compliance and success with mechanical plaque control.

CLINICAL NOTE 12-8 Remember to begin oral hygiene instruction with the patient's current habits in mind. Recommending too much, too soon is ineffective; greater compliance is achieved by starting with the patient's current habits and likes, dislikes, and incrementally working together to achieve ideal home care practices.

IRRIGATION

In the 1960s, irrigation of the oral cavity as an adjunct to plaque control became popular with the marketing of pulsating jet irrigators. These devices provide supragingival irrigation by forcing water between the teeth with a single jet or multiple jets of pulsed beads of water. In a clinical study of 155 college-age women, these devices did not reduce plaque formation and had a minimal effect on gingivitis scores; however, they did reduce calculus formation.[28] Another study reported that only 8.1% of stainable material, plaque and material alba, was removed from the mouths of 10 experimental subjects by water jet irrigation alone. An additional 67.6% was removed by tooth brushing.[29]

Studies reviewed by Ciancio[30] have shown significant decreases in gingivitis when water jet irrigation was used in a regular, at-home, plaque control regimen. Significant results were seen in studies of varying duration, from 6 weeks to 6 months. Improved gingival health was noted regardless of whether a chemical plaque control agent was used during the irrigation. Gingivitis reductions in the range of 25% were noted, and some studies showed comparable results to the beneficial effects of rinsing with the antimicrobial agent chlorhexidine (discussed later in this chapter).

Supragingival irrigation with chlorhexidine showed some additional benefit. Plaque scores were not always reduced by irrigation, corroborating the results of the earlier work, but bleeding of the gingiva was reduced significantly. Ciancio[30] suggested that although plaque biofilm may be minimally affected by irrigation, its toxicity may be altered, explaining the beneficial effects of supragingival irrigation.

The technique for supragingival irrigation is to direct the tip between the teeth at right angles to the interdental papillae and holding it there for several seconds to permit flushing of the proximal surfaces. Then the tip is moved along the gingival margin to the next proximal area. The pressure setting on the irrigator may be gradually increased if the tissue condition permits.[31] This procedure should be performed over a sink to avoid creating a mess with dripping water.

Oral irrigation is associated with bacteremia, occurring in as many as 50% of patients with periodontitis. However, the relationship of bacteremia caused by oral irrigation to infective endocarditis is not known.[31] If there is any question, the patient's physician should be consulted about the use of daily home oral irrigation. Generally speaking, patients who need antibiotic coverage for dental treatment and those with acute conditions, such as pericoronitis, should not use supragingival irrigation. In addition, if irrigation is recommended for periodontal patients after periodontal surgery, it should be postponed for at least 1 month, longer in the case of regenerative surgery, to permit healing of tissues.[7]

Subgingival irrigation can be accomplished with the use of a special soft rubber tip that permits the irrigant to be directed under the gingiva. The tip is slipped gently under the gingiva in areas with deep pockets and irrigant is flushed into the pockets. The pressure for the irrigation unit should be set on low. This technique extends the cleansing action of irrigation beyond the generally accepted 3-mm depth reached with the standard technique. Work remains to be done to elucidate the extent of the effects of subgingival irrigation and whether the addition of antimicrobial agents has any further beneficial effects.[7]

Recommendations

The preponderance of data suggests that supragingival irrigation reduces gingivitis and is an acceptable tool to be recommended in plaque biofilm control programs. It is especially useful for patients who cannot or will not adopt mechanical devices for interproximal cleaning. Commonly used oral irrigation tips are illustrated in Figure 12-13.

CHEMICAL PLAQUE CONTROL

Chemical plaque control has increased in popularity and importance as studies have shown the positive effects of various medicaments on the oral environment. A variety of over-the-counter and prescription agents are available. These agents have known, if variable, abilities to control the growth or regrowth of bacterial plaque microorganisms. No longer are mouthwashes thought to be only cosmetic. Some of these agents can provide significant advantages to periodontal patients, who often have complex gingival architecture that is time-consuming and

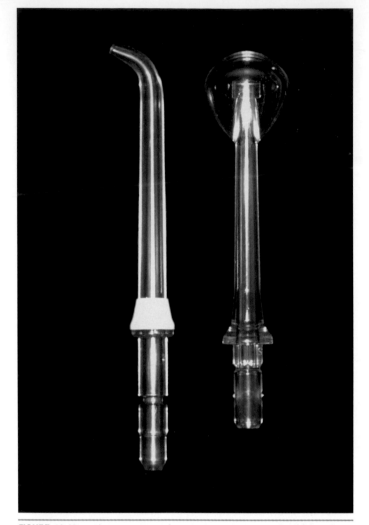

FIGURE 12-13 ■ The supragingival water jet irrigator tip should be placed at a 45-degree angle to the marginal gingiva and the water jet directed through the proximal space for several seconds. There are also tips that permit the patient to clean the tongue with the water spray. (From Newman MG, Takei HH, Klokkevold PR, , et al, eds. *Carranza's Clinical Periodontology.* 11th ed. St. Louis, MO: Elsevier Saunders; 2012.)

difficult to clean solely with mechanical devices. Many have been waiting for the next generation of chemical agents to emerge that would eliminate the need for mechanical plaque removal. Increased understanding of the biofilm nature of dental plaque explains why this silver bullet approach to plaque removal has yet to appear. Plaque biofilm is adherent and interdependent; the colonies of bacteria facilitate growth among the biofilm mass and protect deeper colonies from the effects of chemical agents. Chemical agents can clearly assist in plaque control programs, but they are not a substitute for good mechanical oral hygiene practices.

To provide the most beneficial effects, chemical antiplaque agents should demonstrate several properties[32]:

1. **Antiplaque action**. This activity can be bactericidal (causing cell death) or bacteriostatic (affecting the functioning of the cells to render them less virulent by affecting bacterial adhesion, growth, or metabolism).
2. **Substantivity**. This is the ability to adhere to structures in the oral environment and be released slowly over time, enhancing the duration of effectiveness. The bacterial

population in the mouth recovers rapidly from the assault of many antibacterial agents because they are rapidly cleared by saliva flow and swallowing. Even subgingival application of agents is quickly diluted by the flow of gingival crevicular fluid. Substantive agents, such as chlorhexidine digluconate, possess positively charged ions that adhere to the predominantly negatively charged tissues in the mouth for several hours. They remain in the mouth for some time to exert a continued effect on plaque bacteria.[32,33]

3. **Low toxicity and nonirritating**. Agents must be nontoxic to tissues because they must adhere for a substantial period. Low toxicity allows them to extend their effects on the bacterial population without damaging host tissues.
4. **Low permeability**. The oral mucosal tissue is easily permeated by chemicals. An effective antiplaque agent must have low permeability to allow its retention in the oral cavity.

Chemical antiplaque agents available on the market are primarily toothpastes and mouthwashes. Most are over-the-counter products, but some are prescription items. These products are useful for the dental hygienist in developing a personalized daily plaque control program because they are readily available and patients are often familiar with them through advertising.

CHLORHEXIDINE

The most effective antibacterial agent available today is chlorhexidine, sold by prescription in the United States as a mouthwash containing 0.12% of the active ingredient, chlorhexidine digluconate. This agent reduces plaque and gingivitis in humans.[33,34] Clinical studies of the effectiveness of chlorhexidine were presented in the Proceedings of the World Workshop in Clinical Periodontics in 1989.[35] These indicated that plaque and gingivitis were reduced by 60% in short-term studies and by 55% and 45%, respectively, in separate long-term studies. Chlorhexidine is highly substantive, not being cleared from the mouth for several hours. It acts by altering the bacterial cell wall and interfering with the adsorption of bacteria to teeth. In addition, no changes in the composition of bacteria or the resistance of organisms to this substance have been shown.[36]

Chlorhexidine is now available as a gelatin chip with sustained release (see Chapter 7). In some parts of the world, it is also found in toothpastes and in a spray delivery system. However, the most common use in the United States is as a mouth rinse.

A number of side effects have been reported with the use of chlorhexidine mouthwash. Dark brown staining of the teeth can occur, as seen in Figure 12-14, and increased supragingival calculus formation is common. Some patients have a reversible desquamation of the oral tissue. In addition, chlorhexidine tastes very bitter and patients commonly report altered taste sensations immediately following its use. The mouthwash contains 11.6% alcohol, so patients who are sensitive about using products containing alcohol should be warned.[33,35]

The dental hygienist should recommend the use of chlorhexidine as a mouth rinse, full strength (0.12%), twice daily for 30 seconds using 15 mL of rinse. Long-term use does no harm

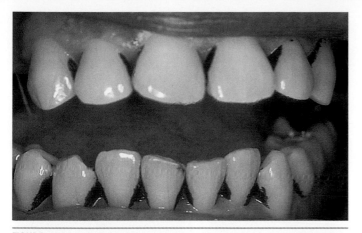

FIGURE 12-14 ■ Chlorhexidine stain in a periodontal patient is dark brown or black. The appearance can be troublesome for patients and discourage them from using the rinses.

other than the cosmetic inconvenience of staining and some reported taste alterations.

Chlorhexidine also reduces gingivitis when used once daily in supragingival irrigation with an oral irrigator in a 1:1 dilution with water (0.06%). It has also been used for subgingival irrigation. Compared with rinsing, chlorhexidine delivery through an irrigation device only enhances plaque and gingivitis reductions by a small amount. The side effects of staining and calculus formation occur with both rinsing and irrigation.[37]

Daily use of a chlorhexidine solution or water in a home irrigator for subgingival application does not appear to have any substantial long-term benefits in the treatment of periodontal disease. Additional research into various delivery methods will eventually confirm the short- and long-term effects, if any, of subgingival irrigation with antimicrobial agents.[31]

Periodontal patients who benefit from the use of chlorhexidine mouthwash are those who cannot or will not control supragingival plaque through mechanical means or who have systemic conditions that may increase their susceptibility to the effects of periodontal infections. In addition, refractory cases and patients who have had periodontal surgery may be helped by chemical plaque control. The dental hygienist, in conjunction with the dentist or periodontist, should recommend the use of chlorhexidine based on the needs of the individual patient. Chlorhexidine at 0.12% strength has been tested extensively and has been accepted by the American Dental Association (ADA) as effective for the control of gingivitis.[31,38]

Essential Oil Mouthwash (Phenolic Compounds)

Mouthwashes containing essential oils—thymol, eucalyptol, menthol, and methyl salicylate—have been shown to reduce plaque and gingivitis by about 30%. These phenolic compounds probably work by altering the bacterial cell wall.[30] These products contain a substantial percentage of alcohol, up to 26.4%, have a strong flavor, and can cause staining. They are available over the counter, which can be advantageous for patients, and they are less costly than chlorhexidine mouthwash. One product has been on the market for many years and carries the ADA seal verifying that 6-month studies have shown that it is effective in reducing gingivitis.[39] These products are popular and can provide a reasonable alternative to chlorhexidine for patients

who would benefit from chemical plaque control to augment their mechanical efforts. Mouth rinses containing phenolic compounds are also effective in helping patients who have undergone periodontal surgery to maintain plaque control during the healing phase.[40] However, these rinses can taste bitter and cause a burning sensation.[30]

Triclosan, another phenolic compound, is also available in the United States. The product is available without prescription in a toothpaste formulation and has shown promising results as an antiplaque, anticalculus, and antigingivitis agent, especially when combined with other agents. Triclosan toothpastes with either zinc citrate or a copolymer of methoxyethylene and maleic acid as the active agent have been shown in numerous studies to reduce plaque by about 25% and gingivitis by about 20%.[33]

Quaternary Ammonium Compounds

Cetylpyridinium chloride, a quaternary ammonium compound, is the active ingredient in commonly available mouthwashes. Some preparations also contain domiphen bromide. These products were shown to reduce gingivitis in some short-term clinical studies of a few hours or days in duration. Their mechanism of action is probably the ability to increase bacterial cell wall permeability, decrease cell metabolism, and reduce cell attachment to tooth surfaces.[30,33] Quaternary ammonium compounds have limited substantivity and are not accepted by the ADA because their ability to reduce gingivitis has not been adequately documented in long-term studies.

Stannous Fluoride

Stannous fluoride has been used extensively in dentistry for its caries-inhibiting effects. Reports in the 1970s and 1980s strongly suggested the possibility that stannous fluoride possesses antiplaque properties. Stannous fluoride alters bacterial cell metabolism and cell adhesion properties in addition to reacting with tooth surfaces for caries prevention. Clinical studies have shown delayed microbial repopulation of periodontal pockets in some cases, but these data have not been confirmed. Stannous fluoride gel has shown antigingivitis effects in extremely inflamed tissue around abutment teeth and orthodontic bands, and when used on a daily basis, may have this additional benefit for teeth. The usual strength for daily home use is 0.4% stannous fluoride delivered in gel or toothpaste form. Some of the available products carry the ADA seal for caries control. None has demonstrated antigingivitis effects of sufficient quantity or duration to carry an additional seal for these effects, but it has been used in combination products that may be useful for periodontal patients for caries control.[33] Tooth staining, as seen in Figure 12-15, is a common side effect of stannous fluoride, and some patients complain of poor taste.

Problem of Delivery to the Site of Disease

The most meticulous supragingival plaque control method does not remove plaque in pockets deeper than about 2 mm.[31,41] Subgingival plaque control is a goal to be desired but not one easily achieved. The dental hygienist accomplishes this during scaling and root planing, but pathologic plaque biofilm begins to grow back quickly. Patients are also limited in achieving subgingival

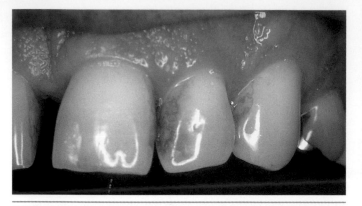

FIGURE 12-15 ■ Stannous fluoride stain in this periodontal patient appears diffuse and less dark than chlorhexidine stain. It can also be a cosmetic problem that discourages compliance.

plaque control because mechanical oral hygiene devices may not reach into pocket depths or may be impossible to apply into pockets. For these reasons, the notion of lavage, flushing or irrigating the periodontal pockets to remove plaque, especially with the use of an antimicrobial agent, is attractive. This procedure can place the antimicrobial agent directly into the site of infection rather than limiting it to supragingival areas.

SUBGINGIVAL IRRIGATION

Subgingival irrigation has been evaluated in a variety of circumstances. It has been delivered by powered oral irrigation devices and by blunt needle and syringe systems. A tip designed to place antimicrobial agents in the pockets is shown in Figure 12-16. A number of agents and regimens have been tested with inconclusive results. Subgingival irrigation can be viewed as an office procedure performed by the dental hygienist at treatment visits, an at-home procedure performed daily by patients, or as a combination of the two.

According to Greenstein,[42] several aspects of irrigation must be considered. These include penetration of drugs into the pockets, relationship to scaling and root planing, and safety.

Irrigation with a syringe fitted with a blunt needle and powered oral irrigation devices have been shown to penetrate into periodontal pockets, at least 3 mm subgingivally. Therefore, it is possible to deliver antimicrobial agents subgingivally to some distance, if not to the base of pockets. When treated with antimicrobial subgingival irrigation, bacterial populations rebound quickly unless the treatment is preceded by scaling and root planing. This observation suggests that scaling and debridement of pockets are essential for any therapeutic effects of irrigation to occur. Negative effects of subgingival irrigation, such as self-inflicted wounds, microbial infections in the tissues, and resistant strains, have not been reported, so the procedure appears to be safe. However, there is no single agent that is recommended for subgingival irrigation and no compelling evidence that the procedure provides significant benefits.[42]

Office-Applied Agents

Antimicrobial agents can be applied subgingivally by the dental hygienist in the office during or after scaling and root planing procedures. This procedure is commonly done with a disposable syringe fitted with a blunt needle or an irrigating pump device with a thin cannula. It can also be accomplished by

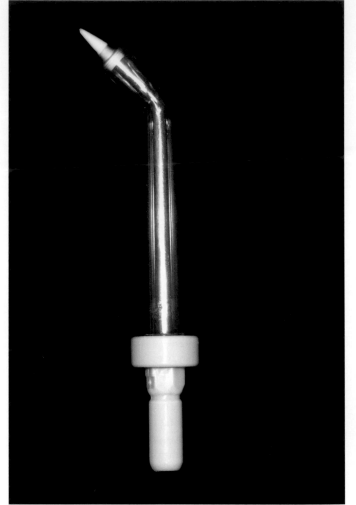

FIGURE 12-16 ■ A subgingival irrigation tip made of soft rubber can be directed into the periodontal pocket to reach several millimeters subgingivally. (From Newman MG, Takei HH, Klokkevold PR, et al, eds. *Carranza's Clinical Periodontology.* 11th ed. St. Louis, MO: Elsevier Saunders; 2012.

running an antimicrobial irrigant through the ultrasonic tip during scaling.[43] In a review of studies of irrigation after scaling and root planing, Shiloah and Hovious[44] affirmed that scaling removed most of the attached and unattached bacterial plaque biofilm. They pointed out that many attempts to improve the results with a variety of subgingival antimicrobial agents immediately after scaling did not yield significant results. Greenstein[42] reached the same conclusion in describing the relationship between scaling and antimicrobial irrigation. There is general agreement that routinely following scaling procedures with irrigation in the dental office, although not harmful, is of questionable benefit.[41,42]

Home-Applied Agents

In contrast to irrigation in the dental office, supragingival and subgingival irrigation performed at home by the patient has demonstrated positive effects on gingival health. Supragingival irrigation using a powered irrigating device has been shown to reduce the number of bleeding sites and the amount of gingivitis significantly over a 6-month period. In this study, irrigation with water achieved almost as good a result as irrigation with diluted chlorhexidine, and both were better than conventional mechanical oral hygiene procedures.[37] Another study tested home irrigation with diluted iodine and found improved gingival health after 8 weeks compared with a no-irrigation control group.[45] This study also included lavage or flushing of pockets in the dental office after scaling and root planing, so it was not possible to determine the specific effects of home irrigation. However, the preponderance of evidence suggests that daily irrigation at home has a greater effect than antimicrobial treatment immediately after scaling, reliably reduces gingivitis, and is safe for use in maintenance regimens.[31,41]

> **CLINICAL NOTE 12-9** Daily irrigation of residual pockets with antimicrobials such as chlorhexidine is effective in maintaining periodontal health when adopted by patients for home use.

ANTICALCULUS AGENTS

A number of toothpastes are available that have as active ingredients anticalculus agents that inhibit the formation of new supragingival calculus. These are commonly referred to as tartar control toothpastes. The active ingredients are soluble pyrophosphates that inhibit amorphous calcium phosphate around the teeth from crystallizing into hydroxyapatite, the most common crystal in calculus. Toothpastes containing zinc citrate also retard calculus formation. A small percentage of patients have sloughing of the epithelium with the use of these products, in which case the product should be discontinued.[31]

Clinical studies show approximately a 20% to 40% reduction in supragingival calculus formation when anticalculus toothpastes are used. Specifically, data from one study of pyrophosphate-containing toothpaste reported a 25.9% reduction in supragingival calculus formation on six lower anterior teeth, a smaller mass of calculus, and calculus formation on fewer sites. The study was made up of 217 subjects and was conducted over 2 months.[46] A similar study evaluating all teeth, not just the mandibular anterior teeth, showed a 32.4% reduction in supragingival calculus formation and a 32.1% reduction in the number of sites of calculus after 6 months of use.[47]

The anticalculus effects of a zinc citrate–containing dentifrice and triclosan-containing dentifrice have been evaluated in clinical studies. The mechanisms of action are less well understood but may be related to the plaque-inhibiting action or some inhibition of crystallization. Zinc citrate dentifrice reduced new supragingival calculus formation by 32.3% and the pyrophosphate paste reduced it by 21.4% compared with the control toothpaste.[47] Triclosan, together with a copolymer, reduced supragingival calculus formation by about 36% compared with the control toothpaste.[48] Other comparison studies have shown similar results[49] and verify that reductions represent decreases in new calculus formation, not reduction of existing calculus.

Although forming less supragingival calculus has desirable cosmetic benefits for many patients and makes less work for the dental hygienist, the health benefits to periodontal patients have not been established. Plaque biofilm is the etiologic agent in periodontal disease; supragingival calculus may only represent inconvenience. It is still important to control supragingival calculus deposits because they are always associated with plaque biofilm and make plaque control more difficult. Reduction in calculus deposition rates can be helpful to the patient

and the dental hygienist but should not be considered a substitute for the oral health benefits of good plaque biofilm control.

PATIENT MOTIVATION

Motivating patients to institute and continue appropriate oral hygiene procedures is a major challenge in dental hygiene practice. Knowledge and behavioral changes begin with education provided to patients by the dental hygienist. Many theories and strategies have been tried to accomplish this task. In the 1970s and 1980s, multiple-appointment education sessions were recommended as a possible improvement on traditional chairside teaching. Two studies compared variations of these teaching strategies; five 30-minute sessions over 14 days were compared with two 60-minute presentations of the same oral hygiene educational materials and a separate study compared one educational session plus two reinforcement follow-up visits. Both strategies significantly reduced plaque over a 2-year observation period; no one method was superior.[50,51] Another study of patients who received oral health education from dental hygienists showed that patients retained more knowledge about self-care and were better motivated than those who had never visited a dental hygienist.[52]

Clearly, the teaching of oral hygiene to achieve plaque biofilm control can be done in a variety of ways. Dental hygienists should determine their preferences and develop a successful style that is unique and knowledge-based so that patients receive the maximum benefit from professional care.

ROLE OF REINFORCEMENT AND LONG-TERM RAPPORT

In a comparison of the Bass and roll brushing techniques, Gibson and Wade[53] expressed their disappointment at the poor performances of the subjects, regardless of the technique they were taught. They emphasized the importance of the dental hygienist teaching and reinforcing good brushing techniques to promote changes in individuals' long-standing habits. Instruction given once or twice was not enough to achieve more than 50% plaque removal. This observation is true for plaque biofilm control education in general.

No matter how great the potential for plaque biofilm removal with all the techniques and devices described here, the dental hygienist plays the key role. Dental hygienists are educated to promote oral health. Several studies have shown that the hygienist can provide these services at less cost than the dentist while maintaining a high quality of health care.[54] The responsibility of the dental hygienist is to assess the individual periodontal patient's needs and educate, customize, motivate, and reinforce the plaque control process for successful periodontal therapy. The knowledge, patience, and time spent on this endeavor will help to restore periodontal patients to health and empower them to maintain it. The dental hygienist spends a significant portion of every practice day in these activities. Patient education remains primarily a chairside activity in the profession and permits patients to take responsibility for their own oral health.

> **CLINICAL NOTE 12-10** The dental hygienist's most important role is educating patients and providing individualized reinforcement for optimal home care.

DENTAL HYGIENE CONSIDERATIONS

- Mechanical procedures are essential for controlling plaque biofilm.
- The goals of plaque biofilm control for periodontal patients are motivation, personal responsibility, mastering complex routines, caries control, and long-term maintenance.
- The best toothbrushing method is one geared toward complete biofilm removal at the gingival margins and as far onto interproximal surfaces as possible.
- Powered toothbrushing is as effective as manual toothbrushing.
- Dental floss is an efficient interproximal cleaner but does not access complex root architecture and furcation areas.
- Interdental brushes and toothpicks can access complex root architecture and furcations.
- Gingival massage does not promote better tissue healing than plaque biofilm removal alone.
- Supragingival and subgingival irrigation are useful in controlling gingivitis when performed at home on a daily basis.
- Subgingival irrigation by the dental hygienist immediately after scaling and root planing does not improve the healing effects of calculus and plaque biofilm from periodontal pockets.
- Chemical antiplaque agents should have proven antimicrobial effects, substantivity, low toxicity, and low permeability.
- Chlorhexidine mouth rinse reliably controls plaque biofilm and reduces gingivitis, although it has significant side effects.
- Essential oil mouth rinses reduce gingivitis and have fewer side effects than chlorhexidine.
- Anticalculus agents reduce the formation of new supragingival calculus.
- Education and motivation must be individualized to permit the patient to take responsibility for periodontal health.
- Patient education and motivation are significant challenges for dental hygienists.

✦ CASE SCENARIO

You have completed a two-session scaling and root planing treatment for Mr. Charles and are discussing with him the periodontal maintenance phase of his care. His periodontal condition has healed and he now presents with 2- to 3-mm probing depths throughout his dentition and 1 to 2 mm of recession on all surfaces of his teeth. Mr. Charles has responded well to treatment and has learned to use interproximal brushes along with using a toothbrush and dental floss. He is very concerned that his periodontal disease will cause him to lose his teeth, as happened to several of his family members.

1. Your discussion with Mr. Charles should include which of the following pieces of information?
   A. Daily plaque control is not as critical as regular visits for maintenance care.
   B. Maintaining the teeth is related more to genetic disposition than daily plaque control.
   C. Daily plaque control is associated with better results for periodontal treatment.
   D. Daily plaque control is not associated with better results for periodontal treatment.

2. The added benefit of using interproximal brushes is
   A. providing Mr. Charles with enough oral hygiene tools.
   B. helping Mr. Charles move away from using dental floss.
   C. reaching into root concavities where floss cannot disrupt the plaque biofilm.
   D. making sure Mr. Charles spends enough time on his plaque biofilm routine.

3. You should be concerned about the generalized recession and exposed root surfaces because Mr. Charles may be at risk for
   A. root caries.
   B. food impaction areas.
   C. recurrent periodontal disease.
   D. aggressive periodontal disease.

STUDY QUESTIONS

Answers and rationales to these questions can be obtained from your instructor.

MULTIPLE CHOICE

1. The goals of a plaque control program for the periodontal patient include all the following EXCEPT one. Which one is the EXCEPTION?
   A. Support for home care practices
   B. Maintenance of gingival and periodontal health
   C. Patient education
   D. Manual flossing

2. Plaque control for periodontal patients includes toothbrushing and the use of an appropriate interdental aid. All periodontal patients must use dental floss.
   A. Both statements are true.
   B. Both statements are false.
   C. The first statement is true, and the second statement is false.
   D. The first statement is false, and the second statement is true.

3. Which of the following toothbrushing methods is focused on the gingival margin?
   A. Bass method
   B. Scrub method
   C. Charters method
   D. All of the above

4. All of the following are true regarding powered toothbrushes EXCEPT one. Which one is the EXCEPTION?
   A. They are at least as effective as manual toothbrushes.
   B. They can be helpful for patients with limited dexterity.
   C. They are essential in maintaining periodontal health.
   D. All of the above are true.

5. Which of the following oral hygiene aids are best suited to areas of furcation involvement?
   A. Dental floss
   B. Powered toothbrushes
   C. Phenol mouthrinse
   D. Toothpicks

6. Irrigation is a useful component of home care for the periodontal patient. Bacteremia has been shown to be associated with oral irrigation.
   A. Both statements are true.
   B. Both statements are false.
   C. The first statement is true, and the second statement is false.
   D. The first statement is false, and the second statement is true.

7. Dental hygiene support for home care for the periodontal patient includes
   A. demonstrating the necessary techniques in the office.
   B. understanding individual patient likes and dislikes relating to oral care.
   C. ongoing encouragement.
   D. all of the above.

8. All of the following are characteristics of chlorhexidine EXCEPT one. Which one is the EXCEPTION?
   A. Substantivity
   B. Anticalculus agent
   C. Taste perversion
   D. ADA-approved for gingivitis treatment

SHORT ANSWER

9. Where should you begin plaque control instruction with a patient who currently brushes once a day and does not perform any interdental hygiene?

10. What would you recommend for a periodontal patient who has large interproximal spaces and dislikes flossing?

Please visit http://evolve.elsevier.com/Perry/periodontology for additional practice and study support tools.

REFERENCES

1. Löe H, Theilade E, Jensen SE. Experimental gingivitis in man. *J Periodontol*. 1965;36:177–187.
2. Loomer PM, Armitage GC. Microbiology of periodontal diseases. In: Rose LF, Mealey BL, eds. *Periodontics: Medicine, Surgery and Implants*. St. Louis, MO: Elsevier Mosby; 2004:69–84.
3. Waerhaug J. Effect of toothbrushing on subgingival plaque formation. *J Periodontol*. 1981;52:30–34.
4. Axelsson P, Lindhe J. Effect of controlled oral hygiene procedures on caries and periodontal disease in adults. *J Clin Periodontol*. 1978;5:133–151.
5. Teughels W, Quirynen M, Jakubovics N. Periodontal microbiology. In: Newman MG, Takei HH, Klokkevold PR, et al, eds. *Carranza's Clinical Periodontology*. 11th ed. St. Louis, MO: Elsevier Saunders; 2012:232–271.
6. Philippot P, Lenoir N, D'Hoore W, et al. Improving patients' compliance with the treatment of periodontitis: a controlled study of behavioral intervention. *J Clin Periodontol*. 2005;32:653–659.
7. Thomas MV. Oral physiotherapy. In: Rose LF, Mealey BL, eds. *Periodontics: Medicine, Surgery and Implants*. St. Louis, MO: Elsevier Mosby; 2004:214–236.
8. Niemi ML, Sandholm L, Ainamo J. Frequency of gingival lesions after standardized brushing as related to stiffness of toothbrush and abrasiveness of dentifrice. *J Clin Periodontol*. 1984;11:254–261.
9. Bass CC. The optimum characteristics of toothbrushes for personal oral hygiene. *Dent Items Interest*. 1948;70:697–719.
10. Gift HC. Current utilization patterns of oral hygiene practices: state-of-the-science review. In: Löe H, Kleinman DV, eds. *Dental Plaque Control Measures and Oral Hygiene Practices*. Washington, DC: IRL Press; 1986:39–71.
11. Jepsen S. The role of manual toothbrushes in effective plaque control: advantages and limitations. In: Lang NP, Attstrom R, Löe H, eds. *Proceedings of the European Workshop on Mechanical Plaque Control*. Carol Stream, IL: Quintessence; 1998:121–137.
12. Raposa, K. Oral infections control: Toothbrushes and toothbrushing. In: Wilkins EM, ed. *Clinical Practice of the Dental Hygienist*. 11th ed. Philadelphia, PA: Lippincott Williams & Wilkins; 2013;386–407.
13. Charters WJ. Eliminating mouth infections with the toothbrush and other stimulating instruments. *Dent Digest*. 1932;38:130–136.
14. Lang NP, Cumming BR, Löe H. Toothbrushing frequency as it relates to plaque development and gingival health. *J Periodontol*. 1973;44:396–405.
15. Stillman PR. A philosophy of treatment of periodontal disease. *Dent Digest*. 1932;38:315–319.
16. Bass CC. An effective method of personal oral hygiene. *J La State Med Soc*. 1954;106:100–112.
17. Forrest JL, Miller SA. Manual versus powered toothbrushes: a summary of the Cochrane Oral Health Group's systematic review. Part II. *J Dent Hyg*. 2004; 78:349–354.
18. Boyd RL, Murray P, Robertson PB. Effect on periodontal status of rotary electric toothbrushes vs. manual toothbrushes during periodontal maintenance. I. Clinical results. *J Periodontol*. 1989;60:390–395.
19. Van der Weijden GA, Timmerman MF, Danser MM, et al. The role of electric toothbrushes: advantages and limitations. In: Lang NP, Attstrom R, Löe H, eds. *Proceedings of the European Workshop on Mechanical Plaque Control*. Carol Stream, IL: Quintessence; 1998:138–155.
20. Graves RC, Disney JA, Stamm JW. Comparative effectiveness of flossing and brushing in reducing interproximal bleeding. *J Periodontol*. 1989;60:243–247.
21. Lang WP, Farghaly MM, Ronis DL. The relation of preventive dental behaviors to periodontal health status. *J Clin Periodontol*. 1994;21:194–198.
22. Axelsson P, Lindhe J, Nystrom B. On the prevention of caries and periodontal disease: results of a 15-year longitudinal study in adults. *J Clin Periodontol*. 1991;18:182–189.
23. Bass CC. The optimum characteristics of dental floss for personal oral hygiene. *Dent Items Interest*. 1948;70:921–934.
24. Perry DA, Pattison GA. An investigation of wax residue on tooth surfaces after the use of waxed dental floss. *Dent Hyg*. 1986;60:16–19.
25. Spolsky VS, Perry DA, Meng Z, et al. Evaluating the efficacy of a new flossing aid. *J Clin Periodontol*. 1993;20:490–497.
26. Boardman TJ. Clinical evaluation of an automatic flossing device vs. manual flossing. *J Clin Dent*. 2001;12:63–66.
27. Christou V, Timmerman MF, Van der Velden U, et al. Comparison of different approaches of interdental oral hygiene: interdental brushes versus dental floss. *J Periodontol*. 1998;69:759–764.
28. Lobene RR. The effect of a pulsed water pressure cleansing device on oral health. *J Periodontol*. 1969;40:667–670.
29. Fine DH, Baumhammers A. Effect of water pressure irrigation on stainable material on the teeth. *J Periodontol*. 1970;41:468–472.
30. Ciancio SG. Powered oral irrigation and control of gingivitis. *Biol Ther Dent*. 1990;5:21–24.
31. Black TL. Chemotherapeutics and topical delivery systems. In: Wilkins EM, ed. *Clinical Practice of the Dental Hygienist*. 11th ed. Philadelphia, PA: Lippincott Williams & Wilkins; 2013:423–435.
32. Cummins D, Creeth JE. Delivery of antiplaque agents from dentifrices, gels, and mouthwashes. *J Dent Res*. 1992;71:1439–1449.
33. Hill M, Moore RL. Locally acting oral chemotherapeutic agents. In: Rose LF, Mealey BL, eds. *Periodontics: Medicine, Surgery and Implants*. St. Louis, MO: Elsevier Mosby; 2004:276–287.
34. Jones CG. Chlorhexidine: is it still the gold standard? *Periodontol 2000*. 1997;15:55–62.
35. Ciancio SG. Non-surgical periodontal treatment. In: Nevins M, Becker W, Kornman K, eds. *Proceedings of the World Workshop in Clinical Periodontics*. Chicago, IL: American Academy of Periodontology; 1989: II-1–II-11.
36. Briner WW, Grassman E, Buckner RY, et al. Assessment of susceptibility of plaque bacteria to chlorhexidine after six months' oral use. *J Periodont Res*. 1986;21(suppl):53–59.

37. Flemmig TF, Newman MG, Doherty FM, et al. Supragingival irrigation with 0.06% chlorhexidine in naturally occurring gingivitis. I: 6 month clinical observations. *J Periodontol*. 1990;61:112–117.
38. Council on Dental Therapeutics accepts Peridex. *J Am Dent Assoc*. 1988;117:516–517.
39. Council on Dental Therapeutics accepts Listerine. *J Am Dent Assoc*. 1988;117:515–516.
40. Zambon JJ, Ciancio SG, Mather ML, et al. The effect of an antimicrobial mouthrinse on early healing of gingival flap surgery wounds. *J Periodontol*. 1989;60:31–36.
41. Ciancio SC, Mariotti A. Antiinfective therapy. In: Newman MG, Takei HH, Klokkevold PR, et al, eds. *Carranza's Clinical Periodontology*. 11th ed. St. Louis, MO: Elsevier Saunders; 2012;482–491.
42. Greenstein G. Subgingival irrigation, an adjunct to periodontal therapy: current status and future directions. *J Dent Hyg*. 1990;64:389–397.
43. Nosal G, Scheidt MJ, O'Neal RO, et al. The penetration of lavage solution into the periodontal pocket during ultrasonic instrumentation. *J Periodontol*. 1991;62:554–557.
44. Shiloah J, Hovious A. The role of subgingival irrigations in the treatment of periodontitis. *J Periodontol*. 1993;6:835–843.
45. Wolff LF, Bakdash MB, Pihlstrom BL, et al. The effect of professional and home subgingival irrigation and antimicrobial agents on gingivitis and early periodontitis. *J Dent Hyg*. 1989;63:222–225.
46. Mallatt ME, Beiswanger BB, Stookey GK, et al. Influence of soluble pyrophosphates on calculus formation in adults. *J Dent Res*. 1985;64:1159–1162.
47. Kazmierczak M, Mather M, Ciancio S, et al. A clinical evaluation of anticalculus dentifrices. *J Clin Prev Dent*. 1990;12:13–17.
48. Lobene RR, Battista GW, Petrone DM. Clinical efficacy of an anticalculus fluoride dentifrice containing triclosan and a copolymer: a 6-month study. *Am J Dent*. 1991;4:83–85.
49. Kohut BE, Rubin MA, Baron HJ. The relative clinical effectiveness of three anticalculus dentifrices. *J Clin Preventive Dent*. 1989;11:13–16.
50. Soderhölm G, Nöbreus N, Attström R, et al. Teaching plaque control. I. A five-visit versus a two-visit program. *J Clin Periodontol*. 1982;9:203–213.
51. Soderhölm G, Egelberg J. Teaching plaque control. II. 30-minute versus 15-minute appointments in a three-visit program. *J Clin Periodontol*. 1982;9:214–222.
52. Uitenbröek DG, Schaub RMH, Tromp JAH, et al. Dental hygienists' influence on the patients' knowledge, motivation, self-care, and perception of change. *Commun Dent Oral Epidemiol*. 1989;17:87–90.
53. Gibson JA, Wade AB. Plaque removal by the Bass and roll brushing techniques. *J Periodontol*. 1977;48:456–459.
54. Schou L. Behavioral aspects of dental plaque control measures: an oral health promotion perspective. In: Lang NP, Attstrom R, Löe H, eds. *Proceedings of the European Workshop on Mechanical Plaque Control*. Carol Stream, IL: Quintessence; 1998:287–289.

CHAPTER 13

Nonsurgical Periodontal Therapy

Phyllis L. Beemsterboer and Dorothy A. Perry

LEARNING OUTCOMES

- Define nonsurgical periodontal therapy.
- Describe the short- and long-term goals of nonsurgical periodontal therapy.
- Identify the techniques and applications for nonsurgical periodontal therapy procedures.
- Describe the process of healing after periodontal debridement procedures, scaling, and root planing.

- Explain the limitations of calculus removal and the expectations for clinician proficiency.
- Discuss the use of lasers in nonsurgical therapy.
- Describe the contributions of magnification with use of loupes, endoscopy, and microscopes to nonsurgical therapy.
- Explain the benefits and indications of antimicrobial adjuncts to nonsurgical therapy.

KEY TERMS

Dentin sensitivity
Dentinal hypersensitivity
Endoscope
Gingival curettage
Hand instrumentation
Hydrodynamic theory of dentinal
   sensitivity

Irrigation
Loupes
Magnification
Microscope
Nonsurgical periodontal therapy
Periodontal debridement
Polishing

Powered instrumentation
Prophylaxis
Root planing
Scaling
Sonic instrumentation
Specific plaque hypothesis
Ultrasonic instrumentation

The initial approach for treating gingival and periodontal diseases is debridement of plaque biofilm and calculus through nonsurgical therapeutic techniques. The term nonsurgical therapy is often considered a misnomer because the procedures performed require the application of sharp blades to cut tissues, which is a form of surgery. However, in periodontology, the term *surgery* is reserved for more invasive cutting procedures. Other terms used to describe nonsurgical periodontal therapy include initial therapy,[1] Phase I therapy,[2,3] etiotropic phase,[2] and periodontal debridement.

In its broadest sense, nonsurgical therapy defines all of the procedures performed to treat gingival and periodontal diseases up to the time of reevaluation, which is when patients begin maintenance care and the need for periodontal surgery to enhance results is determined. Nonsurgical therapy includes the procedures listed in Table 13-1.

This chapter defines the technical procedures applied by dental hygienists and the instruments used for treatment. These are the procedures and instruments required to scale, root-plane, and debride the tooth surfaces of bacterial plaque biofilms and calculus and to remove stains by the application of polishing techniques.[3]

Patient plaque biofilm control is a cornerstone of long-term successful therapy. For this reason, every patient must participate in treatment by adopting a regular and effective biofilm removal regimen. Positive, long-term effects of periodontal therapy are reliably achieved with patient compliance, effective plaque biofilm control, and excellent dental hygiene treatment.[3] These are all aspects of dental hygiene care and are essential in the application of nonsurgical periodontal therapy.

> **CLINICAL NOTE 13-1** Patient plaque biofilm control is a cornerstone of long-term successful nonsurgical therapy.

DEFINITIONS OF NONSURGICAL PERIODONTAL THERAPY

This chapter discusses the biologic basis and rationale for non-surgical therapeutic procedures performed in the dental office. It describes scaling procedures, both hand instrumentation and powered instrumentation, root planing, gingival curettage, and polishing. Treatment frequently requires the use of pain control measures. Elements of dental hygiene care are illustrated in Figures 13-1 to 13-3.

The definitions of procedures must be clear and consistent. Specific definitions accepted in the dental hygiene community

TABLE 13-1	Nonsurgical Periodontal Therapy Appointment Procedures
TECHNIQUE	**APPLICATION**
Oral hygiene instruction for daily plaque biofilm control	Comprehensive techniques Individualized Reinforced at each appointment
Calculus removal	Scaling and root planing techniques Hand or powered instruments Significant component of periodontal debridement biofilm
Supragingival and subgingival plaque biofilm removal	Instrumentation techniques to remove or disrupt subgingival biofilm Identification of plaque-retentive factors Referral for treatment of plaque-retentive conditions such as poorly fitting restorations and malpositioned teeth
Gingival curettage	Instrumentation techniques to alter the environment of the pocket wall, if necessary
Occlusal evaluation	Identification of occlusion-related factors affecting the periodontium
Polishing	Selective procedure for supragingival plaque and stain removal Cosmetic demand
Antimicrobial use	Locally or systemically delivered antimicrobial, antiseptic and antiinflammatory medications

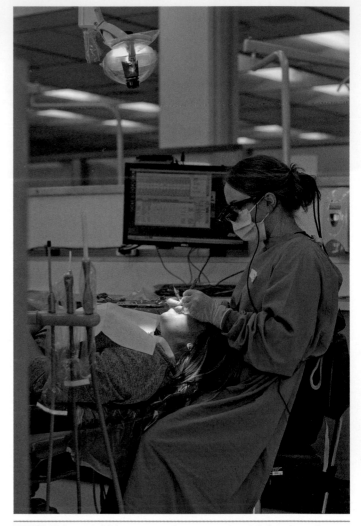

FIGURE 13-1 ■ Dental hygienist performing nonsurgical therapy in the contemporary clinical setting.

are provided for commonly used terminology found in publications and other communications.

SCALING

The American Academy of Periodontology (AAP) defines scaling as "instrumentation of the crown and root surfaces of the teeth to remove plaque, calculus, and stains from these surfaces."[4] However, subgingival scaling is also referred to as simply the removal of subgingival calculus[3] or the more general term, subgingival deposits.[5] Scaling is most commonly thought of as the removal of identifiable deposits of calculus, but associated plaque biofilm deposits are also removed during the procedure. The focus of the application of the instruments is to remove calculus and biofilms; success of treatment at the time of the therapy is assessed by explorer evaluation of root smoothness after scaling procedures to ensure calculus removal.

Scaling may be accomplished with sharp hand instruments or with sonic or ultrasonic instrumentation using powered scaling devices.

ROOT PLANING

Root planing is defined by the AAP as "a treatment procedure designed to remove cementum or surface dentin that is rough, impregnated with calculus, or contaminated with toxins or microorganisms."[6] This procedure focuses not on identifiable deposits of calculus but on the entire root surface associated with the periodontal pocket. The goal of root planing is to remove the surface layer of cementum or dentin that may be impregnated with bacterial lipopolysaccharides (endotoxins) or calculus to create a glassy, hard surface.[5] When the root surfaces feel smooth and hard, the dental hygienist can be confident that the treated pockets are free of deposits and contaminants on and embedded in the root surfaces.[7] Root planing was thought to render root surfaces less prone to the reestablishment of the cause of disease—bacterial plaque biofilm—than scaling alone, but this theory has not been proven. The difference between scaling and root planing is a matter of degree; root planing involves a specific effort to instrument every portion of the root surfaces, not simply identifiable calculus deposits.

The goal of root planing, leaving the roots clean, has not changed, but the extent to which root tissue is scraped away to create a glassy, hard texture has been under scrutiny. There is no evidence that root-planed teeth are easier to maintain or less likely to be associated with periodontal diseases than those that have simply been rendered free of calculus and plaque biofilm.[8]

Root planing, like scaling, may be successfully performed by hand instrumentation or powered scaling devices.

CLINICAL NOTE 13-2 Although there are adjunct procedures that improve periodontal health, there is no substitute for scaling and root planing to remove local irritants to the tissues.

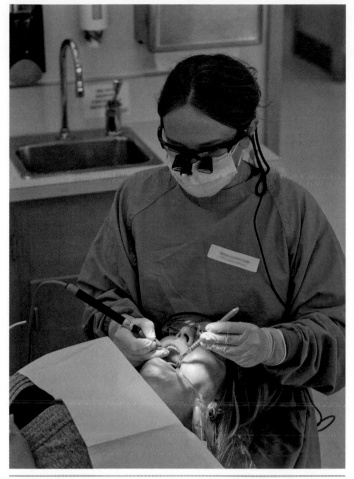

FIGURE 13-2 ■ The use of both ultrasonic instrumentation and magnification to improve vision are important components of dental hygiene practice.

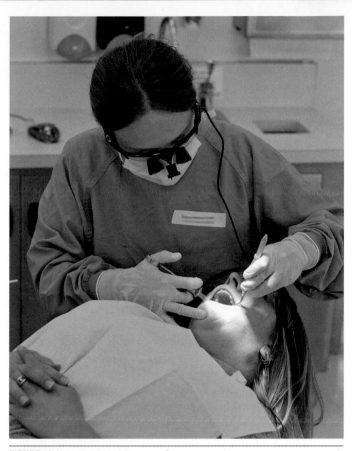

FIGURE 13-3 ■ The dental hygienist has many patient treatment options available for nonsurgical periodontal therapy, including the use of injected local anesthetics for pain control.

PERIODONTAL DEBRIDEMENT

The terms *nonsurgical periodontal therapy* or **periodontal debridement** are used along with the traditional terms of *scaling* and *root planing.* These terms include supragingival and subgingival scaling and root planing and disruption or removal of plaque biofilm, with a minimum of tooth structure removal.[4] They also incorporate removal of plaque biofilm, plaque retentive features, and calculus, both above and below the gingival margin. The goal of periodontal debridement and scaling is to restore the periodontium to health and produce surfaces that are free of various deposits.[6,9]

PROPHYLAXIS

Prophylaxis is a preventive procedure to remove local gingival irritants and includes complete calculus removal followed by root planing. The term is commonly used and has several variations: oral prophylaxis, dental prophylaxis or, simply, prophy. The purpose of prophylaxis is to assist the patient in maintaining and preserving periodontal health. It is usually accomplished during one appointment and has many facets. A comprehensive explanation of periodontal maintenance is found in Chapter 17.

POLISHING AND STAIN REMOVAL

Polishing is the use of polishing agents to remove stains and supragingival plaque biofilm from the teeth. It is most commonly performed by rubber-cup application of polishing agents with a slow-speed handpiece. There are also air devices that polish teeth with a power-driven handpiece that sprays abrasive slurry against the tooth surfaces. The polishing procedure is commonly referred to as a prophylaxis or a prophy, but this term is incorrect. Polishing may have some aesthetic value for patients and may help motivate them to maintain a clean mouth, but it has no proven therapeutic value.

Stains on the teeth are generally considered harmless, so their removal is secondary to the therapeutic and preventive goals of the dental hygienist. Polishing should be performed selectively.[10,11]

Selective polishing is choosing the surfaces to polish on the basis of patient concerns and the presence of plaque biofilm and stains that cannot be removed with normal patient oral hygiene practices. The concept of selective polishing emerged when research on enamel and root surfaces after polishing revealed changes in the hard tissues. In 1976 Wilkins, in her fourth edition of *Clinical Practice of the Dental Hygienist,* introduced the idea of selective polishing and encouraged this modification in treatment.[9] She stressed the critical importance of teaching personal plaque biofilm control rather than performing polishing during the appointment because of the limited amount of time the dental hygienist has with each patient. Providing information about performing effective plaque biofilm control is more valuable than performing what is primarily a cosmetic procedure.

The concerns around polishing grew out of early research that indicated a loss of the tooth surface from the removal of the fluoride-rich surface layer of enamel. However, the minerals in saliva remineralize the tooth surfaces, so surface alterations are only temporary.

Several other concerns about polishing exist. Abrasives used during polishing can scratch amalgam, composite resin, and gold restorative materials. It was once thought that tooth surfaces had to be plaque-free to absorb fluoride during fluoride treatments, so polishing of teeth was performed routinely before office fluoride applications. It is now known that the presence of plaque biofilms does not interfere with the uptake of fluoride by tooth structures. Other concerns include the possibility of creating bacteremia in the patient and possibly damaging the tooth pulps by heat generated from the power-driven prophylaxis angle. Cleaning agents are available for polishing the teeth and are preferable to those that contain abrasives. The contents of any material used for patient care should be read carefully; this is especially warranted when dealing with the myriad choices available for stain removal. Barnes recommended that the least abrasive paste necessary to remove stains was appropriate and if no stain was present a cleaning agent should be employed. One size fits all grit paste ignores the science of abrasion, can cause sensitivity, and damage aesthetic restorations.[5]

Air powder polishing removes most extrinsic stains and soft deposits from the exposed surfaces of the teeth. It works by mechanical abrasion using a slurry of sodium bicarbonate and water. The power and powder-to-water ratio is controlled with a foot pedal and can be increased or decreased as needed. Air powder polishing is especially effective with severe staining, such as that found in cigarette and pipe smokers. Caution must be exercised with this device to prevent damage to exposed root surfaces; thus, its application for periodontal patients is limited. Because this system produces an extensive aerosol, it is contraindicated in patients with infectious diseases, respiratory illnesses, hypertension, or those who are on hemodialysis.[10] The periodontal patient often has multiple exposed root surfaces and caution with the choice of polishing agent is advised.

The term *selective polishing* has been clarified to mean that the clinician selects the appropriate agent based on the presenting needs of the patient. Appearance of the teeth is of great importance to patients, and the polishing procedure can be an excellent way to motivate them to remove plaque biofilm for health as well as appearance.

GINGIVAL CURETTAGE

Curettage had been defined by the AAP as scraping or cleaning the walls of a cavity or surface by means of a curette.[12] It is a commonly misused term, often applied to a variety of procedures from removal of the pocket lining, termed *closed curettage*, to a surgical flap procedure called *open curettage*. Specifically, curettage performed by the dental hygienist (legally permitted in some states), properly termed *gingival curettage*, is limited to closed curettage. It is defined as the removal of the inflamed soft tissue lateral to the pocket wall. A number of clinical trials have confirmed that gingival curettage provides no additional benefit to healing compared with scaling and root planing alone in terms of probing depth reduction, attachment gain, or inflammation reduction. Gingival curettage is thus considered to have little therapeutic value in the treatment of chronic periodontitis and is no longer listed as a method of treatment by the American Dental Association and the AAP.[12]

Inadvertent curettage is a term used to describe accidental and incomplete removal of the pocket lining during scaling and root planing or periodontal debridement procedures. It commonly occurs during nonsurgical periodontal therapy.

GOALS OF NONSURGICAL PERIODONTAL THERAPY

The goals of nonsurgical periodontal therapy must be considered in terms of the immediate treatment goals at the time of the appointment and the long-term goals for the patient. During periodontal debridement procedures, the goal for the dental hygienist is to promote plaque biofilm control and instrument the tooth surfaces until they are clean and smooth, touching all portions of the roots to disrupt plaque biofilm and remove calculus. This end point is best evaluated by explorer detection of smooth surfaces.[3] Calculus removal may be considered a subgoal rather than the primary focus.[3] The goal at the treatment visit is not to render the roots glassy and hard through extensive planing away of tooth structure.

The long-term goal of treatment is to restore gingival health. For periodontal patients, this goal often requires multiple appointments with the dental hygienist. The restoration of gingival health is the sum of good plaque control, complete scaling and periodontal debridement, and sufficient time for healing to occur—several months for complete healing of both the epithelium and connective tissue.[2,3] These goals are summarized in Table 13-2.

CLINICAL NOTE 13-3 The technical skill of the dental hygienist is the critical element in successful nonsurgical periodontal therapy.

TABLE 13-2 Goals of Nonsurgical Periodontal Therapy

	PLAQUE BIOFILM CONTROL	CALCULUS AND BIOFILM REMOVAL (PERIODONTAL DEBRIDEMENT)	EVALUATION
Short-term goals	Provide technique instruction and reinforcement	Complete removal of deposits Clean surfaces	Clean and smooth root surfaces
Long-term goals	Ensure adoption of adequate daily oral hygiene procedures Reinforcement	Regular removal of new deposits at subsequent visits	Tissue health restored Compliance with maintenance regimen (regular evaluation and treatment as necessary)

RATIONALE FOR NONSURGICAL PERIODONTAL THERAPY

The rationale for nonsurgical periodontal therapy is to remove the etiologic agent of disease—bacterial plaque biofilm—and its associated factors. Scaling and root planing is the standard of care for nonsurgical and nonpharmacologic treatment of chronic periodontal diseases. Clinical trials have consistently demonstrated that scaling and root planing reduce gingival inflammation and probing depths and result in gains of clinical attachment in most periodontal patients.[13] There are also secondary influences on periodontal health that must be considered. Calculus, although not an etiologic agent in itself, is virtually always associated with plaque biofilm, and its removal is associated with improved periodontal health.

Anatomic and iatrogenic plaque traps, such as overhanging restorations and malposed teeth, must be considered during nonsurgical therapy. Although these features are primarily plaque biofilm control problems, the dental hygienist should recognize them, design specific plaque control measures, and refer patients for further treatment. Replacement restorations or orthodontic movement of the teeth can simplify plaque biofilm control and help the patient achieve periodontal health. These local factors are described in Chapter 5.

Several issues surround the application of nonsurgical periodontal therapy. The following information is a summary of evidence supporting the provision of nonsurgical periodontal treatment: plaque biofilm and calculus removal, hand instruments and powered instruments, the relative merit of smooth roots, healing after nonsurgical treatment, laser use, and antimicrobial adjuncts.

REMOVAL OF CAUSATIVE FACTORS

Dental hygienists remove the primary etiologic factor of periodontal disease, plaque biofilm, and its associated factors through scaling and root planing, cleaning and smoothing of the roots or, more broadly, periodontal debridement. These procedures are demanding technical activities that require a large share of each therapeutic treatment appointment.

Plaque Biofilm

Plaque biofilm is the primary causative agent in gingival and periodontal diseases. Animal studies provide strong evidence that these destructive diseases occur in the presence of microbes, but not in animals raised in germ-free environments. Although some periodontal destruction has been observed in germ-free (gnotobiotic) animal experiments, it tends to be localized and related to the impaction of foreign objects, such as hairs. Inflammation and tissue destruction in conventionally raised animals with oral biota are vastly more widespread and severe.[5]

Bacteria live in the mouth and are present around diseased teeth. Convincing experimental evidence that plaque microorganisms cause human gingival disease was presented by Löe and colleagues in 1965.[14] The researchers initiated extensive plaque control in a small group of dental students and brought them to a level of excellent periodontal health; then the subjects refrained from oral hygiene procedures for 3 weeks. Within 10 to 21 days, every subject had gingivitis, which resolved in about 1 week when oral hygiene practices were resumed. In addition,

the microbial composition of dental plaque changed from one of gram-positive microbiota to one dominated by gram-negative organisms.

CLINICAL NOTE 13-4 Animal studies, the landmark study on human experimental gingivitis, and much additional evidence prove that plaque biofilm removal is a major part of nonsurgical periodontal therapy. The dental hygienist cannot focus solely on the technical aspects of calculus removal.

As the understanding of plaque biofilm as the pathologic agent has grown, various periodontal diseases have been identified with specific microbial organisms. All plaques are no longer considered intrinsically bad. The specific plaque hypothesis was proposed by Loesche in the 1970s.[15] This classic study has increased the understanding of periodontal disease and the use of appropriate antimicrobial agents to improve treatment results. An excellent example of the application of the specific plaque hypothesis is the treatment of aggressive periodontitis in its juvenile form. In the 1960s, this disease was recognized as different from typical periodontitis because the conventional therapy, which consisted of scaling and root planing in the localized affected areas of the anterior teeth and first molars, could only slow the loss of these teeth. A specific plaque bacterium, *Actinobacillus actinomycetemcomitans*, was identified in these lesions. Therefore, treatment emphasis changed to include both conventional therapy and the use of appropriate antibiotics and resulted in successful restoration of periodontal health with less tooth loss.

Periodontal diseases present similar symptoms, but they likely have different bacterial origins that are not yet fully defined. Eventually, they will be much better understood so that therapies directed toward the specific plaque bacteria in each individual can be used, including the use of more antimicrobial and antiseptic agents.[16]

Although more specific gingival and periodontal diseases are recognized, nonsurgical periodontal therapy focuses on total plaque biofilm removal. The quality of the plaque is more important than the quantity, but plaque biofilm is still the causative agent in disease. Bacteria-specific tests and treatments have been developed and will be more widely used as the understanding of periodontal disease increases.[7]

It is possible to remove all supragingival plaque effectively. To do so, the patient uses oral hygiene procedures and the dental hygienist performs coronal polishing. However, subgingival plaque is not effectively altered by supragingival oral hygiene procedures, especially in deeper pockets of 5 mm or more. Supragingival oral hygiene procedures have limited effects on symptoms associated with deeper pockets, such as bleeding on probing.[17]

Subgingival plaque biofilm removal is essential in nonsurgical therapy to disrupt the established colonies of bacteria and let a younger plaque develop that is less associated with pathologic conditions. Dental hygiene procedures with hand instruments or powered scalers adequately accomplish subgingival plaque biofilm removal. A study published in the 1980s compared the performance of hand instruments with that of ultrasonic tips in the removal of plaque in pockets. Both were effective in removing approximately 67% of the plaque in pockets deeper than 5 mm and the ultrasonic instruments per-formed as well as the hand instruments.[16,17] The AAP consensus report on nonsurgical periodontal therapy suggested that 11% plaque remaining on root surfaces after thorough instrumentation was more likely an accurate figure.[17]

Calculus

Calculus is little more than calcified plaque biofilm. As plaque biofilm ages, the organic matrix and bacterial cells calcify. Calculus adheres to tooth surfaces through pellicular attachment, mechanical locking, and intercrystalline forces. It varies in crystal composition, type of attachment, and degree of difficulty in removal (see Chapter 5). Although calculus is an inert substance, its role appears to be that of plaque biofilm retention, and its removal is associated with a return to periodontal health, as seen in Figure 13-4.

The thoroughness of calculus removal by instrumentation has been studied and shows surprising results. Kepic and colleagues[18] demonstrated residual calculus on most teeth after 45 to 60 minutes of treatment time per quadrant. Even when teeth were instrumented for as long as 39 minutes each, residual calculus was noted regularly in deeper pockets, and totally clean surfaces were achieved only in the 3- to 4-mm range.[19,20] Even the best instrumentation techniques leave some residual deposits on the teeth; however, these very small deposits were also present in the subjects of long-term studies used to verify the effectiveness of nonsurgical periodontal treatment, and they did not appear to cause the treatment to fail.[2,3]

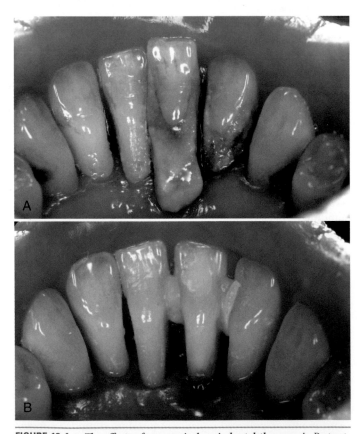

FIGURE 13-4 ■ **The effects of nonsurgical periodontal therapy. A,** Pretreatment documentation for a 45-year-old woman with severe periodontal destruction and calculus accumulation. **B,** Periodontal healing 4 weeks after nonsurgical periodontal treatment. Note the temporary splint placed to limit mobility of teeth #24, #25, and #26.

> **CLINICAL NOTE 13-5** Some residual calculus is likely to remain after dental hygiene treatment, especially in deeper pockets, but patients can probably tolerate some small amount. If the long-term goal of restoring periodontal health has not been achieved after conscientious nonsurgical therapy, the dental hygienist must first suspect residual calculus (and plaque biofilm) and re-treat nonresponding areas. Areas in the periodontium that do not respond to therapy, even after retreatment and evaluation, may benefit from long-term subgingival antimicrobial treatment or surgical intervention.

ROOT SMOOTHNESS

Achieving root smoothness is important for evaluating short-term goals during treatment appointments. The dental hygienist must develop a tactile sense that permits detection of obvious calculus on the teeth. This tactile sense is used to determine the amount of calculus present in the untreated patient, the existence of irritating factors such as overhangs, and the point at which thorough instrumentation (periodontal debridement) is finished at each appointment. Glassy, smooth root surfaces are not end points in treatment. After instrumentation, some roots feel smooth, whereas others have varying degrees of granular roughness. Experience suggests that the roots in an individual patient's mouth will feel equally smooth after thorough instrumentation. This uniform smoothness should be identified. Most importantly, no surfaces should feel rough, as if calculus is still present. Plaque biofilm must also be dislodged from all accessible surfaces. Clearly, this requires clinical experience and judgment on the part of the dental hygienist. Armitage reviewed the reasons dental hygienists and dentists attempt to smooth roots to a glassy, hard texture through root planing. These reasons are[8] as follows:

- Smooth surfaces are easier to clean.
- Smooth surfaces retard plaque formation.
- Rough surfaces mechanically irritate gingival tissues.
- Smooth surfaces promote gingival healing.

> **CLINICAL NOTE 13-6** Explorer-detectable root roughness may not be calculus but merely the texture of the root. Quantifiable research has not shown this roughness to be harmful.

Armitage presented the following information regarding root surface roughness[8]:

1. Slightly rough root surfaces, those that are scaled and cleaned but not planed in a systematic way to remove cementum and leave glassy surfaces, do not accumulate plaque more rapidly than smoother surfaces. The appealing notion that rough surfaces would present more of a plaque control problem for patients is borne out by experience with obvious calculus or overhanging restorations. However, the roughness associated with calculus and poor restorations is far greater than the slightly granular texture of calculus-free root surfaces.
2. Studies evaluating plaque biofilm formation on rough root surfaces are equivocal. Early studies that used visual appraisal of deposits or colony counts on surfaces showed

that smooth surfaces had less plaque biofilm formation; however, root texture was not measured. The only study that attempted to measure root texture with quantifiable profilometer (Micrometrical Manufacturing, Ann Arbor, MI) readings found that the amount of root roughness did not affect plaque biofilm formation.

3. No experimental evidence indicates that rough root surfaces are mechanical irritants and would therefore delay healing.

4. Smooth root surfaces do not appear to promote better or faster healing than rough surfaces. In fact, in some studies, gingivae next to root surfaces that were notched for orientation of researchers after tooth extraction healed uneventfully in the mouth. This indicated that roughness itself had no effect on wound healing.

Because smooth surfaces are clinically associated with the restoration of gingival health, clinicians believe that smooth root surfaces are good. The question remains whether root surfaces need to be glassy smooth. It appears that variation in smoothness is acceptable as long as calculus that makes surfaces feel rough and irregular has been removed and plaque biofilm has been disrupted.

Root roughness has been equated with incomplete instrumentation because of concerns that endotoxins (e.g., lipopolysaccharides) formed by gram-negative bacteria invade the root structure. Removal of endotoxins would require the planing away of diseased cementum. This practice supports the old notion of "necrotic" root surfaces. Much has been learned about the penetration and removal of lipopolysaccharide endotoxins. Studies indicate that endotoxins do not penetrate deeply into cemental surfaces and that retained toxins are associated with missed calculus and plaque rather than diseased cementum. Nyman and colleagues[20] compared these treatment strategies by testing the healing of quadrants after periodontal surgery. One side was treated with conventional root planing and the other with calculus carefully flicked off and root surfaces polished before the tissue was sutured back in place. There was no difference in the healing of the differently treated areas; cementum removal through root planing did not improve healing beyond that achieved by calculus removal and polishing.

These data indicate that toxins are superficially located on root surfaces and easily removed. Extensive root instrumentation is not required beyond the removal of calculus and plaque. Thus, the rationale for root planing to remove root roughness and achieve glassy, smooth root surfaces is no longer valid. Dramatically thinned root surfaces are shown in Figure 13-5. This thinning is an example of overinstrumentation or root planing without rationale.

CLINICAL NOTE 13-7 Conscientious removal of calculus and plaque biofilm with minimum destruction of cementum, termed *periodontal debridement*, is justified. The repeated removal of tooth structure during nonsurgical therapy appointments and subsequent maintenance visits is not a goal of therapy, and it may result in thinned and sensitive root surfaces.

GINGIVAL CURETTAGE

Gingival curettage, also called closed curettage or nonsurgical gingival curettage (truly a misnomer), was traditionally performed to remove inflamed pocket lining for reasons distinct from periodontal debridement. Inflamed pocket lining is composed of thin ulcerated strands of epithelium, with rete pegs extending into the underlying connective tissue and granulation tissue containing disorganized masses of cells. It may also contain dislodged calculus and plaque bacteria. Removal of this tissue was assumed to enhance pocket reduction beyond the results achieved by scaling and root planing alone, providing faster healing and the formation of new connective tissue attachments to the root surfaces. This rationale has been questioned for many years and the procedure is no longer considered standard treatment.[21,22]

No clinical studies have shown greater pocket reduction, more rapid healing, or more new attachment after gingival curettage has been performed compared with scaling and root planing alone.[22] In animal studies, gingival curettage promoted the formation of long junctional epithelium during healing, rather than new connective tissue attachment.[23] Clinical trials reviewed by Kalkwarf[22] indicated that tissue healed through long junctional epithelium rather than connective tissue attachment can be maintained successfully for years, suggesting that this is a satisfactory treatment result.

A number of dental hygiene programs in the United States teach gingival curettage because it is a legally sanctioned duty in many states and may be performed by practitioners in the community.[24] In this era of increased emphasis on nonsurgical therapies, removal of disorganized granulation tissue and ulcerated epithelium from pocket linings remains appealing to many clinicians, even if data do not show improved healing.

CLINICAL NOTE 13-8 The restoration of gingival health is the sum of good plaque control, complete scaling and periodontal debridement, and sufficient time for healing to occur.

HEALING

Healing after scaling, root planing, and gingival curettage occurs as a repair of existing tissues rather than regeneration of tissues lost in the periodontal disease process. After periodontal debridement is performed (unless there are systemic complications) periodontal pockets, alveolar bone, periodontal ligament, and epithelium will heal. Inflammation will be resolved, long junctional epithelial attachment is likely to occur, and recession will often result. Subgingival bacterial plaque biofilm will regrow but, at least initially, it will consist of a younger, less pathogenic bacterial biofilm than that associated with untreated periodontal pockets.

The formation of new bone to replace bone that is lost, new connective tissue attachment to the root surface, and new cementum on the root are not predictable outcomes.

Soft Tissue Healing After Scaling and Periodontal Debridement

Scaling and root planing causes some removal and disruption of the epithelial attachment to the tooth, junctional epithelium, and deeper connective tissue. The epithelial lining of the pocket wall is also often disrupted and partially removed through inadvertent curettage.

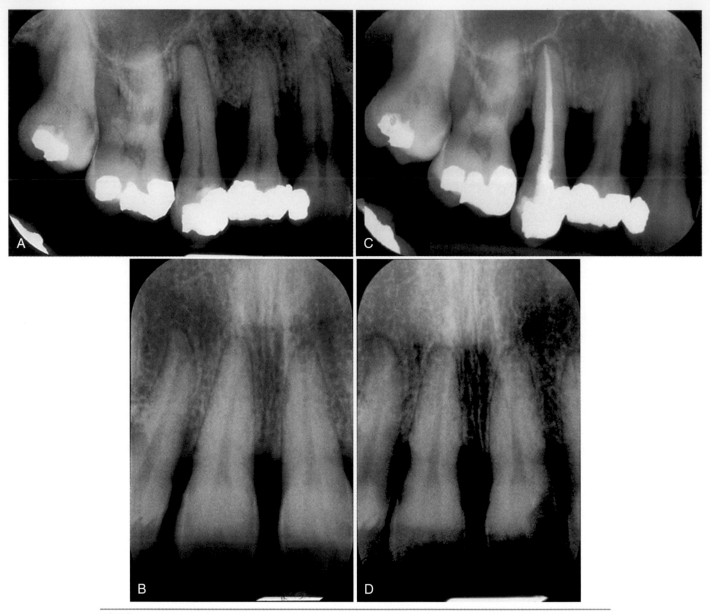

FIGURE 13-5 ■ **Overinstrumentation. A and B,** Pretreatment radiographs of periodontally involved teeth. **C and D,** The same teeth 3 years later, after periodontal therapy and 11 maintenance visits. The roots have been planed to a substantially reduced dimension. This is an example of excessive root planing during the maintenance phase. (Courtesy of Dr. Thomas Bramanti.)

When the junctional epithelium has been injured or separated from the tooth surfaces, as it would be during periodontal debridement, healing can be expected to take approximately 1 week. Animal studies show that hemidesmosomes begin to reattach from the apical end of the junctional epithelium and are intact after 7 days. Normal turnover of cells in the junctional epithelium, which migrate from the apical end to the coronal end, takes about 5 days. Repair after disruption of the junctional epithelium during scaling procedures (not removal, which occurs with surgical excision) is similar to the normal course of events in tissue turnover.[25]

Inflammatory activity occurs in the underlying connective tissue during the disease process and is also a result of treatment. Connective tissue fibers are disrupted and lysed beneath the epithelium. Healing of inflamed connective tissue is complex, requiring many cells and mediators. It takes considerably longer than healing of epithelium—up to several months.[26] New connective tissue fiber attachment to the tooth surface is not a predictable outcome, but the development of an elongated junctional epithelial attachment may result in reduced probe readings. Because of the fragile state of healing connective tissues, probing after treatment should be avoided for 4 weeks.[17]

Repopulation of Microorganisms After Therapy
Scaling and periodontal debridement are effective in reducing the volume of plaque biofilm bacteria in treated sites. The numbers of organisms are reduced dramatically and grow back in different proportions. The bacterial plaque shifts from predominantly gram-negative microbiota to one that is gram-positive, with many fewer motile forms, especially spirochetes. These new microbiota are similar to those found in

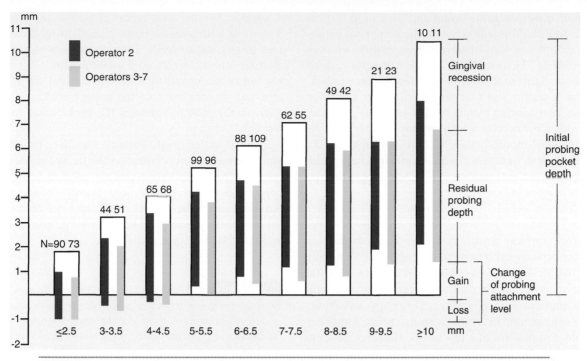

FIGURE 13-6 ■ Average values for gingival recession, residual probing depth, and gain or loss of clinical attachment 24 months after nonsurgical therapy compared with initial probing pocket depth. The mean values for clinician 2 are compared with the mean values for other clinicians, showing slight differences in results. (Used with permission from Baderstein A, Nilueus R, Egelberg J. Effect of non-surgical periodontal therapy. IV. Operator variability. *J Clin Periodontol.* 1985;12:190-200. Copyright 1985 Munksgaard International Publishers Ltd., Copenhagen, Denmark)

periodontally healthy sites. Bacteria repopulate in a specific order, starting with *Streptococcus* and *Actinobacillus* species, followed by *Veillonella, Bacteroides, Porphyromonas, Prevotella,* and *Fusobacterium* species. *Capnocytophaga* species and spirochetes are the last to grow back. The cycle may take as long as 6 months to complete.[8] Repopulation can be expected to vary for many reasons, one of which is clinician differences in complete removal of plaque biofilm and calculus.

Clinical Response

After thorough scaling and periodontal debridement procedures, the expected clinical response is a reduction in pocket depths, changes in attachment, recession, fewer bleeding sites, and less reddened tissue. Minimum amounts of new bone are generated after nonsurgical periodontal therapy. In contrast, bone growth can be seen after surgical interventions. Clinical results from a variety of studies on nonsurgical therapy have generally concluded the following:

- Shallower pockets are reduced less than deeper ones.
- Redness and bleeding are reduced dramatically.
- Healing is greatest 3 to 6 weeks after nonsurgical periodontal therapy.

Changes continue to occur up to 12 months after treatment, at which time the situation stabilizes.[25]

Data suggest that in pockets with initial probe depths of 1 to 3 mm, there is little pocket reduction, attachment loss of up to 0.89 mm after 5 years, and possibly slight recession of less than 1 mm. Pockets with initial depths of 4 to 6 mm tend to be reduced in probe depth by about 1 mm through attachment gain of about 0.5 mm, with recession making up the rest of the difference. Results of these studies vary, with longer studies showing more recession.

Deeper pockets of more than 7 mm showed the greatest pocket reduction, about 1.5 to 3 mm, made up of attachment gain of about 1 mm and the rest made up of recession of swollen gingiva. In the studies reviewed, the number of bleeding sites was reduced by 50% or more and gingival redness was reduced to almost zero after nonsurgical therapy.[25,26]

Baderstein and colleagues[27] found similar results in their study and noted that differences can occur among clinicians. Figure 13-6 shows that overall healing results were similar for all their subjects, but that one clinician generally achieved slightly less recession and possibly more attachment gain. Again, sites with deeper initial probe depths responded with greater improvements, with 2 mm or more reduction.

Attachment gain must be considered carefully. Attachment changes are computed by measuring periodontal probe depths and then adding the distance to a fixed reference point on the tooth, usually the cementoenamel junction. Periodontal probes penetrate the epithelial attachment by 1 mm or more, especially in inflamed tissue.[8] What is considered attachment gain may simply be a more accurate reading of probing pocket depth after healing from treatment. The periodontal probe is less likely to penetrate healed junctional epithelium and intact connective tissue fibers 4 weeks after scaling and root planing than inflamed tissue before treatment. The reevaluation probe depths, measured several weeks after treatment, probably reflect the histologic depth of pockets more accurately than the pretreatment probe depths. The reevaluation depths are important for monitoring the long-term results of treatment and determining whether more extensive periodontal therapy is needed. Results should not be evaluated at less than 3 or 4 weeks after therapy.[21]

Studies have suggested that it may be advantageous to scale the mouth in fewer longer sessions as opposed to the traditional four-quadrant, four-session approach used to treat chronic periodontitis. This would reduce the number of pathogens in the mouth and avoid bacterial repopulation in areas previously treated.[28] However, this approach has not gained wide acceptance. Some of these studies added the use of disinfectant agents to scaling and root planing in an attempt to be more effective in managing plaque biofilm and host response. Additional evidence is necessary to determine whether this full-mouth versus partial-mouth approach is clinically superior.[29] As with any periodontal treatment, numerous factors have to be considered in establishing a treatment plan, and longer therapy appointments may be indicated.

Sensitivity

Dentin, or root surface, sensitivity is commonly created or increased after periodontal treatment procedures. This usually occurs after surgical procedures, but often after periodontal debridement as well. Patients commonly return for a second or third appointment during nonsurgical therapy and report sensitivity to cold or toothbrushing in treated areas. Most sensitivity is mild and resolves in a few weeks. However, in some cases, sensitivity is extreme and inhibits patients' plaque control efforts. This sensitivity can lead to poor therapeutic results and possibly to caries formation. The dental hygienist must be aware of the causes and treatments available for dentin sensitivity and develop strategies to deal with this problem.

Dentin sensitivity, or root sensitivity, is often referred to as dentinal hypersensitivity, an extreme or unexpectedly elevated response to stimuli. Periodontal debridement results in the removal of some cementum and dentin because of the nature of the procedures, which expose some fresh dentin surfaces to the oral environment. Exposed dentin is sensitive, not necessarily hypersensitive, making "root sensitivity" a better descriptor of this condition.[30]

The hydrodynamic theory of dentin sensitivity is the generally accepted explanation for root sensitivity. Dentin can become sensitive when patent dentinal tubules are exposed to the oral environment. Tubules, which are filled with fluid, course from the tooth root surface directly to the pulp chamber of the tooth. The odontoblastic processes extend into the tubules at the pulpal ends. Hydrodynamic forces stimulate pain responses through these open tubules. Stimuli such as cold, sweet, acid (including plaque biofilm acids), drying, and scraping with metal instruments cause a rapid and immediate flow of the tubule contents outward, stimulating the odontoblastic processes and causing pain. The nerve fibers coursing around the odontoblasts are only capable of reacting with pain, so therefore all stimuli cause pain. Heat stimulation causes an inflow of fluid into the pulp chamber, also disturbing the nerve fibers. However, this pain reaction comes from fibers deeper in the pulp and can lead to a dull, aching pain in the jaw. Heat-stimulated pain is not considered dentin sensitivity but is a more serious indication of irreversible pulpal changes.[31,32]

No evidence of the incidence of sensitivity after periodontal therapy procedures is available. However, it is commonly reported anecdotally.[31] Subgingival scaling procedures, including periodontal debridement, caused post-treatment sensitivity to cold blasts of air in half of the subjects in one study, beginning immediately after treatment and diminishing in 3 to 4 weeks.[32] Another case report of postscaling sensitivity over 3 years of maintenance therapy resulted in the extraction of four lower anterior teeth. These teeth, viewed under scanning electron microscopy, showed odontoblastic processes protruding out of the dental tubules into the oral environment. The area was so sensitive that the patient could not tolerate the teeth in the mouth, although the periodontal condition was stable.[33]

Not all scaled teeth become sensitive, probably because scaling creates a smear layer over the treated surfaces. This layer contains crystalline debris (mostly calcium and phosphorus), covers the dentin surface, and greatly reduces fluid flow.[34] Scaling removes the existing smear layer and creates a new one; this layer is fragile and can be removed through toothbrushing and possibly by an acidic diet.[35]

> **CLINICAL NOTE 13-9** The dental hygienist should include a strategy for the treatment of sensitivity at the nonsurgical therapy appointment. If the patient reports more sensitive areas at subsequent appointments, the affected sites should be treated in the office and the patient should be sent home with information and products to help treat the sensitivity.

Several chemicals have been used in the dental office to treat sensitivity. Perhaps the most commonly used preparations are fluorides. A 33.3% paste of kaolin, glycerin, and sodium fluoride has been burnished into sensitive root surfaces for decades. This paste works because the burnishing action creates a smear layer, occluding tubules, rather than because of the precipitation of fluoride-rich crystals on the surface.[36] Calcium hydroxide in a water slurry has also been burnished onto sensitive surfaces and has provided immediate, if short-lived, relief.[37] Again, the burnishing may provide a protective smear layer. Cavity varnishes painted onto exposed surfaces can also provide relief.[37] Both potassium oxalate[38] and ferric oxalate[39] remove the smear layer and precipitate crystals, significantly occluding the dentinal tubules. These effects are relatively short-lived, lasting 1 to 2 weeks.[39]

To complicate the understanding of post-treatment root sensitivity, most roots go through a natural process of crystallization and occlusion of the open dentinal tubules. This process occurs a few weeks after treatment and often diminishes or eliminates postprocedural sensitivity. It is not clear how long a desensitizing agent works or how often it needs to be applied. Informing the patient and providing some form of immediate relief after therapy are often sufficient strategies. Plaque biofilm accumulation is also associated with increased sensitivity, so patients need to be encouraged to use good plaque biofilm control measures, even in sensitive areas. A soft-bristled brush with a light grasp can make plaque control easier for the affected patient.

Patients can use a variety of toothpastes for desensitizing the teeth at home. Some data suggest that pastes containing potassium nitrate or potassium citrate work effectively. Others containing strontium chloride have been available for many years and show evidence of efficacy.[40] One study showed that fluoride toothpastes may work as well as strontium chloride to provide relief.[41] These agents usually require regular use for several weeks. Once patients obtain relief, they are reluctant to give up the product. In the case of strontium chloride products, the clinician must also consider the benefits of regular fluoride use and either recommend products that contain fluoride or find another avenue to apply fluoride, such as office treatments or daily use of a fluoride mouth rinse.

The dental hygienist must have a strategy for helping patients with post-therapy sensitivity. This strategy should include the following:

- Warning the patient before treatment about possible sensitivity
- Treating existing sensitive areas with in-office therapies
- Prescribing home treatments

Often, the passage of time greatly reduces the problem, but these treatments can make the wait less painful and patients more comfortable.

PREDICTIVENESS OF RESULTS

Scaling and periodontal debridement are effective for the treatment of infectious periodontal disease.[6] They reliably result in decreased probing depths and less bleeding, increases in attachment in deep pockets, and a generally healthier oral environment in almost all cases. These results are reliable, even in cases of advanced periodontitis. Baderstein and colleagues[42] reported that outcomes from scaling and root planing were not compromised by the severity of lesions 24 months after treatment, regardless of whether treatment was performed with hand or ultrasonic instruments. Sites with deep initial probing depths showed a high incidence of attachment gain. In another analysis, Claffey and colleagues[43] showed that even deep initial probing depths tended to gain attachment after nonsurgical periodontal therapy. Subjects with higher proportions of attachment gain after therapy had few sites that lost attachment. They also reported that sites with probing attachment loss after 24 months were more frequently associated with bleeding, plaque, suppuration, and residual probing depth than sites that did not lose attachment. However, the predictability of any one clinical parameter has been shown to be low, so the need to record and consider attachment loss measurements was critical in evaluating the results.[44] At best, the predictability of attachment loss over 5 years was 30% for high plaque or bleeding scores and residual probing depth of 7 mm or more was 50% predictive. Probing depth that deepened by 1 mm or more was predictive of attachment loss approximately 80% of the time.[45]

CLINICAL NOTE 13-10 The dental hygienist should monitor patients carefully over time, evaluating probing depths and attachment loss. Even deep pockets can be stabilized through nonsurgical therapy. The presence of plaque biofilm and bleeding over time is a source of concern and should be addressed, but these events are not absolute signs of periodontal disease activity. Increases in probing depths or attachment loss are cause for concern, re-treatment, and possibly referral to a specialist.

TECHNIQUES

HAND INSTRUMENTATION

The use of hand scalers and curettes for instrumentation has a long tradition in periodontal therapy (Box 13-1). Universal curettes and sickles are among the oldest instrument designs. These instruments have cutting edges on both sides of the blade. Sickles have pointed ends and universal curettes have rounded ends. Area-specific curettes were first designed in the 1930s by Clayton Gracey,[46] and several variations exist today. Ultrasonic scaling instruments appeared in the 1960s and were a modification of an ultrasonic instrument designed to cut tooth structure. These instruments could not compete with high-speed drills, so they were modified for use as scalers. New instruments are introduced into the marketplace every year and more will undoubtedly be invented in the future as instrument companies respond to the needs of the dental community.

In addition to design differences between instruments, there are variations in materials. Most curette manufacturers use stainless steel. Carbon steel instruments are also available that hold a sharp cutting edge longer, but they are more brittle than stainless steel. In addition, some manufacturers treat their stainless steel curettes and sickles cryogenically and claim longer lasting sharpness of the cutting edges.

Periodontal instruments, such as scalers and curettes, have a tradition of success in therapeutic settings. Variations in designs and materials permit the dental hygienist to select instruments on the basis of personal preferences and treatment needs, and selections are often guided by what was taught during the educational process.

This section describes commonly used periodontal instruments, but it is not meant to be an inclusive list of the available options. Individual clinicians develop preferences for specific designs and materials.

Universal Curettes

Universal curettes are designed to adapt and instrument all surfaces of all teeth in the mouth. The curette blades have cutting edges on both sides and are usually double ended. Thus, one universal curette can scale around all the teeth in the dentition, explaining why they are called "universal."

Area-Specific Curettes

Area-specific curettes have been available since the 1930s. The first ones, designed by Gracey, are still popular today. Figure 13-7 illustrates a set of Gracey scalers as originally designed. The blades of the Gracey curettes have one cutting edge and are usually double-ended. The curettes are numbered to identify the recommended locations. Gracey 1/2, 3/4, and 5/6 curettes are generally used in the anterior areas, possibly the premolars. Gracey 7/8 and 9/10 curettes are designed to instrument the buccal and lingual surfaces of the posterior teeth. The Gracey 11/12 curette has extra bends in the shank to allow it to adapt to the mesial surfaces of the posterior teeth. The Gracey 13/14 curette adapts to the distal surfaces of the posterior teeth. Two modifications of the Gracey curette design are the Gracey 15/16 and 17/18. These are modifications of the current 11/12 and 13/14 designs that some clinicians believe provide better access to the mesial and distal

BOX 13-1   Evolution of Periodontal Instrument

As early as the tenth century BCE, scholars interested in oral health designed tooth scrapers and named them after themselves. Albucasis created a set of 14 scrapers, a few examples of which exist today. Pierre Fauchard, known as the "Father of Modern Dentistry," made many contributions to dentistry, including designing instruments that he named after himself. Other pioneers in periodontal therapy in the early twentieth century designed and refined scaling instruments and continued the naming tradition. Each refinement was expected to improve the usefulness of the instruments and improve the results of therapy. Hirshfeld, Hartzell, McCall, Bunting, and Gracey are some of the dentists whose instrument designs have outlived them and are still in use today.

John McCall wrote complaining of the crudeness of periodontal instruments in the 1930s and the fact that there seemed to be no philosophy about the most efficient method of instrumentation.[53] He believed that perfection of scaler designs and their use in treatment techniques were the basic requirements for success in periodontal therapy. Another twentieth-century pioneer, John Riggs, is credited with developing instruments that were designed for specific surfaces of the teeth and specific uses during treatment. Riggs' instruments were rustic by today's standards because they lacked contra-angled shanks. Hoe scalers and periodontal files were also introduced in the early twentieth century, but the designs were not refined until C.M. Carr introduced sets that included 18 groups of eight hoes, divided into three classes according to length of shank. Thus, a full set of instruments consisted of 144 hoes and six sickle scalers. Carr's extensive set of working end designs allowed scaling techniques to become more standardized and probably served to encourage others to continue to refine scaler designs. McCall worked to improve the

temper of metal scalers, thus making them stronger. Thomas Hartzell and Austin James refined the designs of Carr and McCall. Clinicians today continue to refine and improve instrument design with the same goal, that of improving therapeutic techniques and restoring periodontal health.[46]

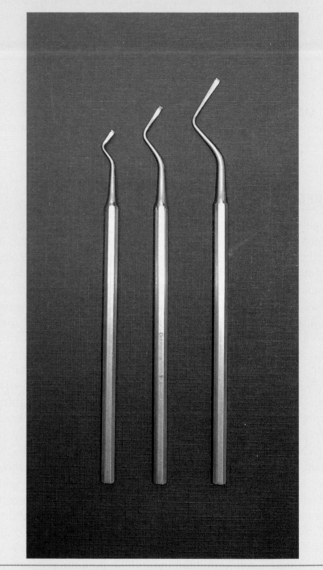

Detail of three hoes. Each working end design is the same, but the shanks vary in length to permit access into pockets of different depths.

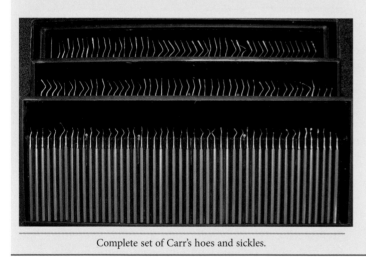

Complete set of Carr's hoes and sickles.

---

surfaces of the posterior teeth on one side of the mouth.

Modifications of the Gracey design have provided area-specific instruments with extended shanks to reach into deeper pockets. Also, a modification of the length and thickness of the blade has resulted in the availability of an area-specific curette series with smaller blades that adapt well to the healthier tissues of maintenance patients.[47] These options permit the dental hygienist to customize the instrumentation approach for specific situations. Examples of some modified Gracey instruments are presented in Figure 13-8.

Special Instruments

Sickle Scalers. Sickle scalers are designed to remove heavy calculus and are primarily used on supragingival calculus. The sickle design ends in a sharp point, making it unacceptable for scaling into periodontal pockets. The sickle has two cutting edges on each blade and can be adapted under the gingiva no more than 1 or 2 mm to break off ledges of calculus. It is a useful instrument when ultrasonic or sonic scaling is not an option. An example of sickle scalers is presented in Figure 13-9.

Hoes, Chisels, and Files. Hoes, chisels, and files are instruments designed for removing heavy calculus. Chisels are push

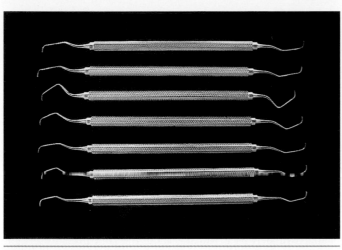

FIGURE 13-7 ■ A set of Gracey instruments as originally designed by Dr. Clayton Gracey in the 1930s. Bottom to top: 1/2, 3/4, 5/6, 7/8, 9/10, 11/12, and 13/14.

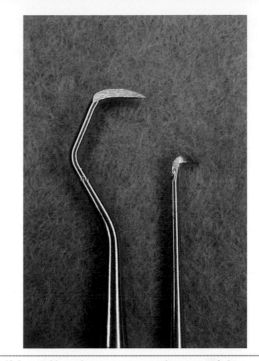

FIGURE 13-9 ■ Sickle scalers come in a wide variety of shapes and shank designs, but all have a characteristic shape with cutting edges on both sides that converge into a strong, sharp point. The sickle is useful for removing supragingival calculus and breaking off heavy ledges of deposits.

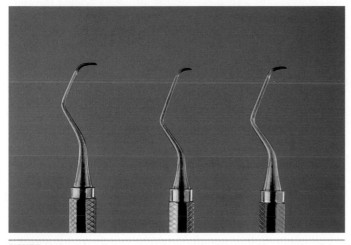

FIGURE 13-8 ■ The Gracey 7/8 instrument in three popular versions *(left to right)*: original design, shorter and thinner blade with a longer shank, and longer shank configuration.

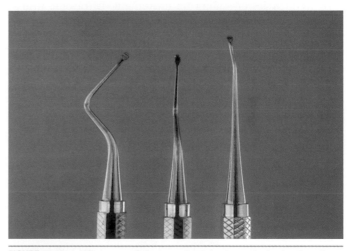

FIGURE 13-10 ■ Files are used for removing tenacious calculus but have been largely replaced by ultrasonic instrumentation.

instruments and hoes and files are pull instruments. All are designed to crush and disrupt heavy deposits of calculus; they are illustrated in Figure 13-10.

Expectation of Competence

The technical skill of the dental hygienist is the critical element in successful nonsurgical periodontal therapy. Variations in instrument design provide the dental hygienist with choices. Few studies have compared how well hand instruments perform calculus removal. Many dental hygienists believe that area-specific curettes work better on all teeth or on teeth with attachment loss. Other clinicians believe that universal curettes are the only acceptable instruments.

One study was initiated to compare conventional area-specific curettes with newly designed area-specific curettes with longer shanks, which are supposed to adapt better in deep pockets. In this study, Nagy and colleagues[47] evaluated 140 root surfaces instrumented for 15 minutes per tooth by standard rigid Gracey curettes or longer shank, rigid Gracey curettes. Probe depths were as great as 7 mm. Both types of curettes

worked equally well. Mesial surfaces were clean to a deeper level than other surfaces, but that was true for both types of curettes. These results indicate that the knowledge and skill of the dental hygienist are far more important than the particular type of instruments used. The type of instruments used should be personal choices.

It is more difficult to scale furcation areas than other surfaces. Calculus is routinely missed even when flaps are laid to permit access for scaling. One study compared scaling results on multirooted teeth with both hand and ultrasonic instruments. Results showed that even experienced clinicians left calculus in furcations most of the time. These clinicians used a variety of hand and ultrasonic instruments and spent 11.4 to 15.1 minutes scaling each tooth. Two points were clarified[48]:

- Experienced clinicians removed more calculus than inexperienced ones.
- Complete calculus removal in molar furcation areas is difficult, if not impossible, to achieve.

SONIC AND ULTRASONIC INSTRUMENTATION: POWERED SCALING

Sonic and ultrasonic instrumentation of tooth surfaces have been dramatically increasing in popularity. Powered instrumentation has the potential to make scaling less demanding, more time-efficient, and more ergonomically friendly.[49] For years, ultrasonic instruments were primarily recommended for heavy deposit removal. It was thought that their use had to be followed by hand instrumentation to remove necrotic root substance completely. As mentioned earlier, this theory is no longer accepted.

Much research has been conducted to evaluate the effectiveness of sonic and ultrasonic instrumentation. It is important to understand how well both sonic and ultrasonic instruments work in achieving the short- and long-term goals of nonsurgical periodontal therapy.

Ultrasonic and Sonic Devices

Ultrasonic scaling devices generate vibrations in the range of 20,000 to 50,000 cycles per second. These are separate units that use magnetostrictive or piezoelectric systems to generate ultra-high frequencies of scaling tip movement. Ultrasonic instruments work by a combination of mechanical forces, irrigation, cavitation, and acoustic streaming forces. Sonic scalers attach directly to the high-speed handpiece and generate vibrations of 3000 to 8000 cycles per second. The technique for using both sonic and ultrasonic instruments requires only that the tip be kept moving rapidly to prevent overheating the tooth and in constant contact with the tooth surface to remove calculus. The motion of the tip can be elliptical or linear, depending on the particular device. No lateral pressure is applied because lateral force applied during powered instrumentation can cause severe root damage.[50-52]

Ultrasonic and sonic scalers have been compared in laboratory settings with extracted teeth. In these settings, both ultrasonic and sonic scalers remove calculus effectively and sonic scalers were at least as effective as ultrasonic scalers for calculus removal, if not slightly better. In terms of root surface roughness and removal of tooth structure, ultrasonic instruments caused slightly less trauma to the roots than sonic instruments. However, all root damage was superficial and localized. Overall, the cemental surfaces were left smooth. In addition, the time required to achieve good results was similar for both types of powered scalers. No damage was seen that would contraindicate the use of either type of scaler.[51] Studies comparing sonic, piezoelectric, and magnetostrictive scalers show nearly equivalent clinical results, despite a wide variation of the relative frequencies and differences in the directional movement of the tips.[53]

Plaque Removal

Ultrasonic instrumentation is remarkably efficient at removing plaque biofilm from root surfaces.[52] Cavitation, the inwardly collapsing bubbles of water that are produced as the stream touches the vibrating tip, appears to have an antimicrobial effect in lysing the bacterial walls and flushing debris out of the pockets. The stream of fluid also reaches the bottom of the pocket, providing a flushing effect during treatment.[54] The removal of plaque biofilms can be readily accomplished with power-driven scalers at a level comparable to that of hand instrumentation.

Endotoxin Removal

In vitro studies verify that ultrasonic instrumentation is as effective as hand instrumentation in removing endotoxins (detoxifying) from root surfaces. Fibroblast attachment occurs equally on diseased root surfaces after either type of instrumentation.[55] Endotoxins (lipopolysaccharides) embedded in the root surface are removed by ultrasonic scaling with overlapping light strokes of approximately 50 g, which is about the same pressure as light probing. Root surfaces treated this way for 0.8 seconds/mm^2 have the same root surface properties as scaled periodontally healthy teeth and no residual endotoxins.[56] Clearly, endotoxins can be removed with ultrasonic scaling; however, they can also be removed with washing, brushing, or lightly scaling the contaminated root surface.

Calculus Removal

Dragoo[57] demonstrated that ultrasonic tips are effective in calculus removal. With the use of a curette efficiency index, in which a score of 1 meant no calculus present and a score of 3 indicated gross amounts, he compared standard ultrasonic tips with newly designed thinner tips and hand curettes. The thinner ultrasonic tips were 16% to 27% more effective in calculus removal than hand curettes and 27% to 46% better than standard ultrasonic tips. All instruments reached to within approximately 1 mm of the apical extent of pockets, and the thin ultrasonic tips appeared to clean more efficiently in the deeper areas.

A number of clinical studies have compared calculus removal with an ultrasonic device to hand instruments. Judges who were blinded to the type of experimental treatment found no difference in post-treatment healing.[58] Other studies have further attempted to establish superiority of power scaling devices over hand instrumentation and have concluded that both approaches are effective for scaling and root planing.[59,60]

Root Smoothness: Short-Term Goal of Nonsurgical Therapy

Root smoothness is the yardstick where by the dental hygienist determines the end point of scaling and root planing. It is a short-term goal of nonsurgical therapy and it is the objective achieved during every treatment. Explorer examination of root surfaces to determine the presence of calculus or root smoothness is a valuable tool for the dental hygienist. Some clinicians prefer to use the periodontal probe for this evaluation. Whatever instrument is used, if clicks and bumps of calculus are felt, the teeth should be instrumented until they are smooth. All the surfaces in a specific patient should be instrumented to approximately the same degree of smoothness. If an area on a root surface feels rougher than other treated areas, missed or residual calculus must be suspected and the area should be treated again. All surfaces should be clean of plaque biofilm and free of calculus. These smooth surfaces do not require that the cementum be shaved off by further systematic instrumentation. All treated dentitions should feel smooth and calculus-free after treatment.

Healing After Treatment: Long-Term Goal of Nonsurgical Therapy

Although laboratory and clinical evaluations of the efficiency of calculus removal are of interest, the important comparison between ultrasonic instrumentation and hand instrumentation is healing after therapy. These comparisons evaluate the long-term goal of nonsurgical periodontal therapy, which is healing of the periodontal tissues, and provide the basis for selecting and determining the future course of treatment for the periodontal patient. Healing after treatment of moderate and advanced periodontitis was reported in studies by Baderstein and colleagues[26,42] in the 1980s; half the mouth was treated by hand instrumentation and the other half by ultrasonic instrumentation. Subsequent examination verified that hand and ultrasonic instruments both achieved the long-term goals of therapy; the type of instrument used was secondary to the excellence of technique.

Specifically, Baderstein and colleagues[44] evaluated 15 subjects with moderately advanced periodontitis over a period of 13 months. Plaque, bleeding, probing depth, and attachment loss were measured. Subjects were given oral hygiene instructions repeatedly during the first month of the study. Instrumentation was performed and subjects were evaluated 1 month after treatment. Monthly clinical assessments were performed for 13 months, and teeth were reinstrumented 2 and 6 months after the first treatment. The percentage of surfaces with plaque was reduced from 65% to 73% to about 12% after the oral hygiene instruction and remained at that level throughout the study. Importantly, the percentage of bleeding surfaces ranged from 77% to 90% before treatment and changed substantially. This percentage was not reduced by oral hygiene instruction alone but by instrumentation to 36% to 41% at 2 months and 8% to 16% by 6 months. That percentage then remained at the 6-month level. Mean probing depths were 4.1 to 4.5 mm at the beginning of the study. Oral hygiene alone reduced probing depths by 0.03 to 0.07 mm. One month after instrumentation, depths were reduced by 0.5 to 0.7 mm and, at 4 months, pockets were reduced by 1.3 to 1.7 mm and remained at that level. Attachment loss also changed over the course of the study. Shallow pockets lost little attachment, as expected, and deep pockets of 7 mm or more gained 1.1 to 1.5 mm in attachment. Quadrants were randomly assigned to hand instrumentation or ultrasonic instrumentation, and an examiner who was blind to the treatments evaluated all the subjects. There was no difference between the results achieved by hand instrumentation and those achieved by ultrasonic instrumentation.

The same researchers also evaluated subjects with more advanced periodontal disease in a study of similar design. Subjects had probe depths of greater than 5 mm, and many depths of 8, 9, and 10 mm were included in the study. The same parameters were evaluated. First, oral hygiene instruction was given. Three months later, the teeth were instrumented and then they were reinstrumented at 6 and 9 months. Subjects were evaluated monthly for 24 months. Plaque was reduced significantly by the oral hygiene instruction and the level remained stable throughout the study. Bleeding initially occurred on 84% to 90% of

the surfaces. Little effect was seen with oral hygiene alone, and the percentage of bleeding sites was reduced to 14% to 18% at 12 months after instrumentation. Mean probing depths were 5.5 to 5.8 mm. They were reduced to 5.1 to 5.3 mm by oral hygiene and further reduced to 3.6 to 3.9 mm 12 months after the first instrumentation. Notable recession was seen over 12 months, 1.6 to 1.8 mm. The attachment loss pattern was similar to that of other studies; shallow pockets lost attachment slightly and deeper pockets tended to gain attachment. The treatment results did not differ between quadrants scaled with hand instruments and those scaled with ultrasonic instruments.[26]

The decision to use ultrasonic instruments rather than or in addition to hand instruments when providing nonsurgical periodontal therapy should be based on the preference of the dental hygienist and the patient.[53] Both treatments are effective and achieve the short- and long-term goals of scaling and periodontal debridement.[61,62]

CLINICAL NOTE 13-11   Both hand and power scalers are effective modalities and achieve the short- and long-term goals of periodontal debridement.

Contraindication

There is one contraindication to treatment with ultrasonic scaling. The electromagnetic field generated in the handpiece can interfere with the functioning of some cardiac pacemakers. Most pacemakers, but not all, are shielded and are not affected by this field. The dental hygienist cannot determine which type of pacemaker the patient may be wearing. In fact, the patient may not know. To ensure that powered scaling will do no harm, ultrasonic instruments should not be used on patients with pacemakers. In addition, dentists and dental hygienists who wear pacemakers should not operate ultrasonic devices.[63] Sonic scalers do not create an electromagnetic field and may be used as a substitute.[53] There are no U.S. Food and Drug Administration (FDA) warnings on these devices but caution should be exercised when the clinician is unsure of the status of the patient's pacemaker.

Aerosols

Infection control is a constant and critical part of dental hygiene practice. The application of universal infection control standards is an absolute requirement of the Occupational Health and Safety Administration (OSHA). These requirements indicate that contaminated splatter and aerosol spray be minimized in dental and dental hygiene practice. Obviously, a rapidly moving, water-cooled device such as an ultrasonic tip will create substantial splatter and aerosol. Aerosols generated by subgingival powered scaling contain blood.[64] The prevention of disease transmission and use of barrier techniques during powered scaling procedures is therefore essential. Dental hygienists and dentists must wear appropriate face masks and protective eyewear when using these devices.[65] High-volume suction devices can significantly reduce the amount of aerosol contamination.[66,67]

Patients rinsing for 30 seconds with an antiseptic mouthwash before ultrasonic scaling reduce recoverable colony-forming bacterial units from aerosols by 93%. Rinsing with a nonantiseptic mouthwash reduces the bacterial counts by 33%.[65] Preprocedural rinsing may help to reduce bacteria, but its effect on viruses is unknown. In addition, blood borne contaminants inoculated into the aerosol and splatter by subgingival ultrasonic scaling are not likely to be affected by preprocedural rinsing. In practice, preprocedural rinsing is not a required component of infection control. If it is adopted by individual dental hygienists or clinics, it must be used for every patient to meet the requirement of universal infection control, not selectively on patients who are known to be infectious.

New and Old Designs for Tips

The studies described earlier demonstrating long-term healing after nonsurgical periodontal therapy compared hand instruments with conventional ultrasonic insert designs that have been available for decades. The results clearly indicated that standard ultrasonic tip designs worked as well as hand instruments.

Until the 1980s, all ultrasonic inserts and sonic tips were fairly thick and blunt. Some were curved in various dimensions. Many dental hygienists found them awkward to use subgingivally. Some dentists and dental hygienists began to sharpen and reshape the tips to make them more adaptable. Sharpening resulted in thinning the diameter of the tips rather than creating a cutting edge. These recontoured tips have been used successfully and safely. Dragoo[57] advocated the use of these recontoured tips exclusively and showed in laboratory experiments that thin, curved tips reached more deeply than traditional designs and cleaned more efficiently than hand curettes. Piezoelectric tips have also been sharpened and reduced in dimension to make them more adaptable. Thin, curved ultrasonic tips now available commercially for use with various ultrasonic units make subgingival access more attainable. Diamond-coated inserts are also available and have shown greater root surface removal and greater residual root surface roughness after use.[68] Caution should be used with any insert during powered scaling. The thinner, curved tips adapt very well into deeper pockets and furcations. The handles of some inserts have been improved, providing an ergonomic benefit to the clinician. The dental hygienist should sample several designs and select those that are the most comfortable and the most efficient.

> **CLINICAL NOTE 13-12** Power-driven instruments may increase efficiency, reduce time spent per tooth, and be less demanding physically for the dental hygienist. Patients occasionally respond negatively to the use of powered scalers, so the use of these devices must be evaluated for each patient.

LASERS

Lasers were introduced into dentistry in the latter half of the twentieth century and have been applied to a growing number of clinical uses. Many are now approved by the FDA for a variety of dental uses.

Each type of laser has specific characteristics and applications as a result of its wavelength and waveform.[69] Laser tissue interactions are dependent on the combination of laser parameters (emission wavelength, amount of electrical power, pulse duration, and amount of energy delivered to the tissue) and the characteristics of the tissue that allow the laser light to be absorbed.

In periodontics, lasers have been used for calculus removal, reduction of subgingival bacterial biota, "sterilization" of periodontal pockets, enhanced root instrumentation, and periodontal surgery. Diode and neodymium:yttrium-aluminum-garnet (Nd:YAG) lasers are absorbed by pigmented granulation tissue and can be used for sulcular debridement. Surgical applications for dental lasers involve photothermal events (light is absorbed by the tissue and the tissue is heated). The most common lasers for soft tissue use are the Nd:YAG, diode, erbium, and carbon dioxide lasers. Nd:YAG lasers have been shown to be safe for use on periodontal soft tissues. They have been evaluated and can be successfully used for gingival curettage to the epithelial lining of the pockets. Some researchers reported that incision and excision of the gingiva, gingivectomy, and biopsy could also be safely performed with these devices.[70,71] However, there is minimal evidence to support the use of lasers for subgingival debridement or the reduction of subgingival microbial levels.

The erbium lasers (Er:YAG and ErCr:YSGG) have also been evaluated for nonsurgical periodontal procedures in a number of studies but have shown mixed results. Er:YAG laser scaling resulted in increased loss of cementum and dentin on extracted teeth.[72] Although a slight benefit in attachment levels has been shown in some studies, further investigation is needed to determine if scaling and root planing can be enhanced with the use of lasers.

Lasers are currently viewed by some as an adjunct in periodontal therapy for removal of soft tissue within the periodontal pocket. With the use of typical clinical indicators such as pocket depth, clinical attachment levels, and plaque index scores, laser scaling has shown results that are equal but not superior to scaling and root planing alone.[71-73] Little evidence exists to support the concept that lasers are more effective than current nonsurgical therapies using hand or powered instruments. Improved healing of periodontal lesions after the use of lasers for periodontal surgery is not supported by research.[72] Lasers are appropriately used as an adjunct to periodontal therapy but are not a substitute for conventional periodontal treatment at this time. Lasers are also used for caries removal and cavity preparation, primarily for minimally invasive restorative procedures.[74]

Lasers are a promising technology with growing numbers of applications in dentistry. Further research will define and provide evidence for specific laser applications in nonsurgical and surgical periodontal therapies.

MAGNIFICATION

There are several technologies available to increase the visibility of the teeth and tissues during periodontal treatment. These options, which provide magnification of the treatment area, are valuable in diagnosis and treatment. **Magnification** is especially valuable for protecting the musculoskeletal system of the clinician because it makes it easier to sit up straight while working and enhances visual acuity. Many dental hygienists have reported improvements in nonsurgical treatment results for patients and decreases in muscle pain and eye fatigue for themselves as a result of the use of loupes, endoscopes, or microscopes.[75]

Loupes, or eyeglass-mounted telescopes, magnify the field of vision up to six times actual size. A variety of loupes are available and each has features that may appeal to the clinician. Loupes should be custom-fitted to the user and are easy to adapt to in the clinical setting. Some individuals complain of the weight on the nose, but most find the improvement in vision and physical posture well worth the adjustment to the working environment.

The dental endoscope allows subgingival visualization and illumination to the working field at magnifications in the range of 24 to 48 times. The clinician views a video monitor that displays the magnified image transmitted by fiberoptics attached to a subgingival probe. The subgingival root surfaces and soft tissues are magnified and illuminated, and the clinician can see into the periodontal pockets for instrumentation and irrigation. Indications for use of the endoscope are nonsurgical therapy, nonresponding cases, patients with deep pockets who refuse surgery or who are not candidates for surgery, and identification of subgingival conditions.[76] The technology is expensive and mastery requires some practice. Clinicians who have adopted this tool report anecdotally that it helps them to improve treatment responses. However, thus far, comparison studies evaluating typical clinical measurements have not found statistically significant results with the use of endoscopy compared with traditional scaling and root planing.[77]

Microscopes are commonly used for magnification and have been adapted for use chairside in dentistry, especially in endodontics and restorative dentistry.

Cost is a factor with any of these magnification devices and adapting to the particular aspects of the technology is challenging for the most accomplished clinicians. However, dental hygienists report benefits, including improved access, better clinical results, and greater clinician comfort because of improved ergonomic factors.[78,79]

ANTIMICROBIAL AGENTS

SYSTEMIC ANTIMICROBIAL AGENTS

Pharmacologic agents are used systemically in certain types of periodontal disease and conditions to help control the disease process. Systemic antibiotics can be used along with nonsurgical instrumentation in a comprehensive treatment plan to reduce the bacterial load and enhance the host's defense to the infectious oral pathogens in chronic periodontitis, aggressive periodontitis, and periodontitis as a manifestation of systemic diseases, such as diabetes mellitus. Antibiotics are prescribed by the dentist for the patient to take orally. Common antibiotics used to treat periodontal diseases are tetracycline, doxycycline, and occasionally penicillin.

The use of antibiotics is based on the patient's medical and dental history, periodontal diagnosis, and evaluation of possible side effects related to the particular drug. Use and overuse of antibiotics worldwide has led to the emergence of resistant microorganisms, so this adjunctive treatment is not to be used indiscriminately. Microbial sampling of infected pockets is recommended to identify the infecting organism and permit selection of the appropriate antibiotic to target that organism.[80] Systemic antibiotics are particularly effective in aggressive forms of periodontitis, refractory periodontitis, or the treatment of multiple sites in advanced disease.[81] These adjuncts to nonsurgical therapy are important aspects of the collaborative care provided by the dentist and dental hygienist. Antibiotic therapy is described in greater detail in Chapter 7 as it relates to specific forms of periodontal disease.

IRRIGATION WITH ANTIMICROBIAL AGENTS

Use of local antimicrobial adjuncts in nonsurgical periodontal therapy has become commonplace. Rinsing with an antimicrobial mouth rinse has negligible effects on subgingival biota. However, antimicrobial agents used for irrigation penetrate to the bottom of the periodontal pockets if applied with a syringe or with irrigation devices with a soft rubber tip or a canula.[82]

Irrigation is the term used to refer to a lavage, or flushing, of pockets during or after periodontal debridement procedures. The bacterial population is vastly reduced through mechanical removal during nonsurgical therapy whether instrumentation is performed with hand or powered scalers. For an antimicrobial agent delivered as an irrigant to have an additional effect, several requirements must be met[82]:

- The agent must reach the site of disease activity, the base of the pockets.
- Antimicrobial agents must be used at bactericidal concentrations.
- Medicaments must be substantive or present long enough to work.

Effective antimicrobial products that have been used as irrigants include 0.12% chlorhexidine, 0.4% stannous fluoride, and 0.05% povidone-iodine.[83,84] It has been shown that irrigation treatment without previous scaling reduces effectiveness so that microbe levels rebound completely in just a few days[82] compared with scaling and root planing, which suppresses microbial populations for 2 to 6 months. Microbial suppression is not increased when a one-time irrigation is used after periodontal debridement.[83] Even a substantive antimicrobial such as chlorhexidine would have to be available in the pocket for many days to interfere with plaque biofilm regrowth after scaling. It would appear that mechanical scaling and root planing is the primary antimicrobial treatment and that one-time, office-applied irrigation is not reliable in augmenting its effects.

Shiloah and Hovious[84] agreed that irrigation during nonsurgical therapy has limited effects but reported improved probing depths after 1 year when ultrasonic periodontal debridement was performed with 0.05% povidone-iodine as an irrigant. This evidence suggests that antimicrobial irrigation

TABLE 13-3 Commonly Used Antimicrobial Agents for Periodontal Diseases

ANTIMICROBIAL	COMMERCIAL AGENT	PRODUCT FORM	COMMENTS
Minocycline	Arestin	Microspheres	Placed with syringe Biodegrades
Doxycycline	Atridox	Gel	Placed with syringe Biodegrades
Chlorhexidine	PerioChip	Disk	Placed with instrument Biodegrades

during nonsurgical periodontal therapy may be beneficial if it is performed under the right conditions. The adjunctive effects of one-time irrigation, if any, may occur in hard to scale areas such as furcations and deeper pockets.[85-87]

LOCAL DELIVERY

Antimicrobial agents incorporated in time-release delivery devices solve the major problem presented by irrigation, that of retaining the drug at the site for many hours or days after scaling and root planing. These delivery systems allow a concentration of a specific drug to be placed in active or nonresponsive periodontal pockets to achieve a therapeutic effect. A number of them are available for use in the form of strips, chips, microcapsules, and gels. Drugs placed by syringe delivery or chips or films placed in the periodontal pocket provide high concentrations of the drug in the local area but low serum concentrations. The drug and its delivery system are gradually resorbed by the body over a few days.

The antiseptic chlorhexidine and the antibiotics tetracycline, minocycline, and doxycycline can be delivered by this route. Each has been evaluated in clinical trials and shown to reduce pocket depths and improve clinical attachment levels by modest amounts, about 1 mm, when placed locally after scaling and root planing.[88-90] These drugs are further described in Chapter 7; those commonly used are listed in Table 13-3.

The positive results of locally delivered agents are encouraging, but the majority of rigorous studies have shown relatively small improvements in pocket depths and attachment levels.[83] These drug delivery systems do not routinely provide a superior result compared with scaling and root planing alone.[90] For these reasons, the indications for local site delivery of antimicrobial agents are limited to severe forms of disease and nonresponsive conditions, including the following:

• Advanced chronic periodontitis
• Refractory periodontitis
• Recurrent periodontal disease

CLINICAL NOTE 13-14 There is no identified agent that is a substitute for scaling and root planing. Home use of locally delivered antimicrobial agents may be beneficial in residual pockets and furcation areas when used regularly by patients.

Ramfjord[21] defined the true measure of the quality of life for periodontal patients as the function and preservation of

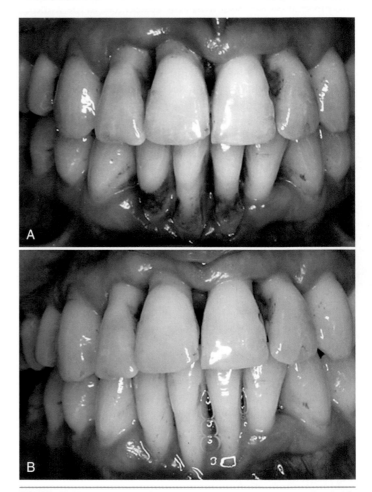

FIGURE 13-11 ■ **Nonsurgical therapy provides consistent and reliable results. A,** A 55-year-old patient with moderate to severe chronic periodontitis characterized by poor plaque biofilm control, 4- to 6-mm probing depths, significant attachment loss in the anterior areas, and heavy deposits of calculus. **B,** The same patient 4 weeks after completion of nonsurgical periodontal therapy.

the teeth in an aesthetic state with a minimum of sensitive teeth.

Meticulous root debridement, coupled with compliance with maintenance regimens, both regular recall visits and daily oral hygiene routines, provide reliable and predictable nonsurgical periodontal therapy; there are adjunctive therapies that can improve treatment results in difficult or unresponsive cases. An example of the effectiveness of nonsurgical periodontal therapy is seen in Figure 13-11.

Root smoothness is a matter of clinical judgment, but it should reflect calculus-free surfaces.

DENTAL HYGIENE CONSIDERATIONS

- Polishing is primarily a cosmetic procedure that should be applied selectively.
- Gingival curettage provides no predictable improvements to healing.
- Dentin sensitivity is a common finding after periodontal debridement procedures and should be treated with office-applied desensitizers and home treatment.
- The appropriate reevaluation time when probing will provide reliable measurements of probe depths and attachment loss is 4 weeks after nonsurgical therapy.
- Shallower probe depths can be expected to reduce in depth about 1 mm after nonsurgical therapy and deeper pockets will resolve by about 2 mm.
- Hand and powered instruments are equally effective for scaling, root planing, and biofilm removal.
- Lasers are used increasingly in dentistry and may have some application in periodontal therapy, but no evidence has shown them to be superior to other treatment techniques at this time.
- Magnification is useful for dental hygienists because it provides an improved view of the working area and permits more ergonomic posture during treatment appointments.

CASE SCENARIO

Ms. Nicholas is a 34-year-old white female. She is reported to be in excellent health, has no history of systemic disease and no medical contraindications to treatment, and currently takes no medications nor does she use recreational drugs. She works at a law firm and is raising a family of two children. Ms. Nicholas has not been to see a dentist for 14 years due to her focus on her education, her growing family, and her career. She knows that she needs to have regular dental and dental hygiene care and is now committed to making it a priority. Ms. Nicholas presents with no active decay, and the only restorations are Class I amalgams on her molars. Her gingiva is reddened and bleeds easily; she has generalized 4- to 5-mm probing depths and 1 mm of recession on the buccal surfaces of her teeth. You identify some supragingival calculus in the lower anterior and find that she has subgingival ledges of calculus in rings around all of her teeth. She asks you what your treatment will include, if it will be painful, and what results will occur.

1. The treatment plan for Ms. Nicholas is likely to include
   A. gross scaling and plaque biofilm removal instructions.
   B. quadrant scaling and root planing and plaque biofilm removal instructions.
   C. full-mouth scaling at one appointment and plaque biofilm removal instructions.
   D. full-mouth scaling and root planing at one appointment and plaque biofilm removal instructions.
2. How long after completing the Phase I therapy should you permit healing to occur before reassessing Ms. Nicholas's periodontal condition?
   A. 1 week
   B. 2 weeks
   C. 3 weeks
   D. 4 weeks

3. How much resolution to the 4- and 5-mm probing pocket depths do you expect to find upon reassessment?
   A. 1 mm
   B. 2 mm
   C. 3 mm
   D. Cannot be predicted
4. Reductions in probing pocket depths are related to
   A. decreased inflammation and shrinkage of the gingival tissues.
   B. decreased penetration of the probe tip at the base of the pocket related to connective tissue healing.
   C. increased penetration of the probe tip at the base of the pocket related to connective tissue healing.
   D. both decreased inflammation and decreased penetration of the probe tip at the base of the pockets.
   E. both decreased inflammation and increased penetration of the probe tip at the base of the pockets.
5. Based on the presence of generalized recession, what additional considerations should you have in mind for future treatment?
   A. Susceptibility to root caries
   B. Susceptibility to coronal caries
   C. Post-treatment root sensitivity
   D. Both caries potential and root surface sensitivity

STUDY QUESTIONS

Answers and rationales to these questions can be obtained from your instructor.

MULTIPLE CHOICE

1. The goal of periodontal instrumentation is to return the periodontium to a state of health. Periodontal health is achieved through surgical therapy techniques.
   A. Both statements are true.
   B. Both statements are false.
   C. The first statement is true, and the second statement is false.
   D. The first statement is false, and the second statement is true.
2. The concept of periodontal pathogens associated with different types of periodontal disease is called
   A. aggressive periodontitis.
   B. nonaggressive periodontitis.
   C. nonspecific plaque hypothesis.
   D. specific plaque hypothesis.
3. Complete calculus removal with hand or powered instruments is a goal for the dental hygienist. Calculus is the etiologic agent in periodontal disease.
   A. Both statements are true.
   B. Both statements are false.
   C. The first statement is true, and the second statement is false.
   D. The first statement is false, and the second statement is true.

4. The term for removal of the inflamed soft tissue wall lining the periodontal pocket is
   A. root planing.
   B. gingival curettage.
   C. selective polishing.
   D. subgingival curettage.

5. Experimental evidence indicates that rough root surfaces are mechanical irritants. Rough root surfaces delay healing.
   A. Both statements are true.
   B. Both statements are false.
   C. The first statement is true, and the second statement is false.
   D. The first statement is false, and the second statement is true.

6. Air powder polishing works by application of a mechanical abrasion slurry of
   A. calcium and phosphorus.
   B. potassium nitrate.
   C. sodium bicarbonate and water.
   D. toothpaste.

7. Root smoothness achieves all of the following EXCEPT one. Which one is the EXCEPTION?
   A. Delays tissue attachment
   B. Enhances self-cleaning
   C. Promotes healing
   D. Retards plaque formation
   E. Sooths irritated tissues

8. Attachment gain after nonsurgical therapy should be measured carefully because inflamed tissues may not provide an accurate reading.
   A. Both the statement and reason are correct and related.
   B. Both the statement and reason are correct but NOT related.
   C. The statement is correct, but the reason is NOT correct.
   D. The statement is NOT correct, but the reason is correct.
   E. NEITHER the statement NOR the reason is correct.

SHORT ANSWER

9. Describe the difference between scaling and root planing.
10. Compare the short- and long-term goals of nonsurgical therapy.

Ⓔ Please visit **http://evolve.elsevier.com/Perry/periodontology** for additional practice and study support tools.

REFERENCES

1. Lindhe J. *Textbook of Clinical Periodontology.* Philadelphia, PA: WB Saunders; 1983:327–352.
2. Carranza FA, Takei HH. The treatment plan. In: Newman MG, Takei HH, Klokkevold PR, et al, eds. *Carranza's Clinical Periodontology.* 11th ed. St. Louis, MO: Elsevier Saunders; 2012:384–386.
3. Perry DA, Takei HH. Phase I periodontal therapy. In: Newman MG, Takei HH, Klokkevold PR, et al, eds. *Carranza's Clinical Periodontology.* 11th ed. St. Louis, MO: Elsevier Saunders; 2012:448–451.
4. American Academy of Periodontology. *Glossary of Periodontal Terms.* 4th ed. Chicago, IL: American Academy of Periodontology; 2001.
5. Matsuda SA, Wilkins EM. Nonsurgical periodontal instrumentation. In: Wilkins EM, ed. *Clinical Practice of the Dental Hygienist.* 11th ed. Philadelphia, PA: Lippincott Williams &Wilkins; 2011:608–638.
6. American Academy of Periodontology; Comprehensive periodontal therapy: a statement by the American Academy of Periodontology. *J Periodontol.* 2011; 82:943–949.
7. Loomer PM, Armitage GC. Microbiology of periodontal diseases. In: Rose LF, Mealey BL, eds. *Periodontics: Medicine, Surgery and Implants.* St. Louis, MO: Elsevier Mosby; 2004:69–84.
8. Armitage GC. *Biologic Basis of Periodontal Maintenance Therapy.* Berkeley, CA: Praxis; 1980:33–115.
9. Wilkins EM. *Clinical Practice of the Dental Hygienist.* 4th ed. St. Louis, MO: Lea & Febiger; 1976.
10. Barnes CM. Extrinsic stain removal. In: Wilkins EM, ed. *Clinical Practice of the Dental Hygienist.* 11th ed. Philadelphia, PA: Lippincott Williams & Wilkins; 2013:689–708.
11. Barnes CM. Shining a new light on selective polishing. *Dimens Dent Hyg.* 2012; 10(3):42. 44.
12. American Academy of Periodontology. Statement regarding gingival curettage. *J Periodontol.* 2002;73:19–1230.
13. Cobb CM. Non-surgical pocket therapy: mechanical. *Ann Periodontol.* 1996;1:443–490.
14. Löe H, Theilade E, Jensen SB. Experimental gingivitis in man. *J Periodontol.* 1965;36:177–187.
15. Loesche WJ. The bacterial etiology of periodontal disease: the specific plaque hypothesis. Clark JW, ed. *Clinical Dentistry.* Philadelphia, PA: JB Lippincott; 1987:1–11.
16. Teughels W, Quirynen M, Jakubovics N. Periodontal microbiology. In: Newman MG, Takei HH, Klokkevold PR, et al. eds. *Carranza's Clinical Periodontology.* 11th ed. St. Louis, MO: Elsevier Saunders; 2012:232–270.
17. Ciancio S. Non-surgical periodontal treatment. In: Nevins M, Becker W, Kornman K, eds. *Proceedings of the World Workshop in Clinical Periodontics.* Chicago, IL: American Academy of Periodontology; 1989; II-1–II-20.
18. Kepic TJ, O'Leary TJ, Kafrawy AH. Total calculus removal: an attainable objective? *J Periodontol.* 1990;61:16–20.
19. Stambaugh RV, Dragoo M, Smith DM, et al. The limits of subgingival scaling. *Int J Periodont Res Dent.* 1981;1:30–41.
20. Nyman R, Westfelt E, Sarhed G, et al. Role of "diseased" root cementum in healing following treatment of periodontal disease: a clinical study. *J Clin Periodontol.* 1988;15:464–468.
21. Ramfjord SP. Long-term assessment of periodontal surgery versus curettage or scaling and root planing. *Int J Technol Assess Health Care.* 1990;6:392–402.
22. Kalkwarf KL. Tissue attachment. In: Nevins M, Becker W, Kornman K, eds. *Proceedings of the World Workshop in Clinical Periodontics.* Chicago, IL: American Academy of Periodontology; 1989;V-1–V-21.
23. Yukna RA. A clinical and histological study of healing following the excisional new attachment procedure in rhesus monkeys. *J Periodontol.* 1976;47:701–709.
24. DeVore CH, Hicks MJ, Whitacre HL, et al. Non-surgical gingival curettage in dental hygiene curricula. *J Dent Educ.* 1993:762–765.
25. Robertson PB, Buchanan SA. Wound healing after periodontal therapy. In: Genco RJ, Goldman HM, Cohen DW, eds. *Contemporary Periodontics.* St. Louis, MO: Mosby; 1990:382–393.
26. Baderstein A, Nilveus R, Egelberg J. Effect of non-surgical periodontal therapy. II: Severely advanced periodontitis. *J Clin Periodontol.* 1984;11:63–76.
27. Baderstein A, Nilveus R, Egelberg J. Effect of non-surgical periodontal therapy. IV: Operator variability. *J Clin Periodontol.* 1985;12:190–200.
28. Mongardini C, Van Steenberghe D, Dekeyser C, et al. One stage full-verses partial-mouth disinfection in the treatment of chronic adult or generalized early-onset periodontitis. I: Long-term clinical observations. *J Periodontol.* 1999;70:632–645.
29. Greenstein G. Full-mouth therapy verses individual quadrant root planing: a critical commentary. *J Periodontol.* 2002;73:797–812.
30. Newbrun E. Dentinal sensitivity. In: Wei S, ed. *Clinical Uses of Fluorides.* Philadelphia, PA: Lea & Febiger; 1985:93–102.
31. Cuenin MF, Scheidt MJ, O'Neal RB, et al. An in vivo study of dentin sensitivity: the relation of dentin sensitivity and the patency of dentin tubules. *J Periodontol.* 1991;62:668–673.
32. Fischer C, Wennberg A, Fischer RG, et al. Clinical evaluation of pulp and dentine sensitivity after supragingival and subgingival scaling. *Endodontic Dent Traumatol.* 1991;7:259–263.

33. Haugen E, Johansen JR. Tooth hypersensitivity after periodontal treatment: a case report including SEM studies. *J Clin Periodontol*. 1988; 15:399–401.

34. Pashley DH, Galloway SE. The effects of oxalate treatment on the smear layer of ground surfaces of human dentine. *Arch Oral Biol*. 1985;30: 731–737.

35. Absi EG, Addy M, Adams D. Dentine hypersensitivity: the effect of toothbrushing and dietary compounds on dentine in vitro: an SEM study. *J Oral Rehabil*. 1992;19:101–110.

36. Pashley DH, Leibach JG, Horner JA. The effects of burnishing NaF/kaolin/ glycerin paste on dentin permeability. *J Periodontol*. 1987;58:19–23.

37. Zaimoglu A, Ayden AK. An evaluation of smear layer with various desensitizing agents after tooth preparation. *J Prosthet Dent*. 1992;68: 450–454.

38. Pillon FL, Romani IG, Schmidt ER. Effect of 3% potassium oxalate topical application on dentinal hypersensitivity after subgingival scaling and root planing. *J Periodontol*. 2004;75:1461–1464.

39. Dragolich WE, Pashley DH, Brennan WA, et al. An in vitro study of dentinal tubule occlusion by ferric oxalate. *J Periodontol*. 1993;64:1045–1051.

40. Tarbet WJ, Silverman G, Fratarcangelo PA, et al. Home treatment for dentinal hypersensitivity: a comparative study. *J Am Dent Assoc*. 1982;105: 7–230.

41. Pearce NX, Addy M, Newcombe RG. Dentine hypersensitivity: A clinical trial to compare 2 strontium desensitizing toothpastes with a conventional fluoride toothpaste. *J Periodontol*. 1994;65:113–119.

42. Baderstein A, Nilveus R, Egelberg J. Effect of non-surgical periodontal therapy. VIII. Probing attachment changes related to clinical characteristics. *J Clin Periodontol*. 1987;14:425–432.

43. Claffey N, Loos B, Gantes B, et al. Probing depth at re-evaluation following initial periodontal therapy to indicate the initial response to treatment. *J Clin Periodontol*. 1989;16:9–233.

44. Baderstein A, Nilveus R, Egelberg J. Effect of non-surgical periodontal therapy. VII. Bleeding, suppuration, and probing depth in sites with probing attachment loss. *J Clin Periodontol*. 1985;12:432–440.

45. Baderstein A, Nilveus R, Egelberg J. Scores of plaque, bleeding, suppuration and probing depth to predict probing attachment loss: 5 years of observation following nonsurgical periodontal therapy. *J Clin Periodontol*. 1990;17:102–107.

46. McCall JO. The evolution of the scaler and its influence on development of periodontia. *J Periodontol*. 1939;10:69–81.

47. Nagy RJ, Otomo-Corgel J, Stambaugh R. The effectiveness of scaling and root planing with curets designed for deep pockets. *J Periodontol*. 1992;63:954–959.

48. Fleischer HC, Mellonig JT, Brayer WK, et al. Scaling and root planing efficacy in multirooted teeth. *J Periodontol*. 1989;60:402–409.

49. Jahn CA, Jolkovsky D. Sonic and ultrasonic instrumentation and irrigation. In: Newman MG, Takei HH, Klokkevold PR, et al, eds. *Carranza's Clinical Periodontology*. 11th ed. St. Louis, MO: Elsevier Saunders; 2012:474–481.

50. Flemmig TF, Petersilka GJ, Mehl A, et al. Working parameter of a magnetostrictive ultrasonic scaler influencing root substance removal in vitro. *J Periodontol*. 1998;69:547–553.

51. Jotikasthira NE, Lie T, Leknes KN. Comparative in vitro studies of sonic, ultrasonic and reciprocating scaling instruments. *J Clin Periodontol*. 1992;19:560–569.

52. Brieninger DR, O'Leary TJ, Blumenshine RVH. Comparative effectiveness of ultrasonic and hand scaling for the removal of subgingival plaque and calculus. *J Periodontol*. 1987;58:9–18.

53. Drisko CL, Cochran DL, Blieden T, et al; Research, Science and Therapy Committee of the American Academy of Periodontology. Position paper: sonic and ultrasonic scalers in periodontics. *J Periodontol*. 2000;71: 1792–1801.

54. Nosal G, Scheidt MJ, O'Neal R, et al. The penetration of lavage solution into the periodontal pocket during ultrasonic instrumentation. *J Periodontol*. 1991;62:554–555.

55. Checchi L, Pelliccioni GA. Hand versus ultrasonic instrumentation in the removal of endotoxins from root surfaces in vitro. *J Periodontol*. 1988;59:398–402.

56. Smart GJ, Wilson M, Davies EH, et al. The assessment of ultrasonic root surface debridement by determination of residual endotoxin levels. *J Clin Periodontol*. 1990;17:174–178.

57. Dragoo MR. A clinical evaluation of hand and ultrasonic instruments on subgingival debridement. 1. With unmodified and modified ultrasonic inserts. *Int J Periodontics Restorative Dent*. 1992;12:310–323.

58. Suppipat N. Ultrasonics in periodontics. *J Clin Periodontol*. 1974;1: 206–213.

59. Obeid R, D'Hoore W, Bercy P. Comparative clinical responses related to the use of various periodontal instrumentation. *J Clin Periodontol*. 2004;31:193–199.

60. Khosravi M, Bahrami ZS, Atabaki BS, et al. Comparative effectiveness of hand and ultrasonic instrumentations in root surface planing in vitro. *J Clin Periodontol*. 2004;31:160–165.

61. Heitz-Mayfiled LJA, Trombellia L, Heitz F, et al. A systemic review of the effect of surgical debridement vs. nonsurgical debridement for the treatment of chronic periodontitis. *J Clin Periodontol*. 2001;29(suppl 3): 92–102.

62. Tunkel J, Heinecke A, Flemmig TF. A systemic review of efficacy of machine-driven and manual subgingival debridement in the treatment of chronic periodontitis. *J Clin Periodontol*. 2002;29:72–81.

63. Adams D, Fulford N, Beechy J, et al. The cardiac pacemaker and ultrasonic scalers. *Br Dent J*. 1982;152:171–174.

64. Barnes JB, Harrel SK, Rivera-Hidalgo F. Blood contamination of the aerosols produced by in vivo use of ultrasonic scalers. *J Periodontol*. 1998;69:434–438.

65. Fine DH, Mendieta C, Barnett ML, et al. Efficacy of preprocedural rinsing with an antiseptic in reducing viable bacteria in dental aerosols. *J Periodontol*. 1992;63:821–824.

66. King TB, Muzzin KB, Berry CW, et al. The effectiveness of an aerosol reduction device for ultrasonic scalers. *J Periodontol*. 1997;68:45–59.

67. Rivera-Hidalgo F, Barnes JB, Harrel SK. Aerosol and splatter production by focused spray and standard ultrasonic inserts. *J Periodontol*. 1999; 70:473–477.

68. Vastardis S, Yukna RA, Rice DA, et al. Root surface removal and resultant surface texture with diamond-coated ultrasonic inserts: an in vitro and SEM study. *J Clin Periodontol*. 2005;32:467–473.

69. Dederich DN, Bushick RD. Lasers in dentistry. *J Am Dent Assoc*. 2004; 135:204–212.

70. Frentzen M, Braun A, Aniol D. Er:YAG laser scaling of diseased root surfaces. *J Periodontol*. 2002;73:524–530.

71. Schwartz F, Sculean A, Berakdar M, et al. Clinical evaluation of an ER:YAG laser combined with scaling and root planing for non-surgical periodontal treatment. *J Clin Periodontol*. 2003;30:26–36.

72. American Academy of Periodontology. Statement on the efficacy of lasers in the non-surgical treatment of inflammatory periodontal disease. *J Periodontol*. 2011; 82(4):513–514.

73. Miyazaki A, Yamaguchi T, Nishikata J, et al. Effects of Nd:YAG and CO2 laser treatment and ultrasonic scaling on periodontal pockets of chronic periodontitis patients. *J Periodontol*. 2003;74:175–180.

74. DenBesten PK, White JM, Pelino JEP, et al. The safety and effectiveness of an Er:YAG laser for caries removal and cavity preparation in children. *Med Laser Appl*. 2001;16:215–212.

75. Osuna T. Improving visualization and ergonomics for the hygienist. *J Practical Hyg*. 2005;14:25–26.

76. Wu JC, Malik A. Maximize your visual acuity. *Dimens Dent Hyg*. 2004;30–35.

77. Avradopoulos V, Wilder RS, Chichester S, et al. Clinical and inflammatory evaluation of perioscopy on patients with chronic periodontitis. *J Dent Hyg*. 2004;78:30–37.

78. Kwan JY. Enhanced periodontal debridement with the use of micro ultrasonic, periodontal endoscopy. *Calif Dent J*. 2005;33:241–248.

79. Sunell S, Rucker LM. Ergonomic risk factors associated with clinical dental hygiene practice. *Probe*. 2003;37:159–166.

80. Ciancio SG. and Mariotti A. Anti-infective therapy. In: Newman MG, Takei HH, Klokkevold PR, et al, eds. *Carranza's Clinical Periodontology*. 11th ed. St. Louis, MO: Elsevier Saunders; 2012:482–491.

81. Slots J, Ting M. Systemic antibiotics in the treatment of periodontal disease. *Periodontol 2000*. 2002;28:106–176.

82. Greenstein G. Subgingival irrigation—an adjunct to periodontal therapy. Current status and future directions. *J Dent Hyg*. 1990;64:389–397.

83. Bonito AJ, Lux L, Lohr KN. Impact of local adjuncts to scaling and root planing in periodontal disease therapy: a systematic review. *J Periodontol*. 2005;76:17–1236.

84. Shiloah J, Hovious A. The role of subgingival irrigations in the treatment of periodontitis. *J Periodontol.* 1993;64:835–843.

85. Heasman PA, Heasman L, Stacy F, et al. Local delivery of chlorhexidine gluconate (PerioChip) in periodontal maintenance patients. *J Clin Periodontol.* 2001;28:90–95.

86. Hallmon WW, Rees TD. Local anti-infective therapy: mechanical and physical approaches. A systematic review. *Ann Periodontol.* 2003;8: 99–114.

87. Hanes PJ, Purvis JP. Local anti-infective therapy: Pharmacological agents. A systematic review. *Ann Periodontol.* 2003;8:79–98.

88. Tonetti MS, Cortellini P, Carnevale G, et al. A controlled multicenter study of adjunctive use of tetracycline periodontal fibers in mandibular class II furcation with persistent bleeding. *J Clin Periodontol.* 1998;25: 728–736.

89. Henderson RJ, Boyens JV, Holborow DW, et al. Scaling and root planing treatment with adjunctive subgingival minocycline. *J Int Acad Periodontol.* 2000;4:77–87.

90. American Academy of Periodontology. Position paper: the role of controlled drug delivery for periodontitis. *J Periodontol.* 2000;71: 125–140.

CHAPTER 14

Periodontal Surgery

Peter M. Loomer and Dorothy A. Perry

LEARNING OUTCOMES

- Describe the rationale for periodontal surgical treatment.
- Recognize the clinical conditions that are most likely to benefit from periodontal surgery.
- Define the types of periodontal surgery:
  - Excisional periodontal surgery
  - Incisional periodontal surgery
  - Access flap procedures
  - Osseous surgery
  - Mucogingival surgery
  - Regeneration surgery
- Describe the healing of tissues after periodontal surgery.
- Define postoperative procedures.
- Describe postoperative instructions for patients receiving periodontal surgery.
- Define the changes and modifications in plaque biofilm control required for patients after periodontal surgery.
- Identify the role of the dental hygienist in the surgical treatment of periodontal disease.

KEY TERMS

Access flap procedures	Incisional periodontal surgery	Periodontal flap surgery
Apically positioned flap	Infrabony pockets	Periodontal plastic surgery
Attachment loss	Intrabony pockets	Periodontal surgery
Biologic width	Mucogingival surgery	Pocket reduction surgery
Excisional periodontal surgery	Osseous defects	Postoperative instructions
Gingivectomy	Osseous surgery	Postoperative procedures
Gingivoplasty	Ostectomy	Regeneration surgery
Guided tissue regeneration	Osteoplasty	Suprabony pockets
Horizontal bone loss	Periodontal dressing	Vertical bone loss

Since the early twentieth century, **periodontal surgery** has been used to help dentists control the progression of periodontal disease. Although advances in root instrumentation techniques and antibiotic therapy have improved the available treatments for periodontal infections, periodontal surgery will continue to be a necessary procedure in the foreseeable future. It is important for the dental hygienist to understand the indications for and contraindications to basic periodontal surgical procedures and to advise patients of the potential therapies available. In many situations, the dental hygienist is the best person to discuss the options for periodontal surgery with the patient and to alert the dentist to the possible need for surgical intervention.

RATIONALE FOR PERIODONTAL SURGERY

Periodontal surgery is indicated to control the progress of periodontal destruction and attachment loss when more conservative nonsurgical treatment is insufficient. The definition of nonsurgical treatment in dentistry is perhaps a misnomer. Surgery is often defined as the practice of treating diseases by instrumentation or manual operations. By this definition, almost all dental procedures would be considered surgery. Dentists often limit the definition of surgery to cutting procedures with sharp instruments, especially scalpels or knives. Even by this definition, most periodontal therapy qualifies as surgery because sharp scalers and curettes cut both hard and soft tissues in the periodontal environment. Scaling and root planing result in intentional cutting of the root surfaces and inadvertent cutting of the surrounding soft tissues. However, they are considered part of nonsurgical periodontal therapy. This chapter limits the definition of periodontal surgery to techniques that intentionally cut into soft tissues to control disease or change the size and shape of tissues.

Periodontal educators have identified a number of goals for periodontal surgery.[1] These goals are defined in Box 14-1. All these goals are valid reasons for recommending periodontal surgery.

ADVANTAGES OF PERIODONTAL SURGERY

The major benefit and indication for periodontal surgery as an adjunct to nonsurgical periodontal treatment is to gain access to the root surface for scaling and root planing. It also improves access for plaque biofilm control. Periodontal surgery results in better access to furcations, complex root surfaces, and infrabony pockets (those apical to the crest of bone, surrounded by bone on one or more sides), areas that are the most difficult to treat by scaling and root planing. Improving access for plaque biofilm control by the patient may require removing tissues or bony forms that block the patient from adequately removing as much biofilm as necessary to control the disease. Other advantages of periodontal surgery include improved access to periodontal abscesses to obtain drainage and the ability to expose root surfaces for restorative dentistry. In addition, numerous new techniques are being used to improve patient aesthetics by altering the position of the gingival margin.[2]

DISADVANTAGES AND CONTRAINDICATIONS OF PERIODONTAL SURGERY

There are a number of disadvantages and contraindications to periodontal surgery. These include the health status or age of the patient and the specific limitations of each procedure.[2] From the patient's perspective, the disadvantages of surgery are usually limited to time, cost, aesthetics, and discomfort.

The dental hygienist is in the unique position to discuss all these concerns with the patient before periodontal surgery is performed. The hygienist is often involved with continuing maintenance procedures, is well known to the patient, or has developed a good rapport with the patient while performing nonsurgical periodontal procedures. By being involved in the patient's decision making process, the hygienist contributes to the patient's understanding and acceptance of the proposed surgical procedure. This contribution may be helpful to the patient in maintaining the teeth.

GENERAL CONSIDERATIONS FOR PERIODONTAL SURGERY

Several things must be considered when periodontal surgical therapy is prescribed. The periodontist usually makes a final decision to proceed with periodontal surgery after sufficient time is allowed for healing after nonsurgical procedures, at least 4 weeks. The amount of pocket reduction observed after these procedures indicates the extent of surgical procedures still required. The patient's concerns and fears must also be considered, and the patient must be fully informed of all factors related to the surgical treatment plan, including what to expect during the procedure and healing process. In prescribing periodontal surgery, the periodontist carefully considers the following:

- Probing pocket depth
- Amount of bone loss
- Importance of the tooth to function and aesthetics
- Patient's level of plaque biofilm control
- Patient's general health[3]

PROBING POCKET DEPTH

A periodontal pocket is a deepened gingival sulcus with an infected root surface covered by an ulcerated epithelial surface, with underlying inflamed connective tissue. The pocket is bound coronally by the gingival margin on one side by the root surface, on the other side by the epithelial surface, and at the base by the junctional epithelium. Studies have shown that scaling and root planing is effective in controlling periodontal disease to probing depths of about 4 mm.[4] Pockets deeper than 5 mm are difficult to instrument and therefore often remain infected, even after the best dental hygiene care. Pockets with probing depths greater than 9 mm suggest extreme loss of attachment, which makes the long-term prognosis for retaining the affected teeth poor.

CLINICAL NOTE 14-1　Periodontal surgery is most successful when treating periodontal pockets with probing depths of 5 to 9 mm.

Probing pocket depth is not always equal to clinical **attachment loss**. The probing depth is the measurement from the crest of the gingival margin to the base of the pocket. The deeper the probing depth, the more difficult is the complete removal of calculus. Therefore, the indication for periodontal surgery is stronger. Attachment loss, rather than probing depth, is measured from the cementoenamel junction to the base of the pocket. If the gingival margin is on the root surface, as when there has been recession, the attachment loss is greater than the probing depth. If the gingival margin is on the enamel surface of the crown, as in gingival hypertrophy, then the attachment loss is less than the probing depth. Attachment loss represents bone destruction, which in turn affects the long-term prognosis of the tooth. The concepts of probing depth and clinical attachment loss are discussed in Chapter 8.

Although surgery may be needed to treat pockets deeper than 5 mm, not all pockets of this depth require surgery. The 5-mm guideline is only the first step in identifying patients who may be helped by periodontal surgery. Patients with moderate pocket depths of 5 to 6 mm may be monitored with a wait-and-see approach to determine whether nonsurgical periodontal therapy and careful maintenance are adequate. If there is no progression of the periodontal disease in these cases, then periodontal surgery is not necessary. However, it is not always safe to wait and see. If the periodontal disease progresses and more attachment loss results, the prognosis for a tooth may worsen. Also, probing measurements are inexact. Measurements may differ by as much as 1 mm because of variations in probing technique. Therefore, to know that the disease is definitely progressing, a 2-mm increase in probing depth (and thus bone loss) must be observed over time. If surgery is postponed, the dentist (and patient) must be willing to risk this 2-mm bone loss.[5]

BONE LOSS

The base of the periodontal pocket is not at the level of the crest of the alveolar bone. There is usually 1 to 2 mm of connective tissue attachment covered by epithelium between the probing depth and the alveolar bone. This area is termed the biologic width[6] and must be considered when estimating the amount of attachment remaining on a periodontally involved tooth.

Bone loss caused by periodontal disease results in osseous defects. These may occur in either a horizontal dimension, where the bone resorbs equally on the mesial and distal surfaces of the teeth, as seen in Figure 14-1, or a vertical dimension, where the resorption is unequal around the teeth, as illustrated in Figure 14-2. Pockets that are coronal to horizontal bone loss are often called suprabony pockets, whereas those that extend apically beyond the crest of the bone are called infrabony pockets.

Vertical bone loss may also occur in a variety of configurations that are usually described by the number of bony walls remaining. When all the walls of the osseous defect are within the bone housing, they may be termed intrabony pockets. These types of bony defects are shown in Figure 14-3.

The amount of bone remaining around a tooth is an important consideration in the decision to perform periodontal surgery. Large amounts of bone supporting a tooth may allow the clinician to take a wait-and-see approach to postpone or avoid periodontal surgery. However, if the amount of bone is already reduced, delaying periodontal surgery may radically decrease the prognosis for the tooth. This rationale is illustrated in Figure 14-4.

Periodontal surgery that includes modification of the bone level or shape is called osseous surgery. The amount of bone remaining is important in determining whether periodontal surgery will be beneficial. If too much bone has been lost through disease or so much bone must be removed during surgery that the tooth will be weakened, osseous surgery becomes a less attractive option for treatment. Other procedures, such as grafting or regeneration techniques, may be required. Generally, osseous surgery performed to correct

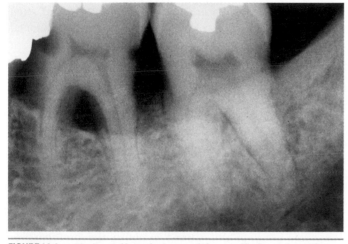

FIGURE 14-1 ■ **Horizontal bone loss around the mandibular molars.** Obvious furcation involvement of the first molar and cervical caries is seen at the mesial and distal cementoenamel junction of the first molar. (Courtesy of University of California, San Francisco, Division of Periodontology.)

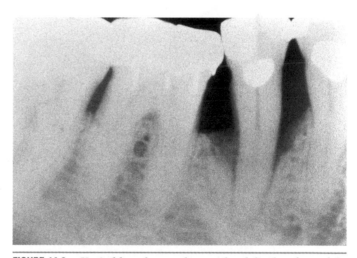

FIGURE 14-2 ■ **Vertical bone loss on the mesial and distal surfaces of the mandibular second premolar.** Although there has been some horizontal bone loss on the adjacent teeth, the bone level is greatly reduced on the premolar, resulting in infrabony pockets.

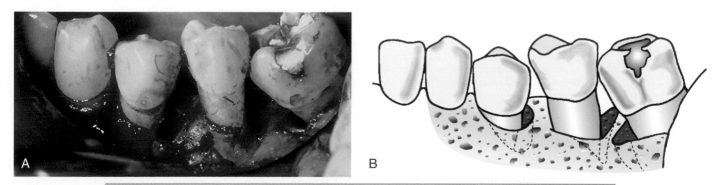

FIGURE 14-3 ■ **Intrabony defects. A,** A two-wall defect on the distal aspect of the first premolar, a one-wall defect on the distal aspect of the second premolar, and a three-wall defect on the mesial aspect of the first molar are evident in this photograph. **B,** The diagram shows the remaining walls of bone around the periodontal pockets. The two-wall defect on the first premolar shows bone destroyed on the distal root surface and the buccal alveolar process; therefore, two bony walls remain. The one-wall defect on the second premolar shows bone destroyed on the distal root surface and on both the buccal and the lingual alveolar processes; therefore, one wall remains. The three-wall defect on the mesial aspect of the molar shows bone destroyed on the root surface, but the alveolar process remains; therefore, three walls of bone remain surrounding the pocket.

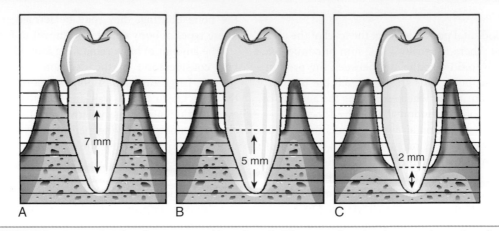

FIGURE 14-4 ■ **Prognosis is based on amount of bone loss. A,** When some bone loss is present, it may be safe to postpone surgery and take a wait-and-see approach; an additional bone loss of 2 mm may not alter the prognosis of the tooth. **B,** When half of the bone has been lost, an additional 2-mm loss can seriously jeopardize the tooth; therefore, surgery is highly recommended. **C,** With advanced bone loss, surgery may be performed in an effort to save the tooth, but the prognosis is poor.

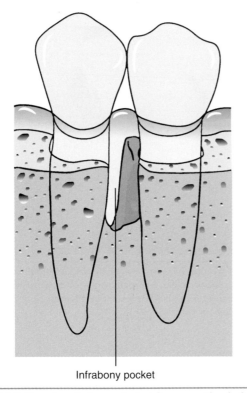

Infrabony pocket

FIGURE 14-5 ■ **Bone loss during periodontal surgery.** The shaded portion shows bone that would need to be removed during surgery to eliminate the bony defect. However, this bone removal would substantially weaken the adjacent tooth, which is a consideration in planning the surgery and can be a contraindication for osseous recontouring.

irregularly shaped defects of the bony support around the tooth is indicated when at least half of the bone support remains, as shown in Figure 14-5.

VALUE OF THE TOOTH

Not all teeth have equal value when considering periodontal surgery. Some periodontally involved teeth cannot be saved, and others are not worth making heroic attempts to treat. Third molars, for example, may not be in a good position for mastication, and they may be extracted without altering the patient's chewing pattern. An abutment tooth for a functioning fixed bridge, however, can be important to the patient, and often every attempt to salvage a particular tooth through periodontal surgery is strongly indicated.

CLINICAL NOTE 14-2 A third or second molar that is unopposed may become supererupted and make it difficult to clean the neighboring tooth. Extraction of supererupted teeth should be considered because these teeth often negatively affect the prognosis of neighboring teeth.

PERSONAL PLAQUE BIOFILM CONTROL OF THE PATIENT

The progression of periodontal disease may increase after periodontal surgery if plaque biofilm is not adequately controlled.[7] Therefore, every patient should establish the best possible supragingival plaque biofilm control before surgical therapy is initiated. If plaque biofilm control is poor, surgical intervention should be postponed or abandoned because it will not prevent the recurrence of periodontal infection and the possible loss of teeth.

AGE AND HEALTH OF THE PATIENT

Patients who are in poor health are not good candidates for periodontal surgery. However, periodontal disease may contribute to poor general physical condition, and periodontists may decide, in concert with the patients' physicians, that periodontal surgery is appropriate. Older patients usually heal as well as younger patients after periodontal surgery, so age in itself is not a contraindication to surgery. The patient's age is an important factor when considering the progress of the periodontal disease. Patients with pocket depths exceeding 5 mm and half their supporting bone lost who are relatively young (younger than 30 years) have an aggressive form of periodontal disease. Surgery is strongly indicated to control this infection. However, older patients (older than 60 years) with the same clinical conditions usually have a more slowly progressing form of the disease. Surgery may be less critical for these patients. It is important to remember that the human life span is increasing. Periodontal surgery, if strongly indicated, should not be denied a patient just because of advanced age. The quality of life of older patients may be significantly improved by controlling periodontal disease and retaining the dentition.

> **CLINICAL NOTE 14-3** Age is not a contraindication for periodontal surgery. Older patients heal as well as younger ones and quality of life must be considered in deciding whether to proceed with periodontal surgery.

PATIENT PREFERENCE

Some patients are reluctant to have periodontal surgery, no matter how strong the indications may be. It is important for patients to know all the ramifications of delaying recommended periodontal surgery and the possible effects on the long-term prognosis of the teeth. All patients must be informed of the alternatives, risks, and benefits of every dental procedure before deciding whether to undergo periodontal surgery. The architecture of gingival tissues resulting after periodontal surgery is more conducive to plaque biofilm control and maintenance. Patients who decide not to have surgery must be willing to undergo more frequent periodontal maintenance procedures and perform more complex subgingival plaque control in an effort to slow the progress of their disease. Even with these additional procedures, patients who decline to have periodontal surgery must understand that their disease will most likely progress and be willing to accept the risk of continued periodontal attachment and tooth loss.

TYPES OF PERIODONTAL SURGERY

Many methods of classifying periodontal surgery have been described. One approach is to name the procedure for the clinician who first described it—for example, the Widman flap. Another approach is to describe how the procedure is performed, as with gingivectomy, which means to remove the gingiva. Lang and Löe proposed a convenient classification of periodontal surgical procedures into five basic categories[8]:

- Procedures for pocket reduction or elimination
- Procedures for access to root surfaces
- Procedures for treatment of osseous defects
- Procedures for correcting mucogingival defects
- Procedures for new attachment

PROCEDURES FOR POCKET REDUCTION OR ELIMINATION

The goal of **pocket reduction surgery** is to reduce periodontal pocket depth by removing soft tissues to a level at which plaque biofilm control and maintenance procedures are effective, usually not exceeding 3 to 4 mm in depth. Methods for pocket reduction include **excisional periodontal surgery** (gingivectomy) and **incisional periodontal surgery** (flap).

Excisional Periodontal Surgery

Excisional periodontal surgery removes the excess tissue from the wall of the periodontal pocket. It is useful for the rapid reduction of gingival pockets. The most basic excisional surgical procedures are termed **gingivectomy**, meaning excision of the gingiva, or **gingivoplasty**, meaning surgical reshaping of the gingival tissues. In practice, both procedures are often performed in combination. Gingivectomy is a reasonably simple surgical procedure that is usually the first consideration for pocket reduction. However, contraindications to gingivectomy are numerous, and there are relatively few cases in which it is the sole therapy required. It is often performed with a special set of surgical instruments, although standard scalpel blades, electrosurgical devices, and dental lasers may also be used.

Indications. The presence of deep periodontal pockets with thick fibrous tissue is the major indication for gingivectomy. Drug-induced gingival hyperplasia is ideally treated by this form of excisional surgery. This condition is often caused by antiseizure medication (e.g., phenytoin), calcium channel blockers to control blood pressure (e.g., nifedipine), or immunosuppressive drugs (e.g., cyclosporine). Other indications include familial gingival hyperplasia and localized crown lengthening for restorative dentistry. Periodontal scaling and root planing, complemented by adequate plaque biofilm control procedures, should be completed 4 to 6 weeks before the surgery to allow tissues to heal. Often, the need for gingivectomy cannot be determined until tissue shrinkage after scaling and root planing has occurred.

> **CLINICAL NOTE 14-4** Edematous, friable, and hemorrhagic tissues are not easily incised and therefore require adequate healing time after scaling and root planing and before surgery.

Procedure. During gingivectomy, the surgeon marks the bottom of the pockets with a periodontal probe or forceps. The gingiva is excised with knives at a 45-degree angle to the gingival surface, keeping the incision within the keratinized gingiva. This practice results in a thin tissue margin at the dentogingival junction. After removal of the majority of the gingival tissues, the underlying exposed connective tissue is refined and trimmed with knives, burs, or other instruments. Exposed root surfaces are carefully examined for residual calculus and roughness and they are cleaned and smoothed as necessary with curettes. Bleeding after surgery is controlled with gauze pads dampened with saline solution, and the surgical area is packed with a periodontal dressing to reduce postoperative discomfort and protect the sensitive underlying connective tissue. Healing is usually uneventful and the gingival epithelium is reestablished 2 weeks after surgery.[9] An example of a gingivectomy procedure is presented in Figure 14-6.

Contraindications. There are many contraindications to excisional surgery, which is why it is rarely used for periodontal pocket reduction. Concerns about this procedure, which are illustrated in Figure 14-7, include the following:

- The primary contraindication is that the procedure does not permit access to infrabony pockets, those below the crest of the alveolar bone, a highly common occurrence in periodontitis.
- A wide wound is created, so healing is relatively slow while the epithelium grows in from the edges of the wound, and there is significant postoperative discomfort.
- The anatomy of the surrounding area may prevent incising the tissues at the proper angle or minimal width of

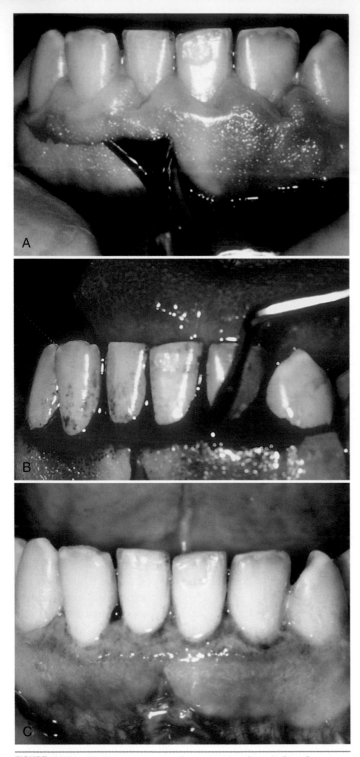

FIGURE 14-6 ■ **Gingivectomy procedure, excisional periodontal surgery.** **A,** The gingivectomy incision is through the keratinized tissue to the root surfaces of the teeth. **B,** The exposed connective tissue is trimmed with a periodontal knife to smooth and shape it to a physiologic form. **C,** Healing of the gingivectomy wound after 1 week. The tissue is reepithelialized by growing in from the margins of the wound.

attached gingiva may prevent keeping the incision within the keratinized tissue.

- The procedure exposes the root surfaces of the teeth, often resulting in unacceptable aesthetics, sensitivity to heat and cold, and susceptibility to root caries.

Incisional Periodontal Surgery

Incisional surgery, commonly called periodontal flap surgery or simply flap surgery, is the procedure of choice when excisional periodontal surgery cannot be performed for pocket reduction. This procedure is called flap surgery because the tissues are pushed away from the underlying tooth roots and alveolar bone, much like the flap of an envelope. Flap surgery includes a variety of techniques for pocket depth reduction. Depending on the clinical circumstances and the preference of the surgeon, the alveolar bone may be resected or modified during the surgical procedure. The usual incisional technique for pocket reduction with flap surgery is called the apically positioned flap because the flap is sutured at a more apical location on the tooth roots to reduce pocket depth.[9]

> **CLINICAL NOTE 14-5** Flap surgery has fewer contraindications than gingivectomy, so incisional procedures are the most common type of surgery performed by periodontists.

Indications. Deepened periodontal pockets, which are contraindicated for gingivectomy, are the primary indication for incisional surgery. Suprabony pockets are often best treated by flap surgery. However, flap surgery also allows access to infrabony pockets, so the procedure is often combined with other osseous surgical procedures to treat existing bony defects.

Procedure. After anesthesia is given, pockets are probed to determine their depths and the bony contours are "sounded" by pushing the periodontal probe through the tissues until the crest of the alveolar bone is detected. The surgeon uses this information to design the incision around the necks of the teeth to retain as much tissue as possible while allowing for pocket reduction. In thick tissues, this incision may be several millimeters away from the root surfaces. Flaps of gingiva are created that are pushed away from the alveolar bone and teeth, usually on the buccal and lingual surfaces, with a periosteal elevator. In this way, the infected epithelium, connective tissue, and granulation tissues can be removed with curettes, scalers, and ultrasonic instruments. The roots are examined for residual calculus and cleaned and smoothed as necessary. The flaps are then readapted at a more apical level to reduce the pockets. At this stage, the surgeon may reduce the bony ledges or may further elevate the flaps past the mucogingival junction to position it for proper adaptation. The surgical wound is closed by suturing the flaps together in the interproximal papillae and closely adapting them around the root surfaces. A periodontal dressing may be applied to help adapt the gingiva to the alveolar bone and assist with pocket reduction by applying pressure to the healing flap. This procedure is illustrated in Figure 14-8.

Contraindications. There are few contraindications to periodontal flap surgery beyond those that preclude any periodontal surgical intervention. The gingival tissues must be wide and thick enough to allow proper incision. Often, the incision must be modified to preserve as much keratinized tissue as possible. Like excisional surgery, apically positioning the gingival flaps exposes the root surfaces. The positioning may have to be altered or compromised for esthetics or in caries-prone patients. Fluoride mouth rinses should be recommended to reduce the potential for root caries.

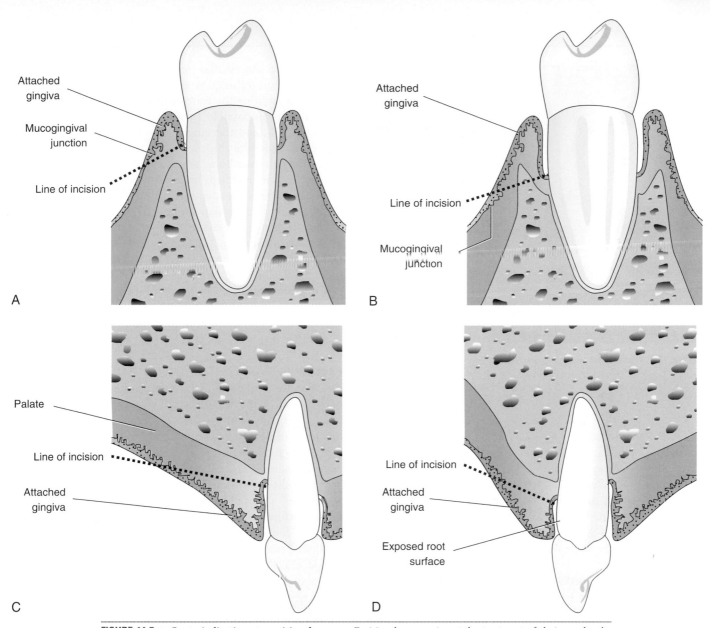

Attached gingiva

Mucogingival junction

Line of incision

A

Attached gingiva

Line of incision

Mucogingival junction

B

Palate

Line of incision

Attached gingiva

C

Line of incision

Attached gingiva

Exposed root surface

D

FIGURE 14-7 ■ **Contraindications to excisional surgery.** Excisional surgery is not the treatment of choice under the following circumstances. **A,** The incision cannot be made entirely through the keratinized gingiva. **B,** Infrabony pockets interfere with the correct line of incision. **C,** The incision would leave a wide wound—for example, on a palatal surface. **D,** Removal of the gingiva could expose long root surfaces that may be unsightly to the patient, sensitive to cold, and susceptible to root caries.

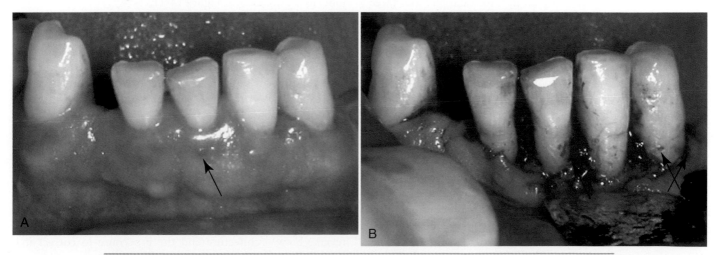

A

B

FIGURE 14-8 ■ **Access flap.** The access flap permits thorough cleaning of root surfaces. In this case, nonsurgical therapy did not result in pocket reduction and adequate healing of the gingival tissues. **A,** Presurgical appearance. Note the reddened and inflamed tissue around the anterior teeth, particularly the swelling on the facial surface of the incisor *(arrow).* **B,** When the flap is reflected, significant calculus remains on all the root surfaces *(arrows).* (Courtesy of Dr. Gary C. Armitage, University of California, San Francisco, School of Dentistry, Division of Periodontology.)

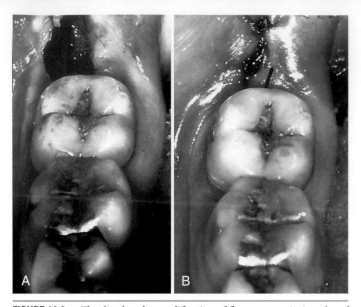

FIGURE 14-9 ■ **The distal wedge modification of flap surgery. A,** A wedge of tissue beneath the separated flaps is removed on the distal aspect of a mandibular second molar. **B,** Flaps sutured to reduce pocket depth.

Special modifications of pocket reduction surgery include combinations of incisional and excisional techniques, such as distal wedge surgery and internal beveled gingivectomy. These techniques are indicated in specific areas, such as the palatal tuberosity region, or where tissues are thick and not easily managed by one method alone.[9] The distal wedge procedure is shown in Figure 14-9. It permits adequate plaque control on the distal surface of the last tooth in the mandibular arch.

PROCEDURES FOR GAINING ACCESS TO THE ROOT SURFACE

The goal of access flap procedures is to provide access to the root surfaces for debridement and to create conditions for reattachment of the gingival tissues to the root. These access procedures include the modified Widman flap,[9,10] the excisional new attachment procedure,[11] and open flap curettage.[12] Most of these procedures are similar and differ only in the details of the technique. The modified Widman flap, for example, uses three incisions to separate the pocket lining from the tooth in a controlled manner, whereas the excisional new attachment procedure usually does not involve elevating the flap past the mucogingival junction. The goal of all these procedures is the same—to gain access to the root surface for plaque biofilm and calculus removal, including scaling and root planing. Pocket reduction by apical positioning is not the goal of access flap procedures.

Access Flap Procedures

Indications. Access flap procedures are used to treat periodontal pockets in aesthetically sensitive areas or where pocket reduction is not desired or indicated. Many periodontists perform access flap procedures instead of pocket reduction procedures because there are few long-term data to show that reducing the pocket depths through surgery extends the life of the teeth.[13] Patients, however, need to be evaluated on an individual basis regarding which type of surgical procedure would provide the most benefit.

Procedure. Access flap techniques are similar to pocket reduction flap techniques except that attention is mainly directed at cleaning the root surfaces and preserving as much gingival tissue as possible. Incisions are made through the crest of the gingiva, and the gingival tissues are reflected only far enough to allow the clinician to see the root surfaces and the crest of the alveolar bone. After complete debridement is performed, the gingival flaps are readapted to re-cover the roots. Although some pocket depth reduction usually occurs through shrinkage after access flap surgery, the major goal is reattachment of the connective tissues to the root surface during healing or creation of a long junctional epithelium resulting in increased attachment for the teeth. Figure 14-10 presents an example of a modified Widman flap procedure.

Contraindications. There are no specific contraindications to access flap procedures. However, the patient should understand that pocket depths may continue to be greater than 3 or 4 mm after therapy.

PROCEDURES FOR THE TREATMENT OF OSSEOUS DEFECTS

Periodontitis, by definition, involves attachment loss of the connective tissue to the root surface of the tooth and loss of alveolar bone. Often, this bone loss creates osseous defects around teeth that make healing unpredictable and result in gingival architecture that is difficult for the patient to maintain with acceptable plaque biofilm control and difficult for the hygienist to maintain with periodic scaling and root planing. During osseous surgical procedures, after reflecting the mucogingival flaps, the periodontist sculpts the alveolar bone with chisels or specially designed dental burs to remove these osseous defects or allow for apical positioning of the flaps.[9] If alveolar bone that contains periodontal fibers that support the tooth is removed, the procedure is termed ostectomy. If only bony ledges or nonsupporting bone are removed, the procedure is termed osteoplasty.[14] As with other surgical procedures, the two procedures are usually performed together to create a bone form that allows the gingival tissues to follow a positive gingival architecture, recreates the anatomic shape of periodontal health, and is free from ledges and craters of bone. A diagram of osseous recontouring is presented in Figure 14-11.

Osseous Defects

Indications. Several changes to the bony architecture from periodontal infections benefit from reshaping the bone with osseous surgery. A primary indication is periodontal pockets that extend below the level of the osseous crest, or infrabony pockets. Also, thick bony ledges are sometimes encountered during pocket reduction surgery that prevent the gingival flap from being adapted at a more apical level. Reverse alveolar bony architecture, a type of bone loss in which the interproximal bone is apical to the facial and lingual bone (the reverse of the configuration in health), permits periodontal pockets to re-form during healing. Correcting this bony deformity is another important indication for osseous surgery.[15] An example of reverse bony architecture and the procedure to correct it is presented in Figure 14-12.

Procedure. After the mucoperiosteal flaps are elevated, bony ledges and craters are modified with burs and chisels to create a positive alveolar form that allows the overlying gingiva

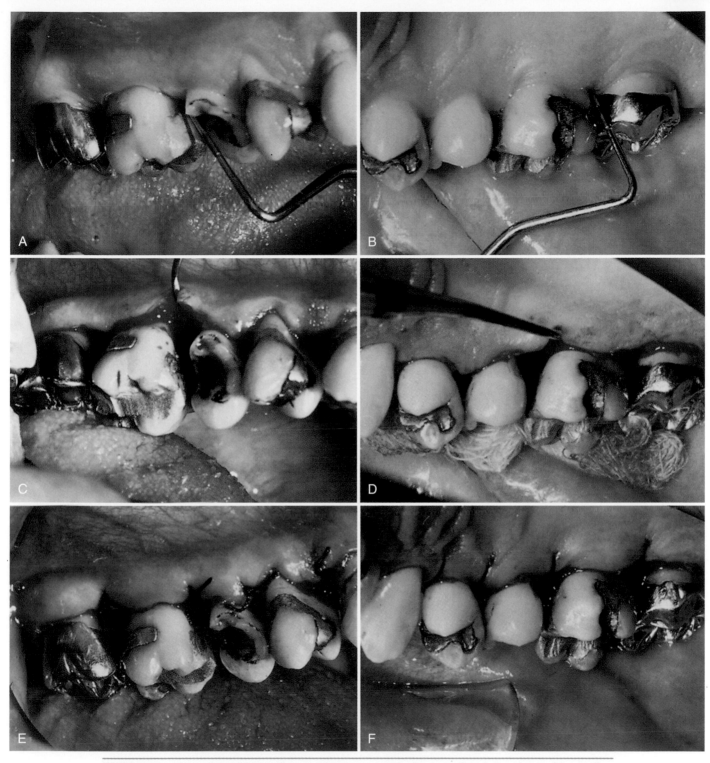

FIGURE 14-10 ■ **The modified Widman flap procedure as an example of an access flap. A,** Buccal view of the maxillary posterior quadrant. A probe is in place showing a 6-mm pocket on the mesial buccal aspect of the first molar. A fractured buccal cusp is seen on the second premolar. **B,** Palatal view of the same area with a probe in place showing a 7-mm pocket on the distal palatal surface of the first molar. **C,** Buccal view of the access flap, with minimal retraction, exposing the root surfaces for debridement. **D,** Palatal view of the same area, showing access to the root surfaces. **E,** Buccal view after debridement, with flaps approximated with interrupted sutures. Flaps are not apically repositioned. The surgical knots are all on the same side, the buccal side. **F,** Palatal view of the sutured flaps.

Continued

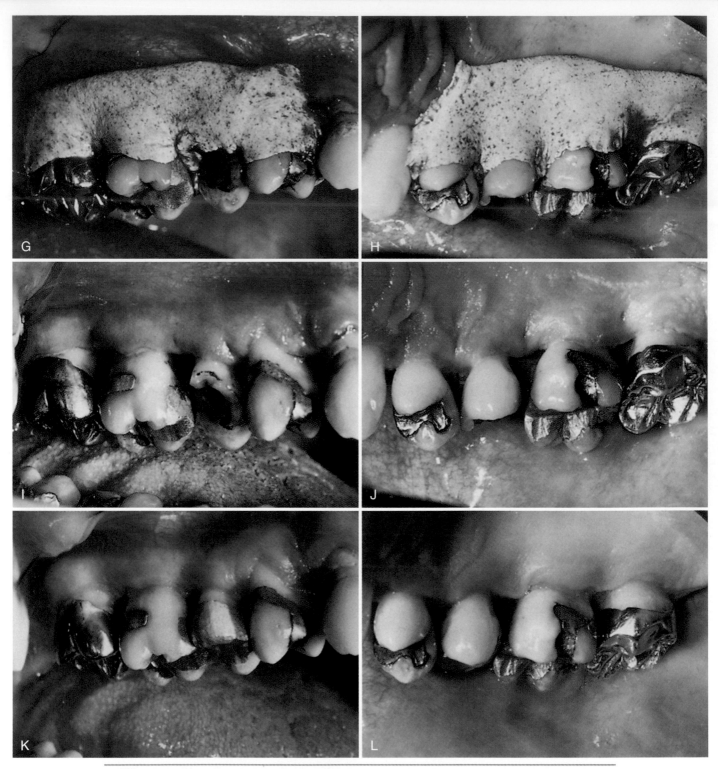

FIGURE 14-10, cont'd ■ **G,** Buccal view of a periodontal pack applied over the wound to adapt the flaps to the root surfaces. **H,** Palatal view with a periodontal pack in place. **I,** Buccal view of the surgery area 1 week later, after removal of the sutures and pack. Accumulated plaque biofilm and food debris have been removed at the postoperative visit. **J,** Palatal view of healing after 1 week. There are tracks on the gingiva from the sutures and the interdental papillary areas have not yet regenerated. **K,** Buccal view of the healed surgery site after 3 months. The contour of the interdental papillae is improved and the second premolar has been restored with a full gold crown. **L,** Palatal view of healing after 3 months shows that the interproximal papillae are not fully recontoured. The healing process can take 1 year or longer. The patient should undergo regular maintenance care, including 3-month recall scaling and use of interproximal home care devices, such as interproximal brushes. (Courtesy of Dr. James F. Coggan.)

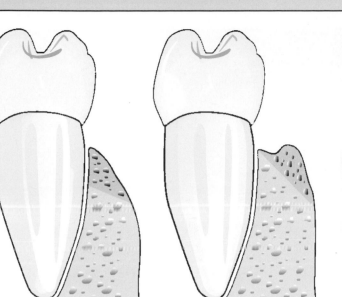

A   B

FIGURE 14-11 ■ **Osseous recontouring. A,** Ostectomy is the removal of supporting bone from the tooth root. The shaded area represents the bone removed. **B,** Osteoplasty is the removal of nonsupporting bone from around the tooth. The shaded area represents the bone removed.

to follow a more physiologic contour. If possible, the walls of bony craters are removed with minimal loss of bony attachment to the tooth. Ledges are thinned and interproximal bony regions are fluted to a form that is more generally found in periodontal health. An interesting case of bone loss associated with a lingual groove, access flap surgery, and bone recontouring is presented in Figure 14-13.

> **CLINICAL NOTE 14-6** Many osseous defects do not lend themselves to osseous recontouring. Either the bony defect is too deep to allow removal of the osseous walls or removing bone from one tooth will weaken the adjacent tooth so much that all of them will have a reduced long-term prognosis. Areas of severe bone loss are often best treated by reducing pocket depths and performing frequent maintenance care.

PROCEDURES FOR CORRECTING MUCOGINGIVAL DEFECTS

Periodontal disease often causes deformities in the oral tissues because of the recession of the marginal gingiva and the development of fissures and clefts. Studies show that patients with poor plaque biofilm control often have recession associated with inflammation and calculus formation and that recession is a common finding among patients with periodontal disease.[16] Recession can lead to extension of the periodontal pocket

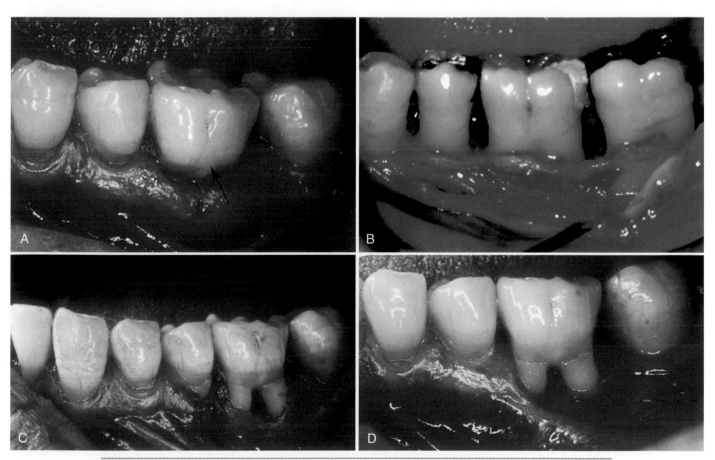

FIGURE 14-12 ■ **Reverse bony architecture and enamel projection. A,** The preoperative appearance of tooth #30. There is a 4-mm probing depth, Class II furcation involvement, and an enamel projection on the buccal surface *(arrow).* **B,** When the flap is reflected, the bone height is clearly seen. **C,** The surgeon has recontoured the bone and opened the furcation site so the patient can access it for good plaque biofilm control. There was no need to remove the enamel projection because the tissue level would be lower after surgery. **D,** Three months after the osseous recontouring, the tissue is healed and the patient is able to keep the area clean. Probing depths have been reduced to 2 mm. (Courtesy of Dr. Gary C. Armitage, University of California, San Francisco, School of Dentistry, Division of Periodontology.)

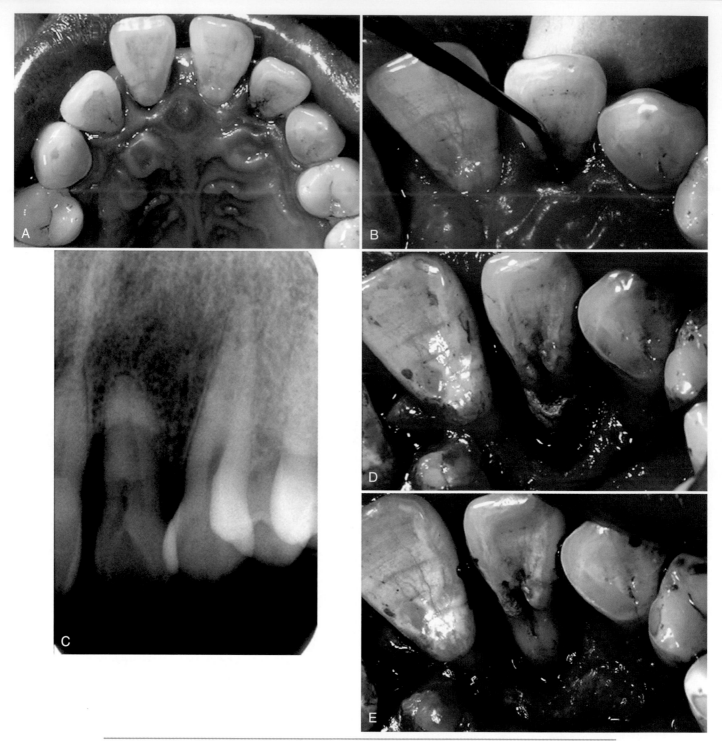

FIGURE 14-13 ■ Access flap and osseous surgery to correct a defect associated with a palatal groove. A, Pretreatment photograph of tooth #7 showing the inflamed tissue surrounding the lingual surface of the tooth. **B,** The probe penetrates easily along the pocket created by plaque biofilm accumulation; the probing depth is 9 mm. **C,** Radiograph showing the extent of bone loss around tooth #7. **D,** When the flap is reflected, the extent of the groove can be seen as well as the large amount of calculus that accumulated on the root. The calculus was not able to be removed during nonsurgical therapy. **E,** With the calculus removed, the extent of the groove can be seen.

beyond the mucogingival junction so that no attached gingiva exists on the tooth surface. These areas are called mucogingival defects and have been implicated in the spread of periodontal diseases into deeper tissues, although this role remains controversial. Mucogingival problems associated with continuing disease are considered for definitive surgical treatment.[17] An example of a mucogingival defect and its corrective surgery is presented in Figure 14-14.

CLINICAL NOTE 14-7 Mucogingival defects may develop after orthodontic treatment when the root surface of the tooth is moved through the alveolar bone. Forceful toothbrushing with a stiff brush used incorrectly can also cause defects, but in these cases, the tissues are healthy and plaque control is often better than average. In addition, some patients appear naturally prone to gingival recession, with no other apparent cause detected.

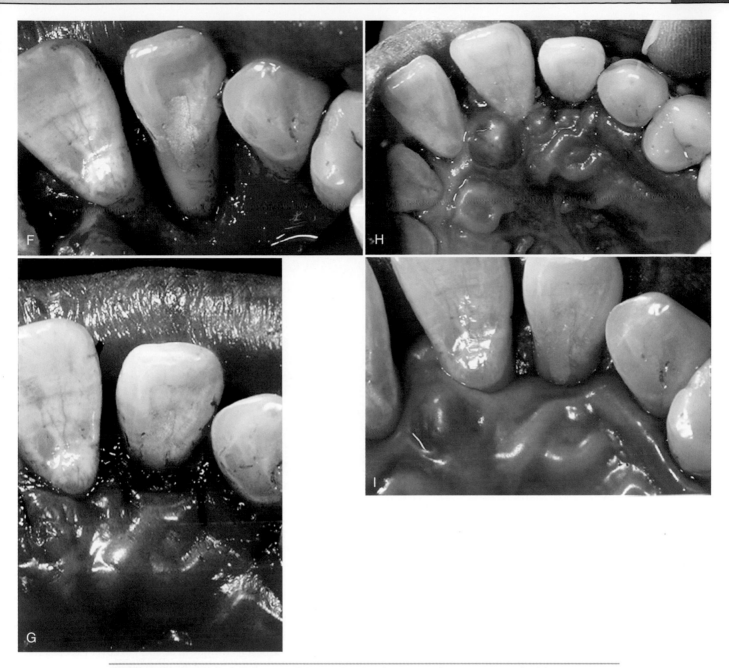

FIGURE 14-13, cont'd ■ **F,** The root was scaled, root-planed, and recontoured to remove as much of the groove as possible, and a tooth-colored restoration was placed to fill the void at the cingulum. The bone was recontoured to reduce the three-wall infrabony pocket. **G,** The flap was repositioned and sutured into place. **H,** One week postoperatively the tissue still looks red. Note that the ungloved finger is the patient holding the lip back for the photograph. **I,** One month postoperatively the tissue has responded well. There is little evidence of inflammation, and probe depths have been reduced to 3 mm. The interproximal papillae are still remodeling. (Courtesy of Dr. Gary C. Armitage, University of California, San Francisco, School of Dentistry, Division of Periodontology.)

Mucogingival surgery includes a variety of **periodontal plastic surgery** procedures to augment the thickness of keratinized gingival tissues, increase the zone of attached gingiva, improve gingival aesthetics by covering recessed root surfaces, or augment edentulous spaces. Although it has been suggested that a wide band of keratinized tissue is required to prevent further recession and the progression of periodontal disease, this belief is supported by little scientific evidence.[18] However, when plaque control is marginal or when a subgingival crown or restoration is planned, most clinicians believe that a broad band of keratinized tissue may help to reduce subsequent inflammation and prevent further recession. Areas of recession are treated by either pedicle grafts or free mucosal grafts, although connective tissue grafts have been increasingly used.[19]

Mucogingival Defects

Indications. Areas of recession that significantly reduce the width of the keratinized gingiva or have progressed beyond the mucogingival junction should be considered for tissue-grafting procedures. Although there is no absolute minimal width of attached gingival tissue, the most often quoted ideal width is 3 mm, particularly if dental restorations will involve manipulation of the gingival tissues.[20] When gingival tissues are thin or receded, mucogingival procedures are sometimes performed

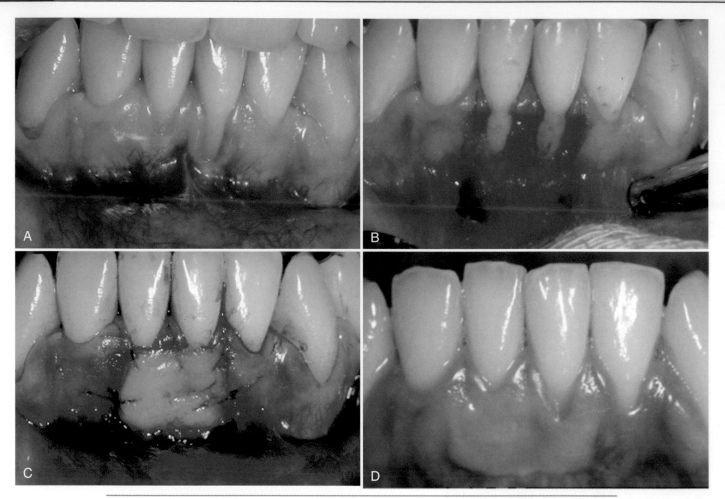

FIGURE 14-14 ■ **Free gingival graft. A,** This area of extensive recession is related to the frenum pull in the area and poor plaque biofilm control. **B,** The extent of bone loss on the facial surfaces of the anterior teeth can be seen when the tissue bed is prepared. **C,** The graft from the palatal donor site is sutured into place. The tissue bed provided nutrients for the graft. **D,** Three months later the graft has healed well and the probe depths have been reduced to 2 mm. Note that the graft tissue retains the more keratinized appearance of the palatal tissue. (Courtesy of Dr. Gary C. Armitage, University of California, San Francisco, School of Dentistry, Division of Periodontology.)

before orthodontic tooth movement, although this approach is controversial. Other indications for surgical intervention to control mucogingival problems are broad labial or lingual frenum attachments near the gingival margin that may result in unsightly diastemata and a shallow vestibular depth that must be deepened to improve the fit and retention of removable dental prostheses.[17]

Procedure. The procedures differ depending on the specific mucogingival problem. The most common procedures are the following:

- Lateral pedicle gingival graft
- Free autogenous gingival graft
- Subgingival connective tissue graft

All these procedures require access to adequate sites for donor graft tissue before they can be performed. An important consideration in all these procedures is preparation of the recipient site for the graft. During the surgery, all inflamed tissues should be trimmed from the recipient area, and the root surface to be covered should be root-planed free of plaque biofilm, calculus, and cementum altered by bacterial endotoxins. The selection of donor tissue to cover the recipient site is a major consideration.

Lateral Pedicle Grafts. The lateral pedicle graft, the sliding of gingival tissue from an adjacent tooth or papilla, has been suggested as the best technique to attempt to cover exposed root surfaces because these grafts bring their blood supply with them. Limitations to pedicle grafts depend largely on the availability of an adequate source of donor tissue adjacent to the area that needs augmentation. The donor pedicle is sharply dissected from the underlying periosteal bed, rotated to the recipient site, and carefully sutured in place. Another important limitation to pedicle grafts is the risk of causing gingival recession to the donor site, particularly if the alveolar bone housing is thin or bony dehiscences are exposed during the surgical procedure.

Free Gingival Grafts. Free gingival grafts have donor sites located somewhere in the mouth away from the site that requires grafting. The most common site for donor tissue is the palate, but edentulous areas are also used. The recipient site is prepared in a manner similar to the pedicle graft site and a donor graft of keratinized epithelium with some underlying connective tissue is removed by surgical excision. The graft is sutured in place and held with firm pressure until the initial blood clot forms to stabilize the graft. It is particularly important that the grafted tissue be immobile for the first week after surgery to allow for the establishment of circulation to the grafted tissue. Healing is usually uneventful, with the primary discomfort coming from the donor site where the epithelium has been removed. Postsurgical hemorrhage is a potential problem at the donor site because the epithelium and underlying connective tissue have been removed and no primary wound closure is possible. It must therefore heal by epithelial growth from the edges of the wound. Postsurgical hemorrhage on the donor site can be controlled with the use of pressure stents or hemostatic surgical dressings, such as resorbable cellulose or collagen pads.

CLINICAL NOTE 14-8 It is important to have a thorough knowledge of the anatomy of the palatal tissues, the usual donor site for graft procedures. Major arteries, usually in close proximity to the second molars, must be avoided. Palatal rugae are generally not included as part of the donor tissue because the recipient site would then take on these anatomic characteristics.

Subgingival (Subepithelial) Connective Tissue Grafts. Grafting of subepithelial connective tissue has become the procedure of choice when root coverage is the objective of mucogingival surgery.[21] Histologic studies of healing free gingival grafts have shown that most of the transplanted epithelium in free grafts is lost and that the genetics of the underlying connective tissue determine the potential for keratinization of healing tissue. Therefore, transplanting only the subepithelial connective tissue rather than the connective tissue and its covering epithelium has many advantages.[17] The donor site wound can be primarily closed by suturing the epithelium in place, greatly reducing postoperative discomfort and bleeding. The tissue color and texture of the healed recipient site are more similar to the preoperative appearance when the migrating epithelium comes from adjacent to the wound site rather than grafted palatal tissue.

Contraindications. Lack of donor tissue is the major contraindication to mucogingival surgery. Although this situation is less of a problem with connective tissue grafting than with either lateral pedicle grafts or free gingival grafts, there are still situations in which minimal or limited tissue is available. Lack of adequate keratinized tissue at the recipient site is a contraindication specific to mucogingival grafting surgery using subepithelial connective tissue grafts because these types of mucogingival procedures do not result in an increase in the width of keratinized tissue. However, this situation can be circumvented by a combination of procedures, such as first grafting tissue for the width of keratinized tissue followed by a second procedure to provide root coverage.

PROCEDURES FOR REGENERATION OF THE PERIODONTIUM

Regeneration surgery includes a variety of surgical techniques that attempt to restore the periodontal tissues lost through disease. By definition, periodontal regeneration is the formation of new alveolar bone, new cementum, and new periodontal ligament on a tooth root surface that was previously diseased.[22] Current techniques include bone grafting and guided tissue

regeneration.[15] Technically, all types of periodontal treatment, including scaling and root planing, have the potential to yield periodontal regeneration. There is some regeneration of connective tissue and epithelium; however, it is not predictable. This category of surgery is reserved for procedures that increase the predictability of the growth of new tissues of the attachment apparatus.

Periodontal Bone Grafting

Transplanting bone to restore that lost from periodontal disease has been attempted for many years. Only in the last 20 years has it been a reasonably predictable procedure, the anatomy of the periodontal defect probably being the most critical factor in determining its success. The classification of periodontal bone grafts is based on the source of graft material.

Autografts. Autografts are created from donor bone from the patient's own body. Bone may be taken from intraoral sites, such as tori, the maxillary tuberosity, or bone removed during osteoplasty. Bone may also come from extraoral sites, such as the iliac crest of the hip or the sternum. Extraoral autogenous bone marrow grafts form large amounts of bone, but problems with obtaining the graft and the possibility of root resorption with fresh bone marrow grafts make them less useful. Intraoral grafts are limited by the small amount of donor material. They have also shown limited osteogenic potential in clinical studies.[23] However, most surgeons still attempt to use as much autogenous bone as possible in an attempt to make bone grafting as biocompatible as possible.

Allografts. Allografts are created from bone that comes from another person. Cadaver bone, obtained from bone banks accredited by the American Association of Tissue Banks, is the most common source of bone allografts used in periodontics. The best clinical results have been obtained with bone that has been freeze-dried and demineralized with hydrochloric acid. The acid decalcification appears to unmask bone morphogenic protein, which some experts suggest increases the osteogenic potential of the graft. Importantly, acid demineralization reduces the risk of disease transmission from the deceased bone donor to the periodontal patient.[24]

Alloplasts. Alloplastic grafts use a variety of synthetic bone minerals. They may be made of hydroxyapatite mineral or ceramics, such as plaster of Paris and tricalcium phosphate. The most successful material appears to be porous hydroxyapatite, although histologic evidence suggests that it functions as a non-irritating filler rather than promoting new bone formation.[25]

Xenografts. Xenografts are created from bone taken from another species, such as bovine (cow) or porcine (pig) bone. Tissues from nonhuman species have strong antigenic reactions with human graft recipients. Until recently, the most successful use of these materials had been as fillers for large osseous defects, using graft material with all organic tissue chemically removed.

Genetic engineering of human tissues and cell cultural cloning techniques will define the future of periodontal surgery and wound healing. Great strides will likely be made in graft techniques in the coming years. More predictable, simpler, and less invasive periodontal regeneration procedures will be possible with improvements in biotechnology.

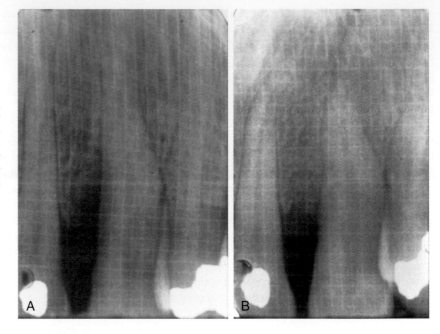

FIGURE 14-15 ■ **Bone graft surgery is an option to fill deep intrabony pockets; it is most successful when three-wall pockets are treated. A,** Preoperative radiograph shows deep vertical bone loss. **B,** Postoperative radiograph taken 1 year later shows substantial increase in the bony support for the tooth. (Gridlines on the films are present to help assess bone levels.) (Courtesy of Dr. Philip R. Melnick, Cerritos, California.)

Indications. Bone grafting can be attempted in infrabony defects that show a potential for regeneration. These are usually defects with sufficient osseous walls to promote healing, ideally three-wall defects. Furcation defects, particularly mandibular molar buccal furcations of Grade II (not through and through), are often good candidates for bone regeneration with osseous grafts. In controlled clinical trials, these types of furcations have been shown to respond more favorably and predictably to periodontal regeneration procedures than other types of furcations.

Procedure. As with all periodontal procedures, meticulous root debridement of the surgical site is imperative. Full-thickness mucoperiosteal flaps are elevated and all granulation tissue removed with curettes. The bone graft material is prepared according to the distributor's instructions or harvested from the donor site and inserted into the defects. The best results appear to be obtained with primary closure of the flaps over the wound site. Radiographs showing the successful result of a bone grafting procedure are presented in Figure 14-15.

Contraindications. There are no specific contraindications to bone fill procedures. The most predictable bone fills occur in clinical cases that have a maximum number of bony walls, improving the chances of success. Some authors believe that root surface demineralization with citric acid may increase success by detoxifying the root surface and exposing collagen fibrils in the cementum.[26] Others have suggested that root surface conditioning with fibronectin, a molecule that promotes connective tissue growth, increases regeneration. Although promising, these procedures have not shown significant improvement in clinical trials.[26]

Guided Tissue Regeneration

An important development in periodontics has been the concept of guided tissue regeneration, or healing by selected cell repopulation. It was long thought that if the right cells were allowed to grow (and the wrong cells inhibited) in a healing periodontal wound site, the potential for regeneration, or growth of a new attachment apparatus, would exist.[27] In a series of well-controlled experiments, researchers have produced new periodontal ligament, alveolar bone, and cementum on previously diseased root surfaces by selectively excluding gingival epithelial cells and fibroblasts. This technique permits the primary healing cells to proliferate from the alveolar bone and periodontal ligament rather than from the growth of epithelium from the gingiva. By placing a barrier membrane that excludes epithelial cells between the periodontal flap and the alveolar bone, only cells from the periodontal ligament space and the medullary bone are allowed to repopulate the site of lost tissue. This approach selectively causes a new attachment apparatus to grow.[17] A number of materials have been suggested for these barriers, including expanded polytetrafluoroethylene (ePTFE) membranes and polylactic acid with citric acid ester membranes.

Indications. Infrabony defects and furcations appear to be the best candidates for guided tissue regeneration. In general, osseous lesions that are likely to respond well to other forms of bone fill or grafting are also the most promising sites for guided tissue regeneration. In some cases, the results are remarkable.

Procedure. Flaps are reflected and, after adequate debridement of the intraosseous lesion, a membrane is placed over the opening in the bone or furcation and fastened to the tooth by suturing or other stabilizing methods. The epithelium is closed over the membrane and the wound is allowed to heal for a period of 30 to 60 days. When nonresorbable ePTFE material is used, the membrane must be removed surgically. The polylactic acid material resorbs through hydrolysis within 6 to 12 months.[28] A guided tissue regeneration procedure is illustrated in Figure 14-16.

CLINICAL NOTE 14-9 Guided tissue regeneration is the most predictable method for regenerating lost periodontal tissues. The most favorable anatomic periodontal defects produce predictable results. Wide Class III furcations and infrabony defects with fewer than two walls are less successful.

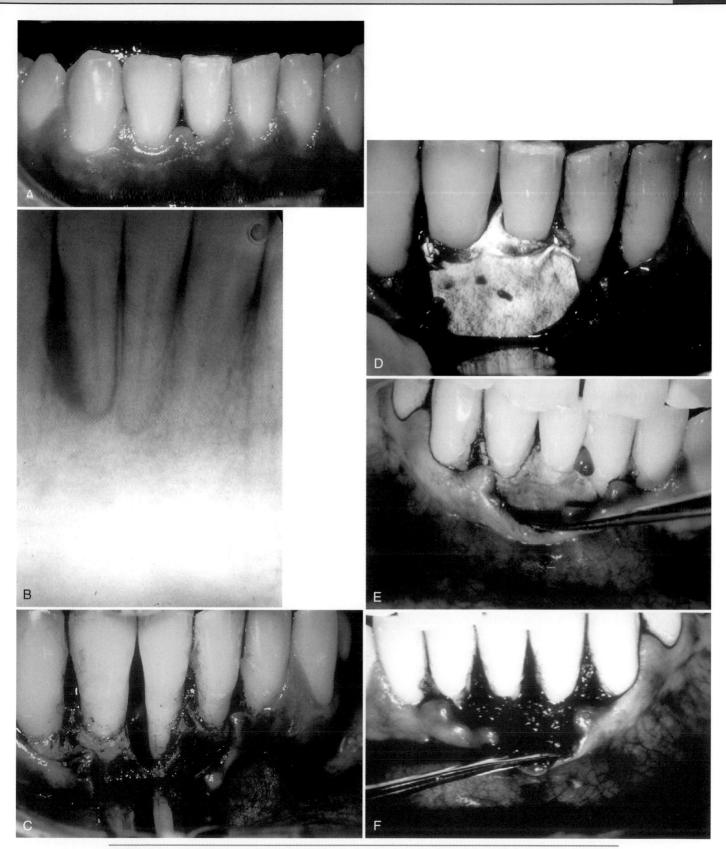

FIGURE 14-16 ■ **Guided tissue regeneration. A,** Preoperative view of a mandibular central incisor with a 9-mm pocket. **B,** Preoperative radiograph showing that the bony defect extends nearly to the apex of the central incisor. **C,** Flap exposing a large, two-wall intrabony defect. **D,** Barrier membrane of ePTFE material sutured over the defect. Flaps will be positioned over this membrane to keep the epithelium from growing into the bony defect. **E,** Membrane surgically exposed after 60 days of healing. **F,** Osteoid (osseous-like) tissue that formed is visible after membrane removal. Flaps will be repositioned and sutured for final healing. (Courtesy of Dr. Gregory J. Conte.)

PROCEDURES IMMEDIATELY AFTER PERIODONTAL SURGERY

A number of procedures are required to complete periodontal surgery. These procedures include closing the wound with the placement of sutures, possibly covering the surgical wound with a protective dressing called a periodontal pack, and providing the patient with postoperative instructions.

SUTURES

Sutures are required to close periodontal surgical wounds and to secure grafts in position. Periodontal surgeons generally use braided black silk sutures, which are easy to see and have good working properties. However, many other types of suture materials are available. Some periodontists prefer resorbable sutures, which have less potential for bacterial adherence. Others use sutures made of synthetic fibers.

Whatever type of suture material is placed, the sutures must be removed in 7 to 14 days. In most cases, that is enough time for wound healing to progress to a point at which sutures are no longer needed. If sutures remain in the tissues much longer than 14 days, they permit plaque biofilm to form in the wound site and produce healing complications. Some synthetic fiber sutures, however, are designed to remain in place for as long as 1 month and are often selected for guided tissue regeneration procedures for exactly this reason. Although resorbable sutures are designed to dissolve in tissue fluids, they do not always dissolve in saliva and may require removal.

> **CLINICAL NOTE 14-10** An infection resulting from sutures retained too long is often called a stitch abscess. This infection appears as a red swollen area and is painful. Extreme inflammation slows healing and reduces the effects of periodontal surgery.

Many techniques are used for suturing periodontal flaps and grafts, ranging from simple stitches, termed interrupted sutures, to complex sling sutures that use the teeth for an anchor, or mattress sutures that allow flaps to be placed in a variety of positions.

Dental hygienists should know the basic rules that guide suture techniques:

1. It is best to tie the suture knots for any type or style of suture on the buccal surface. This placement allows for simple removal because the knot is easy to see and grasp with an instrument when the suture is cut. Thus, it is possible to avoid pulling the knot through the tissues during removal. If a periodontal dressing, or pack, is used, the lingual pack can be removed first, the sutures cut on the lingual surface, and the buccal pack removed. If any of the knots are caught in the buccal dressing, the sutures will pull out easily and not tear the tissue.
2. At least 2 or 3 mm of suture "tail" should be left beyond the knot. This tail allows the suture to be easily found at the postoperative appointment and gives the dentist or dental hygienist something to hold onto when cutting the suture for removal.

3. The location and number of sutures placed must be documented in the chart. This information aids in locating and removing all the sutures to avoid traumatizing the healing wound at the postoperative appointment. It also prevents missing a suture and permitting a stitch abscess to develop.

PERIODONTAL DRESSING

A **periodontal dressing**, or pack, is sometimes placed over the sutures to hold the flaps tightly to the teeth and underlying bone when pocket reduction surgery has been performed. It is also used after excisional surgery, such as gingivectomy, to protect the surgical wound from the oral environment and increase patient comfort during the first week of healing. Although many patients believe that a periodontal pack makes the surgical site more comfortable, some find the pack a nuisance and prefer not to have the dressing placed. The periodontal dressing is a tremendous plaque trap.

Several types of periodontal dressings are available, but the most common type consists of a paste mixture that sets chemically to a firm, rubbery consistency. A light-cured product is available that allows the working and setting times to be more precisely controlled. Whatever dressing is selected, it is mixed according to the manufacturer's instructions and placed in a thin ribbon around the necks of the teeth in the area of surgery but not on the occlusal surfaces. To facilitate retention, the dressing should be compressed into the interproximal spaces for a mechanical lock and the material should not extend coronally to the height of contour of the teeth. Bleeding must be controlled before a periodontal dressing is placed because the pack will not control bleeding. Further more, the periodontal dressing does not prevent plaque biofilm formation. In fact, it prevents plaque biofilm control in the region of the surgery. The use of the periodontal dressing is shown in Figure 14-10, *G* and *H*.

POSTOPERATIVE INSTRUCTIONS AND PROCEDURES

After periodontal surgery, **postoperative procedures** include a prescription for an analgesic and possibly an antibiotic. Many periodontists recommend the use of a disinfectant rinse twice a day to help with plaque biofilm control. A chlorhexidine or essential oil mouthwash may be used to freshen the mouth and inhibit plaque during primary healing in the first week or two after surgery.[17,29]

A number of suggestions and **postoperative instructions** should be given to the patient to ease postoperative discomfort and promote healing. They include the following recommendations:

1. Physical activity should be limited to allow the patient to rest and let the area of surgery heal.
2. Bleeding is usually limited, but if the wound area begins to seep blood after the patient leaves the office, it can usually be controlled with light finger pressure on a gauze sponge in the area of surgery. The patient should be instructed not to rinse because rinsing prolongs the bleeding.
3. A soft diet is usually recommended for the first several days to avoid disturbing the area of surgery or the

periodontal pack, if present. The patient should be urged to eat a nutritious, well-balanced diet to promote healing.

4. Any prescriptions for medications that may have been given should be reviewed with the patient.

5. The patient should be warned that portions of the periodontal dressing may break off before the postoperative appointment. Usually, the dressing has done its job of tightly adapting the tissues to the teeth in the first several hours of healing, and little damage is done if the dressing comes off after the first postoperative day.

6. The patient should be warned that some surgical procedures, particularly osseous surgery, commonly cause swelling. The patient should be told to use an ice pack for short intervals during the first few hours after surgery.

7. The patient should avoid smoking, which will cause the wound to heal more slowly.

8. Home care plaque control instructions should be reviewed carefully with the patient. Plaque biofilm control is more difficult postoperatively, but it leads to better healing. Extra soft toothbrushes, the use of warm water during cleaning, and gentle interproximal cleaning can all be recommended. The unaffected teeth should be cleaned normally. The patient should be shown how to clean the area of surgery and be encouraged to clean once a day, twice if possible. Often, an antiseptic mouthwash, either chlorhexidine or a phenolic rinse, is recommended to help with plaque biofilm control and to freshen the mouth.

9. The patient must be given a list of postoperative instructions that should be reviewed before the patient is dismissed. It is important that the instruction sheet include the telephone number to use if problems arise. The patient should be urged to contact the office if there are any problems or questions. A postoperative visit should be scheduled for about 7 days after the surgery. A sample postoperative instruction sheet is shown in Figure 14-17.

POSTOPERATIVE TREATMENT

The patient should return for a postoperative visit 1 week after periodontal surgery. At this appointment, the patient is examined, the periodontal dressing and sutures are removed, and the surgical site is gently cleaned with a cotton swab that has been moistened with a warm saline solution or a disinfectant mouthwash. The wound is usually well epithelialized by 7 to 10 days after surgery, and the surgeon will rarely redress the area for an additional week.[17] A surgical site with the periodontal dressing, sutures, and accumulated plaque removed after 1 week is shown in Figure 14-10, *I* and *J*.

Home care instructions for plaque biofilm control should be reviewed at this time. The tissue may still be tender from the surgery, so the patient must be instructed to clean the area gently with a soft toothbrush that has been made even softer by soaking in warm water. Because considerable tissue shrinkage and larger spaces between teeth often occur after periodontal surgery, interproximal brushes may be indicated. They should also be used gently. Dental floss should be used carefully during

---

Instructions Following Periodontal Surgery

Activity: Limit your activities to those requiring minimal exertion for the next few days.

Rinsing: Do not rinse your mouth for 24 hours.

Bleeding: Some slight bleeding may occur during the first 4 or 5 hours after the operation. This bleeding is not unusual. If bleeding continues, apply firm pressure for 20 minutes with a piece of gauze. Repeat as necessary. Do not remove the gauze during this period. Do not rinse with water to stop the bleeding. If bleeding persists, call the office.

Discomfort: Some discomfort is to be expected when the anesthesia wears off. If you have been given a prescription, fill it and take the medication as directed. If discomfort persists, call the office.

Eating: Limit yourself to a soft diet immediately after surgery. Avoid chewing in the area of surgery. Do not drink very hot beverages the first day. You may return to your regular diet as soon as you feel comfortable. Highly seasoned or spicy foods may irritate the area of surgery.

Dressing: A dressing material may have been placed around your teeth. It will become hard within about 2 hours and should not be disturbed. Although the dressing may remain in place until your next appointment, small parts may chip off. If a large portion of the dressing comes off, call the office for instructions.

Swelling: Swelling is expected after some procedures. You may use an ice pack on the outside of your face, 15 minutes on and 15 minutes off, for the next 4 hours. If you have excessive swelling in your neck or under your chin, call the office.

Smoking: Do not smoke. Smoking may interfere with the healing process and produce poor results.

Home care: If a surgical dressing is present, brush the top of the dressing lightly with a soft toothbrush. If no dressing is present, gently use a soft toothbrush to clean the area of surgery for the first few days. You may rinse gently with a medicated mouthwash if it was prescribed or warm salt water starting the day after surgery.

IF YOU HAVE ANY QUESTIONS OR CONCERNS, CALL THE OFFICE. Telephone number:

FIGURE 14-17 ■ Sample postoperative patient instructions.

---

the first few weeks after surgery to avoid damaging the healing junctional epithelium and connective tissue attachment in the surgical area.

CLINICAL NOTE 14-11 The importance of postsurgical plaque biofilm control cannot be overemphasized. Poor plaque control after periodontal surgery is the principal reason for slow healing and failure of the surgical treatment. Many clinicians recommend scheduling the patient for several postoperative visits for evaluation of plaque biofilm control during the healing phase.

Teeth in the area of surgery often become mobile as a result of swelling in the periodontal ligament space. The patient should be told that this swelling is normal and that the teeth usually become firm as the tissues heal. Sometimes the dentist may suggest a postsurgical splint to control mobility during the healing process.

Tooth sensitivity, especially to cold, is a common problem after periodontal surgery. Patients should be warned to expect a certain amount of sensitivity. Patients may reduce sensitivity during plaque biofilm control procedures by brushing the teeth with warm water for the first several weeks. Sensitivity is caused by exposure of the root surfaces to the oral environment from apically positioned periodontal flaps, shrinkage of the gingiva during healing, and root planing with cementum removal during the surgical procedure. Dentinal tubules are exposed to the oral environment and hydrodynamic forces may cause pain. The use of home fluoride gels or rinses for the first month after periodontal surgery may alleviate sensitivity. In addition, topical desensitizing office treatments with potassium oxalate or ferric oxalate may help. Desensitizing toothpastes used at home, particularly those containing potassium nitrate, may be effective in controlling postsurgical sensitivity. In most cases, this sensitivity is greatly reduced after 1 to 2 months.[29]

> **CLINICAL NOTE 14-12**   The area of surgery should not be probed for at least 1 month to allow the junctional epithelium to heal and the gingival connective tissue fibers to mature. After 1 month, the region may be gently probed, but healing of the connective tissue fibers is still not complete, so tissues are fragile. Connective tissue continues to heal and remodel for several months.

Periodontal maintenance should be continued at appropriate intervals during the surgical phase of periodontal treatment. Usually, periodontal debridement at intervals of 3 months or less should be continued until all planned surgical procedures are completed and the tissues have healed completely. At that time, a careful assessment of the patient's periodontal health can be made and recall intervals can be gradually increased, if appropriate.

HEALING AFTER PERIODONTAL SURGERY

Healing of the periodontal surgical wound begins shortly after the procedure is completed. A blood clot forms at the surgical site, protecting the wound and allowing the tissue to begin to heal. The blood clot acts as a matrix and scaffolding for healing cells to migrate into the wound area. However, it is essential that the blood clot be as thin as possible because the inflammatory cells associated with wound healing are also required to remove the fibrin clot to complete healing. The inflammatory response needs to be minimized to prevent the destructive forces of the host response from slowing or altering healing (see Chapter 2). Firm pressure is placed on the flap margins after the flaps are sutured to minimize the thickness of the forming clot. The blood clot also provides stability to the wound by binding the displaced flaps to the underlying bone.

The epithelial cells are the first to heal. After an initial stunning effect of about 24 hours, they begin to divide and grow from the wound margins. Epithelial cells migrate about 0.5 to 1.0 mm/day, so in 5 to 7 days the gingival surface of the wound is covered. Epithelial healing is the point at which the wound is

sufficiently protected so that the sutures and pack may be removed. The epithelial cells continue to grow for the next 2 weeks, mainly by thickening the epithelial layer, until normal anatomy is restored. In studies of the healing of periodontal surgical wounds, the junctional epithelium returned to its presurgical appearance in 10 to 12 days.[30]

Beneath the fibrin blood clot, the healing wound exhibits all the classic signs of inflammation, including migrating lymphocytes and macrophages that help to eliminate bacteria and debris in the surgical site. As healing progresses, these inflammatory cells begin to digest the fibrin itself. Connective tissue healing begins after the epithelium has begun to heal and has laid down its basal lamina. Fibroblasts from the connective tissue adjacent to the surgical area begin to divide, proliferate, and migrate into the wound area. Capillaries from the adjacent tissues begin to grow into the site and result in the development of a capillary-rich and heavily cellular healing granulation tissue. The fibroblasts begin to lay down an extracellular matrix of collagen fibers that mature and remodel over the next 2 to 4 weeks. By 2 weeks after surgery, the wound strength approaches presurgical levels. The clinical appearance of an access flap procedure after 1 week is shown in Figure 14-10, *I* and *J*. Healing after 3 months is shown in Figure 14-10, *K* and *L*.

Osseous healing does not begin until late in the healing process. Approximately 1 month after osseous surgery, the wound site is populated with osteoblast cells. At this stage, there is active formation of uncalcified bone matrix, called osteoid. This active tissue may be an effective autogenous grafting material. For this reason, healing tooth extraction sites, 1 or 2 months after tooth removal, are often chosen as a source of donor bone for periodontal bone graft surgery. Calcification continues to increase during the next 6 months. The alveolar bone requires 4 to 6 months to heal and remodel completely. Radiographs of bone at surgical sites usually show significant increases in density 6 to 12 months after surgery.

Gingivectomy wounds require slightly more time to heal than flap procedures because the epithelial cells must migrate relatively long distances from the wound margins. This type of healing is termed *healing by secondary intention* because the large area of fibrin clot must be completely replaced with epithelium, resulting in scar formation. Fortunately, in the oral cavity, scar tissue and gingival tissue both have the same types of cells and collagen fibers. Therefore, healed gingivectomy wounds have the same color and consistency as the normal gingiva.

Free gingival grafts must obtain their nutrients from the underlying recipient site by diffusion for the 2 weeks after surgery. The grafted epithelium usually degenerates and revascularization of the graft begins with anastomosis of the capillaries from the recipient site in 4 to 5 days. After 1 week, the gingival graft areas appear highly inflamed, with a white film of necrotic epithelium. Patients should be warned that this appearance represents the expected healing response and that the gingiva will begin to take on a more normal appearance in the ensuing weeks.

Bone-grafting procedures usually take more time for healing than other osseous procedures. The bone graft material may need to be resorbed before new bone can be formed.

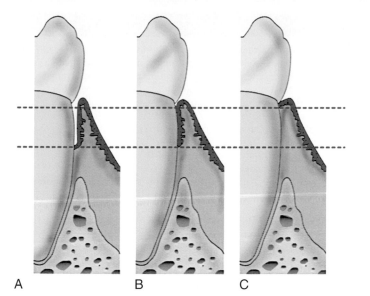

FIGURE 14-18 ■ **Healing of the periodontal tissues to the root surface after periodontal surgery. A,** Preoperative periodontal pocket. **B,** Healing by long junctional epithelium is the more common result. **C,** Healing by new connective tissue attachment is possible but likely only in the most apical regions of the pockets.

Osteogenesis appears to be continuing about 3 weeks after the graft is placed and new periodontal ligament, cementum, and alveolar bone are well formed and functioning in about 3 months. Maturation of the newly formed bone can continue for up to 6 months, or even beyond; thus, radiographs, which are sometimes taken to look at new bone fill, should not be taken before this time.

Healing of the dentogingival junction to a root that was previously exposed to periodontal disease occurs in two ways. A long junctional epithelium may develop that is tightly adapted to the root surface apical to the area of the former pocket. Alternatively, new connective tissue attachment may develop, with new periodontal ligament fibers inserting into re-formed cementum and alveolar bone (regeneration). The purpose of guided tissue regeneration is to encourage new connective tissue attachment and delay growth of oral epithelium into the healing area next to the tooth. In most cases, both types of dentogingival healing occur. Long epithelial attachments form coronally and new connective tissue attachments form only at the most apical levels of the pocket, as illustrated in Figure 14-18. Regeneration and scar tissue formation are described in Box 14-2.

THE ROLE OF THE DENTAL HYGIENIST IN PERIODONTAL SURGERY

The dental hygienist has a significant role in the overall treatment of the periodontal patient, including the surgical phase of therapy. The dental hygienist may be the most appropriate member of the dental team to discuss the advantages and disadvantages of surgical treatment with the patient. The periodontist or dentist is legally charged with the responsibility of informing the patient of the risks, benefits, and alternatives to periodontal surgery. However, the dental hygienist may act as the patient's advocate by asking questions and helping to provide the answers to concerns that the patient is unable to articulate.

The dental hygienist also plays a central role in the postsurgical treatment of the periodontal patient. Postoperative care is often provided by the dental hygienist, including suture and dressing removal, postsurgical biofilm removal, follow-up wound care, and home care instructions. The success of periodontal surgery depends primarily on long-term plaque biofilm control by the patient. This is particularly critical after surgical treatment, when tissues are tender and specialized methods of interdental plaque biofilm control are needed.

In many periodontal offices, the dental hygienist has an important place in the surgical team. The dental hygienist provides presurgical plaque biofilm control, scaling, and root planing therapy, observes and assists during the surgical treatment (and notes the success or failure of specific instrumentation techniques for plaque and calculus removal in deep pockets), and often provides the bulk of postsurgical treatment and follow-up care. A comprehensive understanding of the goals, indications, specific surgical procedures, contraindications, and course of events for these procedures is mandatory to fulfill the obligation of complete informed care of the periodontal patient. These activities are summarized in Table 14-1.

⊚ DENTAL HYGIENE CONSIDERATIONS

- The goals of periodontal surgery are pocket reduction, abscess drainage, correction of mucogingival defects, aesthetic improvement, access for restorative procedures, regeneration of lost tissue, and placement of dental implants.
- Pockets of 5 to 9 mm are the most successfully treated by periodontal surgical procedures.
- Specific considerations in deciding to perform periodontal surgery are pocket depth, bone loss, value of the tooth, plaque biofilm control, health of the patient, and patient preference.
- Pocket reduction surgery includes excisional procedures (gingivectomy and gingivoplasty) and incisional procedures (periodontal flap surgery).
- Osseous surgical procedures combine flap procedures for access with sculpting the bone to restore a physiologic architecture.
- Mucogingival surgery includes a variety of plastic-type surgeries to increase attached gingiva, improve aesthetics, or augment edentulous spaces.
- Regeneration procedures attempt to restore the periodontal tissues destroyed by disease. These include bone-grafting procedures and guided tissue regeneration.
- Guided tissue regeneration permits healing cells to proliferate from bone and periodontal ligament rather than epithelium to more reliably gain new attachment to the tooth more reliably.
- Procedures following periodontal surgery include suturing of tissues, possible use of periodontal dressing, and provision of postoperative instructions.
- Postoperative instructions should be reviewed with the patient and provided in written form. They include limiting physical activity, controlling bleeding with finger pressure if needed, consuming a soft diet, filling and taking prescriptions for analgesics and antibiotics if needed, being aware that swelling may occur, avoiding smoking, and following plaque biofilm instructions.
- The patient should be seen for a postoperative appointment 1 week after surgery. At that time, the dressing and sutures are removed and the patient's plaque biofilm procedures adjusted as needed.

BOX 14-2 Scarring of the Oral Soft Tissues

Despite extensive surgical interventions during periodontal surgery, including incisions made entirely through the gingiva and periosteum to the bone, there is little visible scarring. After periodontal surgery, the gingiva heals with a normal clinical appearance (see Figure 13-10, *K* and *L*). Among oral tissues, this general lack of visible scarring is unique to the gingiva. Scarring is occasionally seen in the attached gingiva but is much more commonly found in other areas, such as the lip or mucosa. Endodontic surgery, such as apicectomy (the removal of the apex of the root and surrounding infected tissue to permit healing of endodontic infections in bone), results in a thin white scar in the alveolar mucosa apical to the gingiva. It is differences in the connective tissue underlying the epithelium that account for this clinical finding.

Healing occurs as *regeneration* of tissues or *repair* of tissues. Regeneration is the process that completely restores injured tissue so that it is indistinguishable in function and appearance from the original. In the periodontium, a wound that only penetrates the epithelium will heal through regeneration. In this type of wound, epithelial cells migrate from the margins of the wound, and the new tissue is identical to uninjured epithelium. Repair is healing that occurs through the formation of a connective tissue scar. It occurs in the periodontium when wounds penetrate into connective tissue or deeper. Scarring is a normal process that is indicative of the loss of mature tissues' ability to regenerate like embryonic tissues.[31]

Healing by repair after an injury is a process to restore tissues to functional integrity. It consists of a series of events that occur in an overlapping manner. These are the early wound-healing or inflammatory phase, the remodeling phase, and the late phase of contraction and scarring.[31]

In the early phase after injury, the body forms a blood clot with a fibrin matrix. With skin wounds, the matrix is called a scab. This matrix permits the growth of cells into the wound area, and 3 or 4 days after the injury, the inflammatory cells, fibroblasts, and immature blood vessels form a highly vascular granulation tissue throughout the matrix. Healing is the gradual replacement of the matrix with functional tissues. The granulation tissue will eventually remodel and establish the healed scar.[31] During the first few days of healing, the fibroblasts also secrete substances that are hydrophilic (attract water), and thus the healing injury appears edematous.

The remodeling phase of healing is the gradual change of the fibrin matrix and granulation tissue to dense organized collagen. It begins with matrix formation and continues long after the wound appears clinically healed, perhaps for months. Reepithelialization, or closure of the surface of the wound, occurs separately but at the same time as the inflammatory and remodeling phases of healing. It does not require vital granulation tissue on which to migrate.[31]

The late phase of healing represents wound contraction and scar formation. As time progresses during healing, the collagen organizes along stress lines, gradually increasing the strength of the healing tissue. As collagen increases, much of the vascularization disappears and the wound appears as a pale white scar. Wound contraction is a phenomenon where by the cells decrease the wound area by drawing together the margins. It occurs independently of epithelial regeneration. Contraction forces are extremely strong and can result in major distortion of tissue, including enough force to bend bone.[31] Often, the result is that even a large wound may contract 90% or more, resulting in a small white line scar.

In the gingival tissues, the collagen is thick and very dense under the attached gingiva. During the latter stages of wound healing, when collagen is organizing into scar tissue, contraction does not occur in this area to the extent that it can in mucosa, where the connective tissue is mostly elastic and has less collagen. Epithelium regenerates over the connective tissue matrix, leaving a healed lesion that is indistinguishable clinically from the original gingival tissue. All the elements of wound healing occur, and the remodeling of the collagen can be seen histologically. The denseness of the underlying collagen and the limited contraction of the wound in the gingiva result in a thin avascular scar, but the scar tissue is clinically indistinguishable from the adjacent normal gingiva. The figure below is an unusual example of scarring of the attached gingiva.

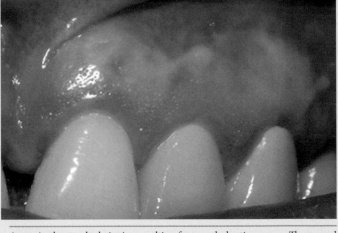

A scar in the attached gingiva resulting from endodontic surgery. The wound margins were not closely adapted together after surgery, causing migration of collagen cells and significant wound contraction, and resulting in a visible scar. Typically, there is no visible scarring after periodontal surgery. For an example of healing of an attached gingiva, see Figure 13-10, *J* to *L*. (Courtesy of Dr. David W. Rising.)

TABLE 14-1   The Responsibilities of the Dental Hygienist in Periodontal Surgery

PRESURGICAL	SURGERY	POSTSURGERY
Nonsurgical treatment Oral hygiene procedures, including patient motivation Scaling and root planing Caries control	Assisting	Postoperative procedures Suture removal Dressing removal Plaque biofilm control
Knowledgeable resource for patient questions	Assessing plaque biofilm control needs	Assessing and reviewing plaque control procedures
	Providing appropriate plaque control education and tools	Treating postoperative sensitivity Providing regular maintenance care

★ CASE SCENARIO

Mr. Herbert had extensive periodontal surgery 2 weeks ago that included all the posterior teeth on the mandibular right side of the mouth. The surgery consisted of the reflection of flaps and osseous contouring to correct the reverse architecture in the area. He came back for his first postoperative appointment 1 week ago and his sutures were removed. The periodontist has now referred him to you for follow-up care.

1. You need to be very conscious of Mr. Herbert's plaque biofilm control because
   A. healing areas are tender.
   B. different oral hygiene aids may need to be taught.
   C. the architecture of the gingiva and bone in the surgical site will be changed.
   D. all of the above.

2. Mr. Herbert is likely to have teeth in the area of surgery that are quite mobile because of swelling in the periodontal ligament space during the healing phase.
   A. Both the statement and the reason are correct and related.
   B. Both the statement and the reason are correct but NOT related.
   C. The statement is correct, but the reason is NOT correct.
   D. The statement is NOT correct, but the reason is correct.
   E. NEITHER the statement NOR the reason is correct.

3. You should NOT probe the surgical area for several weeks because
   A. the tissue will reepithelialize in 7 to 10 days.
   B. the bone is regenerating in the residual pockets.
   C. the junctional epithelium is elongated and fragile.
   D. the connective tissue will heal in 4 or more weeks.

4. Root sensitivity is often experienced by patients after periodontal surgery for all the following reasons EXCEPT one. Which one is the EXCEPTION?
   A. Exposure of root surfaces
   B. Exposure of dentinal tubules
   C. Changes in diet due to surgery
   D. Shrinkage of the gingiva during healing

STUDY QUESTIONS

Answers and rationales to these questions can be obtained from your instructor.

MULTIPLE CHOICE

1. The types of periodontal surgery in which the periodontist shapes the alveolar bone with chisels or burs to remove bony defects are called procedures for
   A. creation of a new attachment.
   B. access to the root surface.
   C. treatment of osseous defects.
   D. pocket reduction or elimination.
   E. correction of mucogingival defects.

2. The types of periodontal surgery that increase the predictability for growth of new tissues of the periodontal apparatus are called procedures for
   A. access to the root surface.
   B. guided tissue regeneration.
   C. treatment of osseous defects.
   D. pocket reduction or elimination.
   E. correction of mucogingival defects.

3. Periodontal surgery is most successful when pocket depths are between 5 and 9 mm. Indications for periodontal surgery are more affected by measurements of clinical attachment loss than by those of pocket depths.
   A. Both statements are TRUE.
   B. Both statements are FALSE.
   C. The first statement is TRUE, and the second statement is FALSE.
   D. The first statement is FALSE, and the second statement is TRUE.

4. Regenerative periodontal surgical procedures
   A. selectively encourage the growth of cells of the attachment apparatus.
   B. selectively discourage the growth of cells of the attachment apparatus.
   C. selectively encourage the growth of the cells of the epithelium of the closely approximated flaps.
   D. selectively discourage the growth of the cells of the epithelium on the surface of the excisional wound.

5. The most common oral site for donor tissue for free gingival graft procedures is the
   A. palate.
   B. tongue.
   C. lingual mucosa.
   D. fresh extraction site.

6. Surgical sites should not be probed for at least 1 week after surgery because the collagen fibers have not had sufficient time to heal to be able to resist the penetration force of the probe.
   A. Both the statement and the reason are correct and related.
   B. Both the statement and the reason are correct but NOT related.
   C. The statement is correct, but the reason is NOT correct.
   D. The statement is NOT correct, but the reason is correct.
   E. NEITHER the statement NOR the reason is correct.

7. The primary reason to perform excisional periodontal surgery is to provide access to root surfaces for debridement. Debridement during surgery is necessary because it is very difficult to remove all the calculus and plaque on root surfaces during the presurgical phase.
   A. Both statements are TRUE.
   B. Both statements are FALSE.
   C. The first statement is TRUE, and the second statement is FALSE.
   D. The first statement is FALSE, and the second statement is TRUE.

8. The most important clinical measure of bone loss is
   A. recession.
   B. probing depth.
   C. attachment loss.
   D. "sounding" for bone.

SHORT ANSWER

9. List the general factors that must be considered before periodontal surgery.

10. Why is thorough Phase I therapy, including scaling, root planing, and oral hygiene instruction, completed at least 4 weeks prior to periodontal surgery?

Please visit **http://evolve.elsevier.com/Perry/periodontology** for additional practice and study support tools.

REFERENCES

1. Ramfjord SP, Ash MM. *Periodontology and Periodontics*. Philadelphia, PA: WB Saunders; 1979.

2. McDonnell HT, Mills MP. Principles and practice of periodontal surgery. In: Rose LF, Mealey BL, eds. *Periodontics: Medicine, Surgery, and Implants*. St. Louis, MO: Elsevier Mosby; 2004:358–404.

3. Green E, Parr RW, Taggart EJ. *Surgery in Periodontal Maintenance Therapy*. San Francisco, CA: Praxis; 1984:8–22.

4. Stambaugh RV, Dragoo M, Smith DV, et al. The limits of subgingival scaling. *Int J Periodontics Restorative Dent*. 1981;1:31–41.

5. Green E, Parr RW, Taggart EJ. *Surgery in Periodontal Maintenance Therapy*. San Francisco, CA: Praxis;1984:44–61.

6. Maynard JG, Wilson RDK. Physiologic dimensions of the periodontium significant to the restorative dentist. *J Periodontol*. 1979;50:170–174.

7. Lindhe J, Westfelt E, Nyman S, et al. Healing following surgical/non-surgical treatment of periodontal disease: a clinical study. *J Clin Periodontol*. 1982;9:115–128.

8. Lang NP, Löe H. Clinical management of periodontal diseases. *Periodontology 2000*. 1993;2:128–139.

9. Tibbetts LS, Ammons Jr WF. Resective periodontal surgery. In: Rose LF, Mealey BL, eds. *Periodontics: Medicine, Surgery, and Implants*. St. Louis, MO: Elsevier Mosby; 2004:502–552.

10. Ramfjord SP, Nissle RR. The modified Widman flap. *J Periodontol*. 1974;45:601–608.

11. Yukna RA. Longitudinal evaluation of the excisional new attachment procedures in humans. *J Periodontol*. 1978;49:142–144.

12. Smith DH, Ammons WF, Van Belle GA. Longitudinal study of periodontal status comparing osseous recontouring with flap curettage. *J Periodontol*. 1980:51:367–375.

13. Moskow B. Longevity: a critical factor in evaluating the effectiveness of periodontal therapy. *J Clin Periodontol*. 1987;14:237–244.

14. Friedman N. Periodontal osseous surgery: osteoplasty and ostectomy. *J Periodontol*. 1955;6:257–269.

15. Ammons WF Jr. Treatment of molar furcations. In: Rose LF, Mealey BL, eds. *Periodontics: Medicine, Surgery, and Implants*. St. Louis, MO: Elsevier Mosby; 2004:553–571.

16. Joshipura KJ, Kent RL, DePaola PF. Gingival recession: intra-oral distribution and associated factors. *J Periodontol*. 1994;65:864–871.

17. Glover ME. Periodontal plastic and reconstructive surgery. In: Rose LF, Mealey BL, eds. *Periodontics: Medicine, Surgery, and Implants*. St. Louis, MO: Elsevier Mosby; 2004:405–487.

18. Wennstrom JL. Lack of association between width of attached gingiva and development of soft tissue recession: a five-year longitudinal study. *J Clin Periodontol*. 1983;10:206–221.

19. Langer B, Calagna LJ. The subepithelial connective tissue graft: a new approach to the enhancement of anterior cosmetics. *Int J Periodont Restorative Dent*. 1982;2:23–33.

20. Maynard JG, Wilson RDK. Physiologic dimensions of the periodontium significant to the restorative dentist. *J Periodontol*. 1979;50:170–174.

21. Cabrera PO. Connective tissue grafting: an option in reconstructive periodontal surgery. *J Am Dent Assoc*. 1994;125:729–737.

22. Mellonig JT. Periodontal regenerative surgery. In: *Periodontal Disease Management*. Chicago, IL: American Academy of Periodontology; 1994: 385–397.

23. Ellegaard B, Low H. New attachment of periodontal tissues after treatment of intrabony pockets. *J Periodontol*. 1971;42:648–652.

24. Mellonig J, Prewett A, Moyer M. HIV inactivation in a bone allograft. *J Periodontol*. 1992;63:979–983.

25. American Academy of Periodontology. *Periodontal Regeneration: Report of the Research, Science and Therapy Committee*. Chicago, IL: American Academy of Periodontology; 1993.

26. Garrett JS, Crigger M, Egelberg J. Effects of citric acid on diseased root surfaces. *J Periodontal Res*. 1978;13:155–163.

27. Caffesse RG, Kerry GJ, Chaves ES, et al. Clinical evaluation of the use of citric acid and autologous fibronectin in periodontal surgery. *J Periodontol*. 1988;59:565–569.

28. Gottlow J, Nyman S, Karring T, et al. New attachment formation in the human periodontium by guided tissue regeneration: case reports. *J Clin Periodontol*. 1986;13:604–616.

29. Klokkevold PR, Takei HH, Carranza FA. General principles of periodontal surgery. In: Newman MG, Takei HH, Klokkevold PR, et al, eds. *Carranza's Clinical Periodontology*. 11th ed. St. Louis, MO: Elsevier Saunders; 2012: 525–534.

30. Takata T, Nikai H, Ijuhin N, et al. Ultrastructure of regenerated junctional epithelium after surgery of rat molar gingiva. *J Periodontol*. 1986;57: 776–783.

31. Bertolami CN, Messadi DV. Complications associated with wound healing. In: Kaban LB, Pogrel MA, Perrott DH, eds. *Complications in Oral and Maxillofacial Surgery*. Philadelphia, PA: WB Saunders; 1997: 41–53.

CHAPTER 15

Dental Implants

Fritz Finzen and Dorothy A. Perry
Based on the original work by Kamran Haghighat

LEARNING OUTCOMES

- Describe the common types of dental implants.
- Discuss the indications and contraindications for dental implant therapy.
- Explain why titanium is the best biomaterial available for use in dental implants.
- Define the concept of osseointegration.

- Compare and contrast the bone and soft tissue interfaces of implants and the natural dentition.
- List the criteria for success used in implant therapy.
- Describe the maintenance protocol for implant patients.
- Evaluate the elements of appropriate home care regimens for patients with implants.

KEY TERMS

Abutment screw
Biocompatibility
Biomaterials
Cover screw
Endosseous implant
Failing implant
Immediate loading
Implant abutment

Implant biologic width
Implant fixture
Jumping distance
Loading
Nonsubmerged protocol
Osseointegration
Peri-implant disease
Peri-implant mucositis

Peri-implantitis
Submerged protocol
Subperiosteal implant
Superstructure
Titanium
Transosteal implant

Since their introduction, dental implants have revolutionized the way dentistry is practiced. Today, many teeth that previously needed heroic treatment efforts to preserve them are now extracted and replaced with implants. Dental implants have undoubtedly been the most significant breakthrough in dentistry over the past 40 years and they have become an integral part of dental practice.

A multitude of dental implant systems are currently used in the rehabilitation of edentulous and partially dentate patients. The majority of the implants used in clinical dentistry are the root form type, **endosseous implants,** which are based on the principle of **osseointegration.** The term *osseointegration* was coined by Professor P.I. Bränemark to describe an intimate lattice that is formed between titanium implant surfaces and bone. From the late 1960s to the mid-1970s, dental implant systems were not osseointegrated and were not viewed favorably by the community because they were considered unpredictable. The observations and findings of Bränemark, Albrektsson, and colleagues, together with the long-term survival data of osseointegrated dental implants, have changed this perception so that the procedure has become a highly predictable and valuable option in the replacement of missing teeth.[1-4]

Today, in excess of 50 implant systems are available, with innovations being proposed and instituted by different manufacturers through intense competition. However, many of these newer systems lack the longitudinal research necessary before patient application. Ideally, longitudinal trials of 5 years or longer are required to forecast the validity of emerging treatment concepts adequately. The American Dental Association provides an acceptance program for endosseous implants through its Council on Dental Materials, Instruments, and Devices.[5] Accepted implants have shown success for a minimum of 5 years in clinical trials of 50 or more patients.

TYPES OF IMPLANTS

The most commonly used dental implant is the osseointegrated root form dental implant. Subperiosteal and transosteal types are also still seen, but much less frequently. All are described in this chapter because they are still seen in clinical practice. However, the focus is on the most common and successful implant, the endosseous osseointegrated root form dental implant.

SUBPERIOSTEAL IMPLANTS

The **subperiosteal implant** is a custom-made cast framework that is placed beneath the periosteum over the alveolar bone. It can be used in either the maxilla or mandible. The frame rests

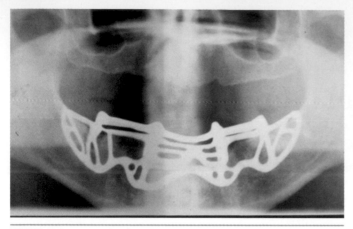

FIGURE 15-1 ■ Example of a subperiosteal implant as it appears in a panographic radiograph.

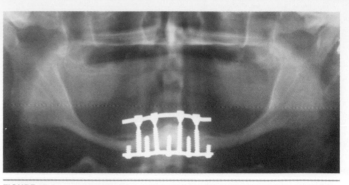

FIGURE 15-2 ■ Example of a transosteal implant as it appears in a panographic radiograph. (Courtesy of Dr. Frederick C. Finzen.)

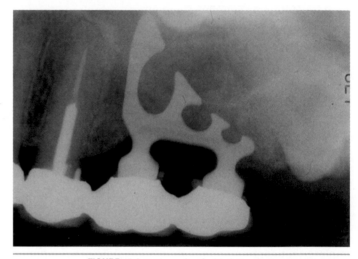

FIGURE 15-3 ■ Example of a blade implant.

on the jawbone, with no evidence of direct union with the bone in most cases. Posts of varying number, based on the prosthetic design, protrude through the soft tissues to provide anchorage for the denture or fixed prosthesis. A radiograph of a subperiosteal implant is presented in Figure 15-1.

TRANSOSTEAL IMPLANTS

Transosteal implants traverse the mandible in an apicocoronal direction. They protrude through the gingival tissues into the mouth for prosthesis anchorage. A stabilization plate is placed along the inferior border of the mandible. Posts are in turn attached to this plate and traverse the mandible to provide anchorage for the prosthesis. Their use is limited to the mandible, where they are commonly referred to as staple implants.

The interfacial adaptation between the subperiosteal and transosteal implants and bone resembles that of scar tissue with no direct bone anchorage. This creates a compromised arrangement under occlusal loads. An example of a transosteal implant is presented in Figure 15-2.

ENDOSSEOUS IMPLANTS

Endosseous implants, which come in a variety of different shapes, are placed within bone. They are broadly divided into blade and root form types. The root form variety is either screw- or cylinder-shaped, with different lengths, diameters, and manufacturer-specific design characteristics. The blade implant is no longer used because it has a high incidence of complications and failures. An example of a blade implant is shown in Figure 15-3.

Root form endosseous implants provide direct osseous anchorage through formation of an intimate lattice between the implant surface and bone. They are the most predictable and acceptable implant type used in clinical practice. These implants are used extensively for replacing missing teeth in partially and totally edentulous patients. Examples of several root form endosseous implants are presented in Figure 15-4.

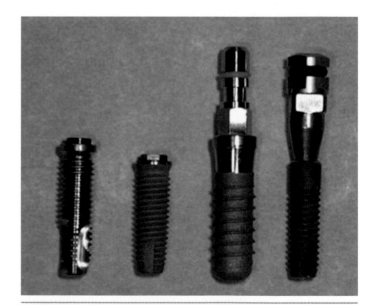

FIGURE 15-4 ■ **A selection of titanium root form endosseous implants.** The two on the right are shown with placement tools.

CLINICAL NOTE 15-1 The most common type of implant seen in dental practice is the root form endosseous implant to which an abutment and fixed prosthesis are attached.

OSSEOINTEGRATION

The definition of osseointegration has evolved through the development of more refined methods of studying the interface between the implant and surrounding bone. The precise nature

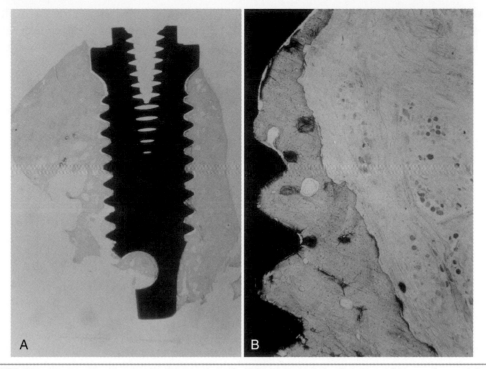

FIGURE 15-5 ■ **Peri-implant supporting tissues seen at the light microscopic level. A,** View of the root form with bone growth surrounding the titanium. **B,** Higher magnification showing bone apposition directly next to the titanium surface. (Used with permission from Bernard G, Carranza FA, Jovanovic S. Biologic aspects of dental implants. In: Newman MG, Takei HG, Carranza FA, eds. *Clinical Periodontology.* 9th ed. Philadelphia, PA: WB Saunders; 2002.)

of this integration is not fully understood. Originally, because of limitations in histologic techniques at the light microscope level, the term was defined as a direct implant to bone union without any intervening soft connective tissue,[3,4] a condition that resembles that of functional ankylosis.[6] A light microscopic view of osseointegration is presented in Figure 15-5. With the advent of scanning electron microscopy, more direct analysis of the interface is possible and osseointegration is more clearly understood. Scanning electron microscopy of the interface reveals a narrow nonmineralized zone, approximately 20 to 40 nm, between the bone and the implant, containing chondroitin sulfate glycosaminoglycans.[7]

The definition of osseointegration, as proposed by Bräne-mark, is a "direct structural and functional connection between ordered, living bone and the surface of a load-bearing implant."[8] This definition is based on clinical and radiographic implant stability rather than true interfacial arrangement, as observed histologically. Because implant integration involves soft and hard tissues, the term *stably integrated* implant has been suggested to describe implant integration better.[9]

Longitudinal observation of the bone-implant interface has also demonstrated that because of the dynamic nature of bone, 100% integration never develops, and the bone to implant contact is both time-dependent and influenced by implant surface characteristics. The amount of bone to implant contact varies among different implant systems (because of surface characteristics) and ranges from 30% to 70%.[10] However, the exact amount of bone to implant contact required for success has not been determined.

Other than its application in the dental field for tooth replacement, the concept of osseointegration has been applied

in maxillofacial prosthodontics for correction of deformities and in orthopedics for joint and limb replacement.

The biologic processes involved in attainment and maintenance of implant integration depend on factors that include biomaterials and biocompatibility, implant design (e.g., length, diameter, shape, surface), bone factors, and surgical and loading considerations.[2]

BIOCOMPATIBILITY

Biocompatibility of a material is defined as allowing "close contact of living cells at its surface, which does not contain leachables (molecules that separate off the surface) that produce inflammation and which does not prevent growth and division of cells in culture."[11] Biocompatible materials are called biomaterials. Many different types of materials are considered biomaterials, including gold, stainless steel, cobalt-chromium alloys, bioactive glasses, niobium, hydroxyapatite, tricalcium phosphate, polymers, zirconium, and titanium. However, not all are compatible as an implant material.

Any implanted material is considered a foreign body. Unlike living tissue, the body recognizes all implanted metals as unnatural (nonself). Metals in contact with tissue fluid are prone to degradation and dissolution by corrosion. Exchange of protons with biologic molecules leads to antigen formation and cellular uptake. This reaction can prove toxic to cells and may inhibit growth and function. For example, fibroblast and osteoblast cells show growth inhibition with most metals other than titanium. Thus, commercially pure titanium has become the standard in osseointegration.

Titanium is a highly reactive yet biocompatible metal. It is the material of choice in osseointegration because it rapidly forms a layer of surface oxides, 0.3- to 0.5-mm thick, most notably of titanium oxide, when exposed to air or fluid (including tissue fluid). Unique to the mode of oxide formation on titanium is that no metal ion reaches the surface to be released. The oxide layer prevents corrosion on the surface so that tissue integration can occur. The tissue ground substance in the vicinity of the implant contains proteoglycans and other adhesion proteins that adhere to specific receptors in the oxide layer. Other advantages of titanium are that it is lightweight and possesses enough strength to withstand occlusal forces.

CLINICAL NOTE 15-2 Titanium is the most commonly used and most successful material for implants.

IMPLANT DESIGN AND SURFACE CONDITIONS
Length
The range of implant lengths varies among manufacturers. Most conventionally used implants are between 8 and 14 mm long; this range conforms to natural root lengths. Selection is based on the available bone height at the implant site and proximity to vital structures, such as nerve trunks and blood vessels.[12]

Diameter
Implant diameters range from 3 to 6 mm. The selection of a particular diameter is based on the width of the jaw ridge at the implant site. The jaw ridge is narrower in the lateral incisor region so narrower implants are used there, whereas wider implants can be used in the molar region. The wider implants provide a larger surface area, which increases the implant stability in areas with limited bone height.

Shape
The most dominant shape of endosseous implants used today is cylindrical. Implants are solid and most exhibit a threaded surface design. The thread pitch varies among implant systems and can influence the initial stability and force distribution to the surrounding bone. There are also hollow implants available with no threads.

Surface
Since the introduction of the original machined-surface implants, a variety of surface topographies and thread designs have been introduced. The initial stability of the implant is, in part, dependent on the surface texture.[13] The rate of bone apposition and growth and the amount of bone to implant contact are influenced by implant surface characteristics. Many studies have demonstrated that a higher bone to implant contact is attained around rough-surfaced implants. Methods for producing roughened implant surfaces include grit blasting, acid etching, plasma spraying, and using additive surfaces such as hydroxyapatite coating. An increased rate of bone growth and amount of surface contact with bone allows for better transfer of forces to bone, facilitates earlier **loading** protocols (placement of restorations on the implants), and permits better success in areas with poorer bone quality. Biomaterials research has been underway to develop surface modifications to improve bone inductive characteristics and to make these treatments even more predictable.

STATE OF HOST SITE AND BONE FACTORS
The amount of bone to implant contact achieved at the time of implant placement is related to the quantity and quality of bone and determines fixture stability. There is variability in the amount of cortical and cancellous tissue within the arch and between the maxilla and mandible. The volume density of cortical bone is three to four times that of cancellous bone. Cancellous bone therefore contributes less to implant stability at placement. Resorption of the alveolus is a natural sequelae to tooth loss. The extent of the resorptive process is dependent on the history of trauma or infection, the length of time since the loss occurred, and loading by removable prostheses. The quality of bone is also influenced by systemic conditions, such as osteoporosis, and social factors, such as smoking. Therefore, the shape and quality of bone must be considered when planning for implant therapy.[14]

LOADING CONSIDERATIONS
There are no fixed guidelines for the length of healing time after surgery and before prosthetic loading of implants. Bränemark originally advised 3 months for the mandible and 6 months for the maxilla. The difference in healing times reflects the variation in bone characteristics.[4] Movement of the implant more than 100 μm during the healing phase may result in fibrous tissue encapsulation of the implant rather than osseointegration, a result that does not provide long-term functional occlusal load. In cases in which the functional load can be controlled and the implant is determined as stable at the time of placement, **immediate loading** (placement of a restoration at the time of the implant surgery) is compatible with attaining osseointegration.[15]

INDICATIONS AND CONTRAINDICATIONS FOR IMPLANT THERAPY
INDICATIONS
The clinical situations in which osseointegrated implant-retained prostheses are used have expanded enormously. A diverse range of scenarios with varying degrees of complexity can be managed with the use of implants. These include the replacement of a single-tooth, treatment of partially and completely edentulous patients,[16] and correction of maxillofacial deformities. Single-tooth replacement with an implant-supported prosthesis is considered to be a highly predictable and effective alternative to conventional prosthodontics procedures, such as fixed partial dentures (bridges), which often require preparation of healthy neighboring teeth. Specific indications for dental implants may include the following:
- Treatment of patients with strong gag reflexes to eliminate palatal coverage by removable prostheses
- Long span bridges
- Free end removable partial dentures
- Alternative to periodontally compromised teeth for bridge abutments
- Hopeless periodontally or endodontically involved teeth
- Orthodontic anchorage

Examples of implant-supported prostheses are presented in Figures 15-6 through 15-9.

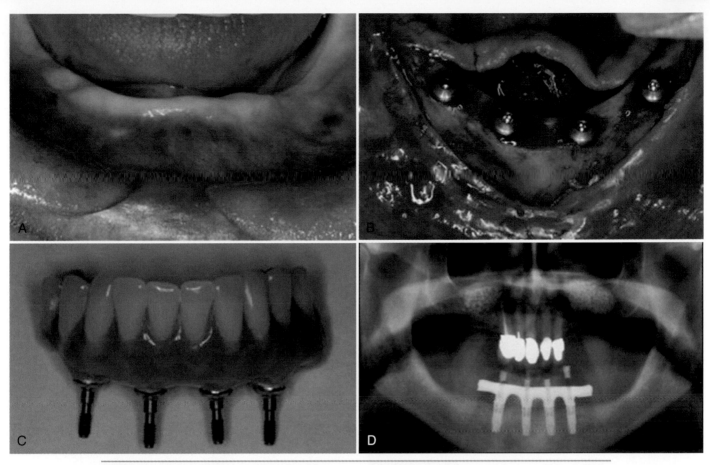

FIGURE 15-6 ■ Example of a mandibular fixed denture supported by four endosseous implants. A, The mandibular ridge as it healed after implant placement. B, The flaps reflected to expose the implants. C, The denture with abutments to attach to the implants. D, Panographic radiograph of the denture in place, attached to the implant fixtures. Note the restored natural teeth in the maxillary arch.

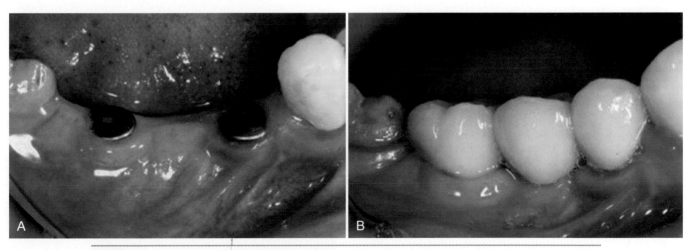

FIGURE 15-7 ■ Example of an implant-supported fixed partial denture. A, The implant fixtures. B, The restoration in place when the implants are loaded.

CONTRAINDICATIONS

It has been speculated that the presence of certain systemic, local, and social factors may affect the outcome of therapy. Age is not a contraindication for dental implants. Treatment should be delayed in younger patients until growth is near completion because, unlike the natural dentition, implants remain stationary during dentoalveolar growth. Similarly, increasing age in older persons has no adverse effect on osseointegration as long as associated medical conditions are well controlled or modified.[16,17]

Conditions that increase the patient's susceptibility to infection, such as uncontrolled diabetes, may result in a higher incidence of peri-implantitis and implant failure.

Osteoporosis, an age-related disease characterized by decreased bone mass and increased susceptibility to fractures, affects 20 million Americans, 80% of whom are older women.

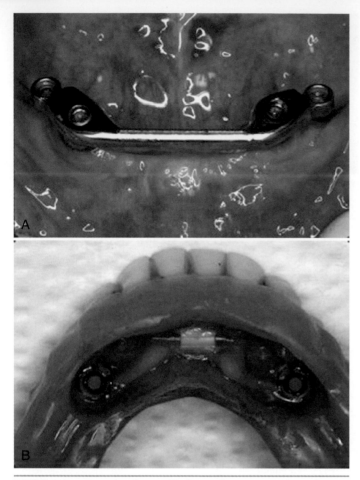

FIGURE 15-8 ▪ **Example of a mandibular implant-supported overdenture. A,** Two implants have been placed connected by a bar. **B,** The undersurface of the denture has attachments for connecting to the bar.

Hormone replacement therapy and osteoporosis do not appear to influence implant survival in this population.[16,18] Therapy with bisphosphonates has recently been attributed to an increased risk of jaw osteonecrosis and patients who have been treated with IV bisphosphonates are particularly at risk. Consultation with the patient's physician is recommended before implant therapy for patients receiving anticoagulant therapy because they are at risk for hemorrhage during surgical procedures. Patients on steroid therapy may have steroid-induced complications.[16]

The microbial pathogens associated with periodontal disease around natural teeth are also associated with disease progression around dental implants. Pathogenic bacteria associated with sites that exhibit active disease around teeth in partially dentate patients can colonize the peri-implant tissues.[19-21] Effective treatment and control of any periodontal disease before implant therapy is essential, and implants should only be considered in patients who demonstrate commitment to good home care and maintenance routines.

CLINICAL NOTE 15-3 The periodontal pathogens that can infect the tissues around implant fixtures are the same pathogens associated with periodontal disease around natural teeth.

The adverse effects of smoking on osseointegration and implant survival have been shown in many studies. Although

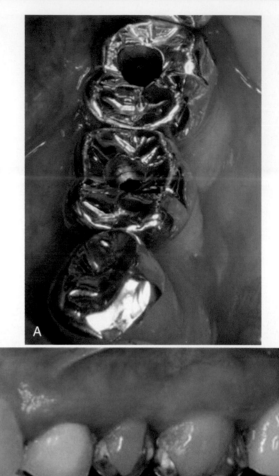

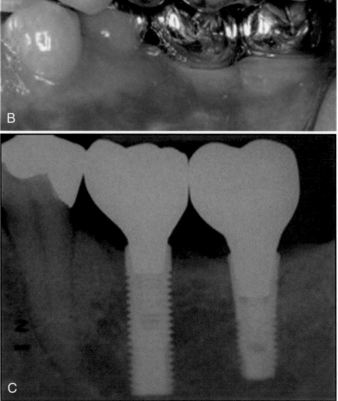

FIGURE 15-9 ▪ **Examples of screw-retained, implant-supported crowns. A,** The crowns in place on the fixtures; the holes are access for the screws that attach the restoration to the abutment. **B,** Lateral view of the crowns in place. **C,** Radiographic view of the implant-supported crowns.

smoking is not an absolute contraindication to implant therapy, it increases the risk of peri-implantitis and implant failure.[16] A smoking cessation protocol before implant surgery and during the healing period improves the treatment outcome.

TEETH AND IMPLANTS

The natural dentition is surrounded by the periodontium, comprising the gingiva, cementum, alveolar bone, and periodontal ligament (PDL). The gingival sulcus is 1 to 3 mm deep in health; the base of the sulcus is formed by the coronal aspect of the junctional epithelium (JE). The JE is attached to the root surface by hemidesmosomes and a basal lamina. The cells of the JE have a high turnover rate and can migrate on the root surface to reestablish an attachment or form a new one. This occurs after trauma, inflammation and bone loss, restorative procedures that impinge upon the epithelial–connective tissue attachment zone (biologic width), and periodontal surgery.

The peri-implant soft tissue is shaped after abutment connection or, in the case of single-stage implant systems, forms around the transmucosal portion of the fixture (the section that extends from the bone into the oral cavity). The collagen fibers are aligned parallel to and organized in a circular arrangement around the supracrestal portion of the implant.[22] There is no cemental layer over the implant surface, so fiber insertion is not possible. Initial observations by Gould and colleagues,[23] and many subsequent studies, have demonstrated that peri-implant soft tissue adheres to the titanium collar of the implant by a hemidesmosomal and basal lamina attachment mechanism, analogous to that of the JE to enamel attachment.[1]

The PDL provides anchorage in the alveolus for natural teeth and allows physiologic mobility and proprioceptive sensation from the dentition. The connective tissue fibers of the PDL attach to the alveolar bone and cementum perpendicularly and adapt to variations in occlusal load. The PDL space is highly vascular and a major source of undifferentiated mesenchymal cells, which play a pivotal role in regenerative and adaptive processes. Resorption and apposition of the surrounding bone and widening of the PDL space under different physiologic conditions, such as those seen in orthodontic tooth movement and occlusal trauma, are also functions of the PDL.

Implants acquire their stability and anchorage through osseointegration. There is no PDL so proprioceptive feedback is minimal, although proprioceptive mechanisms in the surrounding hard and soft tissues exist. Once osseointegrated,

orthodontic movement of implants is not possible, and it is important to control the forces applied to implants for maintenance of the integrated interface. Unfavorable loading of implants is one etiologic factor for bone loss around implants.[10]

> **CLINICAL NOTE 15-4** The bone and implant surface form a direct connection. There is a junctional epithelial attachment to the implant and a poorly organized connective tissue attachment apical to it. However, there is no periodontal ligament nor any connective tissue fibers attaching to the implant fixture.

The biologic width around teeth—that is the dimension of the epithelial and connective tissue attachments—is approximately 2 mm. A similar implant biologic width has also been described for the peri-implant mucosa, which comprises a 2-mm long JE and a 1-mm zone of connective tissue.[16] The connective tissue zone is poorly organized and exists between the JE, which is typically attached to the prosthetic component, called the implant abutment, and bone. The implant abutment extends from the implant through the soft tissues (transmucosally) and can be temporary (to allow soft tissue healing) or permanent. The implant abutment is connected to the implant fixture (the root analogue device in the bone) by an abutment screw.

The osseous crest around natural teeth in health follows the outline of the cementoenamel junction at a distance of 1 to 2 mm apically on the root surface. The location of the crestal bone level around implants depends on the implant design and may vary from 0.5 to 3 mm from the top of the implant fixture. These characteristics are compared in Table 15-1 and demonstrated diagrammatically in Figure 15-10.

SUCCESS CRITERIA

The clinical success of implant therapy is assessed by radiographic imaging, evaluation of implant mobility, and observing the surrounding soft tissue. Refinements to these conventional techniques include the use of digital and subtraction radiography, computed tomography, and devices that record the implant interface contact. Although evaluation of implants includes assessment of soft tissue parameters, such as probing depths, this criterion is considered to be of limited value around implants and remains controversial.[1] Criteria commonly used to determine implant success are outlined in Box 15-1.

TABLE 15-1   Comparison of Teeth and Implants in Health

	TEETH	IMPLANTS
Gingival sulcus depth	Shallow	Depth dependent on implant type and prosthetic component length
Gingival fibers	Inserted into supracrestal root cementum	Fibers arranged parallel to implant
Location of crestal bone	1-2 mm from cementoenamel junction	Dependent on implant design; ranges 0.5-2.5 mm from implant shoulder or to first thread
Connective tissue attachment	Sharpey's collagen fibers inserted into alveolar bone and cementum	Bone-implant interface has no fiber insertions; filled with chondroitin sulfate glycosaminoglycans
Mobility	Physiologic as a function of PDL	No PDL; rigid fixation similar to that of functional ankylosis
Proprioception	Receptors within PDL	No receptors within interface

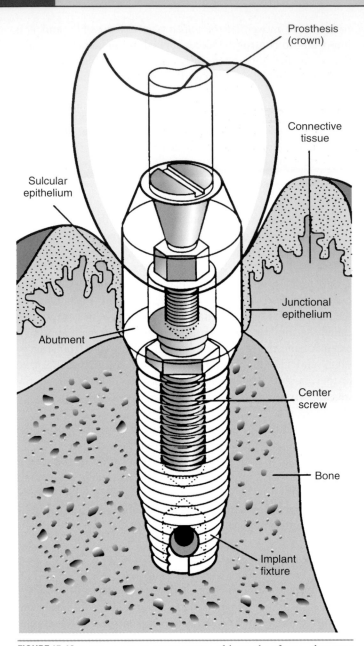

FIGURE 15-10 ■ Diagrammatic representation of the implant fixture, abutment, and crown as they relate to the surrounding tissues.

Labels: Prosthesis (crown); Connective tissue; Sulcular epithelium; Junctional epithelium; Abutment; Center screw; Bone; Implant fixture

BOX 15-1   Criteria for Implant Success[1,24]

1. No peri-implant radiolucency
2. Absence of mobility
3. Bone loss not greater than one third of implant
4. Provide functional service for 5 years in 85% of cases in the anterior maxilla and 90% in the anterior mandible; after 10 years, 80% success in the maxilla and 85% in the mandible
5. Absence of persistent or irreversible signs or symptoms such as pain, infection, neuropathies, paresthesia, and violation of the mandibular canal
6. Bone loss < 0.2 mm annually after first year of service
7. Implant design allows restoration satisfactory to patient and dentist
8. Absence of continuous marginal bone loss
9. Absence of persistent soft tissue complications
10. Probing depth < 4 to 5 mm; bone loss < 4 mm
11. No mechanical failure

Most of the implant systems available for clinical application demonstrate high success rates. The reliability of this treatment has made it a common modality in dental practice and dental hygienists routinely provide maintenance care for implants.

SURGICAL PROCEDURES

There are guidelines for the placement of osseointegrated endosseous implants to ensure high success rates and predictability of this treatment modality. Knowledge of the basics of implant surgery will help the dental hygienist communicate effectively with patients. The following is a brief outline of contemporary surgical issues and protocols.

Implant surgery is highly technique-sensitive and many factors are critical in achieving predictable, long-term results. Trauma to bone during implant recipient site preparation through overheating or use of excessive force must be avoided to ensure treatment success.[1] Bone cells are irreversibly damaged if heated above 47° C for 1 minute, so copious irrigation with a coolant is required during surgery when creating the recipient site in the bone for the implant. There is no recommended aseptic protocol for implant surgery[25] because the outcome of therapy is similar when implant placement is performed under aseptic and clean conditions.

Implant immobility throughout the healing period, ranging from 3 to 6 months, encourages successful osseointegration rather than a fibrous union at the implant-bone interface. For this reason, a two-stage surgical approach was initially recommended to minimize the potential for a functional load on the implant during the healing phase. With the introduction of a single-stage implant surgical protocol, and further research into the application of two-stage implant systems with the use of a single-stage surgical protocol, similar results and implant success rates for soft tissue and bone healing have been shown.[26,27]

After a thorough examination and planning process that includes appropriate radiographs, study casts, and fabrication of surgical guides (stents), implants are placed with the use of a submerged or nonsubmerged protocol. The ideal location and angulation of the implant should be consistent with planned prosthetic **superstructure** (restorations).

SUBMERGED (TWO-STAGE) PROTOCOL

As the name suggests, the **submerged protocol** requires two surgical procedures before the fabrication of the restorations that will be placed on the implants. The first surgery places the implant fixture within bone, followed by a second surgery 3 to 6 months later to uncover the implant so it can be accessed through the mucosa. Examples of implant surgery and prosthetic results are presented in Figures 15-6 through 15-9.

First Surgical Procedure

After anesthesia is administered, a crestal incision is made in the soft tissue along the crest of the alveolar ridge and a flap is reflected in the location where the implant is to be placed. With the aid of a surgical stent, drills specific for the implant system of choice are used under copious saline solution irrigation to prepare the endosseous implant recipient site(s) to the predetermined length and diameter. Guide pins are used to verify the angulations and distances between implants or between the implant and surrounding teeth. Implants are either slowly threaded into place in the case of screw design implants or gently tapped in place in the case of nonthreaded cylindrical designs. The implants are inserted into the prepared sites until they are completely seated. The internal aspect of the implant is protected from ingrowth of tissue by placing a device called a cover screw on top of the implant. The flap is then repositioned and sutured to obtain closure over the implant so that it is submerged under the gingiva. The two-stage submerged protocol is illustrated in Figure 15-11.

Postoperative Procedures

The patient should not wear dentures over the implant site for 2 to 3 weeks after surgery to avoid pressure on the implant. The area should be cleansed with a 0.2% chlorhexidine mouthwash twice daily and the use of systemic antibiotics should be considered to minimize the chance of infection.

Second Surgical Procedure

After a healing period of 3 months for implants placed in the mandible and 6 months for those placed in the maxilla, the second surgical procedure is performed. Submerged implants are exposed by either making small incisions or using circular punches over the implants to gain access to the cover screws and exchange them for healing abutments. Healing abutments are transmucosal posts that allow healing and adaptation of the peri-implant soft tissues to take place. An example of a healing implant in place after second-stage surgery is seen in Figure 15-12.

Restorative Procedures

Restorative procedures can usually begin after 3 to 4 weeks of soft tissue healing.

NONSUBMERGED (SINGLE-STAGE) PROTOCOL
Surgical Procedure

The surgical approach for the nonsubmerged protocol for implant placement is similar to that described for the two-stage submerged procedure except that after implant placement, the tissues are closed around the specially designed transmucosal portion of the implant or around the healing abutment. This eliminates the need for a second surgery to uncover the implant, which may reduce both treatment time and patient discomfort. Figure 15-13 presents an example of the single-stage protocol.

Additional Procedures

Often, intraoral soft and hard tissue deformities prevent implants from being placed in the desired location for the best restorative results. These deformities can occur from trauma, congenital abnormalities, cystic and neoplastic lesions, infections, or periodontal disease. Additional regenerative treatment to restore both soft and hard tissues may be necessary before or concurrent with implant placement. These procedures may include soft tissue augmentation to increase the thickness or amount of keratinized tissue, bone grafting, guided tissue regeneration, or a combination of these procedures. To satisfy the goals of implant dentistry, hard and soft tissues need to be present in adequate volumes and quality.

OTHER IMPLANT PLACEMENT PROTOCOLS

IMMEDIATE IMPLANT PLACEMENT AFTER TOOTH EXTRACTION

Generally, there is a lack of uniformity in the interpretation of the terms *immediate*, *delayed*, and *late* with regard to timing of implant placement. These terms are defined in Table 15-2.

The surgical procedures described thus far are in reference to delayed or late implant placements. These terms imply that the implant surgery is performed after an adequate healing period of the extraction socket has taken place. Immediate placement of implants is performed at the time of tooth extraction, as illustrated in Figure 15-14. The reason for extraction of a tooth determines whether immediate implant placement should be considered. The presence of infection and lack of bone to achieve primary stability of the implant contraindicates immediate placement. However, immediate placement after extraction of teeth for periodontal reasons, which constitutes an infected site, shows results similar to those of healthy sites.[28]

The shape of a single-rooted tooth, and therefore the socket of that extracted tooth, is not the same as that of a cylindrical endosseous implant. Immediate placement of implants into extraction sockets leaves a gap between the nonengaged implant surface and the inner aspect of the socket wall. This distance is referred to as the jumping distance. It is not known how wide a space can be tolerated and still permit normal healing. Studies suggest that gaps of 1 to 2 mm can fill with bone without the use of adjunctive grafting materials.[29] The degree of fill and the rate of bone apposition are influenced by the surface characteristics of the implant.

IMMEDIATE LOADING OF IMPLANTS

The issue of the prolonged healing period required for osseointegration, and thus the need for patient compliance to wear a temporary removable prosthesis, has been overcome by immediately providing a fixed, provisional implant-supported crown after implant placement. This is termed *immediate loading* and has been applied to edentulous jaws, partially edentulous cases, or single implants. If multiple implants are placed, the temporary restorations are typically splinted together to minimize movement and promote even load distribution. Single implant provisional restorations are restored out of occlusion to limit the functional load that may be transmitted to the implant fixture. Immediate loading of an implant placed in an extraction site is illustrated in Figure 15-15.

PROSTHETIC CONSIDERATIONS

The direction and magnitude of forces distributed along the long axis of the implant, which in turn are transmitted to the surrounding bone, are critical in both attainment and maintenance of osseointegration. Prosthetic restorations must be designed to avoid an excessive load on implants to protect them from bone loss and prosthetic component failure. Treatment of

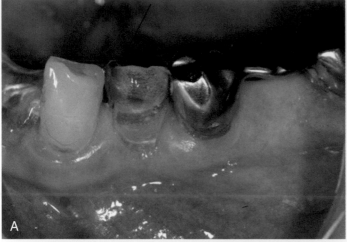
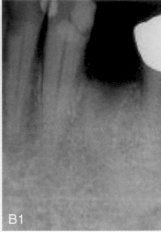
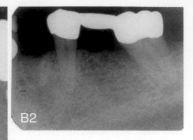
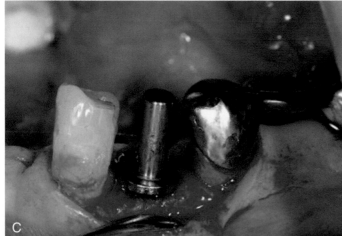
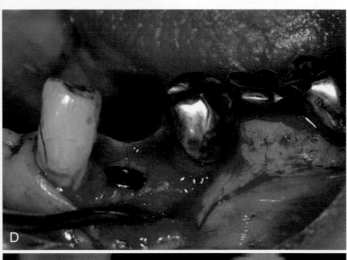
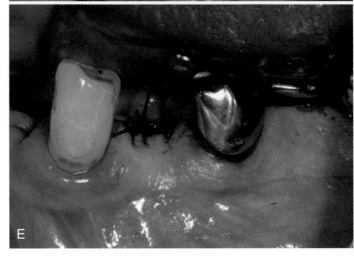
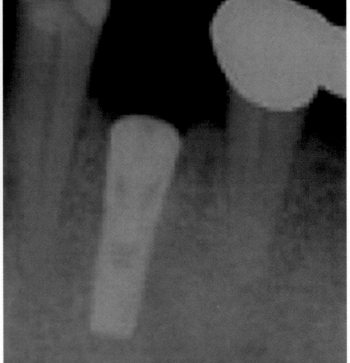

FIGURE 15-11 ■ **Implant placement surgery, submerged technique. A,** Preoperative view of tooth #21. A surgical stent *(arrow)* is used to guide the implant placement. **B,** Preoperative radiographs *(1 and 2)* show adequate volume and quality of bone. **C,** Flaps reflected and guide in place to verify correct implant position after initial osteotomy preparation. **D,** Flaps reflected to show implant placed within the bone. **E,** Flaps repositioned and sutured in place to cover the implant. **F,** Postoperative radiograph confirming good positioning of the implant fixture.

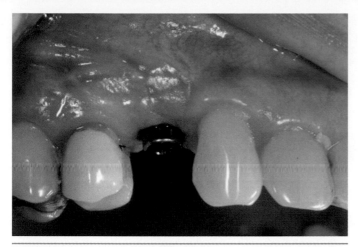

FIGURE 15-12 ■ Example of a healing abutment in place after second-stage surgery to uncover the implant fixture.

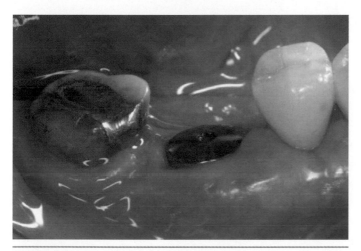

FIGURE 15-13 ■ **Nonsubmerged, single-stage implant 2 weeks after placement.** The cover screw is not submerged and the tissues heal around the transmucosal portion of the implant.

TABLE 15-2	Classification of Timing of Implant Placement
	TIMING OF IMPLANT PLACEMENT
Immediate	At the time of extraction
Delayed	6-10 weeks after extraction
Late	6 months or longer after extraction

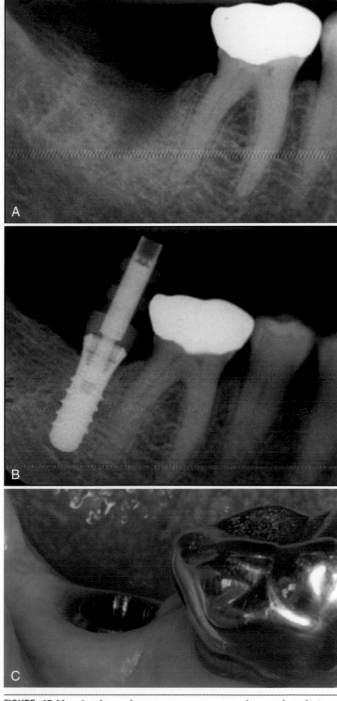

FIGURE 15-14 ■ **Implant placement surgery, nonsubmerged technique. A,** Radiographic view of fresh extraction site. **B,** Radiographic view of implant fixture after several months of healing. Note the adequate healing of bone in the extraction site. **C,** Implant fixture in healed site ready for loading.

patients exhibiting parafunctional habits, such as clenching and bruxism, should be undertaken with caution. An occlusal guard should be considered to help protect the implants after delivery of the prosthesis.

Restorations are either cemented in place or screw-retained. Screw-retained restorations have the advantage of being retrievable, if required, to permit treatment of the implant or address prosthetic complications. However, both implant location and aesthetic demand may favor the use of the cement-retained restorations. The abutment is attached to the implant with a conventional screw system, but the crown is cemented on to the abutment, typically with temporary cement so that it can be removed if necessary.

MAINTENANCE

PARAMETERS OF EVALUATION FOR PATIENTS WITH IMPLANTS

The purpose of regular periodic clinical evaluation of patients is to detect early disease activity and to provide individualized

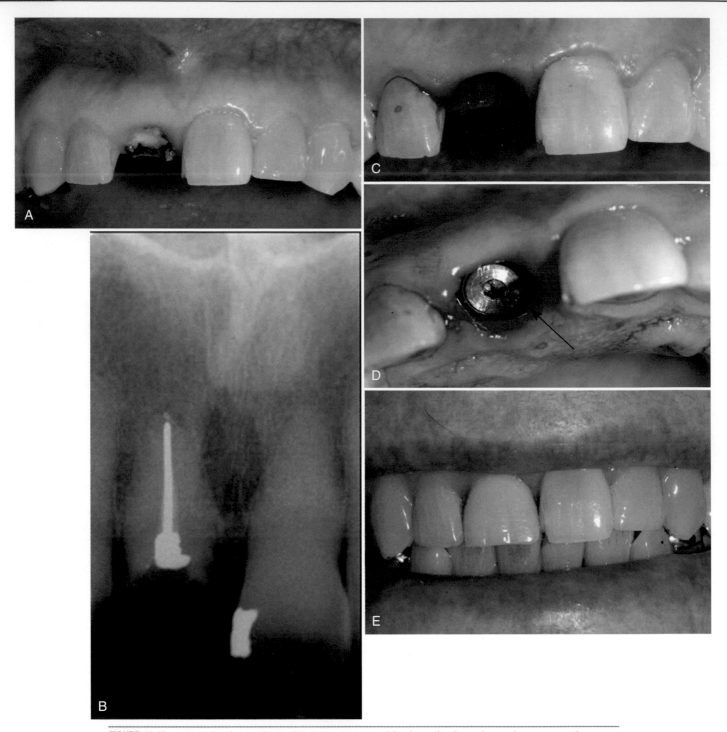

FIGURE 15-15 ■ **Example of immediate placement surgery and loading after loss of a tooth crown. A,** The patient presented having lost the crown of tooth #8 as a result of recurrent caries after endodontic therapy. **B,** Preoperative radiograph shows no signs of infection and adequate bone beyond the apex of the root for implant stabilization. **C,** Atraumatic extraction of the root was performed. **D,** Implant fixture is immediately placed inside the extraction socket. Note the *jumping distance (arrow)* between the implant and the inner socket wall. **E,** Immediate loading was done on the implant the day of surgery.

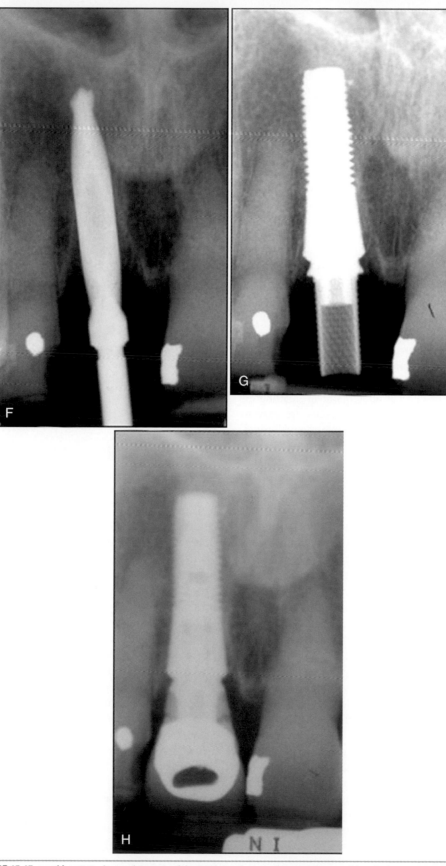

FIGURE 15-15, cont'd ■ **F,** Radiographic view of the guide in place verifying implant position during surgery. **G,** Radiographic view of implant in place. **H,** Radiographic view of completed restoration.

maintenance protocols. Many of the parameters used for the evaluation of natural teeth may be used in patients with implants; however, some of these data are of little value.

> **CLINICAL NOTE 15-5** The dental hygienist is responsible for assessing implants with the same techniques used for natural teeth: mobility, probing depths, bleeding, plaque and calculus.

Mobility

Healthy implants are osseointegrated and do not exhibit clinical signs of mobility. The absence of PDL around implants creates a rigid bone-implant interface, the maintenance of which is key for the long-term success of implants. The presence of clinical mobility, as detected by conventional methods, is an indication of loss of integration and implant failure. Mobility of prosthetic components is usually a result of the loosening or fracture of screws at the implant abutment or abutment crown (if screw-retained) interface.

Probing

A periodontal probe is used to measure probing pocket depths and clinical attachment levels around natural teeth; these measurements provide important information regarding progression of disease or success of periodontal therapy. Increasing probing depth and loss of clinical attachment are pathognomonic for periodontal disease.[30] Probing depths are easy to measure around implants, but their interpretation is limited. Probing force, examiner variability, probe design, gingival health,[31] and obstructing factors, such as crown contours and calculus, influence the extent of probe penetration. Also, inherent differences in the arrangement of the tissues around implants and natural teeth make interpretation of the collected data difficult. Probing pocket depth measurements do not reflect the histologic levels of attachment because probes invariably penetrate the JE and, if it is inflamed, penetrate into the connective tissue.[30,32] Perhaps because of the lack of connective tissue attachment into the implant surface, as seen in the cementum of natural teeth, probes penetrate the attachment with more ease around implants. Studies have indicated that the probe tip penetrates closer to bone in inflamed peri-implant tissues than in healthy sites and that there is a tendency toward deeper probe depths around implants.[33] Probing values representative of health have not been defined, but depths of approximately 3 mm[34] or less than 4 to 5 mm[9,35] are considered consistent with health because patients are able to maintain these depths with daily oral hygiene.

Another complicating factor is that probing depths are dependent on individual implant design, such as abutment height and depth of fixture within bone, and they are therefore system-specific. Most important, it is reported that clinical probing depths around implants do not correlate with the loss of osseointegration and bone loss caused by occlusal overload.[36] For these reasons, many do not regard probing as a valuable diagnostic tool when implants are evaluated.

The use of plastic periodontal probes around implants has been advocated by many to reduce the chances of inadvertently scratching the implant surface.[16] There is no evidence supporting damage caused by probing to the peri-implant tissues. However, not probing during the first 3 months after loading is

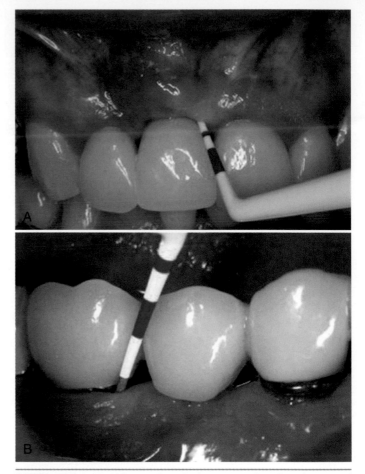

FIGURE 15-16 ■ Use of a graduated plastic periodontal probe around implants. **A,** Anterior adaptation. **B,** Posterior adaptation.

advised so that healing is not disturbed. Probing around implants is illustrated in Figures 15-16 and 15-17.

Indices

Probing around implants provides an assessment of inflammatory parameters, such as bleeding and suppuration. In the natural dentition, the absence of bleeding on probing is considered a good indicator of periodontal health.[37] Conflicting reports have appeared in the literature with regard to bleeding on probing around implants as an indicator of disease activity. One study found no correlation between bleeding on probing and histologic, microbiologic, or radiographic changes around implants,[38] whereas others have reported that healthy sites are characterized by complete absence of bleeding on probing. However, healthy implant sites have been shown to exhibit a greater tendency to bleed during probing than well-maintained teeth.[31]

Other indices that can be applied to implants include gingival and plaque indices to evaluate the patient's oral hygiene status. The important point is to maintain compliance with plaque control to minimize tissue inflammation.[16]

Radiographic Imaging

Periapical radiographs and panoramic images are used in conjunction with standard clinical examination to assess bone levels available for implant sites. Unfortunately, these images provide only a two-dimensional view of the alveolar bone. After

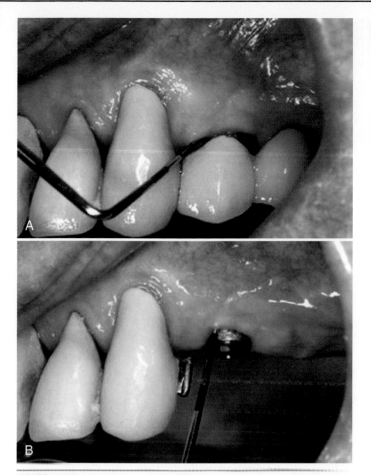

FIGURE 15-17 ■ **Probing may be difficult because of the superstructure design. A,** The probe angulation is exaggerated to permit the tip access to the abutment with the superstructure in place. **B,** The prosthetic superstructure needs to be removed periodically to obtain more accurate probing measurements.

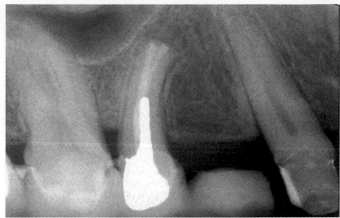

FIGURE 15-18 ■ This periapical radiograph shows limited space between the apices of the teeth for implant restoration of the missing tooth. Note that although the radiograph reveals this concern regarding assessing the suitability of the site for implant restoration, the width of the bony ridge cannot be assessed with a two-dimensional radiograph.

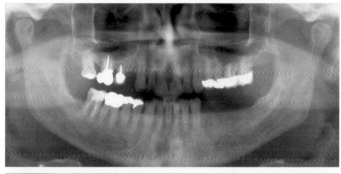

FIGURE 15-19 ■ The panographic view of the oral cavity helps in evaluating patients for implant restoration by showing the location of vital structures (e.g., the nerve trunk in the mandible), the mental foramen, and the maxillary sinuses.

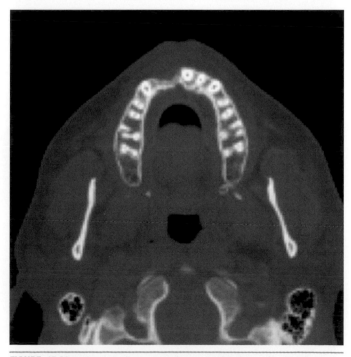

FIGURE 15-20 ■ Computed tomography is useful for evaluating bone for implant restoration. Cortical bone appears as a white line around the maxillary teeth. Note the deficient ridge width in the #7 to #8 area. The white lines on the side are cortical bone at the level of the scan.

implants are placed, images are used to assess the height of proximal bone, the presence of anatomic structures (e.g., the maxillary sinus), anomalies, or pathologic lesions. Correct seating of restorative components can be verified on images after second-stage uncovering of the implant and after placement of the restoration. Examples of the information obtained from radiographic images are presented in Figures 15-18 and 15-19.

More advanced imaging techniques are available to give accurate measurements of bone width and bone quality by providing a three-dimensional view of the implant area. These cross-sectional and tomographic images can be obtained with the use of computed tomography, as shown in Figure 15-20, special tomographic devices, and digital subtraction radiography techniques, which enable quantitative and qualitative assessment of changes in bone density. The classification of bone quality and quantity is an indicator of the amount of bone available for implant placement.[14] The quality of bone, however, is better assessed at the time of surgery.

The amount of the peri-implant bone should be evaluated periodically to monitor the osseointegration status. The criteria for implant success includes bone loss not exceeding 0.2 mm annually after the first year after loading and the absence of peri-implant radiolucencies or associated conditions. Examples of radiographic information correlated with clinical findings are presented in Figures 15-21 through 15-23.

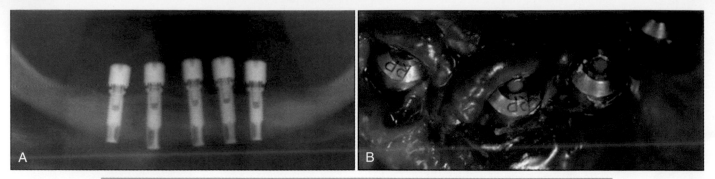

FIGURE 15-21 ■ **Issues related to implant technique. A,** Radiograph showing incomplete seating of the healing abutments after implant uncovering. **B,** This resulted in severe inflammation of the peri-implant tissue as a result of plaque biofilm accumulation.

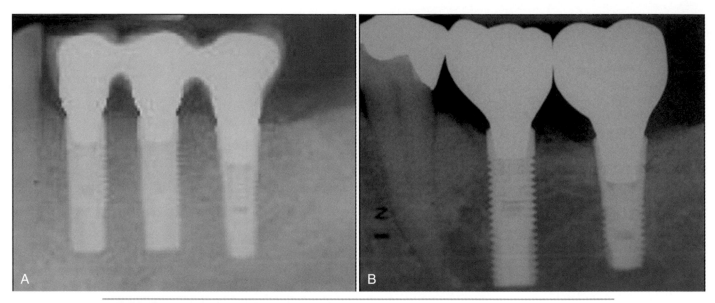

FIGURE 15-22 ■ **Healing of bone after implant surgery. A,** Excellent proximal bone level between implants. **B,** Another example of a satisfactory healing result.

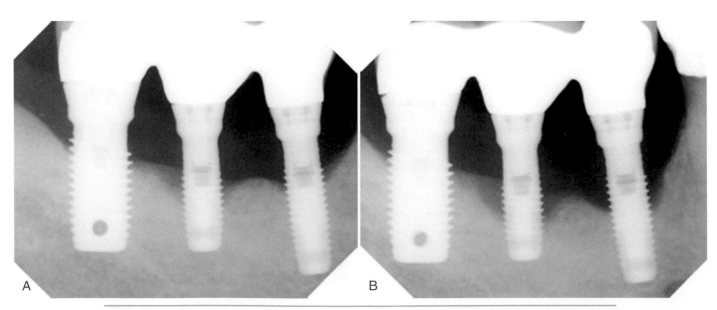

FIGURE 15-23 ■ **Follow-up radiographs can also reveal problems. A,** This patient had significant bone loss. **B,** Six months later, more than 0.2 mm of bone loss had occurred. Note the saucer-shaped defect which is characteristic of bone loss around implants.

These signs are evaluated through radiographic follow-up, which is recommended for implant sites at 6, 12, and 36 months and then every 2 to 3 years thereafter unless clinical symptoms are seen. Some periodontists continue radiographic examination every 3 months for the first year after restoration and then annually thereafter to ensure that the bone levels are stable.

Soft Tissues

The need for keratinized tissue around implants remains controversial. Adequate health and stability of tissues around teeth can be maintained in patients with good oral hygiene practices who exhibit minimal or no keratinized tissue. Given the differences that exist in the soft tissue structural organization around teeth and implants, the question arises about generalizing the same evidence to peri-implant tissues. Factors to consider when determining whether the attached gingiva is adequate include presence of inflammation, existence of gingival recession, oral hygiene status and patient compliance, relationship between the gingiva and alveolar bone, tooth position within the arch, presence of restorations, aesthetic demands, and presence of tooth sensitivity.

There is no direct evidence to support the idea that keratinized peri-implant tissue is associated with better implant success rates than nonkeratinized tissue. As the application of dental implants continues to increase, the functional and psychological improvements achieved from their use continue to be important, but aesthetic demands have catapulted to the forefront in the goals of therapy. Aesthetic demands may dictate that keratinized tissue be present at the implant site. If needed, surgery to increase the width of the attached gingiva can be performed before implant placement, at the time of implant surgery, or at second-stage surgery to uncover the fixture. Attempting this surgery after the implant is in function is less predictable.[39] The results of surgery to increase keratinized tissue are illustrated in Figure 15-24.

PERI-IMPLANT DISEASE

DEFINITIONS

As established by the First European Workshop of Periodontology (Switzerland, 1993), **peri-implant disease** is a collective term for inflammatory reactions in the tissues surrounding an implant. **Peri-implant mucositis** describes a reversible inflammatory reaction in the soft tissues surrounding a functioning implant. It has not been established that if untreated, it will progress to peri-implantitis. **Peri-implantitis** is a term for inflammatory reactions that affect soft and hard tissues around the implant leading to deepening of probing pocket depths and loss of supporting bone on functioning implants. Despite the loss of supporting bone, mobility may not be evident clinically because osseointegration of portions of the implant surface is retained. Peri-implant mucositis and peri-implantitis are associated with bleeding on gentle probing, redness and, rarely, pain. If this condition is left untreated, it will ultimately progress to its failure.[40] Peri-implantitis occurs in about 4% to 19% of implants.[41] The term **failing implant** is not synonymous with peri-implantitis and refers to an implant that has lost osseointegration and is no longer an effective prosthetic anchor.

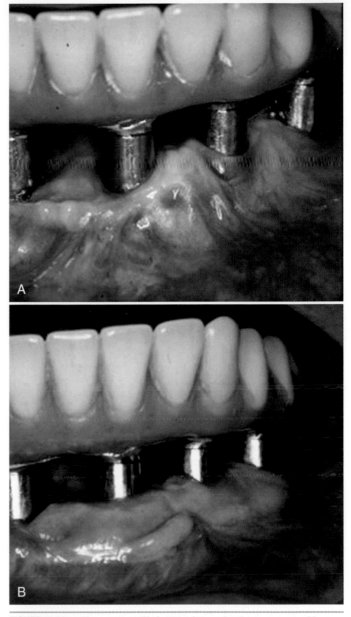

FIGURE 15-24 ■ The amount of keratinized tissue has been augmented by performing a gingival graft to facilitate maintenance for the peri-implant tissues. **A,** Before graft surgery. **B,** Keratinized tissue around the implants after surgery.

Peri-implant mucositis and peri-implantitis are illustrated in Figures 15-25 and 15-26.[42]

> **CLINICAL NOTE 15-6** Peri-implantitis is characterized by increasing probe depths, bleeding, and bone loss. Regular assessment of implants is important to monitor for this condition.

MICROBIOLOGY

As with teeth, plaque biofilm is the primary microbial etiologic factor in peri-implantitis. Numerous studies have demonstrated similarities between the clinical and microbiologic features of peri-implantitis and periodontitis.[43,44]

The microbiota around implants in edentulous patients form early and appear to remain stable in the long term.[45] The microbiota of implants differ between partially and fully

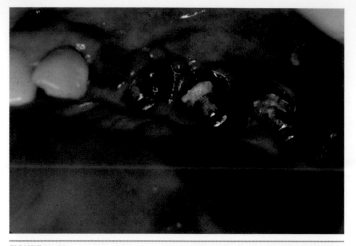

FIGURE 15-25 ■ **Peri-implant mucositis.** Peri-implant mucositis is a reversible process characterized by inflammation within the peri-implant tissues. Note the calculus formation on the abutments.

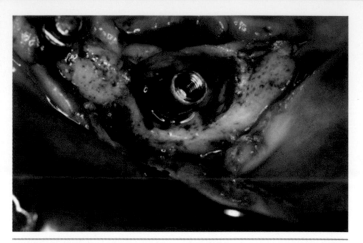

FIGURE 15-27 ■ **Peri-implant bone.** This clinical view of a healthy implant with flaps reflected shows the well-circumscribed saucer shape of the bone around the fixture.

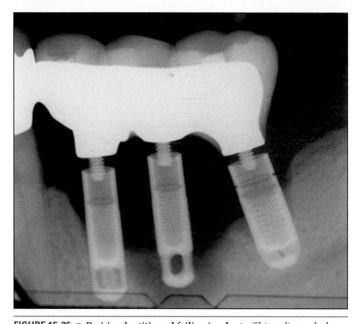

FIGURE 15-26 ■ **Peri-implantitis and failing implants.** This radiograph shows three implants with advanced bone loss in a patient with uncontrolled diabetes mellitus. Clinically, the implants are mobile, have increased probing depths, and the tissues bleed.

PROGRESSION OF INFLAMMATION IN IMPLANTS

As a result of inherent anatomic differences between implants and teeth, and despite similar etiologic factors, progression of inflammatory disease around implants appears to be more rapid than around natural teeth. Periodontal disease is a site-specific disease; pocket formation and bone loss can affect a localized site on a tooth that may lead to angular or horizontal osseous defects. In contrast, implants lack connective tissue fiber insertion, so the only attachment mechanism involves the basal lamina and hemidesmosomes of the epithelium. Inflammation within the peri-implant tissues have a tendency to spread circumferentially and progression to bone may result in angular osseous defects radiographically, whereas clinically it assumes the shape of a well-circumscribed saucer, as shown in Figure 15-27.

RECOGNITION AND TREATMENT

Early implant failures are typically considered to be biologic, occurring within weeks or a few months after placement. They result from failure to achieve osseointegration (possibly because of inherent host tissue factors), bacterial contamination of wounds, poor surgical technique, or instability of the implant at placement. Late implant failures result from factors that cause breakdown of osseointegration. Causative factors may include mechanical overload, fatigue failure of components, and peri-implant infection. Examples of implant failure are presented in Figure 15-28.

Given the microbial association, antimicrobial therapy has been proposed as an important part of treatment for peri-implantitis. Treatment options include a combination of local or systemic antimicrobial therapy, debridement that involves thorough removal of plaque biofilm and calculus, implant surface decontamination, and regeneration of defects. Application of local antibiotics is shown in Figure 15-29.

Access to the "diseased" implant surface is usually achieved through surgical intervention. If defects around implants are amenable to surgical correction, this will involve bone grafting and regenerative therapy. After debridement of the site and implant surface decontamination, repair or regeneration of the osseous defect may be attempted, with the understanding that

edentulous patients. Teeth in partially dentate patients are a source of biota that colonize implants within 2 weeks of exposure in the oral environment. Subgingival sites in healthy implants are populated by high percentages of coccoid cells and nonmotile rods with few spirochetes, whereas *Actinobacillus actinomycetemcomitans, Porphyromonas gingivalis,* and *Prevotella intermedius* have been cultured from implants in patients with minimal visible plaque biofilm but who had not had maintenance visits for 6 months or more.[21] Clearly, the composition of the microbiota before implant placement determines the biota associated with the implants. Patients with untreated periodontitis are at higher risk for development of peri-implantitis than those with controlled periodontal conditions. These findings emphasize the importance of regular maintenance visits for all patients with implants to help prevent the formation of mature pathogenic bacterial plaque biofilm.

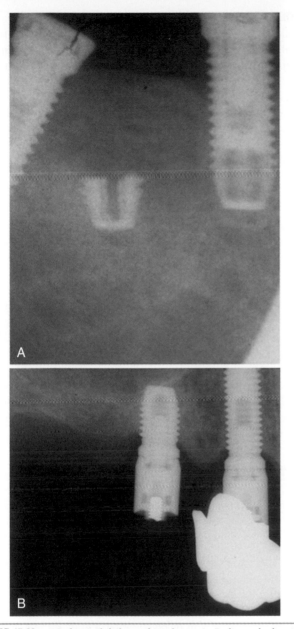

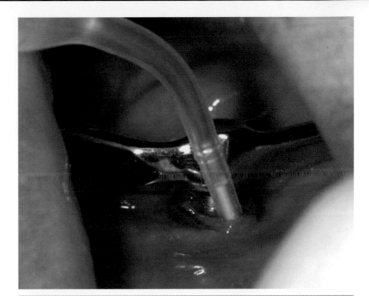

FIGURE 15-29 ■ Locally delivered antimicrobial agents are often used as adjunct therapy to mechanical calculus and plaque biofilm removal around implants.

FIGURE 15-28 ■ **Mechanical failure of implants. A,** Radiograph showing a fractured implant. **B,** Implant fixture with a screw fracture from overload.

TABLE 15-3	Assessments for Implant Maintenance Care	
PROCEDURE	**COMMENT**
Evaluate tissue for tone color, consistency, size, and texture	Look for signs of tissue inflammation
Check for mobility	May not be possible with splinted implants
Probe and record implant sulcus depth	Use plastic probes only; four measurements per implant
Remove and clean superstructure if possible	May not occur at every visit with fixed superstructures
Assess and remove calculus	Ensure complete removal
Radiograph implant area	Done at frequent intervals to check bone levels as determined by dentist
Record assessments	Reference data for other appointments

the final bone-implant interface may not be osseointegrated and may only comprise a close adaptation of grafted bone and the implant surface.

DENTAL HYGIENE CARE

Regular dental hygiene care is an important component of the long-term success of implant therapy. The dental hygienist is responsible for assessing patients with implants, providing maintenance care, and educating and reinforcing home care procedures. This can be particularly challenging because many of these patients do not have a history of compliance and have lost teeth because of neglect and periodontal disease. Implants are now a successful and commonly performed procedure, so the dental hygienist must expect to see many patients with single or multiple implants, whether in general or specialty practice.

ASSESSMENT

Regular assessment of implants is required in addition to assessments of the remaining natural dentition. Dental hygiene care may be performed slightly less frequently in compliant patients with well-maintained implants, but recall intervals for assessment and treatment should not exceed 6 months. Table 15-3 lists the assessments recommended for the dental hygienist to perform for patients with implants. Generally, patients with implants should be seen and evaluated about every 3 months for the first year after restoration of implants.[16]

MAINTENANCE VISITS

Plaque biofilm and calculus removal for dental implants is performed with instruments that are not abrasive to the titanium components. Conventional stainless steel instruments and ultrasonic devices scratch the softer titanium abutments, causing roughness and making them more plaque biofilm retentive. Plastic, nylon, titanium, graphite, or gold-plated curettes and air abrasive devices can be used safely around implants.[46] Ultrasonic instruments should be avoided to prevent damage to implant surfaces.[16] Implants may be polished to remove plaque biofilm and stains, but coarse polishing compounds should be avoided. Tin oxide with rubber cups is a good choice for polishing around implants. The use of plastic scalers on implant surfaces is shown in Figure 15-30.

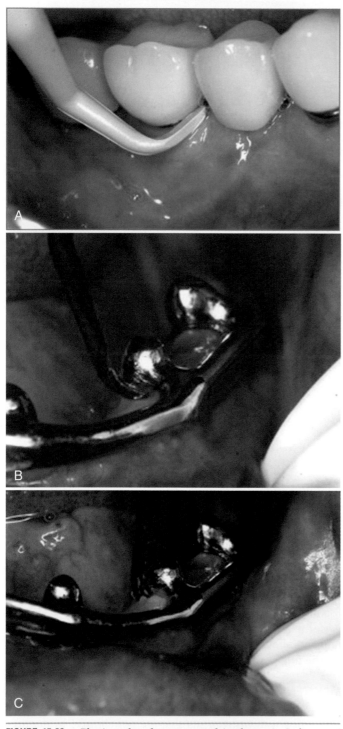

FIGURE 15-30 ■ **Plastic scalers for use around implants. A,** Scalers must be manipulated around the superstructure to reach the abutment surface. **B,** Scaling around implant and bar fixtures is a challenge. **C,** The scaler adapted subgingivally around the abutment.

HOME CARE

Excellent home care practices are as essential as regular professional maintenance care in the long-term success of implant therapy because there is a direct cause and effect association between plaque biofilm accumulation and the initiation of peri-implant disease. Home care procedures must be initiated and regularly assessed before implant treatment begins as a criterion for the suitability of patients to receive implants. The cause of tooth loss among a large number of patients with implants is periodontal disease, and it has been shown that these patients are more prone to future breakdown.[47] An effective customized home care and preventive regimen for these patients is critical to achieve optimal plaque biofilm control and consequent treatment success.

The variety of available home care devices includes a host of manual and powered toothbrushes, interdental aids, and oral irrigation devices. Examples are seen in Figures 15-31 through 15-33. The choice of toothbrush is based on the individual's manual dexterity and the type of implant prosthetic superstructure. Soft toothbrushes or single-tufted brushes are effective for plaque biofilm removal around implant abutments that secure removable prostheses. Implant-supported overdentures can be easily removed by the patient or hygienist to clean implant abutments and peri-implant tissues and to facilitate cleansing of the dentures. Patients must be instructed in thorough daily inspection and cleaning of all removable prostheses.

> **CLINICAL NOTE 15-7** Plaque biofilm control around implants can be difficult and requires careful attention. The dental hygienist plays an important role in ensuring that patients develop the skills to perform thorough plaque control procedures.

Patients with implants and natural teeth must both brush the teeth and clean the interproximal surfaces. Interdental aids are just as useful for interproximal plaque removal around fixed implant-retained prostheses as for around natural teeth. Rubber tip stimulators, wooden or plastic interdental cleaners, manual and powered interproximal brushes, and a variety of flossing cords are available. Patients require individualized instruction in the correct application of these devices to the implants and peri-implant tissues to reduce the chances of iatrogenic damage to both the tissue and implant component surfaces.

Although there is no evidence to suggest that powered devices are superior to manual devices for achieving effective plaque biofilm control, patients with limited dexterity may benefit from the use of these devices and others may simply prefer them. Oral antimicrobial rinses containing chlorhexidine gluconate or phenolic compounds may also be useful for individuals with physical impairments.

The use of subgingival irrigation devices as adjuncts to routine brushing can be recommended with caution so that the delicate peri-implant tissues are not damaged. The effects from subgingival irrigation do not appear to be of clinical significance around dental implants, although studies have shown subgingival delivery of chlorhexidine to be slightly more effective for the reduction of plaque biofilm and bleeding of the peri-implant tissues than rinsing.[48]

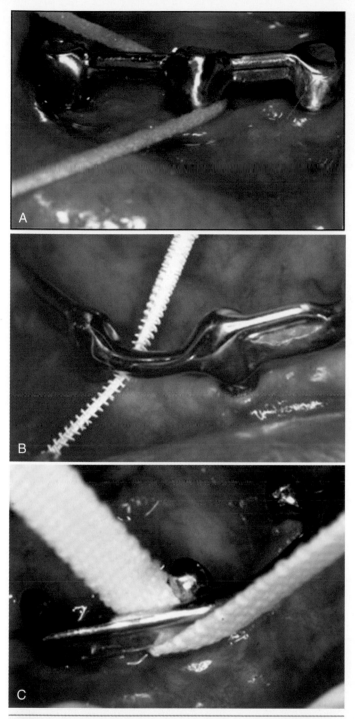

FIGURE 15-31 ■ **Home care aids—floss. A,** Thick floss around an abutment. **B,** Plastic floss under a bar. **C,** Thick strips of floss are also efficient for cleaning.

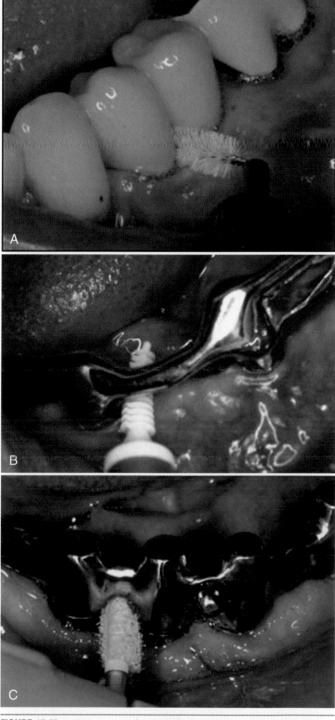

FIGURE 15-32 ■ **Home care aids—interdental brushes. A,** Interdental brush adapted between implant restorations. **B,** Interdental brushes are useful under bars when space permits. **C,** Small interdental brushes can fit well between implants.

ROLE OF THE DENTAL HYGIENIST

Early detection of pathologic conditions improves the chances of treating and maintaining dental implants with appropriate therapy. Available evidence and clinical experience suggest that maintenance visits should occur every 3 or 4 months during the first year after implant placement. Recall intervals should not extend beyond 6 months, even for the most compliant patients. At every recall visit, thorough assessment will permit modification to the home care practices and maintenance intervals on the basis of the oral health of the patient. Even shorter recall intervals may be indicated if 3 months is too long to maintain optimal implant health. The significance of regular dental hygiene care can be seen in Figure 15-34.

Motivation and compliance are crucial elements of treatment success for patients with implants. The dental hygienist plays a central role in educating and motivating the patient about all aspects of implant treatment. This responsibility reduces barriers to compliance, customizes home care routines, and contributes to the success of implant therapy.

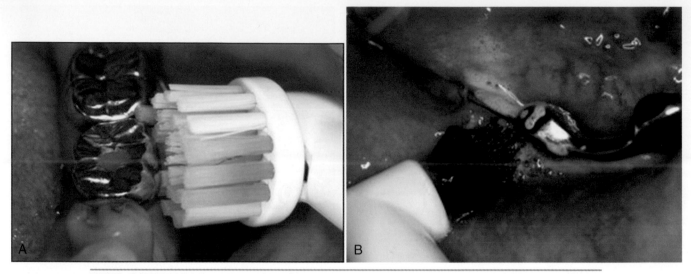

FIGURE 15-33 ■ Home care aids—toothbrushes. A, Mechanical toothbrushes can be easier for patients to use than manual brushes. **B,** Rotary interproximal brushes adapt well around implants.

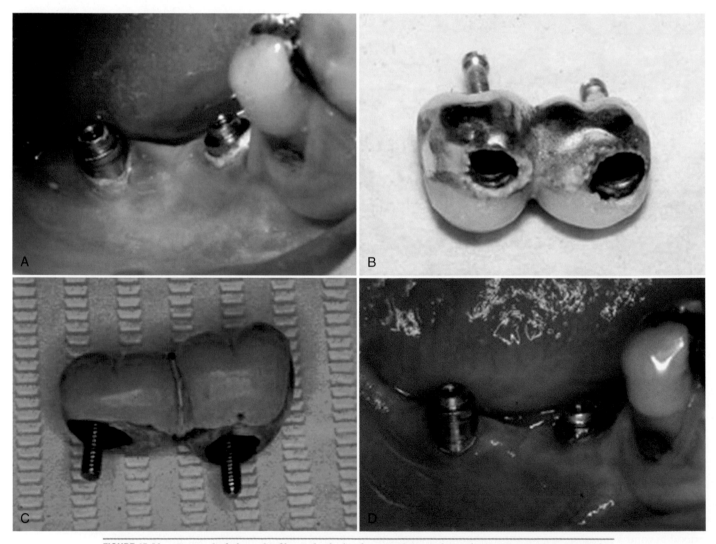

FIGURE 15-34 ■ Removal of plaque biofilm and calculus from implants and prosthetic components is essential to eliminate peri-implant inflammation. A, Inflamed tissue surrounding two implants. Note the calculus and plaque biofilm around the abutments. **B,** The restoration is also coated with plaque biofilm and calculus. **C,** The restoration after cleaning. **D,** The tissues 1 week after cleaning and reinforcement of home care procedures for the patient.

◎ DENTAL HYGIENE CONSIDERATIONS

- Dental implants are a highly successful and increasingly common treatment modality that dental hygienists will encounter often in clinical practice.
- Osseointegration is the formation of an intimate lattice between the titanium implant and bone; it creates a firm abutment for supporting prostheses.
- The most commonly placed implants are endosseous root form implants made of the biomaterial titanium.
- The soft tissue attachment to an implant is an epithelial attachment of hemidesmosomes and basal lamina. There is no PDL or fiber attachment.
- Implants are placed surgically by use of either a submerged (two-stage) procedure or a nonsubmerged (single-stage) procedure. They can also be placed immediately after tooth extraction. Surgical technique is critical to implant success.
- Lack of mobility is a critical factor in the success of implants.
- Assessments of healed implants include mobility evaluation, probing, radiographs, and plaque biofilm and calculus evaluations. Probing is the least useful assessment tool for implants.
- Peri-implant disease includes reversible peri-implant mucositis and more serious peri-implantitis, which can result in loss of the implant.
- The microbiota associated with implants are similar to normal oral biota.
- Dental hygiene care consists of regular assessments, maintenance care, and helping patients maintain excellent home care programs.
- Maintenance visits should occur at least every 3 months but this interval may be extended slightly if the patient is extremely compliant.

✶ CASE SCENARIO

Ms. Caldwell is a 21-year-old African American female, in excellent health, who has congenitally missing lateral incisors replaced by implants. She is in college and has a very active lifestyle. Ms. Caldwell's oral hygiene is good; she brushes well but does not floss regularly and she has a limited budget, like most college students. There is slight localized gingivitis around the implants and on the lingual surfaces of her lower molars. She has no subgingival calculus, normal sulcus depths, no recession, and a light accumulation of supragingival calculus on the mandibular anterior lingual surfaces.

1. The patient does not need to come in as regularly because she has good enough oral hygiene and no subgingival calculus.
   A. Both the statement and the reason are correct and related.
   B. Both the statement and the reason are correct but NOT related.
   C. The statement is correct, but the reason is NOT correct.
   D. The statement is NOT correct, but the reason is correct.
   E. NEITHER the statement NOR the reason is correct.
2. Localized inflammation around the implants and the mandibular molars suggests that
   A. Ms. Caldwell needs to floss better.
   B. Ms. Caldwell needs to brush better.
   C. Ms. Caldwell needs diet counseling.
   D. Ms. Caldwell needs to brush and floss better.

3. Probing should be performed around implants to establish base measurements of the distance between the gingival margin and the bone integration level of the implant. Probing depths around implants of 3 to 5 mm or less are consistent with periodontal health.
   A. Both statements are true.
   B. Bothe statements are false.
   C. The first statement is true, and the second statement is false.
   D. The first statement is false, and the second statement is true.
4. You should recommend a short interval for Ms. Caldwell's recall because she is on a limited budget.
   A. Both the statement and the reason are correct and related.
   B. Both the statement and the reason are correct but NOT related.
   C. The statement is correct, but the reason is NOT correct.
   D. The statement is NOT correct, but the reason is correct.
   E. NEITHER the statement NOR the reason is correct.
5. When might Ms. Caldwell be able to extend the recall interval?
   A. In 4 months
   B. In 3 months
   C. When tissue inflammation is resolved
   D. When she has demonstrated better plaque control

STUDY QUESTIONS

Answers and rationales to these questions can be obtained from your instructor.

MULTIPLE CHOICE

1. Dental implants with the highest success rates are made of
   A. titanium.
   B. tin oxide.
   C. hydroxyapatite.
   D. aluminum oxide.
2. Which type of implant provides direct osseous anchorage through formation of a lattice between surface and bone?
   A. Transosteal
   B. Endodontic
   C. Endosseous
   D. Subperiosteal
3. According to the American Dental Association Council on Dental Materials, Instruments and Implants, accepted implants have demonstrated success in clinical trials of at least 50 patients for a minimum of
   A. 1 year.
   B. 3 years.
   C. 5 years.
   D. 10 years.
4. The term *loading* refers to which aspect of implant therapy?
   A. Size and shape of the implant
   B. Bulk of the bone at the implant site
   C. Placement of the implant into the bone
   D. Placement of abutments and restorations on implants for function

5. Which modality is always acceptable for cleaning implant abutments?
   A. Sonic scaling
   B. Ultrasonic scaling
   C. Air-powder polishing
   D. Rubber cup polishing

6. Periodontal pathogens associated with failing implants are similar to those found in periodontal disease around natural teeth. Any signs and symptoms of periodontal inflammation should be addressed with thorough cleaning and plaque biofilm control.
   A. Both statements are true.
   B. Both statements are false.
   C. The first statement is true, and the second statement is false.
   D. The first statement is false, and the second statement is true.

7. Patients with implants may require special instructions and devices for plaque biofilm control because the shapes of the fixtures, abutments, and prostheses can be very complex.
   A. Both the statement and the reason are correct and related.
   B. Both the statement and the reason are correct but NOT related.
   C. The statement is correct, but the reason is NOT correct.
   D. The statement is NOT correct, but the reason is correct.
   E. NEITHER the statement NOR the reason is correct.

8. Recall intervals for patients with implants can be the same as for patients without implants. Implants tend to accumulate biofilm and calculus quickly, but these are easy for patients to remove.
   A. Both statements are true.
   B. Both statements are false.
   C. The first statement is true, and the second statement is false.
   D. The first statement is false, and the second statement is true.

SHORT ANSWER

9. What are the symptoms of a failing dental implant?
10. What are the two critical elements of patient compliance for the implant patient?

Please visit http://evolve.elsevier.com/Perry/periodontology for additional practice and study support tools.

REFERENCES

1. Fiorellini J, Kao DWK, Wada K, et al. Periimplant anatomy, biology, and function. In: Newman MG, Takei HH, Klokkevold PR, et al, eds. *Carranza's Clinical Periodontology*. 11th ed. St. Louis, MO: Elsevier Saunders; 2012:626–634.
2. Albrektsson T, Bränemark PI, Hansson HA, et al. Osseointegrated titanium implants: requirements for ensuring a long-lasting, direct bone-to-implant anchorage in man. *Acta Orthop Scand*. 1981;52:155–170.
3. Bränemark PI, Adell R, Breine U, et al. Intra-osseous anchorage of dental prostheses, I. Experimental studies. *Scand J Plast Reconstr Surg*. 1969;3:81–100.
4. Bränemark PI, Hansson BO, Adell R, et al. Osseointegrated implants in the treatment of the edentulous jaw: experience from a 10-year period. *Scand J Plast Reconstr Surg*. 1977;16(suppl):1–132.
5. Donovan TE, Chee WW. ADA acceptance program for endosseous implants. *J Calif Dent Assoc*. 1992;20:60–62.
6. Schroeder A, van der Zypen E, Stich H, et al. The reactions of bone, connective tissue, and epithelium to endosteal implants with titanium-sprayed surfaces. *J Maxillofac Surg*. 1981;9:15–25.
7. Albrektsson T, Hansson HA. An ultrastructural characterization of the interface between bone and sputtered titanium or stainless steel. *Biomaterials*. 1986;7:201–205.
8. Listgarten MA, Lang NP, Schroeder HE, et al. Periodontal tissues and their counterparts around endosseous implants. *Clin Oral Implants Res*. 1991;2:1–19.
9. Cochran D. Implant therapy I. *Ann Periodontol*. 1996;1:707–791.
10. Stanford CM, Brand RA. Toward an understanding of implant occlusion and strain adaptive bone modeling and remodeling. *J Prosthet Dent*. 1999;81:553–561.
11. Wilson J, Pigott GH, Schoen FJ, et al. Toxicology and biocompatibility of bioactive glasses. *J Biomed Mater Res*. 1981;15:805–817.
12. Fugazzotto PA. Shorter implants in clinical practice: rationale and treatment results. *Int J Oral Maxillofac Implants*. 2008;23:487–496.
13. Carlsson L, Rostlund T, Albrektsson B, et al. Implant fixation improved by close fit: cylindrical implant-bone interface studied in rabbits. *Acta Orthop Scand*. 1988;59:272–275.
14. Lekholm U, Zarb GA. Patient selection and preparation. In: Bränemark PI, Zarb GA, Albrektsson B, eds. *Tissue Integrated Prosthesis: Osseointegration in Clinical Dentistry*. Chicago, IL: Quintessence; 1985:199–209.
15. Misch CE, Wang HL, Misch CM, et al. Rationale for the application of immediate load in implant dentistry, I. *Implant Dent*. 2004;13:207–217.
16. Klokkevold PR, Cochran DL. Clinical evaluation of the implant patient. In: Newman MG, Takei HH, Klokkevold PR, et al, eds. *Carranza's Clinical Periodontology*. 11th ed. St. Louis, MO: Elsevier Saunders. 2012:635–648.
17. Oates T, Stanford C, Huynh-Ba G, et al. Systemic factors affecting implant survival? *Int J Oral Maxillofac Implants*. 2011;26:469–470.
18. Friberg B. Treatment with dental implants in patients with severe osteoporosis: a case report. *Int J Periodont Restorative Dent*. 1994;14:348–353.
19. Mombelli A. Microbiology and antimicrobial therapy of peri-implantitis. *Periodontol 2000*. 2002;28:177–189.
20. Mombelli A, Lang NP. Microbial aspects of implant dentistry. *Periodontol 2000*. 1994;4:74–80.
21. Mombelli A, van Oosten MA, Schurch E Jr, et al. The microbiota associated with successful or failing osseointegrated titanium implants. *Oral Microbiol Immunol*. 1987;2:145–151.
22. Hansson HA, Albrektsson T, Bränemark PI. Structural aspects of the interface between tissue and titanium implants. *J Prosthet Dent*. 1983;50:108–113.
23. Gould TRL, Westbury L, Brunette DM. Ultrastructural study of the attachment of human gingiva to titanium in vivo. *J Prosthet Dent*. 1984;52:418–420.
24. Klokkevold PR. Implant-related complications and failures. In: Newman MG, Takei HH, Klokkevold PR, et al, eds. *Carranza's Clinical Periodontology*. 11th ed. St. Louis, MO: Elsevier Saunders. 2012:1182–1192.
25. Scharf DR, Tarnow DP. Success rates of osseointegration for implants placed under sterile versus clean conditions. *J Periodontol*. 1993;64:954–956.
26. Buser D, Weber HP, Bragger U, et al. Tissue integration of one-stage ITI implants: 3-year results of a longitudinal study with hollow-cylinder and hollow-screw implants. *Int J Oral Maxillofac Implants*. 1991;6:405–412.
27. Bernard JP, Belser UC, Martinet JP, et al. Osseointegration of Bränemark fixtures using a single-step operating technique: a preliminary prospective one-year study in the edentulous mandible. *Clin Oral Implants Res*. 1995;6:122–129.
28. Novaes AB Jr, Marcaccini AM, Souza SL, et al. Immediate placement of implants into periodontally infected sites in dogs: a histomorphometric study of bone-implant contact. *Int J Oral Maxillofac Implants*. 2003;18:391–398.
29. Knox R, Caudill R, Meffert R. Histologic evaluation of dental endosseous implants placed in surgically created extraction defects. *Int J Periodontics Restorative Dent*. 1991;11:364–375.
30. Armitage GC, Svanberg GK, Löe H. Microscopic evaluation of clinical measurements of connective tissue attachment levels. *J Clin Periodontol*. 1977;4:173–190.

31. Armitage GC. Clinical evaluation of periodontal diseases. *Periodontol 2000.* 1995;7:39–53.

32. Listgarten MA, Mao R, Robinson PJ. Periodontal probing and the relationship of the probe tip to periodontal tissues. *J Periodontol.* 1976;47:511–513.

33. Lang NP, Wetzel AC, Stich H, et al. Histologic probe penetration in healthy and inflamed peri-implant tissues. *Clin Oral Implants Res.* 1994;5:191–201.

34. Adell R, Lekholm U, Rockler B, et al. A 15-year study of osseointegrated implants in the treatment of the edentulous jaw. *Int J Oral Surg.* 1981;10:387–416.

35. Balshi TJ. Hygiene maintenance procedures for patients treated with the tissue integrated prosthesis (osseointegration). *Quintessence Int.* 1986;17:95–102.

36. Isidore F. Clinical probing and radiographic assessment in relation to the histological bone level at oral implants in monkeys. *Clin Oral Implants Res.* 1997;8:255–264.

37. Lang NP, Joss A, Orsanic T, et al. Bleeding on probing: a predictor for the progression of periodontal disease? *J Clin Periodontol.* 1986;13:590–596.

38. Adell R, Lekholm U, Rockler B, et al. Marginal tissue reactions at osseointegrated titanium fixtures. I. A 3-year longitudinal prospective study. *Int J Oral Maxillofac Surg.* 1986;15:39–52.

39. Fu J-H, Lee A, Wang H-L. Influence of tissue biotype on implant esthetics. *Int J Oral Maxillorfac Implants.* 2011;26:499–508.

40. Mombelli A. Prevention and therapy of peri-implant infections. In: Lang NP, Karring T, Lindhe J, eds. *Proceedings of the 3rd European Workshop of Periodontology.* Berlin, Germany: Quintessence; 1999:281–303.

41. Lekholm U, Gunne J, Henry P, et al. Survival of the Bränemark implant in partially edentulous jaws: a 10-year prospective multicenter study. *Int J Oral Maxillofac Implants.* 1999;14:639–645.

42. Ellington J-E, Stanford C, Huynh-Ba G, et al. Peri-implantitis–associated bone loss and its maintenance. *Int J Oral Maxillofac Implants.* 2011;26:700–709.

43. Rams TE, Roberts TW, Tatum H Jr, et al. The subgingival microbial flora associated with human dental implants. *J Prosthet Dent.* 1984;51:529–534.

44. Rams TE, Link CC Jr. Microbiology of failing dental implants in humans: electron microscopic observations. *J Oral Implantol.* 1983;11:93–100.

45. Bower RC, Radny NR, Wall CD, et al. Clinical and microscopic findings in edentulous patients 3 years after incorporation of osseointegrated implant-supported bridgework. *J Clin Periodontol.* 1989;16:580–587.

46. Sato S, Kishida M, Ito K. The comparative effect of ultrasonic scalers on titanium surfaces: an in vitro study. *J Periodontol.* 2004;75:1269–1273.

47. Haffajee AD, Socransky SS, Goodson JM. Clinical parameters as predictors of destructive periodontal disease activity. *J Clin Periodontol.* 1983;10:257–265.

48. Felo A, Shibly O, Ciancio SG, et al. Effects of subgingival chlorhexidine irrigation on peri-implant maintenance. *Am J Dent.* 1997;10:107–110.

CHAPTER

16

Periodontal Emergencies

Dorothy A. Perry and Phyllis L. Beemsterboer

LEARNING OUTCOMES

- Define the role of the dental hygienist in the recognition and treatment of periodontal emergencies.
- Describe the etiology of periodontal abscesses.
- Compare and contrast the signs, symptoms, and treatment considerations in patients with gingival, periodontal, and periapical abscesses.

- Describe the distinguishing features of necrotizing ulcerative gingivitis.
- List the identifying features of pericoronitis.
- Outline the treatment for necrotizing ulcerative gingivitis and oral herpetic lesions.
- Describe the symptoms and oral lesions of acute herpetic gingivostomatitis.

KEY TERMS

Acute herpetic gingivostomatitis
Acute periodontal abscess
Chronic periodontal abscess
Combination abscess
Endodontic abscess

Gingival abscess
Herpetic whitlow
Necrotizing ulcerative gingivitis
Necrotizing ulcerative periodontitis
Operculum

Periapical abscess
Pericoronitis
Periodontal abscess
Purulence
Suppuration

Knowledge of emergency situations and treatment priorities assists patients in receiving the timeliest and most appropriate care. The dental hygienist must recognize conditions that are variations of a normal clinical presentation. In the case of periodontal emergencies, delayed therapy can result in additional discomfort for the patient, with possible consequences of increased bone loss and damage to other periodontal tissues. Treatment of all periodontal emergency conditions requires cotherapy with the dentist or periodontist. To identify these conditions, the dental hygienist must take a careful medical and dental history before beginning any procedure.

PERIODONTAL ABSCESSES

A **periodontal abscess** is an inflammation of microbial origin that is associated with accumulations of **suppuration** or **purulence** (pus) in the periodontal tissues. The pus is often referred to as exudate or purulent exudate. Such infections have rapid onset and are usually characterized by pain, swelling, and discomfort. The periodontal abscess is caused by microbiota that have become established in the tissue as a result of trauma, advancing disease process, or incomplete scaling and root planing. The response of the tissue to this inflammatory process depends on the patient's resistance. Individual factors, such as systemic disease, can affect the clinical situation and worsen

the acute condition. There are three basic types of abscesses: periodontal, gingival, and periapical. Each type may be acute or chronic—although the chronic periodontal abscess is likely an acute abscess that drains—and there are combination abscesses.[1]

> **CLINICAL NOTE 16-1** There are three basic types of abscesses: periodontal, gingival, and periapical.

ACUTE PERIODONTAL ABSCESSES

Acute periodontal abscesses are associated with preexisting periodontal disease. They may occur around any tooth in the mouth when the periodontal pocket becomes occluded, often as a result of a foreign object. An exacerbated inflammatory reaction then occurs. If the pocket can drain through a sulcus or a fistula (opening in the tissue), the infection can stabilize and be considered in a chronic state.[1] Stabilization will not occur if a foreign object, such as a peanut skin, popcorn hull, or berry seed, remains in the pocket.

Acute periodontal abscesses appear as shiny, red, raised, and rounded masses on the gingiva or mucosa.[2] They can point and drain through the tissue or drain through the pocket opening. Pus is usually seen around the opening of the abscess, but not always. In these cases, visual examination is not sufficient to recognize the abscess and finger pressure is required to express pus into the oral cavity so it can be seen. Examples of acute abscesses are shown in Figure 16-1.

Treatment Considerations

Treatment of acute periodontal abscesses consists mainly of drainage and the use of antibiotics or antimicrobial agents. The abscess must be treated immediately to alleviate pain and prevent spread of infection. It may be drained through the pocket opening or by access through an incision. Drainage through the pocket opening is usually possible. The teeth in the affected area are scaled and root-planed when the patient is anesthetized and curettage may be performed to remove granulation tissue. Postoperative instructions call for rest, fluid intake, and warm salt water rinses (1 tsp of salt in a glass of warm water) to help reduce swelling. Follow-up treatment, often involving periodontal surgery, is required to eliminate the problem.[4]

The initial treatment of the abscess through the pocket is often the responsibility of the dental hygienist. However, sometimes flap surgery is required at the initial appointment to obtain access for complete debridement. This treatment is performed by the dentist or periodontist. Antibiotics and pain medications are not usually required.[4] If the patient has a fever or if lymphadenopathy is present, antibiotics should be prescribed. The antibiotic recommended can be an analogue of tetracycline because these drugs have the ability to create high titers in the gingival sulcus and inhibit collagenase in the host.[5]

> **CLINICAL NOTE 16-2** Healthy gingival biota are predominantly gram-positive and aerobic. Periodontal abscesses are predominantly gram-negative and anaerobic.

CHRONIC PERIODONTAL ABSCESS

Chronic periodontal abscesses resemble acute periodontal abscesses; in fact, they may be indistinguishable.[1] These abscesses are characterized by an overgrowth of pathogenic organisms that result in suppuration. Chronic abscesses are usually painless because they drain into the oral cavity, either through the opening of the pocket or through a sinus tract. On careful questioning, patients often recount previous experiences of pain and swelling, probably caused by acute episodes of infection.[2]

The chronic periodontal abscess exhibits suppuration that exudes into the oral cavity on digital pressure through the pocket or sinus tract. The associated gingival tissue is red and swollen. As long as the chronic abscess is draining, it is unlikely to be painful, so patients tolerate the condition or do not realize it is occurring. The dental hygienist must understand that suppuration that exudes from the periodontium indicates a chronic abscess and requires appropriate treatment. An example of a chronic abscess with a sinus tract through the tissue is presented in Figure 16-2.

Treatment Considerations

The treatment of chronic periodontal abscesses is similar to the treatment of acute periodontal abscesses. The affected tooth crown and root surfaces must be scaled and root-planed, curettage performed, local antimicrobial therapy completed if needed, and the patient seen for follow-up care to evaluate the need for further periodontal treatment, often including

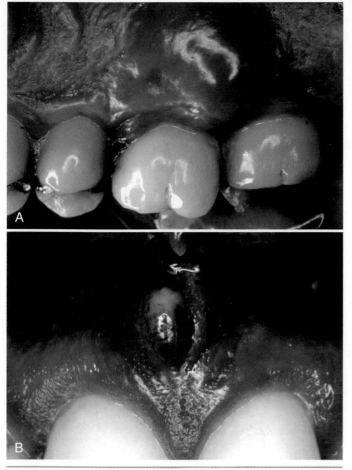

FIGURE 16-1 ■ **Acute periodontal abscess. A,** Clinical appearance of an acute periodontal abscess. There is marked swelling of the periodontal tissues. Clinically, the tissue appears shiny, reddened, and raised. The patient had severe pain. **B,** Acute periodontal abscess associated with a central incisor with a large fistulous track. The fistula drained periodically, thus relieving the swelling and pain for a short time. The fistula then closed temporarily and the swelling and pain recurred. (**A** courtesy of Dr. Philip R. Melnick.)

The most common symptom of acute periodontal abscess is pain. Other symptoms include the following:
- Swelling
- Deep red to blue discoloration of the affected tissue
- Tooth sensitivity to pressure
- Tooth mobility

The patient may also report that the tooth feels "high" in the occlusion because it may become slightly extruded as a result of swelling of the periodontal ligament.[1] Radiographs may be helpful in locating a preexisting area of bone loss, which may be the origin of the abscess. However, the infection moves through the tissue in the direction of least resistance so that the external features may appear at some distance from the affected tooth. The opening of a fistula or sinus along the lateral aspect of the tooth in the adult dentition is usually indicative of a periodontal abscess. However, it may be the result of a periapical abscess. In the primary dentition, a sinus opening on the lateral aspect of the tooth is usually associated with a periapical rather than a periodontal abscess.[2]

The microbiota in the acute periodontal abscess are predominantly gram-negative and anaerobic. In contrast, healthy gingival biota are predominantly gram-positive and aerobic.[3]

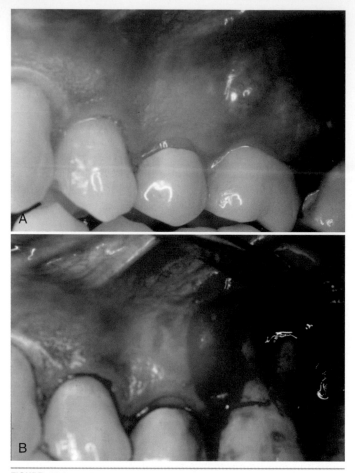

FIGURE 16-2 ■ **Chronic periodontal abscess. A,** Inflammatory exudate drained continuously through the opening of the pocket. **B,** On surgical opening of the defect, an extensive furcation involvement was seen. (Courtesy of Dr. Philip R. Melnick.)

periodontal surgery.[4] The patient must be made aware of the chronic condition, informed about possible acute episodes if no further treatment is performed, and encouraged to cooperate with meticulous maintenance therapy.

> **CLINICAL NOTE 16-3** Patients often do not know that rapid bone loss occurs during acute episodes of infection, placing the teeth in jeopardy. The dental hygienist must educate patients to seek treatment immediately when abscess symptoms occur so that teeth can be preserved.

TOOTH LOSS ASSOCIATED WITH PERIODONTAL ABSCESSES

Periodontal abscesses do not necessarily result in tooth extraction. A classic retrospective study of 114 patients treated and maintained at a university periodontology clinic, all having had moderate to severe periodontal disease, suggested that teeth that develop periodontal abscesses can be treated successfully and maintained for years. Over the 13-year study, 109 periodontal abscesses occurred. Symptoms of the infected teeth were pain, swelling, exudate, and fistulous tracts. In total, 45% of teeth were extracted, but 55% of the teeth were treated and maintained for an average of 12.5 years; the range was 5 to 29 years.[6] For this reason, it is important for the dental hygienist

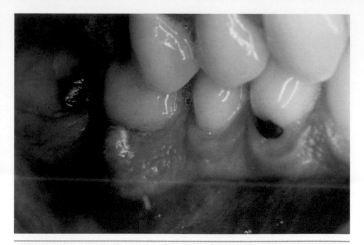

FIGURE 16-3 ■ **Gingival abscess.** This gingival abscess appeared as a localized area of swelling away from the sulcus. It was painful for the patient. (Courtesy of Dr. Philip R. Melnick.)

to recognize periodontal abscesses and refer them for immediate treatment.

> **CLINICAL NOTE 16-4** Exudate is a material such as fluid or cellular debris that has escaped from blood vessels and been deposited in or on tissue surfaces.

GINGIVAL ABSCESS

Gingival abscesses are primarily distinguished from acute periodontal abscesses by taking a good medical and dental history. Gingival abscesses often occur in disease-free areas, and they may be related to forceful inclusion of some foreign object into the area. Usually, gingival abscesses are found on the marginal gingiva and are not associated with any abnormality of the deeper tissues.[1] A gingival abscess is shown in Figure 16-3.

The gingival abscess typically appears as a shiny raised area of acute inflammation that may be painful. The swelling, although it may be quite large, is usually confined to the marginal gingiva.[2] A suppurative lesion is usually evident on the gingival tissues.[1]

TREATMENT CONSIDERATIONS

The gingival abscess must be drained and irrigated. The treatment is usually performed by the dentist or periodontist. It is incised, drained, and irrigated with warm water. Warm salt water rinses should be recommended for postoperative therapy. After treatment of the abscess, scaling and root planing of the teeth should be performed, usually the next day. If the reduced lesion is still large, it may require excision.[4]

ENDODONTIC ABSCESS

An endodontic abscess is sometimes difficult to distinguish from an acute periodontal abscess. The facial pain and tenderness to the tooth are similar in both cases. Endodontic abscesses result from infection through caries, traumatic fracture of the tooth, or trauma from a dental procedure.[1] In addition, pulpal infection of a tooth can spread to the pulp from an adjacent infected tooth through the lateral canals.[7] Most commonly, microorganisms are spread from a carious lesion into the pulp through the dentinal tubules. The microorganisms colonize in the pulp and produce a variety of toxins that result in pulp cell death. Bacteria and their metabolic products then exit the apical foramen and can cause abscess formation.[8]

The endodontic abscess often appears on radiographs as a rounded radiolucency at the apex of the tooth. In this case it may be correctly termed a periapical abscess. However, early in abscess formation, the radiographic changes are much more subtle. Some abscesses drain through a sinus duct through the cortical bone and some drain through the periodontal ligament, making them less identifiable on radiographs. Draining endodontic abscesses can resemble acute periodontal abscesses because their symptoms are similar.[1]

In evaluating an abscess to determine whether it is periodontal or endodontic, it is helpful to know that 85% of tooth pain is pulpal and 15% is periodontal. In addition, many endodontically abscessed teeth test as nonvital, which is a good distinguishing clue. However, some populations of patients, such as those being treated in the office of a periodontist, are much more likely to have periodontal abscesses than pulpal abscesses. Pain may be the feature that distinguishes periapical abscesses from periodontal abscesses. Periapical pain is characterized as sharp, severe, intermittent, and difficult to localize. In contrast, periodontal pain is usually constant, localized, and less severe. Table 16-1 summarizes the characteristics of periodontal and endodontic abscesses.

TREATMENT CONSIDERATIONS

Treatment of endodontic abscesses requires endodontic therapy or extraction of the tooth. It is extremely important that patients with endodontic lesions receive treatment. In addition to causing severe pain, untreated endodontic abscesses can lead to abscesses of the brain[9] or fasciitis of the neck or chest wall.[8] These extensions of infection into deeper tissues can be life-threatening.[10] An example of a treated endodontic lesion is presented in Figure 16-4.

COMBINATION ABSCESSES

An abscess is an infectious process that can spread from the pulp to the periodontium or from the periodontal pocket to the pulp. These circumstances lead to combination periapical and periodontal abscesses.

Combination abscesses have some combination of the signs and symptoms of both types of abscess and may be difficult to diagnose. Periodontal and periapical abscesses can cause extensive damage to the surrounding periodontium because symptoms can be intermittent, causing patients to delay treatment. These abscesses require extensive therapy, both periodontal and endodontic, and often result in tooth loss. The radiographic appearance of a combination abscess is presented in Figure 16-5.

CLINICAL NOTE 16-5 It is important for the dental hygienist to recognize periodontal abscesses and refer them for immediate treatment.

TABLE 16-1 Characteristics of Periodontal and Endodontic Abscesses

	TYPE OF PAIN	TOOTH VITALITY	RADIOGRAPHIC IMAGE
Periodontal abscess	Constant Localized Severe, sharp	Vital	Bone loss No apical radiolucency
Endodontic abscess	Intermittent Hard to localize Extremely severe	Usually nonvital	Apical radiolucency common Widened PDL and other subtle changes can sometimes be seen

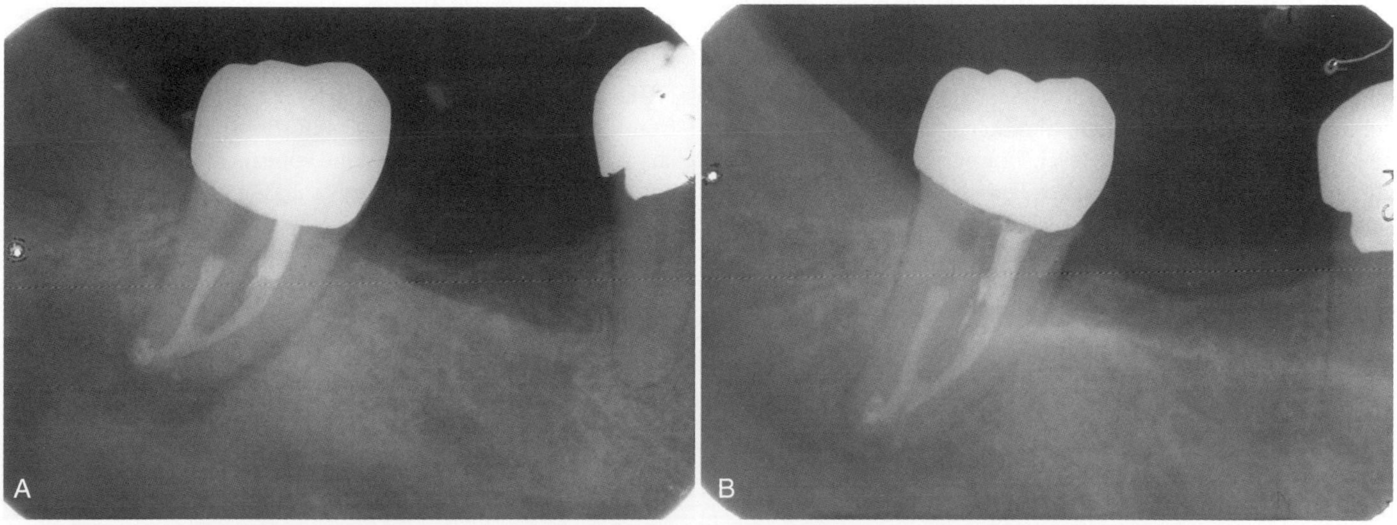

FIGURE 16-4 ■ Periapical abscess. A, Radiographic appearance of an endodontic abscess. Radiolucency is seen at the apex of the root immediately after treatment. **B,** Radiographic appearance of the healed endodontic lesion 1 year after treatment. (Courtesy of Dr. Harold Goodis.)

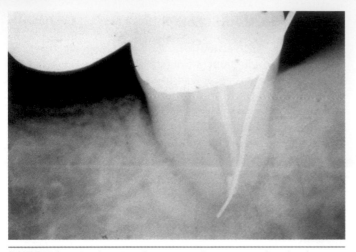

FIGURE 16-5 ■ Combination abscess. A combination periodontal and periapical abscess. Gutta percha points have been inserted through the periodontal pocket to the oral cavity. They penetrate all the way to the apex of the roots. Widening of the periodontal ligament space can also be seen. (Courtesy of Dr. Harold Goodis.)

PERICORONITIS

Pericoronitis is an abscess associated with a partially or fully erupted tooth that is covered completely or partly by a flap of tissue called an **operculum**. The most commonly affected tooth is the mandibular third molar, but maxillary third molars and other teeth that are the most distal in the arch are also associated with the condition. Pericoronitis is generally seen in young adults[1] and has been a serious problem for military personnel, most of whom are 17 to 26 years old. Leone and Edenfield[11] reported that 20% of the military dental emergencies in World War II and 16% of those treated during the Vietnam conflict were pericoronitis. The military population incidence of pericoronitis was reported to be 1.9 cases of pericoronitis per 100 recruits.

The symptoms of acute pericoronitis are swelling of the operculum and other gingiva associated with the most distal tooth in the arch, redness, and extreme pain. The tissue may be so swollen that it interferes with mastication because it may be compressed during chewing.[1] Trismus (muscle spasm) may also occur. (For a description of trismus, see Chapter 11.) The patient may also have a fever and purulent exudate occurs in about half of cases. Of 25 patients in a military population, few bled on palpation and none had a fever. However, pain, swelling, and redness were present in every case. Pericoronitis may be a recurring situation. Two thirds of the 25 patients reported a previous incident of pericoronitis.[11]

TREATMENT CONSIDERATIONS

Treatment for pericoronitis varies according to the severity of the case, whether it is a recurrence, and whether there are systemic complications. Treatment usually requires multiple visits.

Initial therapy is palliative and symptomatic to make the patient more comfortable. After a topical anesthetic is applied, the infected area must be debrided, usually by flushing with warm water or chlorhexidine. It may not be possible to manipulate the tissue very much, and debridement with instruments may not be tolerable at the first visit. After this initial debridement, the patient should be instructed to rest, use warm salt water rinses, and drink fluids to avoid dehydration. Antibiotics should be prescribed if the patient has a fever.[12]

The patient should return the next day. At that time, the tissue is usually considerably improved. At the second visit, the area should be flushed and instrumented if possible. More thorough patient education and plaque biofilm removal can be provided.

After the acute condition has resolved, the patient should be evaluated by the dentist for further treatment. Extraction of the third molar, which is often only partially erupted, may be required. If the tooth is to be retained, the operculum can be surgically removed to obtain a more normal gingival contour.[1,12]

> **CLINICAL NOTE 16-6** Pericoronitis is an acute inflammation of an operculum and is usually found in young adults.

NECROTIZING ULCERATIVE GINGIVITIS

Necrotizing ulcerative gingivitis (NUG) is an opportunistic infection of the gingiva that is associated with stress, lifestyle, and some chronic illnesses and conditions, such as blood dyscrasias, human immunodeficiency virus infection, and Down syndrome. The disease was first described by Vincent in the late nineteenth century. It was so common among troops fighting in the trenches in Europe during World War I that it was named "trench mouth" and was thought to be communicable. Now it is primarily seen in young adults under severe stress and individuals who are immunocompromised. NUG is not communicable.[1]

NUG is a recurring disease with a complex bacteriology consisting of a large proportion of spirochetes and gram-negative organisms. The bacteria invade the tissue and cause the characteristic pseudomembranous appearance of the disease.[1,13] Recurrent NUG can result in attachment loss. When this occurs, the more appropriate name for the disease is **necrotizing ulcerative periodontitis**.

CHARACTERISTICS OF NECROTIZING ULCERATIVE GINGIVITIS

NUG has specific clinical characteristics that distinguish it from other forms of acute oral infections. The involved papillary gingiva becomes necrotic and appears cratered or punched-out. The surface of the gingiva has a pseudomembranous coating made up of necrotic bacteria and tissue. The gingiva is reddened and painful. The lesions may be localized to specific areas or generalized throughout the mouth, and patients often have a strong and offensive breath odor, described as fetid (fetor oris). The three most reliable criteria for recognizing the disease were best described by Stevens and colleagues,[14] as follows:

- Acute necrosis and ulceration of the interproximal papillae
- Pain
- Bleeding

A study conducted by Falker and colleagues[15] of patients with NUG who attended a dental school clinic described the

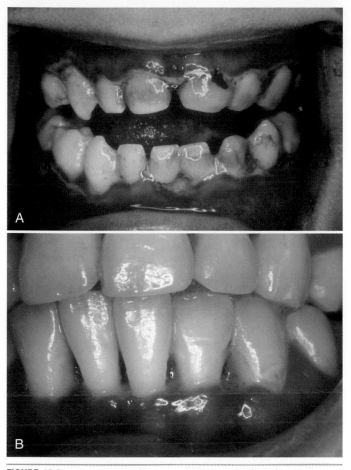

FIGURE 16-6 ■ **Necrotizing ulcerative gingivitis. A,** Clinical appearance of NUG in a 17-year-old male patient. Heavy plaque accumulation and pseudo-membrane formation are seen. The condition was complicated by heavy plaque biofilm accumulation because it was too painful for the patient to brush properly. **B,** This case of NUG is also very painful. The cratering of the papillae and the pseudomembrane are present. Note that there is some attachment loss around these teeth, so this disease is more properly called necrotizing ulcerative periodontitis. (**A** courtesy of Dr. Philip R. Melnick.)

distribution of signs and symptoms of NUG. Necrotic papillae, pain, and bleeding occurred 100% of the time. Fetid breath odor occurred in 97% of cases, pseudomembrane in 87%, lymphade-nopathy in 61%, and fever in 39%. Smoking appeared to be a risk factor associated with NUG because 83% of patients who had symptoms smoked. NUG is illustrated in Figure 16-6.

TREATMENT CONSIDERATIONS

Patients with NUG usually seek treatment for acute pain. Treatment requires the following approaches[12]:

- Alleviation of acute inflammation and treatment of chronic conditions
- Alleviation of systemic symptoms, such as fever and malaise
- Correction of conditions that contribute to the initiation or progress of the disease

Treatment progresses over a few days during the acute phase of the disease because the pain prevents the patient and the dental hygienist from thoroughly cleaning the affected areas. The recommended treatment sequence requires several visits. The goal of treatment is to reduce the microbial load and remove necrotic tissue to assist healing.[1,12]

The first visit requires a limited amount of debridement, only what the patient can tolerate. The use of ultrasonic instruments and topical or local anesthetics may be helpful in removing sloughing tissue, loose debris, and supragingival plaque biofilm and calculus.[1] Subgingival scaling and root planing are contraindicated at this time because of the possibility of extending the infection to deeper tissues and causing bacteremia. Careful oral hygiene instruction should be provided. The dentist may prescribe systemic antibiotics if the patient has a fever or lymphadenopathy.[12]

The second treatment should occur 1 or 2 days later. In this short time, the condition usually improves enough to permit more thorough debridement and better home care. Subgingival scaling may be performed if the patient's sensitivity permits.[12] The third visit should occur 3 to 5 days after the first visit so that debridement can be completed. Any defective restoration margins should be smoothed or replaced to minimize plaque biofilm retention.

During the course of emergency management of NUG, the patient should be instructed to rest, drink plenty of fluids, avoid spicy foods, rinse with warm salt water as needed, and refrain from smoking. If antibiotics have been prescribed, the patient should be strongly urged to fill the prescription and follow the treatment regimen.[1,12]

After emergency treatment is completed, the patient should be evaluated by the dentist or periodontist. All factors related to plaque biofilm retention should be addressed. The disease often leaves cratered papillae that may require surgical correction. Maintenance therapy should be provided at frequent intervals to minimize the risk of recurrence.[12,15]

ACUTE HERPETIC GINGIVOSTOMATITIS

Acute herpetic gingivostomatitis is the oral manifestation of primary infection with the herpesvirus, usually herpes simplex virus 1 (HSV-1). Approximately 10% to 20% of patients with initial infection with HSV-1 are symptomatic.[1,12] Historically, acute herpetic gingivostomatitis has been seen primarily in infants and children. The disease is now more commonly found in young adults in their 20s and 30s, possibly representing primary infection with genital herpesvirus, herpes simplex virus 2 (HSV-2). Primary herpetic gingivostomatitis in adolescents and older adults is usually caused by HSV-1 but may be the initial manifestation of HSV-2. Many patients with primary herpetic infections become carriers of the disease through recurrent expressions of the virus as herpes labialis.[16]

The painful herpetic ulcers in the mouth associated with primary infection often cause reduction in food and fluid intake, which can be critical to health. This highly infectious disease requires education of patients, families, and office staff to prevent its spread. Dental and dental hygiene care should be postponed until the condition has subsided so that the clinician removes the risk of self-inoculation and does not spread the area of infection in the patient.

Acute herpetic gingivostomatitis is characterized by a set of systemic and intraoral symptoms. The disease is commonly associated with prodromal symptoms, such as fever, malaise, headache, irritability, and lymphadenopathy.[13] A good medical

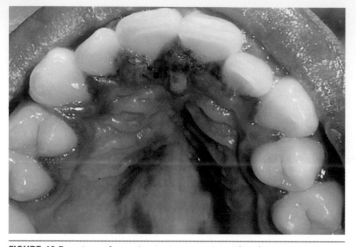

FIGURE 16-7 ■ Acute herpetic gingivostomatitis. This disease appears as a generalized infection characterized by vesicle formation and reddened tissue. Tissue changes were seen around all of the anterior teeth. There was severe gingival pain that caused this patient to seek treatment. (Courtesy of Dr. Gary C. Armitage.)

and dental history and interview may be necessary to identify the prodromal symptoms when suspicious oral lesions are seen.

Oral lesions begin as small yellow vesicles. These vesicles coalesce to form larger round ulcers with gray centers and bright red borders. The vesicles and ulcers may be present on any of the oral mucous membranes, including the lips, tongue, gingiva, and buccal mucosa, and appear generally throughout the oral cavity.[2] The patient may have serious, even extreme, pain. Recognition of the disease is based on knowledge of the appearance of the ulcers and on questioning the patient about systemic manifestations. Diagnostic tests can be used to confirm the presence of the virus, but they are not routinely performed.

After the primary infection has occurred, the herpesvirus travels through the nerves to reside in neuronal ganglia. There it can become active again and recur most commonly in the form of herpes labialis. These secondary lesions occur in about one third of the world's population and are triggered by sunlight, trauma, fever, or stress.[2] Figure 16-7 presents an example of primary herpetic gingivostomatitis.

TREATMENT CONSIDERATIONS

The treatment of acute herpetic gingivostomatitis is supportive because the disease runs its course in 7 to 10 days. Gingival inflammation can be reduced by plaque biofilm removal if the patient can tolerate the discomfort. The patient should do this at home rather than in the office because of the possibility of transmission of the virus to the dental hygienist and other workers. Even if the hygienist has been previously exposed to herpesvirus, the possibility of initiating herpetic whitlow from an inadvertent puncture exists. *Whitlow* is the term for the herpetic lesion that occurs most often on the fingers of the dentist or dental hygienist where the inoculation of herpesvirus occurred.[12] Use of all personal protective equipment is imperative.

The patient should be encouraged to maintain an adequate diet, perform oral hygiene as much as possible and, if necessary, use over-the-counter topical anesthetics to control the discomfort.[12] Chlorhexidine rinses may also be helpful.[1] Topical anesthetics should be used cautiously to avoid anesthetizing the throat, a feeling can that can be frightening, especially for children.[16] For more controlled delivery, topical anesthetics can be swabbed on the lesions rather than rinsed or sprayed.

◎ DENTAL HYGIENE CONSIDERATIONS

- It is the professional responsibility of the dental hygienist to be familiar with the identification and initial treatment of periodontal emergencies. Recognizing emergency conditions as quickly as possible helps to limit the destructive processes, start timely care, and restore patients to comfort and function.
- The most common symptom of acute periodontal abscess is pain.
- Acute periodontal abscesses are exacerbations of periodontal disease that should be treated quickly to minimize further destruction of periodontal support.
- Periodontal abscesses can be treated successfully and do not necessarily mean that teeth will be lost.
- Gingival abscesses usually occur in otherwise healthy periodontia and are related to injury or embedded foreign objects.
- Endodontic abscesses must be treated to avoid possible life-threatening spread of infection.
- Abscesses may be combinations of periodontal and endodontic lesions.
- NUG is an opportunistic gram-negative and spirochetal infection characterized by necrotic pseudomembrane, punched-out papillae, and terrible breath odor.
- Acute herpetic gingivostomatitis is a reaction to infection by one of the herpesviruses. The infection runs its course in about 2 weeks and is extremely contagious.

★ CASE SCENARIO

Mr. Sanchez, who is a regular recall patient of yours in the office of Dr. Engle, a periodontist, arrives for his 3-month recall appointment complaining of intermittent swelling of the gingiva associated with tooth #3. He relates that this has been going on for about 3 weeks, that it hurts when the swelling is large, and that it stops hurting when the swelling goes away. Your assessment reveals a reddened gingiva on the buccal surface of tooth #3 that spreads out to the adjacent teeth and probing depths on the direct buccal surface of 6 mm. This is an increase from Mr. Sanchez's previous visit 3 months earlier when you recorded a probing depth of 3 mm in the chart. As you press gently on the tissue, a yellow exudate emerges from the pocket.

1. The most likely cause of this condition is
   A. pericoronitis.
   B. acute periodontal abscess.
   C. chronic periodontal abscess.
   D. combination periodontal-endodontic abscess.

2. Mr. Sanchez is relating the symptoms of a periodontal abscess because evidence of infection was not present in the area 3 months ago.
   A. Both the statement and the reason are correct and related.
   B. Both the statement and the reason are correct but NOT related.
   C. The statement is correct, but the reason is NOT correct.
   D. The statement is NOT correct, but the reason is correct.
   E. NEITHER the statement NOR the reason is correct.
3. You advise Mr. Sanchez to seek immediate treatment in the future should the condition recur because rapid bone loss occurs with periodontal abscesses.
   A. Both the statement and the reason are correct and related.
   B. Both the statement and the reason are correct but NOT related.
   C. The statement is correct, but the reason is NOT correct.
   D. The statement is NOT correct, but the reason is correct.
   E. NEITHER the statement NOR the reason is correct.
4. Mr. Sanchez reports that the tooth has become sensitive. This suggests that he might have
   A. recession.
   B. periodontal abscess.
   C. exposed root surfaces.
   D. endodontic involvement.
5. Acute or chronic periodontal abscesses have all the following symptoms EXCEPT one. Which one is the EXCEPTION?
   A. Swelling
   B. Tooth mobility
   C. Tooth sensitivity
   D. Fever and malaise
   E. Reddened tissue in the area

STUDY QUESTIONS

Answers and rationales to these questions can be obtained from your instructor.

MULTIPLE CHOICE

1. The periodontal abscess is characterized by all of the following symptoms EXCEPT one. Which one is the EXCEPTION?
   A. Pain
   B. Swelling
   C. Bleeding
   D. Tenderness
2. The microbiota found in the acute periodontal abscess are predominantly
   A. gram-positive and aerobic.
   B. gram-negative and aerobic.
   C. gram-positive and anaerobic.
   D. gram-negative and anaerobic.
3. An acute periodontal abscess can occur as the result of all of the following EXCEPT one. Which one is the EXCEPTION?
   A. Antibiotic usage
   B. Dental procedures
   C. Subgingival scaling
   D. Retained popcorn hull or berry seed

4. What is the term for an abscess that is found on the marginal gingiva and is not involved in the deeper periodontium?
   A. Pericoronitis
   B. Gingival abscess
   C. Periapical abscess
   D. Acute periodontal abscess
   E. Chronic periodontal abscess
5. What is the term for an abscess that is the result of a pulpal infection from caries or trauma?
   A. Pericoronitis
   B. Gingival abscess
   C. Periapical abscess
   D. Acute periodontal abscess
   E. Chronic periodontal abscess
6. The presence of pain can assist the clinician in distinguishing a periodontal abscess from a periapical abscess because periapical pain is difficult to localize.
   A. Both the statement and the reason are correct and related.
   B. Both the statement and the reason are correct but NOT related.
   C. The statement is correct, but the reason is NOT correct.
   D. The statement is NOT correct, but the reason is correct.
   E. NEITHER the statement NOR the reason is correct.
7. An acute periodontal abscess presents as red, raised, and shiny. Suppuration is always found in patients with acute periodontal abscesses.
   A. Both statements are true.
   B. Both statements are false.
   C. The first statement is true, and the second statement is false.
   D. The first statement is false, and the second statement is true.
8. Which of the following oral conditions are contagious?
   A. Acute pericoronitis
   B. Chronic periodontitis
   C. Herpetic gingivostomatitis
   D. Necrotizing ulcerative gingivitis

SHORT ANSWER

9. Describe the clinical characteristics of necrotizing ulcerative gingivitis?
10. What is the recommended treatment approach for acute herpetic gingivostomatitis?

Please visit **http://evolve.elsevier.com/Perry/periodontology** for additional practice and study support tools.

REFERENCES

1. Kerns DG. Acute periodontal conditions. In: Rose LF, Mealey BL, eds. *Periodontics: Medicine, Surgery, and Implants.* St. Louis, MO: Elsevier Mosby; 2004:200–213.
2. Carranza FA, Camargo PM. The periodontal pocket. In: Newman MG, Takei HH, Klokkevold PR, et al, eds. *Carranza's Clinical Periodontology.* 11th ed. St. Louis, MO: Elsevier Saunders; 2012:127–139.
3. Newman MG, Sims TN. The predominant cultivable microbiota of the periodontal abscess. *J Periodontol.* 1979;50:350–354.
4. Melnick PR, Takei HH. Treatment of periodontal abscess. In: Newman MG, Takei HH, Klokkevold PR, et al, eds. *Carranza's Clinical Periodontology.* 11th ed. St. Louis, MO: Elsevier Saunders; 2012:443–448.

5. Ciancio SC, Mariotti A. Antiinfective therapy. In: Newman MG, Takei HH, Klokkevold PR, et al, eds. *Carranza's Clinical Periodontology*. 11th ed. St. Louis, MO: Elsevier Saunders; 2012:482–491.

6. McLeod DE, Lainson PA, Spivey JD. Tooth loss due to periodontal abscess: a retrospective study. *J Periodontol*. 1997;68:963–966.

7. Kureishi A, Chow AW. The tender tooth. Dentoalveolar, pericoronal, and periodontal infections. *Infect Dis Clin North Am*. 1988;2:163–182.

8. Macfarlane TW. Plaque-related infections. *J Med Microbiol*. 1989;29: 161–170.

9. Saal CJ, Mason JC, Cheuk SL, et al. Brain abscess from chronic odontogenic cause: report of a case. *J Am Dent Assoc*. 1988;117: 453–455.

10. Umeda M, Shibuya Y, Komori T. Necrotizing fasciitis caused by dental infection: a retrospective analysis of 9 cases and a review of the literature. *Oral Surg Oral Med Oral Pathol Oral Radiol Endod*. 2003;95:283–290.

11. Leone SA, Edenfield MJ. Third molars and acute pericoronitis: a military problem. *Mil Med*. 1987;152:146–149.

12. Klokkevold P. Treatment of acute gingival disease. In: Newman MG, Takei HH, Klokkevold PR, et al, eds. *Carranza's Clinical Periodontology*. 11th ed. St. Louis, MO: Elsevier Saunders; 2012:437–442.

13. American Academy of Periodontology. *Glossary of Periodontal Terms*. 4th ed. Chicago, IL: American Academy of Periodontology; 2001.

14. Stevens AW, Cogen RB, Cohen Cole S, et al. Demographic and clinical data associated with acute necrotizing ulcerative gingivitis in a dental school population. *J Clin Periodontol*. 1984;11:487–493.

15. Falker WA, Martin SA, Vincent JW, et al. A clinical, demographic and microbiologic study of ANUG patients in an urban dental school. *J Clin Periodontol*. 1987;14:307–314.

16. Balciunas BA, Overholser CD. Diagnosis and treatment of common oral lesions. *Am Fam Physician*. 1987;35:206–220.

Results of Periodontal Therapy

Perhaps the most gratifying aspect of dental hygiene care for periodontal patients is that it works well. Periodontal treatment often results in the development of lasting partnerships between the dental hygienist and patients. Part V defines this relationship and describes the results of therapy. The following questions are addressed in Part V:

CHAPTER 17   How do periodontal patients stay healthy after the treatment sequence?

CHAPTER 18   What is the prognosis for patients who have periodontal treatment provided by the dental hygienist?

17

Periodontal Maintenance and Prevention

Gwen Essex
Based on the original work by Mari-Anne L. Low

LEARNING OUTCOMES

- Explain the effectiveness of periodontal maintenance therapy in the prevention of disease, disease progression, and tooth loss.
- Describe the elements of a successful maintenance program.
- State five major objectives of periodontal maintenance.
- Define the importance of patient compliance.
- Describe strategies to improve compliance with recommended maintenance intervals and oral hygiene regimens.

- List the principal aims and components of the maintenance appointment.
- Recognize the signs of recurrent periodontitis and assess the factors that contribute to its development.
- Describe the causes of root surface caries and therapeutic approaches to prevent development of this common problem.
- Explain the theory, causes, and management of dentin sensitivity.

KEY TERMS

Compliance
Dentin sensitivity and hypersensitivity
Fluoride therapy

Gingival recession
Periodontal maintenance
Recall

Recurrent periodontitis
Root caries
Xerostomia

Preventing recurrent disease and maintaining oral health are of fundamental importance for the success of periodontal therapy. Chronic gingival inflammation can resolve if the local etiologic factors are removed during the active phase of periodontal treatment. However, the long-term stability of results and the prevention of recurring disease require regular supervision in an effective periodontal maintenance program. **Periodontal maintenance** is "the continuing periodic assessment and prophylactic treatment of the periodontal structures that permit early detection and treatment of new or recurring abnormalities or disease,"[1] commonly referred to as **recall**, periodontal maintenance therapy, supportive periodontal therapy, or the maintenance phase of periodontal treatment.

The overall goal of dentistry is to attain and maintain healthy and functional dentitions and oral tissues for a lifetime. Within this context, the primary objective of periodontal maintenance is to preserve the stable state achieved during the active phase of periodontal therapy. This chapter focuses on issues that are relevant to maintenance, including the following:

- Effectiveness of periodontal therapy in arresting the progression of periodontitis and preventing tooth loss
- Objectives of periodontal maintenance
- Importance of patient compliance with recommended recall schedules and plaque biofilm control regimens
- Components of the maintenance appointment
- Recurrence of periodontal disease

- Significance of caries in the periodontal maintenance population and the appropriate use of fluorides in caries prevention
- Sensitivity of dentin after periodontal therapy and recommended treatment

Providing preventive, educational, and therapeutic services for maintenance care is a challenging task. As a primary care provider in the treatment of periodontal disease, the dental hygienist retains significant responsibility for maintenance after the patient has completed active periodontal treatment. Periodontal maintenance emphasizes the important link between preventive oral health care and dental hygiene care aimed at achieving optimum oral health. As the public becomes increasingly aware of the importance of oral health, the role of the dental hygienist in providing maintenance care and patient education continues to grow.

SEQUENCE OF PERIODONTAL THERAPY

Periodontal maintenance plays a critical role within the spectrum of periodontal therapy. Periodontal therapy consists of a series of three phases of treatment, as outlined in Figure 17-1:

- Initial, or hygienic, phase including the reevaluation phase (Phase I)
- Surgical phase (Phase II)
- Maintenance phase (Phase IV)

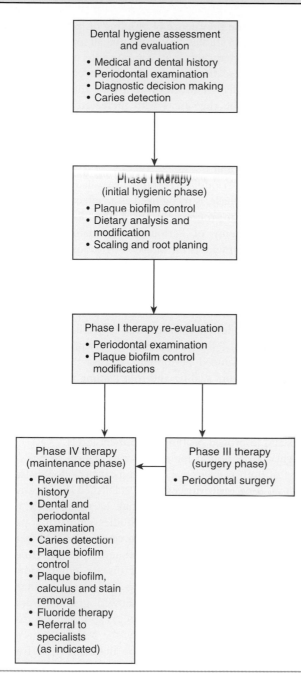

FIGURE 17-1 ■ The periodontal treatment plan. (Modified from McCullough C, Tavtigian R. Perio trends: diagnosis and treatment planning. *Access.* 1993;7:27.)

The initial phase consists of individualized oral hygiene instruction and supragingival and subgingival debridement of bacterial plaque biofilm and calculus. During the reevaluation, a second assessment of the periodontal condition is performed to determine the results of initial therapy and whether additional periodontal intervention is required. The maintenance program is initiated immediately after reevaluation to ensure the stability of results attained in the initial phase. During this period, corrective surgical and restorative procedures are performed as indicated. The aim of the surgical phase is to provide reconstructive or surgical therapy to improve the periodontal condition further and increase the ability of the patient to perform adequate daily oral hygiene.

> **CLINICAL NOTE 17-1** Periodontal patients must be informed that maintenance following active therapy is critical in maximizing the results of treatment. It is helpful to refer to the maintenance phase and future care throughout the active therapy phase to increase understanding of their importance to successful therapy.

EFFECTIVENESS OF PERIODONTAL THERAPY

The major objective of periodontal therapy is to arrest the progression of periodontal disease by eliminating or reducing the local microbial etiologic factors—that is, removal of the pathogens that illicit the inflammatory response in the host. Overwhelming evidence shows the effectiveness of periodontal therapy in preventing disease, slowing the progression of disease, and minimizing tooth loss caused by the periodontal disease process. Many longitudinal studies show that periodontal therapy is effective in maintaining teeth in a state of health, function, and comfort for many years.[2] In contrast, untreated periodontal disease progresses, with a continual loss of the periodontium over time.[3] Ultimately, this chronic destruction is responsible for tooth mortality. Furthermore, the stability of results obtained through active periodontal therapy requires a regular maintenance program.

PREVENTION OF DISEASE

Successful prevention of gingivitis and periodontitis begins with good personal oral hygiene and periodic professional maintenance care to minimize or eliminate the etiologic factors that lead to the pathogenic state. As an oral health educator and clinician, the dental hygienist is an essential provider of preventive services in the initial phase of periodontal therapy and during periodontal maintenance care. Hence, the dental hygienist must recognize the benefits of periodontal therapy, maintenance care, and effective plaque biofilm control in order to select appropriate treatment modalities and effectively educate patients about the prevention of gingival and periodontal diseases.

Epidemiologic and clinical studies have provided strong evidence to correlate poor personal oral hygiene care and the presence of gingivitis. A landmark study by Löe and colleagues[4] and Theilade and associates[5] described heavy plaque biofilm accumulation and generalized mild gingivitis in patients with a normally healthy periodontium after 9 to 21 days without any personal oral hygiene. The observed experimental gingivitis was reversed when daily plaque biofilm control procedures were reinstituted. These results provide the foundation on which plaque biofilm control is based. To encourage and support the patient in maintaining a clean and healthy oral environment, the dental hygienist should emphasize the significance of personal oral hygiene and review appropriate plaque biofilm control techniques during each maintenance visit.

> **CLINICAL NOTE 17-2** Many patients come to maintenance appointments expecting a lecture about flossing. It is far more effective to provide individualized instruction based on findings during your assessment than simply to provide general principles of plaque control.

Gingivitis is associated with the occurrence of periodontal disease. Both human and laboratory animal studies have shown that gingivitis does not always proceed to periodontitis; however, periodontitis is always preceded by gingivitis.[3] Therefore, the recognition and treatment of gingivitis are vital to the goals of maintenance therapy.

Both effective personal oral hygiene and professional maintenance therapy are critical to the prevention of periodontal disease. Despite their benefit in resolving gingivitis, daily oral hygiene procedures alone have limited effects on periodontal disease. Evidence suggests that supragingival plaque biofilm control alone can reduce inflammation associated with gingivitis; however, improvement in probing depths and clinical attachment from plaque biofilm control alone is minimal in patients with periodontitis.[6] This limited clinical improvement may be a result of the unpredictable effect of supragingival plaque biofilm control in altering the subgingival microbiota in pocket depths greater than 5 mm. However, scaling and root planing have a significant effect on subgingival biota and probing depths.[7-10] This observation reinforces the importance of professional subgingival mechanical instrumentation at regular intervals in conjunction with personal oral hygiene to maintain periodontal health.

PREVENTION OF DISEASE PROGRESSION

The periodontal response after effective nonsurgical and surgical therapy favors the reestablishment and maintenance of periodontal health. Numerous studies have shown that removing supragingival and subgingival bacterial deposits can resolve inflammation and halt disease progression.[6] In addition, significant advances in understanding the complex causes of periodontal disease and a wider selection of therapeutic modalities have contributed to successful periodontal treatment.

Commonly, several forms of therapy are combined to disrupt the pathogenesis of periodontal disease. Current periodontal therapies and the clinical benefits provided are shown in Table 17-1.

Research has verified the effect of periodontal therapies on clinical parameters such as bleeding on probing, loss of clinical attachment, and changes in gingival color and form. For example, two longitudinal studies evaluated the effects of four types of periodontal therapy—coronal scaling, root planing, modified Widman surgery (flap surgery to provide access for scaling and root planing), and flap surgery with osseous resection—on the prevalence of bleeding on probing and suppuration.[11,12] Both studies confirmed that all four therapies, followed by maintenance care at 3-month intervals, reduced the prevalence of these disease indicators. However, coronal scaling alone was less effective in sites with greater than 5-mm pocket depths. It may be that areas with increased probing depths continued to exhibit greater inflammation because adequate debridement was more difficult without surgical intervention. Maintenance care at 3-month intervals promoted the long-term results of all therapies.

Nonsurgical periodontal therapy, also called Phase I therapy, or the hygienic phase, is recognized as an effective treatment to arrest or retard the progression of early periodontal disease. The American Academy of Periodontology defines nonsurgical periodontal treatment as the phase of periodontal therapy that includes plaque biofilm control, plaque biofilm removal, supragingival and subgingival scaling, root planing, and the use of chemical adjuncts.[13] Several longitudinal studies confirmed the effectiveness of nonsurgical periodontal therapy for early intervention of periodontal disease when it is followed by regular maintenance visits.[6] Research conducted in a patient group with moderate to advanced periodontal disease treated with oral hygiene instruction, scaling and root planing, and elimination of plaque biofilm retentive factors demonstrated the short-term effects of initial periodontal therapy. When examined 3 to 5 months after therapy, patients had reduced probing pocket depths and improved probing attachment levels.[9]

Regular periodontal maintenance is critical to the lasting success of both nonsurgical and surgical periodontal therapy. Numerous long-term studies have established the effectiveness of frequent maintenance care to halt or significantly reduce the rate of disease progression. Studies comparing patients who received maintenance care three to six times per year with patients who received maintenance care only once per year clearly showed the arrest of disease progression with frequent recall visits. Patients who underwent maintenance care visits only once per year showed gradual worsening of plaque biofilm and gingival indices, probing depths, and clinical attachment loss.[14-16] Clearly, the benefits achieved by active periodontal therapy must be maintained by frequent maintenance care to prevent further deterioration of the periodontium.

CLINICAL NOTE 17-3 It is the responsibility of the dental hygienist to help maintenance patients understand the benefits of regular professional care and daily personal plaque biofilm control.

PREVENTION OF TOOTH LOSS

Many long-term studies have shown the effectiveness of periodontal therapy and maintenance care in reducing the number of teeth extracted because of end-stage periodontal destruction. Several researchers have documented tooth loss in longitudinal studies of individuals either receiving or not receiving periodontal treatment, including maintenance therapy.[17,18] Tooth mortality rates in treated individuals ranged from 0.6 to 2.2 teeth lost over 10 years. By comparison, individuals with untreated periodontitis lost five to six teeth over 10 years.[19] For more detailed information regarding prognosis, see Chapter 18.

TABLE 17-1	Available Periodontal Therapies and Potential Clinical Benefits
PERIODONTAL THERAPIES	**CLINICAL BENEFITS**
• Nonsurgical periodontal therapy: scaling and root planing • Periodontal surgery • Irrigation with antimicrobial medications • Subgingival sustained-release drug delivery systems • Systemic antimicrobial therapy	• Resolution of inflammation • Elimination of infection • Reduction of pocket depths • Arrested disease progression • Prevention of tooth loss • Enhanced patient comfort • Healthy gingival appearance

The dental hygienist should use easily understandable terms and statements to help motivate patients. For example, sharing the dramatic improvement in tooth retention for a patient in ongoing care in a patient-friendly manner may help gain patient compliance.

EFFECTIVENESS OF PERIODONTAL MAINTENANCE

The long-term success of periodontal and maintenance therapy has been documented in both prospective and retrospective studies.[0] These studies demonstrated that surgical and nonsurgical periodontal therapies were effective in halting the destructive disease if routine professional maintenance was followed. Maintenance care must begin soon after active therapy and must occur at 3- to 4-month intervals. Conversely, periodontal therapy without comprehensive maintenance care resulted in higher rates of loss of attachment than expected without treatment.[20] In fact, alveolar bone loss and tooth mortality rates in unmaintained individuals have been reported to be twice those observed in patients receiving maintenance therapy.[21] Furthermore, regular effective plaque biofilm control by the patient, in addition to proper maintenance care by the clinician, is necessary to maintain the results of periodontal therapy.[17] Poor oral hygiene permits an environment for opportunistic reinfection by pathogenic microbes, possibly resulting in disease progression.

CLINICAL NOTE 17-5 Patients maximize their investment of time, money, and effort by committing to maintenance care. The benefits of treatment are diminished without maintenance and the disease process may begin again.

DETERMINANTS OF SUCCESSFUL PERIODONTAL MAINTENANCE

The success of periodontal treatment relies on surgical and nonsurgical procedures for thorough root debridement and long-term maintenance through periodic professional therapy and daily personal oral hygiene. There are several integrated factors that contribute to the success of periodontal maintenance, as listed in Table 17-2.

TABLE 17-2 Determinants of Successful Periodontal Maintenance

FACTORS	RATIONALE
• Collaboration among periodontist, dentist, and dental hygienist is established.	• This ensures that all oral care providers understand the patient's goals, the treatment plan, and case prognosis.
• Partnership between patient and oral health care team is created.	• This facilitates a positive relationship and favorable outcome.
• Patient accepts responsibility for oral health.	• Success relies on the patient's commitment to achieve and maintain oral health.
• Maintenance of periodontal health is influenced by patient's overall condition.	• Factors to be considered include the nature and severity of periodontal disease, systemic health, mental health, and host response to therapy.

OBJECTIVES OF PERIODONTAL MAINTENANCE

The overall objective of periodontal maintenance is to prevent the development of new or recurrent periodontal disease through supervised care and to preserve a functional and comfortable dentition for life. Specifically, there are five underlying objectives[22]:

- Preservation of clinical attachment levels
- Maintenance of alveolar bone height
- Control of inflammation
- Evaluation and reinforcement of personal oral hygiene
- Maintenance of optimal oral health

PRESERVATION OF CLINICAL ATTACHMENT LEVELS

Monitoring the gain or loss of clinical attachment levels and probing depths is necessary to assess periodontal health. A gain of clinical attachment and improved probe depth measurements are common findings after active periodontal therapy. However, long-term results are highly dependent on patient **compliance** with maintenance care and the frequency of maintenance visits. For poorly maintained patients with insufficient plaque biofilm control, clinical inflammatory parameters soon resemble those observed before treatment and deeper probe depths, indicating the continued loss of attachment and alveolar bone, are common.[17]

Reductions in probe depths after periodontal therapy result from healing at the epithelial attachment and reduction of gingival swelling.[8] Therefore, increasing probe depths are the most valuable and practical measurements to predict clinical attachment loss during maintenance therapy. They are more predictable than increased plaque biofilm scores, bleeding sites, or amount of suppuration.[23]

Evaluation of the stability of periodontal health requires thorough documentation of probe depths and clinical attachment levels. These measurements are essential for monitoring patient periodontal status during the maintenance phase. However, there are no national guidelines recommending the frequency of these comprehensive evaluations. Suggestions include evaluation at annual or biannual intervals or at every maintenance visit.[24] Despite this lack of standardization of the comprehensive evaluation, every recall appointment must include a periodontal evaluation, regardless of whether it is a comprehensive or a monitoring assessment. The monitoring examination has been described as a "directed" assessment in which all sites are evaluated for inflammatory changes, with problem sites recorded. Thus, comparisons with baseline data can be made and significant changes identified.

CLINICAL NOTE 17-6 Regular periodontal probing and assessment of clinical attachment loss is the most reliable means of determining the current health of the periodontium for maintenance patients. Assessments should be completed at each appointment, even if the entire assessment is not recorded.

MAINTENANCE OF ALVEOLAR BONE HEIGHT

Periodontal disease is characterized by the progression of gingival inflammation into deeper periodontal structures, resulting in the loss of alveolar bone support for the teeth. Periodic radiographic examinations are required to compare bone changes over time. Radiographs provide important data that can be used to evaluate the long-term stability of alveolar bone height during maintenance therapy. However, radiographic image records of alveolar crestal height reflect only historical bone loss, not active bone destruction; therefore, they are a necessary record of therapy but not a substitute for monitoring clinical parameters.

CONTROL OF INFLAMMATION

Maintenance of satisfactory periodontal health requires control of inflammation and prevention of recurrent disease. Toward this end, personal oral hygiene is one of the most important aspects of periodontal maintenance. Studies of supervised maintenance programs that focused on refinement of personal oral hygiene skills showed that improved gingival and periodontal conditions were achieved in compliant subjects.[25] In contrast, Lindhe and colleagues[26] showed that maintenance patients with imperfect plaque biofilm control continued to exhibit loss of periodontal attachment. Other studies have shown that patients with imperfect plaque biofilm control could maintain clinical attachment levels as long as regular, professional, subgingival instrumentation was performed.[27] Poor oral hygiene alone, resulting in marginal gingival inflammation in maintenance patients, may not lead to increased periodontal destruction. Evidence-based review confirms that routine professional care, including disruption of the subgingival microbial biofilm ecosystem, plays a vital role in conjunction with daily oral home care in maintaining a stable periodontium.

EVALUATION AND REINFORCEMENT OF PERSONAL ORAL HYGIENE

Daily personal oral hygiene, in conjunction with professional maintenance care, is the foundation of preventive periodontics. Each maintenance visit must include an evaluation of the patient's oral home care and personalized instruction on proper plaque biofilm control techniques, as indicated by current assessments. It has been shown that in patients who had 2 years of professionally monitored plaque biofilm control emphasizing meticulous oral hygiene, the subgingival microbiota changed to one associated with health.[26] Although perfect supragingival plaque biofilm control is an unrealistic goal for most patients, the amount of plaque biofilm can be reduced to levels tolerated by the body. This change can prevent the reestablishment of gingivitis or reinfection by opportunistic periodontal pathogens. Using behavioral modification and motivational techniques, the dental hygienist plays a role in plaque biofilm control education that is equally as important and demanding as the more technical aspects of maintenance therapy.

MAINTENANCE OF OPTIMAL ORAL HEALTH

An essential component of the maintenance program is the evaluation of the overall health of each patient. Updating the patient's medical record is imperative to identify any systemic conditions that may complicate or contraindicate dental and dental hygiene care. In addition to the periodontal examination, assessment of oral soft tissues, restorations, caries, sensitive teeth, occlusion, and dental prostheses must be performed each time the patient is seen for a maintenance visit. All these assessments are essential elements of the preventive and therapeutic services provided by the dental hygienist during maintenance therapy, and each contributes to helping patients achieve optimal oral health.

COMPLIANCE WITH PERIODONTAL MAINTENANCE

The overall success of periodontal therapy depends significantly on patient compliance with recommended recall schedules and personal oral hygiene regimens. Many studies show that patients who comply with maintenance recommendations have better periodontal health and overall prognoses than patients who forgo maintenance care.[27] Periodontal patients must be made aware that continued maintenance care and personal plaque biofilm control are essential elements of successful treatment. Failure to comply with these regimens can lead to further periodontal destruction and possibly to tooth loss. In essence, periodontal disease can be arrested and controlled, but not cured. Compliance requirements seem demanding, but for most individuals, the benefits of compliance far outweigh the risks of periodontal disease and tooth loss.

CLINICAL NOTE 17-7 Periodontal treatment is never finished; it is ongoing throughout the patient's lifetime.

COMPLIANCE WITH RECOMMENDED MAINTENANCE INTERVALS

Numerous studies verify that periodontal health is maintained in individuals who comply with suggested maintenance intervals, regardless of the type of surgical or nonsurgical therapy received.[6] In contrast, patients who do not comply or who comply erratically have increased periodontal deterioration. Typically, patients who comply erratically show an increased loss of periodontal attachment,[28] require more corrective surgical procedures,[29] and tend to lose more teeth.[18]

Large variations are seen in studies describing patient compliance with recommended maintenance therapy. In private periodontal practices, 16% to 95% of patients complied with 3-month maintenance intervals.[29,30] University-based studies reported relatively low percentages of maintenance schedule compliance, ranging from 11% to 45%.[31,32] These discrepancies, like compliance, may have many causes and are not easily explained. However, it appears that obtaining patient cooperation is a major challenge for dental hygienists.

The reasons patients do not comply with maintenance schedules are complex, because each individual has different needs and experiences. Some of these reasons are detailed in Box 17-1. In general, noncompliance is seen more commonly in patients who do not perceive chronic diseases to be life-threatening.[32] It is the dental hygienist who must take the time to identify the factors that will be personally motivating for each patient and individualize instruction.

COMPLIANCE WITH RECOMMENDED ORAL HYGIENE REGIMENS

Bacterial plaque biofilm is the primary etiologic agent of gingivitis and periodontal disease, and it is well established that meticulous oral hygiene can prevent both dental caries and periodontal disease. Adequate plaque biofilm control is a major determinant of successful periodontal therapy. Daily mechanical plaque biofilm control with a variety of cleaning aids is the responsibility of the patient. However, the dental hygienist is responsible for educating patients and motivating them to perform these tasks.

Reported rates of compliance with suggested oral hygiene procedures vary, but they are often disappointing. A survey of patients in a private dental practice showed approximately equal proportions of patients claiming to be highly, moderately, and poorly compliant.[33] Other findings suggest that at most, 51% of patients claim high compliance, 38% report moderate compliance, and 11% are noncompliant 30 days after oral hygiene instruction.[34] Patient compliance with the use of interproximal cleaning devices appears no better, with less than 50% compliance.[35]

CLINICAL NOTE 17-8 Compliance with plaque biofilm control regimens is often temporary, so the dental hygienist should reinforce daily oral hygiene practices at each dental hygiene visit.

Periodontal patients report that oral hygiene procedures are cumbersome and time-consuming. Improved plaque biofilm control may be achieved in these patients by introducing an electric toothbrush, which they perceive as faster and simpler than manual brushing.[36] Compliance with suggested oral hygiene regimens may also be directly related to the number of cleaning aids recommended at the maintenance visit. When more oral hygiene aids are recommended, decreased compliance is observed.[37] The dental hygienist should therefore avoid giving instruction for every possible aid at one time and instead create a plan for implementation of recommended tools over time.

CLINICAL NOTE 17-9 Patients can be easily overwhelmed when confronted with too many tools and techniques for daily oral care routines. Prioritize a treatment plan and work on one or two new behaviors, allowing the patient to master one before adding another. This approach will build patient confidence and increase compliance.

STRATEGIES TO IMPROVE PATIENT COMPLIANCE

Strategies to increase compliance start with increasing the patient's knowledge. The importance of periodontal maintenance, the benefits of preventive therapy, an appreciation of

TABLE 17-3 Recommendations to Improve Patient Compliance

STEP	RATIONALE
1. Simplify	Speaking at the patient's level of understanding enhances communication efforts; patients tend to remember what is told to them first; the simpler the required behavior, the more likely it is that the patient will comply.
2. Accommodate	Recommendations should be tailored to the patient's needs and lifestyle; satisfied patients tend to comply more than dissatisfied patients.
3. Remind patients of appointments	Patients must recognize the importance of frequent recall appointments to maintain periodontal health.
4. Keep records of compliance	Noting the patient's history of compliance with recommended maintenance schedules and plaque control regimens provides legal documentation as well as a guideline for behavior modification.
5. Inform	Written specifications of the recommended regimens can be reminders for patients.
6. Provide positive reinforcement	Positive feedback enhances compliance more than a negative approach.
7. Identify	If noncompliance is suspected in a patient, the consequences of failure to comply should be discussed before therapy is initiated.

(From Wilson TG. Compliance: a review of the literature with possible applications to periodontics. *J Periodontol.* 1987;58:709.)

improved oral health, and the dental hygienist's commitment to maintaining a caring attitude and providing the highest quality professional services should be emphasized. Recommendations to improve compliance are listed in Table 17-3.[32]

Research suggests that the highest patient dropout rate occurs during the first year of maintenance therapy. Up to 35% of patients who received periodontal therapy thought that treatment was complete after the initial phase, before maintenance even began.[38] Therefore, special attention should be given to patients at the initiation of treatment and again at the commencement of periodontal maintenance to emphasize the importance of compliance and establish a positive long-term relationship.

Economic considerations are a common source of concern about suggested maintenance intervals. Socioeconomic status, educational level, and perception of oral health may affect a patient's attitude toward purchasing oral health care services. The cost of maintenance appointments is often a primary determinant of patient compliance. A survey of noncompliant maintenance patients in a private periodontal practice showed that many were concerned about the long-term expense of treatment.[32] This concern may reflect a lack of appreciation for the cost-effectiveness of maintenance care. Because chronic periodontal disease is often asymptomatic, disease progression goes unnoticed. Subsequent re-treatment can be much more expensive than maintenance in terms of financial cost and tooth loss. The dental hygienist can correct these misconceptions and help patients understand the preventive and cost-effective aspects of maintenance care.

The popularity of healthy lifestyles and physical fitness has skyrocketed and health concerns have become a part of mainstream American life. The promotion of physical and mental health and well-being focuses on prevention. This requires individuals to make decisions leading to healthier lifestyles. The promotion of oral health is a part of this trend. The media, federal and state governments, employers, health professionals, family, and friends greatly influence an individual's attitude toward health. Because oral health is often a reflection of systemic health, the dental hygienist is in an excellent position to encourage patients to maintain both their oral and physical health. As evidence continues to emerge suggesting a link between periodontal and systemic diseases, patients' awareness of oral health as an essential component of overall well-being will increase. Moreover, evidence suggests that health-related behavior, including compliance, is often dictated by the individual's beliefs about health.[38] Hence, an appreciation of oral health is likely to improve compliance and ultimately help achieve success in periodontal maintenance.

As a health professional, the dental hygienist is obligated to educate and motivate patients continually to comply with recommendations for good oral health. The establishment of a partnership between the patient and the dental hygienist is essential to facilitate this learning relationship. Dental hygienists have sometimes been perceived as indifferent to patient concerns.[32] Maintaining a caring attitude and good rapport encourages patients to ask questions and express their fears and concerns regarding therapy. Dental hygienists should take advantage of opportunities to teach and provide a better understanding of maintenance therapy; this understanding, in turn, promotes patient compliance.

THE MAINTENANCE APPOINTMENT

Regular professional maintenance visits are the cornerstone of periodontal maintenance. The following are the principal aims of the maintenance appointment:

- To evaluate the stability of results after active therapy
- To remove bacterial plaque biofilm accumulations on the tooth surface thoroughly
- To eliminate all factors that favor the persistence of pathogenic bacteria
- To evaluate and reinforce plaque biofilm control

To achieve these objectives, the maintenance visit consists of a medical history update, a complete periodontal and dental examination, a radiographic examination if needed, a review of personal oral hygiene, and removal of supragingival and subgingival plaque biofilm and calculus. The maintenance visit is outlined in Box 17-2. On average, the maintenance appointment lasts 1 hour and generally provides sufficient time for thorough and proper care.[39] However, the length of the appointment can be adjusted depending on the needs of the patient. The next section describes the components of a periodontal maintenance appointment, commonly referred to as a maintenance visit or periodontal recall.

BOX 17-2 Periodontal Maintenance Appointment

Assessment Procedures
Medical and Dental History Update
- Review chart before seating patient
- Identify recent illnesses, current health status and medications, and other pertinent information
- Determine vital signs

Oral and Dental Examination
- Examine extraoral and intraoral soft tissues for pathologic conditions
- Detect caries, assess restorations, and evaluate prostheses

Periodontal Evaluation
- Measure probing pocket depths
- Measure gingival recession
- Record specific sites of bleeding on probing
- Assess tooth mobility
- Classify furcations
- Evaluate sites of mucogingival involvement

Radiographic Examination
- Obtain and review necessary radiographs

Plaque Control Evaluation
- Assess quantity and location of existing plaque biofilm
- Educate, motivate, and reinforce plaque biofilm control

Therapeutic Procedures
Oral Hygiene Instruction
- Review toothbrushing and interdental cleaning techniques
- Reinforce importance of daily oral hygiene care

Periodontal Debridement
- Remove plaque biofilm and calculus deposits from supragingival and subgingival tooth surfaces

Plaque Biofilm and Stain Removal
- Polish teeth to remove plaque and stains
- Floss interproximal areas

Fluoride Therapy
- Apply topical fluoride preparations as necessary
- Recommend home fluoride preparations as needed

Sensitivity Therapy
- Apply topical antisensitivity preparations as needed
- Recommend and dispense toothpaste for sensitive teeth as needed

Referrals
Dental Specialists
- Refer patient to dentist to address additional dental needs
- Refer patient to periodontist for further periodontal evaluation and treatment

Maintenance Intervals
- Establish appropriate interval for periodontal maintenance on an individual basis

---

COMPONENTS OF THE MAINTENANCE VISIT

MEDICAL AND DENTAL HISTORY UPDATE

Before seeing the patient, the dental hygienist should review the patient's chart to determine the patient's medical history, dental history, need for antibiotic premedication, record of compliance, and any special circumstances that may affect the dental hygiene care plan. The time necessary for this review is brief, but it is important to be familiar with each patient's background and needs.

The periodontal maintenance appointment must begin with a verbal and written update of the patient's medical history, dental history, current medications, and vital signs. Changes in health conditions may also require modifications of the dental hygiene care plan. In addition, a review of the patient's dental history and specific dental concerns may alert the dental hygienist to conditions that require special attention.

ORAL AND DENTAL EXAMINATION

A thorough extraoral and intraoral examination of the soft tissues to detect pathologic conditions is a routine component of each maintenance visit. If an abnormality is identified, the dental hygienist is responsible for providing detailed documentation and obtaining an evaluation by the dentist.

A complete dental examination that includes caries detection, restorative assessment, and prosthesis evaluation is performed during each maintenance appointment. Recognition of conditions that may be detrimental to the patient's periodontal health is an indispensable skill and an important responsibility of the dental hygienist. Factors that may cause adverse periodontal conditions include defective restorations, overhanging margins, open contacts, overcontoured crowns, and poorly fitting removable prostheses. All oral conditions that appear to deviate from normal should be brought to the attention of both the patient and the dentist. In addition, even excellent restorations and prostheses may cause plaque biofilm retention and problems with oral hygiene. These special problems can be identified and the patient can be taught techniques to clean such areas.

PERIODONTAL EVALUATION

Before any therapy is performed, assessment of the patient's current periodontal status is mandatory. The clinical parameters that are evaluated include the following:

- Probing pocket depths
- Clinical attachment loss
- Gingival recession
- Bleeding on probing
- Suppuration
- Tooth mobility
- Furcations
- Mucogingival involvement

Probing Pocket Depths

Periodontal probing is a valuable tool for the assessment of periodontal health. Evaluation of probing depths serves to complement the initial visual assessment of the gingival tissues. The periodontal probe is used to measure the normal sulcus and periodontal pocket depths from the base of the sulcus to the gingival margin. Six measurements are taken for each tooth on the distobuccal, buccal, mesiobuccal, distolingual, lingual, and mesiolingual surfaces. To permit changes to be monitored over time, a complete periodontal charting is performed at least once a year. Measurements obtained at maintenance intervals that deviate from this baseline must be documented in the patient's chart.

Research shows that changes in clinical attachment are more accurately represented in measurements of attachment loss than by probing depths.[40] Determination of attachment loss is made from a fixed reference point on the tooth surface, such as the cementoenamel junction or the margin of a restoration to the base of the pocket. For a complete discussion of measuring attachment loss, see Chapter 8. This procedure is time-consuming but important to include in practice.

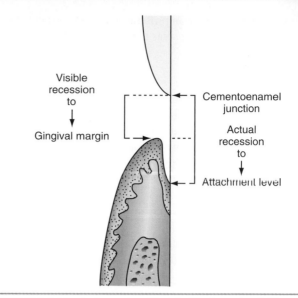

FIGURE 17-2 ■ Gingival recession. The left side shows the visible recession measured from the cementoenamel junction to the gingival margin. The right side shows the actual recession measured from the cementoenamel junction to the base of the sulcus. (Modified from Wilkins EM. The gingiva. In: Wilkins EM, ed. *Clinical Practice of the Dental Hygienist*. 11th ed. Baltimore, MD: Lippincott Williams & Wilkins; 2013.)

Gingival Recession

Gingival recession is apparent when the root surface is clinically exposed as a result of apical migration of the junctional epithelium and loss of marginal gingiva, as illustrated in Figure 17-2. It represents increased attachment loss, but it is not equivalent to the measurement of loss of attachment. Recession is measured from the cementoenamel junction to the gingival margin, and when added to probing depths in the area, it provides an estimate of total clinical attachment loss. The exposed root surfaces in the areas of recession are of special concern because of the increased risk for dentin sensitivity or hypersensitivity and carious lesions. The dental hygienist must carefully assess all areas of recession for these conditions.

Bleeding on Probing

Specific sites that elicit bleeding on gentle probing during the examination should be noted. Bleeding on probing is a reliable indicator of pocket inflammation and is a good, but not perfect, predictor of active disease.[41] In contrast, the absence of bleeding on probing indicates periodontal health in patients who are undergoing maintenance care.[42]

Suppuration

Suppuration is the formation of pus that is visible at the entrance of the pocket when light pressure is placed on the external gingival surface. It is also referred to as exudate or purulent exudate. Pus is an accumulation of inflammatory cells and serum proteins. The amount and rate of suppuration and its very presence are related to the severity of inflammation; the presence of pus indicates that the site requires treatment. Sites with bleeding or suppuration show some or all of the characteristic signs of inflammation: redness, swelling, heat, and pain. These sites must be treated during the maintenance visit and the patient possibly rescheduled for further treatment. A record of sites that showed bleeding on probing at previous visits helps to identify consistent problem areas that require further therapeutic intervention.

Tooth Mobility

Tooth mobility must be routinely evaluated during maintenance visits because increasing mobility may signify a pathologic condition. Causes of mobility include the following[43]:

- Inflammation of the periodontal ligament
- Loss of periodontal support
- Trauma from occlusion (described in detail in Chapter 11)

Furcation Involvement

Furcation involvement is defined as loss of clinical attachment and supporting bone to a multirooted tooth beyond the division of the roots. This situation complicates maintenance therapy. The status of furcations is evaluated with a periodontal probe or a curved Nabers probe and must be assessed at every maintenance appointment. Successful long-term maintenance of furcations is possible[44]; however, frequent maintenance visits and conscientious daily home care in the furcation area are required. Instrumentation of these areas by the dental hygienist and daily plaque biofilm removal by the patient are technically demanding tasks. The dental hygienist must spend more time treating the furcation areas because they are less accessible to debridement techniques and teaching the patient specific home care techniques, such as the use of toothpicks or interproximal brushes. The patient must also make special efforts to clean these areas.

Mucogingival Involvement

Extension of the pocket beyond the mucogingival junction and into the alveolar mucosa represents mucogingival involvement. Although the attached gingiva is absent, maintenance of periodontal health and attachment for the tooth is possible if adequate plaque biofilm control is achieved.[45] In comparison, gingival inflammation and further recession may occur if personal and professional oral hygiene care are neglected. Therefore, charting of mucogingival involvement and instruction in careful plaque biofilm control for these areas are necessary steps at all maintenance appointments.

RADIOGRAPHIC IMAGING

The need for radiographic images during the maintenance program varies with each patient. The frequency of imaging varies on the basis of age, risk for disease, and signs and symptoms.[46] Indications for radiographs include caries activity, increased periodontal destruction, and suspected pathology.[47] It has been suggested that a full-mouth series of radiographs should be taken every 2 to 4 years during maintenance care for comparison with previous films. This practice permits the detection of changes in alveolar bone height, repair of osseous defects, signs of trauma from occlusion, periapical conditions, and caries. Vertical posterior bitewing images are often preferred in periodontics to provide both caries detection and a better image of alveolar bone levels. These films may be taken annually if the patient's disease status is less stable and warrants evaluation.

EVALUATION OF PLAQUE BIOFILM CONTROL

After the periodontal examination is completed, a plaque biofilm evaluation is necessary to determine the patient's effectiveness in maintaining a clean oral environment. Plaque biofilm accumulation is easily seen when disclosing agents are used. The use of disclosing agents serves two purposes. First, a plaque biofilm score can be calculated, which can be recorded in the patient's chart and compared at subsequent maintenance visits to help motivate compliance with home care regimens. Second, the patient can be shown existing plaque biofilm as an educational tool to demonstrate oral hygiene techniques. At the very least, a written description in the chart of the amount and location of plaque biofilm, as well as the reported patient daily oral care practices, is necessary.

THERAPEUTIC PROCEDURES

The extent of therapy performed at the maintenance visit depends on the information gathered during the assessment phase of the appointment. Personalized oral hygiene instruction must always be provided. In addition, with the goal of total plaque biofilm and calculus removal in mind, meticulous instrumentation, often with both ultrasonic and hand instruments, must be performed to remove subgingival and supragingival deposits. Rubbercup polishing may be necessary to remove extrinsic stains not removed by prior instrumentation. Fluoride therapy and treatment for tooth sensitivity may also be required as an adjunct to the periodontal maintenance visit.

Oral Hygiene Instruction

Oral hygiene instruction is an essential component of every preventive maintenance program. Both toothbrushing and interdental cleaning techniques should be emphasized to reinforce the importance of disrupting plaque biofilm accumulations on all surfaces of the teeth every day. Wide variation exists in the ability of each patient to maintain optimal oral cleanliness, so each oral hygiene regimen must be unique to the specific patient. As discussed earlier, behavioral modification techniques are often necessary to improve compliance. Continuing positive reinforcement and encouragement, often involving several maintenance appointments, can motivate patients to maintain improved oral hygiene.

Patients who have continued gingival inflammation despite compliance and plaque biofilm control efforts may benefit from the use of chemotherapeutic agents, such as chlorhexidine. A 0.12% chlorhexidine gluconate solution is both safe and effective to decrease the accumulation of supragingival bacterial plaque biofilm and prevent gingivitis.[48] Because the side effects include tooth staining and increased supragingival calculus formation, the long-term use of chlorhexidine may be impractical. However, greater substantivity of this chemotherapeutic agent compared with phenolic and plant alkaloid mouthwashes[49] justifies its use for some patients with increased periodontal problems.

Periodontal Debridement

Thorough removal of plaque biofilm and calculus deposits is achieved through scaling and root planing. After active therapy, the periodontal tissues generally exhibit increased health characterized by tight adaptation around teeth and more shallow probing depths; however, residual pockets may complicate the scaling procedures.[27] Effective removal of subgingival deposits in pocket depths of 3 mm or less is possible; however, complete debridement of subgingival surfaces in pocket depths of 5 mm or greater is less reliable.[50] In areas with deeper pockets or furcation involvement that cannot be maintained in health, surgical therapy may be required. Because subgingival instrumentation is technically demanding, sufficient time must be allotted to perform thorough debridement. Often, areas with increased probing depths or bleeding on probing should be addressed first to permit efficient use of time during the maintenance appointment. Selective use of local anesthesia may be necessary.

Polishing

Typically, polishing the teeth with a rubber cup and prophy paste, or a cleansing agent, has followed scaling, root planing, and other periodontal procedures. The purpose is to remove acquired pellicle, bacterial plaque biofilm, and extrinsic stains completely from the clinical crowns of the teeth, providing smooth and shiny tooth surfaces.[51] Complete removal of pellicle and bacterial plaque biofilm provides a positive aesthetic experience that may motivate the patient to maintain good oral hygiene habits. However, the therapeutic value of polishing is limited because pellicle begins to form within minutes and plaque biofilm accumulates again about 1 to 2 hours later. Similarly, the removal of stains is a cosmetic procedure because extrinsic stain is not considered an etiologic factor in gingivitis or periodontal disease.

CLINICAL NOTE 17-10 Plaque and stains are mostly removed during instrumentation. Polishing is best reserved for areas that still present with stain, reserving more time for patient education.

Many patients equate polishing to "cleaning the teeth" and expect this procedure at the conclusion of the maintenance appointment. There is minimal therapeutic benefit to routine polishing. It should be limited to stain removal after instrumentation[51] and should not take time away from the procedures necessary to maintain oral health.

Fluoride Therapy

Exposed root surfaces are a frequent consequence of periodontal therapy and increase the risk of **root caries** and the development of dentin sensitivity. The cariostatic benefits of fluoride in the inhibition of demineralization and the enhancement of remineralization is well documented and strongly support the professional application of topical fluoride preparations. Although the effectiveness of **fluoride therapy** for dentin sensitivity is less predictable, application of a concentrated sodium fluoride paste has been recommended and may provide some relief of pain.[52] Dentin sensitivity and its management are discussed later in this chapter.

RECOMMENDATIONS AND REFERRALS

At the conclusion of the maintenance appointment, a recommendation is made for the recall interval. This interval must be based on the patient's individual needs and on assessments made during the maintenance visit. In addition, a time frame for the maintenance program helps each patient understand and anticipate the requirements of compliance. Recommendations and referrals to appropriate specialists for additional periodontal therapy or other specific dental needs should be made at this time.

CLINICAL NOTE 17-11 It is difficult to determine the most appropriate interval for maintenance appointments, especially if the general condition is good and there is only localized pocketing remaining. It is a good practice to plan treatment for the least healthy areas of the mouth because they represent the most likely areas for recurrence of disease.

ESTABLISHING INTERVALS FOR PERIODONTAL MAINTENANCE

Research supports the need for frequent maintenance therapy and oral hygiene instruction to prevent periodontal disease and dental caries.[14,15] At the end of each periodontal maintenance appointment, the dentition is free of bacterial plaque biofilm and calculus. This condition facilitates the patient's efforts to maintain a clean oral environment. In addition, the maintenance appointment provides continued opportunities to reinforce oral hygiene skills and motivate patients to establish good daily habits.

There are no absolute rules regarding the appropriate intervals for periodontal maintenance. The interval is determined by the individual needs of each patient, including systemic factors and the ability to perform adequate home care. Information gathered during the assessment phase of the maintenance appointment provides the basis for determining the interval until the next maintenance visit. These factors are listed in Box 17-3. Clinical findings show the patient's current periodontal status. If the degree of inflammation is high, more frequent maintenance visits are warranted.

In general, the first maintenance visit consists of debridement and plaque biofilm control instructions, but not probing, and it occurs 2 to 4 weeks after periodontal surgery. After this initial monitoring, the interval may be lengthened to 3 months.[22,39] Several studies suggest that 2- to 4-month intervals are adequate to maintain the stability of results of treatment and prevent progression of disease. These recommendations for scheduled maintenance visits should be considered only as guidelines because the value of maintenance is derived from the customized nature of the program.

BOX 17-3 Factors for Determining the Interval Between Periodontal Maintenance Visits

- Probing depths
- Bleeding on probing
- Effectiveness of patient plaque biofilm control
- Age
- Medical history
- Dental history
- Periodontal history
- History of compliance with maintenance
- Compliance with oral home care regimen

RECURRENCE OF PERIODONTAL DISEASE

When periodontal disease recurs it is termed **recurrent periodontitis**. Several factors may contribute to the failure of maintenance of periodontal health, including the following:

- Insufficient patient plaque biofilm control
- Incomplete removal of bacterial plaque biofilm and calculus during therapy
- Presence of faulty restorations
- Prostheses that favor the reestablishment of disease
- Lack of patient compliance with recommended maintenance procedures
- Systemic conditions that negatively affect the oral cavity

The underlying factor in each case of treatment failure is the reestablishment of the pathologic subgingival biofilm, which results in continued pocket inflammation. In general, disease recurrence is localized to one or a few sites, although a generalized recurrence may also develop.[22]

Some patients do not respond to treatment, although optimal plaque biofilm control and thorough root debridement are performed. This condition can be a form of aggressive periodontitis that affects about 8% to 13% of the adult population with periodontitis.[53] It is not known why these individuals do not respond favorably to conventional periodontal treatment regimens.

Recognition of the signs of recurrent periodontitis is a primary responsibility of the dental hygienist when providing maintenance care. The following signs of recurrent disease, further described in Table 17-4, can be observed when evaluating the periodontal status of the patient:

- Increasing probing pocket depths, which are indicative of clinical attachment loss
- Recurrent bleeding on probing
- Chronic gingival inflammation
- Gradual increases in radiographic bone loss
- Gradual increases in tooth mobility

Re-treatment of areas with recurrent disease has the same goal as initial periodontal therapy—to achieve and maintain stable periodontal health. The re-treatment phase usually begins with scaling and root planing of the reinfected sites[22] to debride the subgingival environment of all bacterial plaque biofilm and calculus. Approximately 4 to 6 weeks after re-treatment, a complete periodontal reevaluation is necessary to determine the results, prognosis, and treatment recommendations. If residual calculus remains and inflammation persists, surgical therapy may be necessary to provide access to eliminate the infection, reduce periodontal pockets, or repair the periodontium. Other treatment options for disease control include microbiologic monitoring and antibiotic therapy. Referral to a periodontist should be considered as these needs arise.

ROOT CARIES IN THE PERIODONTAL MAINTENANCE POPULATION

Root surface caries is a fundamental concern in the periodontal population because loss of clinical attachment results in exposed, susceptible root surfaces. Root caries is a soft progressive lesion of the root surface that involves bacterial plaque biofilm and microbial invasion. Teeth that might be maintained for years can be lost quickly to root caries. The carious lesion usually

TABLE 17-4 Symptoms and Causes of Recurrence of Disease

SYMPTOM	POSSIBLE CAUSES
Increased mobility	Increased inflammation Poor oral hygiene Subgingival calculus Inadequate restorations Deteriorating or poorly designed prostheses Systemic disease modifying host response to plaque
Recession	Toothbrush abrasion Inadequate keratinized gingiva Frenum pull Orthodontic therapy
Increased mobility with no change in pocket depth and no radiographic change	Occlusal trauma caused by lateral occlusal interference Bruxism High restorations Poorly designed or worn-out prostheses Poor crown-to-root ratio
Increased pocket depth with no radiographic change	Poor oral hygiene Infrequent recall Subgingival calculus Poorly fitting partial dentures Mesial inclination into edentulous space Failure of new attachment surgery Cracked teeth Grooves in teeth New periodontal disease
Increased pocket depth with increased radiographic bone loss	Poor oral hygiene Subgingival calculus Infrequent recall visits Inadequate or deteriorating restorations Poorly designed prostheses Inadequate surgery Systemic disease modifying host response to plaque biofilm Cracked teeth Grooves in teeth New periodontal disease

(From Merin RL. Supportive periodontal treatment. In: Newman MG, Takei HH, Klokkevold PR, et al, eds. *Carranza's Clinical Periodontology*. 11th ed. St. Louis, MO: Elsevier Saunders; 2012:746-755.)

BOX 17-4 Predisposing Conditions for Root Surface Exposure

- Periodontal disease
- Periodontal surgery
- Malocclusion
- Orthodontic treatment
- Mechanical trauma (e.g., toothbrush abrasion)

begins on the cemental surfaces of the root, at or near the cementoenamel junction, and proceeds to invade the underlying and peripheral dentin.[54] *Actinomyces viscosus* is the predominant organism in bacterial plaque biofilm samples covering carious root surfaces. Although their specific roles are unknown, a variety of microbial organisms are associated with root caries, with some microbes different from those typically found in lesions on smooth surfaces.[55] Exposed root surfaces are a prerequisite for root caries. Various conditions that cause recession are listed in Box 17-4.

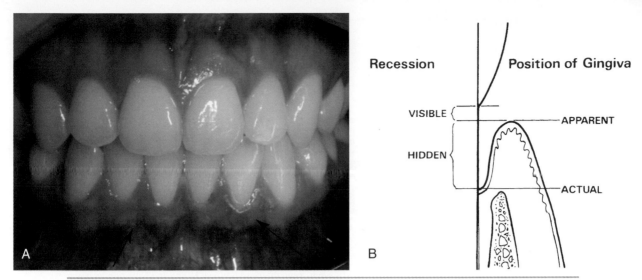

FIGURE 17-3 ■ **The position of the gingiva in periodontal health and disease. A,** An attached gingiva in a healthy periodontium covers the cemental surface, preventing root caries development. Arrows indicate the mucogingival junction. **B,** Visible and hidden gingival recession exposes the cementum, increasing the risk of root caries development. (From Newman MG, Takei HH, Klokkevold PR, et al, eds. *Carranza's Clinical Periodontology.* 11th ed. St. Louis, MO: Elsevier Saunders; 2012.)

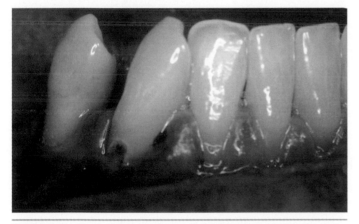

FIGURE 17-4 ■ **Root caries lesion in a periodontal patient.** Appropriate maintenance care requires both plaque biofilm control and caries prevention.

In periodontal health, the cemental root surface is covered by gingival tissues and functions as a major component of the periodontal attachment apparatus, as shown in Figure 17-3. However, in periodontal disease and other conditions that lead to gingival recession, the cementum becomes exposed as the junctional epithelium migrates apically and the gingival margin recedes. As a result, the loss of periodontal attachment and the subsequent exposure of cementum to the oral environment increase the risk for development of root caries, as shown in Figure 17-4. Additionally, root caries may exist in periodontal pockets, especially around crown restorations.

PREVALENCE OF ROOT CARIES

Root caries has received increased attention within the last two decades because people are keeping their teeth longer. Comparisons of prevalence data are difficult as a result of variation in study design, but evidence confirms that a large proportion of adults exhibit root caries.[56] A survey from 1988 to1991 found that 25% of adults in the United States had at least one decayed or filled root surface.[57] Importantly, the

prevalence of root caries increases markedly with age, as shown in Figure 17-5, ranging from 7% to 56%, with men having more root caries than women. The significance of root caries will continue to increase as the U.S. population ages and people retain their teeth for a lifetime.

> **CLINICAL NOTE 17-12** Root caries prevention is an important consideration for maintenance patients. Teeth with treated periodontal conditions that have good prognoses can be lost in a matter of weeks or months due to root caries.

RISK INDICATORS OF ROOT CARIES

Generally, root caries is believed to be a multifactorial disease with many risk factors, often referred to collectively as the caries balance. Loss of gingival attachment is considered a significant risk factor along with age, number of teeth, presence of coronal caries, level of oral hygiene, water fluoridation, and years of education. Incidence data from one study of seniors suggested that periodontal pockets greater than 3 mm deep and existing teeth with root caries were good predictors of risk. These factors are detailed in Table 17-5. Performance of a caries risk assessment that includes sampling the microbial population in the saliva to determine the presence and amount of cariogenic bacteria is a valuable tool in proactively identifying and managing a patient at moderate to high risk of development of caries. Patients at high risk for caries can be aggressively treated with chlorhexidine rinses to reduce the amount of cariogenic bacteria and then encouraged to use appropriate fluoride therapy and diet modifications.[58]

XEROSTOMIA

The protective role of saliva in the oral cavity is well documented. Its functions include antimicrobial activity, control of

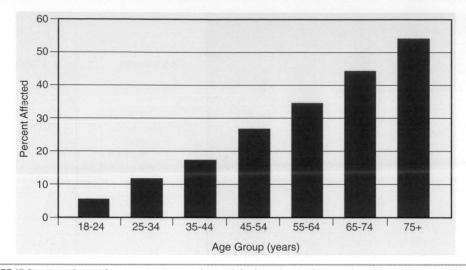

FIGURE 17-5 ■ **Prevalence of root caries.** Survey of U.S. adults from the Third National Health and Nutrition Examination Survey (NHANES III-Phase I): 1988-1991. (Winn DM, Brunelle JA, Selwitz RH, et al. Coronal and root caries in the dentition of adults in the United States, 1988-1991. *J Dent Res.* 1996;75(special issue):642-651. Reprinted with permission from the *Journal of Dental Research.*)

TABLE 17-5	Potential Risk Factors for Root Caries	
RISK FACTOR	**GROUP OF INTEREST**	**RELATIVE RISK**
Age	Older individuals	Increased
Fluoride	Consumers of fluoridated water	Decreased
Coronal caries	High number of coronal caries	Increased
Root caries	High number of root caries	Increased
Oral hygiene	Presence of plaque biofilm and calculus	Increased
Loss of attachment	Presence of gingival recession	Increased
Number of teeth	High retention of teeth	Decreased
Pockets > 3 mm	High number of deeper pocket depths	Increased
Recent illness	Compromised systemic health	Increased
Tobacco use	Smokers and users of smokeless tobacco	Increased
Level of education	High level of education	Decreased
Level of anxiety	High level of anxiety	Increased
Social integration	High social integration	Decreased
Sugar consumption	High intake of sugared foods	Increased

(From Beck J. The epidemiology of root surface caries. *J Dent Res.* 1990;69:1219-1220.)

BOX 17-5	Medications Associated with Causing Xerostomia

- Antiacne drugs
- Antianxiety agents
- Antihypertensives
- Antihistamines
- Antidepressants
- Muscle relaxants
- Antipsychotics
- Decongestants
- Parkinsonism drugs
- Diuretics
- Antiinflammatory analgesics
- Antinauseants (motion sickness medications)

pH, and removal of food debris from the oral cavity. Without these protective functions the adverse effects of **xerostomia** (dry mouth) can lead to difficulties with speaking, eating, swallowing, and wearing dentures. Additionally, xerostomic individuals have an increased risk of *Candida* infections, dental caries, and periodontal disease.[59]

Xerostomia is a relatively common finding that may be related to numerous conditions, including systemic disease (e.g., diabetes, Sjögren's syndrome, immunocompromised states), head and neck radiation therapy, drug therapy, dehydration, stress, and anxiety. Several medications that cause xerostomia are listed in Box 17-5. Individuals with xerostomia complain of changes in both the quantity and quality of the saliva, which may or may not be related to decreased salivary gland function.

An important role of the dental hygienist is to recognize the signs and symptoms of xerostomia. The oral mucosa of a xerostomic patient may appear red, dry, and sticky. Angular cheilitis, characterized by cracking at the corner of the mouth and other infections, may also be present. The saliva may appear to be stringy or foamy with little or no pooled saliva in the floor of the mouth.[59] Dental caries in individuals with xerostomia are often located at the cervical margins or incisal edges of the teeth. Both primary and recurrent caries may also arise at the margin of existing restorations. Signs and symptoms of xerostomia are presented in Table 17-6.

Therapeutic management of xerostomia involves the use of salivary substitutes or salivary stimulants. Temporary relief of symptoms may be achieved with the use of water, glycerin preparations, or artificial saliva as salivary substitutes. Stimulation of natural salivary flow with sugarless candy and chewing gum or medications is useful for individuals with limited functional salivary glands, such as patients undergoing head and neck radiation therapy.

> **CLINICAL NOTE 17-13** Xerostomia is uncomfortable, and many patients seek to relieve the symptoms by consuming products that contain sugar, such as lozenges or hard candies. It is very important to provide relief options that do not put the patient at even greater risk for caries.

Prevention of dental caries is extremely important in xerostomic individuals because of their reduced salivary flow. Strategies for minimizing the risk of caries include frequent dental visits, topical fluorides, and diet control that includes monitoring the frequency of ingestion of fermentable carbohydrates.[60] Recommendations for topical fluorides in xerostomic individuals are listed in Table 17-7.

TABLE 17-6 Signs and Symptoms of Xerostomia

SIGNS	SYMPTOMS
Dry sticky mucosa	Difficulty with eating
Stringy or foamy saliva	Difficulty with swallowing
Little or no pooled saliva on floor of mouth	Difficulty with speaking
	Difficulty with wearing
Difficult to express saliva from major salivary glands	dentures
	Burning sensation associated with oral candidiasis
Caries at cervical margin, incisal edge, or margins of restorations	Changes in taste
	Difficulty with eating spicy or acidic foods
Erythematous mucosa	
Angular cheilitis	

(From Greenspan D. Xerostomia: diagnosis and management. *Oncology.* 1996;10:7-11.)

TABLE 17-7 Topical Fluoride Treatment for Xerostomic Patients

	FLUORIDE RINSE (0.5% SODIUM FLUORIDE)	FLUORIDE GEL (1.1% NEUTRAL SODIUM FLUORIDE)
Mode of application	Swish in mouth Expectorate on completion	Apply with toothbrush or use custom-made plastic tray
Frequency of use	Once or twice daily	Once or twice daily
Length of use	1 minute	2 to 3 minutes

(From Greenspan D. Xerostomia: diagnosis and management. *Oncology.* 1996;10:7-11.)

CLINICAL DETECTION OF ROOT CARIES

An examination for caries during the maintenance appointment is important because of the increased vulnerability of the root surfaces in the periodontal maintenance population. Clinically, early root caries appear as multiple discolored areas that are tan or brown. In advanced stages, these lesions coalesce and form ill-defined areas that may progress apically and may also encircle the root. Active lesions feel soft and appear shallow (<2 mm deep) and are usually covered with bacterial plaque biofilm. In contrast, arrested root caries is characterized by a dark brown to black discoloration and a hard texture. This texture is most likely the result of a remineralized surface layer and a mineralization front advancing into demineralized dentin. The clinical characteristics of root caries are described in Table 17-8. Because root caries can develop on any root surface, both clinical and radiographic examinations are essential for caries assessment. Unlike coronal caries, root caries does not generally produce any pain or discomfort.[60]

PREVENTION AND CONTROL OF ROOT CARIES

The prevention of root caries in the periodontal maintenance population is important because of the high prevalence and incidence rates of exposed root surfaces in this population. The dental hygienist is in a key position to educate patients about the risks and prevention of root caries. The principal strategies to prevent the development of root caries involve the following[61,62]:

- Increasing the remineralization of teeth through fluoride therapy
- Reducing the number of microorganisms through effective plaque biofilm control and antimicrobial agents
- Modifying caries risk by selecting noncariogenic foods
- Limiting the frequency of consuming fermentable carbohydrates
- Improving salivary flow

These strategies are based on the balance between pathologic factors and protective factors in caries development. This balance is illustrated in Figure 17-6.

FLUORIDE THERAPY

Systemic and topical fluoride therapies are significant components of any caries prevention program to increase the resistance of teeth to carious attack.

Fluoride Therapy

Fluoride works by inhibiting demineralization of the tooth surface, enhancing remineralization, and inhibiting bacterial activity. Evidence now indicates that the primary anticaries benefits of fluoride are achieved through its topical application

TABLE 17-8 Clinical Characteristics of Root Caries

COLOR	DISTRIBUTION	TEXTURE	DEPTH	PRESENCE OF PLAQUE	PAIN, DISCOMFORT
Active caries: Tan or brown	Early caries: Multiple discolored areas	Active caries: Soft	Active caries: Shallow (<2 mm deep)	Often	Rare
Arrested caries: Dark brown or black	Advanced caries: Ill-defined area of coalesced lesions	Arrested caries: Hard			

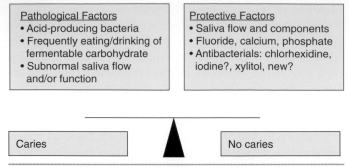

Pathological Factors	Protective Factors
• Acid-producing bacteria	• Saliva flow and components
• Frequently eating/drinking of fermentable carbohydrate	• Fluoride, calcium, phosphate
• Subnormal saliva flow and/or function	• Antibacterials: chlorhexidine, iodine?, xylitol, new?

| Caries | ▲ | No caries |

FIGURE 17-6 ■ **The caries balance.** There is an important balance between pathologic factors and protective factors in the initiation and progression of dental caries. Understanding this balance and educating patients about these factors is an important component of dental hygiene care. This is particularly important with periodontal maintenance patients who are seen frequently and over many years. (Courtesy of Dr. John D. B. Featherstone, University of California, San Francisco, School of Dentistry, Department of Preventive and Restorative Dental Sciences. First published in *Dimensions of Dental Hygiene*.)

rather than from systemic intake.[63] This is in contrast to the previous belief that fluoride incorporation in tooth mineral during the development of the teeth was the major caries-inhibiting effect of fluoride.

Generally, a multiple fluoride approach is the most effective in the inhibition of root caries. This approach includes the use of fluoride at home, in the dental office, and in the community. Common fluoride delivery systems include dentifrices, mouth rinses, topical solutions and gels, and communal water supplies. When devising a therapeutic fluoride program for the periodontal patient, the dental hygienist must tailor recommendations to the individual's needs and environment.

Limited clinical data are available on the ability of conventional fluoride systems to prevent and reverse root caries. The benefits of daily, high-concentration fluoride application in solution or gel form have been explored primarily in individuals receiving therapeutic head and neck radiation. Combination fluoride therapy in these severely xerostomic patients consists of a series of professionally applied fluoride solutions or gels and daily home use of a 1.1% sodium fluoride gel or fluoride rinse.[63] This fluoride treatment program is effective in controlling root caries, but may be more than is needed by periodontal maintenance patients.

Water Fluoridation

Fluoride in drinking water reduces dental caries, but is not sufficient to provide complete protection against cariogenic bacteria. The primary mechanism of action of fluoridated water is through topical delivery.[63] Systemic ingestion of fluoride plays a very limited role in caries prevention.

The benefits of fluoride in preventing root caries are well documented in studies of communities with nonfluoridated and fluoridated water supplies. For example, lifelong consumption of optimally fluoridated water effectively decreases the prevalence of root caries in adults. Water fluoridation at five times the optimal level decreased the prevalence of root caries in lifelong adult residents of one community.[64] In addition, exposure to fluoridated water for 30 to 40 years reduced the incidence of root caries in the older adult population.[65] Clearly,

community water fluoride levels are an important consideration in the prevention of root caries.

> **CLINICAL NOTE 17-14** When considering all the potential sources of fluoride for an individual patient, it is important to ask about bottled water use because most bottled water is not fluoridated. Patients consuming primarily bottled water do not receive the same topical benefit of community fluoridation as those who consume tap water on a regular basis.

Fluoride Rinses

Little controlled clinical research has been done on the use of home fluoride rinses by individuals at risk for root caries. One clinical trial evaluated the effect of a daily fluoride rinse on root caries in an unsupervised home fluoride program.[66] After 3 years of use of a 0.05% sodium fluoride rinse, a 16% decline in the incidence of root caries in older adults was observed.[67] The rationale for unsupervised home use of fluoride rinses is based on self-application of high-frequency, low-concentration or low-frequency/high-concentration fluoride agents to prevent the development of root caries and arrest the progression of existing lesions. The fluoride rinses currently approved for use are 0.2% sodium fluoride used once per week, 0.05% sodium fluoride used daily, and 0.2% acidulated phosphate fluoride used daily.[61] These fluoride rinses can be obtained either over the counter or by prescription, depending on the fluoride content. The regular use of daily fluoride rinses is frequently recommended by dental practitioners for all patients undergoing periodontal maintenance because of the anticaries potential of this treatment.

Fluoride Solutions and Gels

High-concentration topical fluoride solutions and gels can be useful adjuncts to a caries prevention program. They are available in both professionally applied and self-applied formulations. However, the cariostatic benefits of these fluoride delivery systems for the periodontal population is not well established. The clinical data to support the efficacy of topical fluoride solutions or gels in the prevention of root caries are found in studies of patients receiving head and neck radiation therapy; both 1.1% sodium fluoride and 0.4% stannous fluoride were found to be effective.[68] Evidence from animal studies is strong and, combined with the limited clinical data, supports the use of fluoride therapy for periodontal patients.

Professional topical fluoride gels and solutions provide concentrated fluoride application at recall appointments. Currently, topical fluoride solutions or gels are approved for use in the United States in three regimens:
- 1.23% acidulated phosphate fluoride
- 2% neutral sodium fluoride
- 8% stannous fluoride

The two most commonly used office fluorides, 1.23% acidulated phosphate fluoride and 2% neutral sodium fluoride, in solution or gel form, can be applied at maintenance visits. It is recommended that the fluoride be applied directly to the teeth for 4 minutes using cotton pellets or a gel and tray system. Animal studies have shown that periodic application of each

TABLE 17-9 Fluoride Use for Periodontal Patients

	METHOD OF ACTION	STRENGTH	APPLICATION
PATIENTS WITH HIGH RISK FOR CARIES			
Office-based use: High concentration, prescription formulations	Strengthen surface mineral	1.23% acidulated phosphate fluoride— 12,300 parts per million (ppm) 2.0% neutral sodium fluoride (9,000 ppm)	Daily gel application for 4 min; may also be swabbed
Additive to office-based therapy: Home use—lower concentration, prescription or over-the-counter formulations	Strengthen surface mineral	1.1% neutral sodium fluoride—5,000 ppm 0.4% stannous fluoride—1,000 ppm (remineralization function)	Daily brush-on or tray application for 4 min
PATIENTS WITH LOW RISK FOR CARIES			
Home use: Over-the-counter preparations			
Fluoride dentifrice	Remineralization	0.24% neutral sodium fluoride—1,100 ppm or 0.76% monofluorophosphate—1,100 ppm	For use with normal toothbrushing once or twice per day
Fluoride rinses	Remineralization	0.05% neutral sodium fluoride—250 ppm	Rinse for 1 min and expectorate; ideally, before bed and after regular plaque control routine

form of fluoride, including a 0.4% stannous fluoride formulation with 0.3% acidulated phosphate fluoride, is effective in reducing root caries. However, a significantly greater decrease was observed with the 2% sodium fluoride and 1.23% acidulated phosphate fluoride systems.[68] This observation suggests that standard office-applied gel and tray systems may be best used for in-office programs. Table 17-9 provides an overview of fluoride products.

Daily topical fluoride application at home provides additional protection for high-risk patients against the development of root caries. The following are three gel formulations commonly available:

- 0.5% acidulated phosphate fluoride
- 1.1% sodium fluoride
- 0.4% stannous fluoride

After thorough plaque biofilm removal by the patient, the fluoride gel is applied daily, either by direct brushing onto the tooth surface for 1 minute or with the use of disposable or custom-made trays for 4 minutes.

Fluoride Dentifrices

A wealth of research since 1945 has supported the ability of fluoride in dentifrices to control dental caries in children and adolescents. Over the past 20 years, the prevalence of dental caries in children in the United States has declined partly because of the almost universal use of fluoride dentifrice. Fluoride-containing dentifrices currently accepted for use by the American Dental Association consist of either a 0.24% sodium fluoride or 0.76% sodium monofluorophosphate formulation. Recommendations for the use of fluoride dentifrices by patients who are at moderate to high risk for caries entail brushing once or more per day with a fluoride-containing toothpaste.[69]

Less is known about the specific value of fluoride dentifrices in the prevention of root caries in adults. One longitudinal study of noninstitutionalized adults compared a 0.24% sodium fluoride dentifrice with a placebo in the prevention of root caries. After 1 year, the data showed a significant decline in the incidence of both coronal and root caries in the group that used fluoride-containing toothpaste.[70] Another study found that a sodium fluoride dentifrice reduced root caries by more than 65%.[61]

In summary, the anticaries activity of fluoride is well documented in both laboratory and clinical studies. Despite a lack of clinical research to outline clearly a fluoride therapy program for the periodontal maintenance population at risk for root caries, evidence supports the use of combination fluoride therapies to inhibit the development of dental caries. The dental hygienist must tailor fluoride therapy to the needs and abilities of the patient. All maintenance patients should use fluoride toothpaste in combination with other office- and home-applied agents prescribed according to susceptibility and caries incidence. Also, along with fluoride considerations, the patient's individual oral hygiene status and diet must be considered.

ORAL HYGIENE

Overwhelming evidence shows that oral microorganisms are one of the primary etiologic agents for all dental caries, although the specific bacteria present may vary among the types of carious lesions.[60] The amount of cariogenic bacteria associated with root caries can be minimized through meticulous personal plaque biofilm control.

DIET MODIFICATION

Diet plays a major role in the development of dental caries. For example, a sucrose-rich diet highly favors caries formation. Dietary carbohydrates such as glucose, sucrose, fructose, or cooked starch provide the substrate for cariogenic bacteria to produce organic acids. These acids promote demineralization of the tooth structure. Nutritional analysis to evaluate dietary habits and recommendations for diet modification are essential elements of prevention education for caries-prone individuals. The dietary recommendations for periodontal patients described here apply to all individuals and represent a strategy for reducing the risk for dental caries.

BOX 17-6 Nutritional Counseling for the Periodontal Patient

1. Recommend eating a healthy balanced diet, including a variety of foods.
2. Advise avoiding caries-producing foods, snacks, and beverages (i.e., foods with a high sucrose content).
3. Encourage limiting consumption of sucrose-containing foods to mealtime and restricting between meal snacks.
4. Suggest a list of foods and beverages to include and avoid in the diet.
   • Include fresh fruits and vegetables and noncardiogenic sweeteners.
   • Avoid candy, sugar-containing sodas, and dried fruits.
5. Develop a personalized meal plan tailored to the patient's lifestyle, financial resources, cultural preferences, and religious customs.

The dental hygienist plays a major role in assessing the dietary habits of patients who are at risk for dental caries and can provide suggestions for less cariogenic foods and beverages. In addition to providing nutrition education and counseling, the dental hygienist can motivate and encourage patients to maintain a balanced diet to promote their overall oral and systemic health. Patients must accept responsibility for modifying their dietary habits and must be committed to the caries prevention program.

Nutritional Counseling

Effective techniques to assess a patient's dietary habits include a 24-hour recall or a detailed food diary. Together, the dental hygienist and patient can evaluate the diet history and set nutritional goals. Simple, well-defined, and concise nutritional guidelines should be tailored to each patient's needs, as suggested in Box 17-6. Except for the restriction of a few foods and eating practices, a caries-prevention diet is based on the same recommendations as those for a healthy balanced diet.[71] Thus, the goal is to obtain all the necessary nutrients to maintain health and resistance to disease. Patients can help identify substitutes that are appealing and satisfying. They will be more receptive to diet modifications if they understand the role of diet in oral health and if they actively participate in diet planning. Continued evaluation, modification, and positive reinforcement of the patient's dietary habits during the maintenance phase may enhance patient acceptance of and compliance with the personalized dietary program and contribute to overall health.

DENTIN SENSITIVITY IN THE PERIODONTAL MAINTENANCE POPULATION

Understanding the theories, causes, and management of dentin sensitivity is important for every dental hygienist because this condition is such a common occurrence in periodontal patients. Dentin sensitivity is characterized by sharp intermittent pain of short duration or by dull chronic pain. It can affect any number of teeth, and its occurrence is difficult to predict on susceptible surfaces. Pain is caused by various stimuli, such as cold, heat, sweet or sour foods, oral hygiene practices, or dental instruments. It is estimated that one in seven adult patients has

dentinal sensitivity and that nearly 40 million Americans experience sensitivity at some point.[72]

The terms *dentin sensitivity* and *dentin hypersensitivity* are often used interchangeably to describe the pain evoked on stimulation of exposed dentinal surfaces. Technically, the term *sensitivity* simply denotes a normal response to stimulation of newly exposed dentin, whereas *hypersensitivity* refers to excessive sensitivity. *Dentin sensitivity*[73] or *dentin hypersensitivity*[74] are the terms used for describing the response to thermal and other stimuli affecting exposed dentin in periodontal patients.

THEORIES OF DENTINAL PAIN TRANSMISSION

The hydrodynamic theory is the most commonly accepted explanation of sensitivity of the dentinal surface to external stimuli.[75] Stimulation of open dentinal tubules at the root surface causes fluid movement within the tubules. This movement transmits a signal to the nerves in the pulp chamber, resulting in pain. Closing off the exposed dentinal tubules prevents fluid movement and inhibits pain transmission. This principle is the basis of treatments used today for relieving dentinal sensitivity.

FACTORS CONTRIBUTING TO THE DEVELOPMENT OF DENTIN SENSITIVITY

Mechanical, chemical, thermal, or bacterial stimuli can cause tooth pain. Common mechanical causes are toothbrushing, touching with fingers or other objects, and drying. Chemical stimuli are usually acidic or sweet substances. Patients occasionally report dentin sensitivity with the use of tartar control toothpastes containing pyrophosphates. Acids from bacterial plaque biofilm can cause pain and periodontal patients commonly report that hot and cold stimuli induce pain.[74]

Exposure of the root surfaces or loss of enamel is necessary for dentin sensitivity to occur. Periodontal maintenance patients commonly have exposed root surfaces because of histories of periodontal attachment loss, often as a result of periodontal treatment. Research has shown a direct relationship between an increased incidence of sensitivity and the extent of root surface exposure in patients after periodontal surgery. However, not all exposed dentin is painful or the result of periodontal treatment. Gingival recession is observed in normal aging, with malpositioned teeth, and as a result of improper toothbrushing techniques. Whatever the cause, various factors affect the nature of sensitivity, including patient age, the rate of exposure, and the effect of naturally occurring or environmental desensitizing mechanisms. Some patients with very little gingival recession complain of sensitivity, whereas others with major recession have no pain.

Often, scaling and root planing elicits dentin sensitivity. This effect is not surprising because scaling and root planing removes cementum covering the root surface, exposing the dentinal tubules. Pain may not occur immediately because a smear layer of microcrystalline debris initially covers the dentinal surface. However, after approximately 7 days, the smear layer dissolves and sensitivity can occur.[75] Periodontal surgery also often exposes the dentinal tubules, leading to sensitivity.

Individuals vary in the extent and resolution of dentin sensitivity after periodontal treatment. Toothbrushing habits, intake of acidic foods, and rate of plaque biofilm development all affect sensitivity. Fortunately, sensitivity resulting from scaling and root planing most often decreases about 2 weeks after treatment. Spontaneous remission of sensitivity is thought to occur 20% to 45% of the time without therapeutic measures.[76] Theories about the decrease in sensitivity include possible occlusion of the dentinal tubules by newly formed calculus, formation of reparative dentin within the pulp chamber of the tooth, and precipitation of intratubular crystals from salivary minerals.[74,75]

MANAGEMENT OF DENTIN SENSITIVITY

Patients undergoing periodontal maintenance often experience pain when eating or drinking hot or cold foods and when dental instruments are applied to the root surfaces. The dental hygienist must respond to these needs, explain the condition, and provide a therapeutic regimen. In addition, it is important to minimize patient discomfort during maintenance visits by avoiding unnecessary instrumentation or drying of sensitive surfaces.

Desensitizing agents are categorized into two types, chemical and physical, and are available for home use or in-office application, as described in Table 17-10. Generally, these treatments provide some reduction of sensitivity, but results vary in degree of pain relief and duration of results. In-office therapy to treat dentinal sensitivity is successful in 20% to 40% of hypersensitive teeth and results are usually seen within 4 to 8 weeks.[74]

Plaque Biofilm Control

A simple, important, but often overlooked method to reduce sensitivity is improving daily plaque biofilm control. Bacterial plaque biofilm is commonly observed in areas that are sensitive because of periodontal surgery. Patients with poor plaque biofilm control have more sensitivity[77] and are often reluctant

TABLE 17-10 Chemical and Physical Agents Used to Treat Dentin Sensitivity

MODE OF ACTION	AGENTS
CHEMICAL	
Antiinflammatory	Corticosteroids
Protein-precipitating	Silver nitrate, zinc chloride, strontium chloride, formaldehyde
Tubule-occluding	Calcium hydroxide, potassium nitrate, fluorides, sodium citrate, iontophoresis with 2% sodium fluoride, potassium oxalate
PHYSICAL	
Tubule-sealing	Composites, resins, varnishes, sealants, glass ionomer cements, laser sealing of tubules
Physical protection	Soft tissue grafts

(Modified from Scherman A, Jacobsen PL. Managing dentin hypersensitivity: what treatment to recommend to patients. *J Am Dent Assoc.* 1992;123:59. Copyright 1992 American Dental Association. All rights reserved. Adapted 2006 with permission.)

to clean sensitive areas thoroughly. The dental hygienist can educate the patient about bacterial plaque biofilm acids and their contribution to sensitivity and reinforce the importance of meticulous daily oral hygiene.

Chemical Desensitizing Agents

Common therapeutic measures for treating hypersensitive dentin are the use of specific toothpastes, gels, or rinses at home and the application of chemical agents in the dental office. Home remedies and office treatments can provide effective combination therapy to relieve or reduce the condition. On the basis of their mode of action, chemical agents are classified into four categories:

- Antiinflammatory agents
- Protein-precipitating agents
- Tubule-occluding agents
- Tubule sealants

Home Use Agents. The use of a desensitizing dentifrice is the easiest first step in managing dentin sensitivity. Several toothpastes are available that are simple to use and noninvasive. These agents promote compliance because almost everyone brushes their teeth. Potassium nitrate, strontium chloride, and sodium citrate are the active ingredients in desensitizing dentifrice formulations. The low concentration of these desensitizing agents allows for dispensation without a prescription. Studies have shown that potassium nitrate and potassium oxalate are effective in reducing the pain of dentin sensitivity within 4 to 6 weeks.[76] Products that combine desensitizing agents with fluoride are preferred because they provide both desensitizing action and caries control.

Fluoride preparations are also used for home treatment of dentin sensitivity but with varying effects. Unfortunately, they do not seem to have long-term effects.

No clinical studies have compared fluoride compounds, so the best therapeutic agent for the treatment of dentin sensitivity is largely a matter of personal preference. It is important to recommend home use of fluoride agents and desensitizing toothpastes to provide patients with both pain relief and caries prevention.

Office Therapies. Professional application of high-concentration fluoride products is a common remedy for dentin sensitivity in the dental office. After the sensitive tooth is isolated, a 2% sodium fluoride paste can be massaged into the exposed surface with a wooden applicator or cotton swab.[52] A kaolin- and glycerin-based 33.3% fluoride paste has also been used in this manner.

For in-office desensitizing materials, 3% potassium oxalate and ferric oxalate have been found to be effective.[76] Either can provide immediate relief, but the relief is likely to last only a few days. Application is simple; the area is dried with cotton swabs and the compound is applied for 2 minutes.

Physical Desensitizing Agents

If chemical desensitizing agents do not provide relief, physical techniques, such as application of dentin bonding agents, including composite resins, varnishes, sealants, glass ionomer cements, and soft tissue grafts, can be used.[74] These procedures seal or cover the dentinal tubules. Composite resin with a glass ionomer liner is also used to cover exposed root surfaces.

TREATMENT RECOMMENDATIONS

The management of dentin sensitivity can seem daunting because of the many desensitizing treatments available and their variable efficacy. In addition, dentin sensitivity often improves with the passage of time. A recommended treatment plan to reduce dentin sensitivity is described in Table 17-11. Treatment begins with a complete examination to exclude other possible sources of pain.[52] Patient education and good home care are major steps in the control of sensitivity because bacterial

TABLE 17-11 Treatment Recommendations for Dentin Sensitivity

STEP	RATIONALE
1. Perform thorough assessment and evaluate cause.	Other sources of pain should be eliminated.
2. Explain problem and causes.	Informing the patient of the causes of sensitivity provides reassurance that the problem usually improves.
3. Reinforce proper and effective oral hygiene techniques to eliminate bacterial plaque biofilm.	Correction of easily preventable causes may eliminate discomfort and prevent root caries and periodontal disease progression.
4. Provide dietary advice and counseling.	Diet modification may decrease onset of sensitivity.
5. Recommend daily use of desensitizing toothpaste (2- to 6-week trial).	This is a simple and generally effective form of therapy.
6. Provide in-office application of oxalate or fluoride products (2- to 10-week trial).	In-office therapy may provide immediate pain relief to be complemented by home therapy.
7. Recommend physical therapeutic agents and refer patient to dentist for treatment.	Sealing or covering dentinal tubules can be useful if other therapies do not relieve pain.

(From Scherman A, Jacobsen PL. Managing dentin hypersensitivity: what treatment to recommend to patients. *J Am Dent Assoc.* 1992;123:60.)

plaque biofilm is a known cause. Dietary counseling may be helpful if patients consume large quantities of acidic or sugary foods and beverages. Foods to be avoided or used in moderation include citrus fruit juices, apple juice, wine, and ciders.[74]

Treatment should begin with a conservative approach to pain relief. Daily use of desensitizing toothpaste by the patient and in-office treatment with potassium oxalate or fluoride are the first steps in the treatment of dentinal sensitivity. If the discomfort persists after 2 to 6 weeks, other products should be tried. If these are not effective after several weeks, the dentist can place physical agents, such as a composite resin with a glass ionomer base. The dental hygienist must recognize that a favorite desensitizing agent may not work on everyone, so trying different agents may be helpful for nonresponding patients.

Patient education is an important part of the successful treatment of dentin sensitivity. At the beginning of periodontal therapy, the patient should be advised of the risk of sensitivity and the availability of treatments. Patients who are warned about this problem will not be surprised when sensitivity develops and may be more willing to accept treatment alternatives.

ROLE OF THE DENTAL HYGIENIST IN PERIODONTAL MAINTENANCE

The prevalence of periodontal disease is well documented in epidemiologic studies of the U.S. dentate population (see Chapter 3). With the aging population and people keeping their teeth longer, treatment of periodontal disease has become increasingly important to dental hygienists, dentists, and the general public. Periodontal health is greatly dependent on routine professional care, so the demand for preventive and therapeutic periodontal services is likely to increase. The dental hygienist is the primary provider of periodontal maintenance care to the public, and this role is critical in the long-term success of therapy.

The contemporary role of the dental hygienist in periodontal and maintenance therapy has been described as a periodontal co-therapist with both the dentist and the patient. This interrelationship is depicted in Figure 17-7. In collaboration with

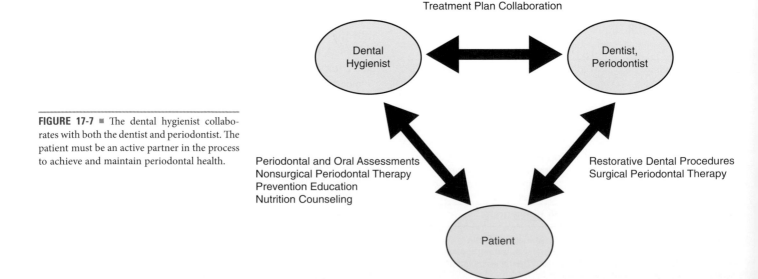

FIGURE 17-7 ■ The dental hygienist collaborates with both the dentist and periodontist. The patient must be an active partner in the process to achieve and maintain periodontal health.

the dentist, the dental hygienist has the goal of providing the highest quality oral health care in a single collaborative approach. The dental hygienist also functions as a co-therapist with the patient, providing the knowledge, skills, and support necessary to achieve successful long-term oral health for the individual.

The patient must be an active partner with the dental hygienist to achieve and maintain periodontal health. The dental hygienist must be an effective communicator and an attentive and careful listener. Patients recognize the dental hygienist's commitment to provide the highest quality care and build trust and confidence in the partnership. Patients will then work with the dental hygienist to take responsibility for their own oral health. The role of the dental hygienist is a broad one that combines outstanding clinical skills, collaboration with other health professionals, and being an educator and partner with the patient to achieve periodontal health.

SIGNIFICANCE OF PERIODONTAL MAINTENANCE

The vital role of periodontal maintenance in preserving periodontal health and the prevention of new or recurrent disease after active therapy is indisputable. Clinical evidence confirms the efficacy of frequent monitoring and maintenance care to achieve the goal of a healthy dentition for a lifetime. This goal is the ultimate measure of success for periodontal patients. To achieve this success, a collaborative effort between patient, dental hygienist, dentist, and periodontist is mandatory. Without a firm commitment from each, maintenance of optimal oral health is far more difficult. An example of successful periodontal maintenance care is presented in Figure 17-8.

The effectiveness of maintenance therapy is dependent on patient compliance. Adherence to both professional and personal plaque biofilm control recommendations is essential for a successful outcome. If the importance of continued maintenance therapy and daily home care is recognized and reinforced, patients are more likely to understand and accept their crucial role in maintaining their own periodontal health.

A well-defined and well-executed maintenance protocol is the foundation of an effective long-term periodontal maintenance program. The components are as follows:

- Compliance
- Assessment
- Prevention
- Treatment

Patients must comply with recommended visit schedules. In general, most periodontal patients benefit from a 3-month maintenance interval, although more frequent visits are sometimes necessary; individual assessment of the appropriate maintenance interval is critical.

Reinforcement of the patient's oral hygiene practices is an indispensable component because plaque biofilm is well

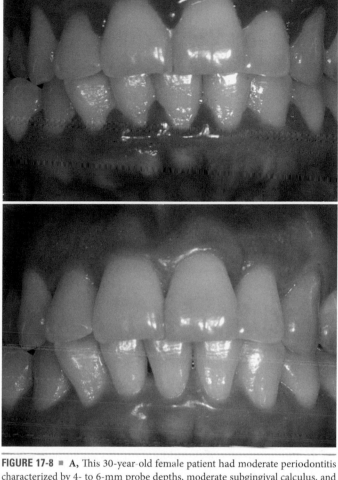

FIGURE 17-8 ■ **A,** This 30-year-old female patient had moderate periodontitis characterized by 4- to 6-mm probe depths, moderate subgingival calculus, and extensive gingival inflammation with recession and heavy accumulation of plaque biofilm and calculus. After nonsurgical therapy, the patient was maintained on 3-month recall intervals. **B,** Patient's appearance after 2 years of periodontal maintenance. The periodontal pocketing has resolved and the patient maintains excellent plaque biofilm control. Note the healthy appearance of the gingiva. (Courtesy of Dr. Gary C. Armitage, University of California, San Francisco, School of Dentistry, Division of Periodontology.)

established as the cause of periodontal disease. Periodic supervised care permits early detection and treatment of new or recurrent disease. Each periodontal maintenance visit also provides the opportunity to motivate patients and prevent and treat complications, such as dentin hypersensitivity and root caries. Finally, thorough debridement of the entire dentition is necessary to eliminate all bacterial accumulations and calculus deposits to create a healthy oral environment. These elements, as part of a periodontal maintenance program, lead to good oral health for the patient and provide a sense of satisfaction and reward for the dental hygienist.

DENTAL HYGIENE CONSIDERATIONS

- Periodontal therapy is effective in restoring the health and function of the teeth only in conjunction with a regular maintenance program.
- The objectives of periodontal maintenance are preservation of clinical attachment, maintenance of alveolar bone height, control of inflammation, evaluation and reinforcement of daily oral hygiene procedures, and maintenance of optimal oral health.
- Compliance is defined as adopting recommended home care procedures and returning for regular dental hygiene maintenance visits.
- The maintenance appointment consists of review of the medical and dental history, thorough examination of the oral soft tissues and teeth, radiographic assessment, plaque biofilm control evaluation, oral hygiene instruction, periodontal instrumentation, caries prevention, hypersensitivity control, and establishment of the next recall appointment.
- Recall intervals must be individualized but are usually every 2 to 4 months.
- Recurrent periodontitis is common, emphasizing the significance of maintenance care.
- Periodontal patients are at risk for root caries and must be provided appropriate fluoride therapy, oral hygiene instruction, and diet recommendations of proper foods and frequency of ingestion.
- Dentin hypersensitivity is often a problem for periodontal maintenance patients and can be addressed by using appropriate in-office and home desensitizing agents.
- Appropriate maintenance care is crucial to the long-term success of periodontal therapy.

★ CASE SCENARIO

Mrs. Rachliff completed her treatment plan with the periodontist for four quadrants of periodontal surgery and is now seeing you for maintenance care. She had flap surgery with osseous recontouring in the posterior areas and papilla preservation procedures in the anterior. All of her surgical treatment was completed 4 weeks ago, and she is very happy with the aesthetic result. She has 2- to 3-mm probing depths in the posterior sextants with 4 mm of recession and residual probing depths of 3 to 5 mm in the anterior with no recession. Mrs. Rachliff wants to know why it is harder to clean her teeth now, if the results of the treatment will last, why her teeth are sensitive, and how often she will need to come in for maintenance care.

1. Periodontal surgery often causes some increases in attachment loss, leading to exposed root surfaces. Exposure of complex root anatomy on teeth makes it harder for patients to remove plaque biofilm.
   A. Both statements are true.
   B. Both statements are false.
   C. The first statement is true, and the second statement is false.
   D. The first statement is false, and the second statement is true.

2. Periodontal therapy is most successful when patients return
   A. annually for maintenance appointments.
   B. annually for maintenance appointments and adopt recommended home care routines.
   C. at a customized interval based on your assessments for maintenance appointments.
   D. at a customized interval based on your assessments for maintenance appointments and adopt recommended home care routines.

3. Dentin hypersensitivity is often seen after periodontal surgery because newly exposed root surfaces may have exposed patent dentinal tubules that react to heat, cold, and tactile stimulation.
   A. Both the statement and reason are correct and related.
   B. Both the statement and reason are correct but NOT related.
   C. The statement is correct, but the reason is NOT correct.
   D. The statement is NOT correct, but the reason is correct.
   E. NEITHER the statement NOR the reason is correct.

4. Maintenance therapy requires careful assessments, including periodontal pocket probing. Probing should only be performed on maintenance patients 2 weeks after surgery is completed and the maintenance phase is begun.
   A. Both statements are true.
   B. Both statements are false.
   C. The first statement is true, and the second statement is false.
   D. The first statement is false, and the second statement is true.

STUDY QUESTIONS

Answers and rationales to these questions can be obtained from your instructor.

MULTIPLE CHOICE

1. The best indicator for establishing an appropriate maintenance interval for a periodontal patient is
   A. slowed progression of attachment loss.
   B. compliance with the prescribed interval.
   C. lack of clinical signs of inflammation on examination.
   D. evidence of improved personal plaque biofilm control.

2. The effectiveness of maintenance therapy is supported by evidence indicating that
   A. a regular maintenance program is not needed to ensure long-term success.
   B. maintenance therapy will decrease disease progression, but prevention of tooth loss is more uncertain.
   C. untreated periodontal disease progresses, with a continual loss of periodontal attachment over time.
   D. supragingival plaque biofilm control alone can improve probing depths and clinical attachment in patients with periodontitis.

3. The most predictable measurement of increasing clinical attachment loss in maintenance patients is
   A. bleeding on probing.
   B. increased probing depths.
   C. higher plaque biofilm scores.
   D. decreased alveolar bone height.
   E. increased amounts of suppuration.

4. Personal oral hygiene procedures should be instituted and reinforced at each periodontal maintenance appointment. For the best results, each oral hygiene aid with potential to assist the patient should be demonstrated and recommended for adoption.
   A. Both statements are true.
   B. Both statements are false.
   C. The first statement is true, and the second statement is false.
   D. The first statement is false, and the second statement is true.

5. Periodontal patients are at risk for root caries because the loss of clinical attachment results in susceptible root surfaces.
   A. Both the statement and reason are correct and related.
   B. Both the statement and reason are correct but NOT related.
   C. The statement is correct, but the reason is NOT correct.
   D. The statement is NOT correct, but the reason is correct.
   E. NEITHER the statement NOR the reason is correct.

6. All of the following medications can cause xerostomia EXCEPT one. Which one is the EXCEPTION?
   A. Antidepressants
   B. Antifungals
   C. Antihypertensives
   D. Antipsychotics
   E. Antiinflammatories

7. The first periodontal maintenance appointment after surgery should occur within
   A. 24 to 48 hours.
   B. 2 to 4 days.
   C. 2 to 4 weeks.
   D. 2 to 4 months.

8. Fluoride rinses are not recommended for the periodontal maintenance patient because systemic water fluoridation is more effective for root caries.
   A. Both the statement and reason are correct and related.
   B. Both the statement and reason are correct but NOT related.
   C. The statement is correct, but the reason is NOT correct.
   D. The statement is NOT correct, but the reason is correct.
   E. NEITHER the statement NOR the reason is correct.

SHORT ANSWER

9. What are the five objectives of periodontal maintenance?
10. Why does scaling and root planing sometimes result in root surface sensitivity?

Please visit http://evolve.elsevier.com/Perry/periodontology for additional practice and study support tools.

REFERENCES

1. American Academy of Periodontology. *Glossary of Periodontal Terms.* 4th ed. Chicago, IL: American Academy of Periodontology; 2001:39–42.
2. McGuire MK. Prognosis versus actual outcome: a long-term survey of 100 treated periodontal patients under maintenance care. *J Periodontal.* 1991;62:51–58.
3. Löe H, Morrison E. Epidemiology of periodontal disease. In: Genco RJ, Goldman HM, Cohen DW, eds. *Contemporary Periodontics.* St. Louis, MO: CV Mosby; 1990:106–116.
4. Löe H, Theilade E, Jensen SB. Experimental gingivitis in man. *J Periodontol.* 1965;36:177–187.
5. Theilade E, Wright WH, Jensen SB, et al. Experimental gingivitis in man. II. A longitudinal clinical and bacterial investigation. *J Periodontal Res.* 1966;1:1–13.
6. Greenstein G. Periodontal response to mechanical non-surgical therapy: a review. *J Periodontol.* 1992;63:118–130.
7. Slots J, Mashimo P, Levine MJ, et al. Periodontal therapy in humans. I. Microbiological and clinical effects of a single course of periodontal scaling and root planing, and of adjunctive tetracycline therapy. *J Periodontol.* 1979;50:495–509.
8. Morrison EC, Ramfjord SP, Hill RW. Short-term effects of initial, non-surgical periodontal treatment (hygienic phase). *J Periodontol.* 1980;7:199–211.
9. Badersten A, Nilveus R, Egelberg J. Effect of non-surgical periodontal therapy. I. Moderately advanced periodontitis. *J Clin Periodontol.* 1981;8:57–72.
10. Badersten A, Nilveus R, Egelberg J. Effect of non-surgical periodontal therapy. II. Severely advanced periodontitis. *J Clin Periodontol.* 1984;11:63–76.
11. Kalkwarf KL, Kaldahl WB, Paul KD, et al. Evaluation of gingival bleeding following 4 types of periodontal therapy. *J Clin Periodontol.* 1989;16:601–608.
12. Kaldahl WB, Kalkwarf KL, Patil KD, et al. Evaluation of gingival suppuration and supragingival plaque biofilm following 4 modalities of periodontal therapy. *J Clin Periodontol.* 1990;17:642–649.
13. American Academy of Periodontology. *Proceedings of the World Workshop in Clinical Periodontics.* Chicago, IL: American Academy of Periodontology; 1989:1–11, 21.
14. Axelsson P, Lindhe J. Effect of controlled oral hygiene procedures on caries and periodontal disease in adults. *J Clin Periodontol.* 1978;5:133–151.
15. Axelsson P, Lindhe J. Effect of controlled oral hygiene procedures on caries and periodontal disease in adults: results after 6 years. *J Clin Periodontol.* 1981;8:239–248.
16. Axelsson P, Lindhe J, Nystrom B. On the prevention of caries and periodontal disease: results of a 15-year longitudinal study in adults. *J Clin Periodontol.* 1991;18:182–189.
17. Merin RL. Results of periodontal treatment. In: Newman MG, Takei HH, Klokkevold PR, et al, eds. *Carranza's Clinical Periodontology.* 11th ed. St. Louis, MO: Elsevier Saunders; 2012:746–755.
18. Wilson TG, Glover ME, Malik AK, et al. Tooth loss in maintenance patients in a private periodontal practice. *J Periodontol.* 1987;58:231–235.
19. Löe H, Anerud A, Boysen H, et al. The natural history of periodontal disease in man: rapid, moderate and no loss of attachment in Sri Lankan laborers 15 to 45 years of age. *J Clin Periodontol.* 1986;13:431–440.
20. Philstrom BL, McHugh RB, Oliphant TH. Molar and nonmolar teeth compared over 6 1/2 years following two methods of periodontal therapy. *J Periodontol.* 1984;55:499–504.
21. Becker W, Becker BE, Berg LE. Long-term evaluation of periodontal treatment and maintenance in 95 patients. *Int J Periodont Restorative Dent.* 1984;4:54–71.
22. Caffesse RG. Maintenance therapy: preventing recurrence of periodontal diseases. In: Genco RJ, Goldman HM, Cohen DW, eds. *Contemporary Periodontics.* St. Louis, MO: CV Mosby; 1990:483–492.
23. Badersten A, Nilveus R, Egelberg J. Scores of plaque biofilm, bleeding, suppuration and probing depth to predict probing attachment loss: 5 years of observation following nonsurgical periodontal therapy. *J Clin Periodontol.* 1990;17:102–107.
24. Hicks MJ, Uldricks JM, Whitacre HL, et al. A national study of periodontal assessment by dental hygienists. *J Dent Hyg.* 1993;67:82–92.

25. Dahlén G, Lindhe J, Sato K, et al. The effect of supragingival plaque biofilm control on the subgingival microbiota in subjects with periodontal disease. *J Clin Periodontol.* 1992;19:802–809.

26. Lindhe J, Socransky S, Nyman S, et al. Critical probing depths in periodontal therapy. *J Clin Periodontol.* 1982;9:323–336.

27. Greenwell H, Bissada NF, Wittwer JW. Periodontics in general practice: professional plaque biofilm control. *J Am Dent Assoc.* 1990;121:642–646.

28. Axelsson P, Lindhe J. The significance of maintenance care in the treatment of periodontal disease. *J Clin Periodontol.* 1981;8:281–294.

29. Schmidt J, Morrison E, Kerry G, et al. Patient compliance with suggested maintenance recall in a private periodontal practice. *J Periodontol.* 1990;61:316–317.

30. Wilson T, Glover M, Schoen J, et al. Compliance with maintenance therapy in a private periodontal practice. *J Periodontol.* 1984;55:468–473.

31. Knowles JW, Burgett FG, Nissle RR, et al. Results of periodontal treatment related to pocket depth and attachment level: eight years. *J Periodontol.* 1979;50:225–233.

32. Wilson TG. Compliance: a review of the literature with possible applications to periodontics. *J Periodontol.* 1987;58:706–714.

33. Boyer EM, Nikias MK. Self-reported compliance with a preventive dental regimen. *Clin Prev Dent.* 1983;5:3–7.

34. Strack BB, McCullough MA, Conine TA. Compliance with oral hygiene instructions. *Dent Hyg.* 1980;54:181–184.

35. Johansson L, Oster B, Hamp S. Evaluation of cause-related periodontal therapy and compliance with maintenance care recommendations. *J Clin Periodontol.* 1984;11:689–699.

36. Hellstadius K, Asman B, Gustafsson A. Improved maintenance of plaque biofilm control by electrical toothbrushing in periodontitis patients with low compliance. *J Clin Periodontol.* 1993;20:235–237.

37. Heasman PA, Jacobs DJ, Chapple IL. An evaluation of the effectiveness and patient compliance with plaque biofilm control methods in the prevention of periodontal disease. *Clin Prev Dent.* 1989;11:24–28.

38. Kuhner MK, Raetzke PB. The effect of health beliefs on the compliance of periodontal patients with oral hygiene instructions. *J Periodontol.* 1989;60:51–56.

39. Merin RL. Supportive periodontal treatment. In: Newman MG, Takei HH, Klokkevold PR, et al, eds. *Carranza's Clinical Periodontology.* 11th ed. St. Louis, MO: Elsevier Saunders; 2012:746–755.

40. Ramfjord SP. Indices for prevalence and incidence of periodontal disease. *J Periodontol.* 1959;30:51–59.

41. Lang NP, Joss A, Orsanic T, et al. Bleeding on probing: a predictor for the progression of periodontal disease? *J Clin Periodontol.* 1986;13:590–596.

42. Chaves ES, Caffesse RG, Morrison EC, et al. Diagnostic discrimination of bleeding on probing during maintenance periodontal therapy. *Am J Dent.* 1990;3:167–170.

43. Wilkins EM. Periodontal examination procedures. In: Wilkins, EM, ed. *Clinical Practice of the Dental Hygienist.* 11th ed. Baltimore, MD: Lippincott Williams & Wilkins; 2013:223–243.

44. Manson JD, Eley BM. Management of bone defects and furcation involvement. In: Derrick DD, ed. *Outline of Periodontics.* 2nd ed. Cornwall: Butterworth; 1989:189–195.

45. Kennedy JE, Bird WC, Palcanis KG, et al. A longitudinal evaluation of varying widths of attached gingiva. *J Clin Periodontol.* 1985;12:667–675.

46. American Dental Association. Frequently asked questions. (http://www.ada.org/1444.aspx).

47. Gruber, JM. Dental radiographic imaging. In: Wilkins EM, ed. *Clinical Practice of the Dental Hygienist.* 11th ed. Baltimore, MD: Lippincott Williams & Wilkins; 2013:158–192.

48. Grossman E, Reiter G, Sturzenberger OP, et al. Six-month study of the effects of a chlorhexidine mouthrinse on gingivitis in adults. *J Periodont Res.* 1986;21(suppl):33–43.

49. Siegrist BE, Gusberti FA, Brecx MC, et al. Efficacy of supervised rinsing with chlorhexidine digluconate in comparison to phenolic and plant alkaloid compounds. *J Periodont Res.* 1986;21(suppl):60–73.

50. Low SB, Ciancio SG. Reviewing nonsurgical periodontal therapy. *J Am Dent Assoc.* 1990;121:467–470.

51. Barnes CM. Extrinsic stain removal. In: Wilkins, EM, ed. *Clinical Practice of the Dental Hygienist.* 11th ed. Baltimore, MD: Lippincott Williams & Wilkins; 2013:689–708.

52. Trowbridge HO, Silver DR. A review of current approaches to in-office management of tooth sensitivity. *Dent Clin North Am.* 1990;34:561–581.

53. Novak KF, Novak MJ. Aggressive periodontitis. In: Newman MG, Takei HH, Klokkevold PR, et al, eds. *Carranza's Clinical Periodontology.* 11th ed. St. Louis, MO: Elsevier Saunders; 2012:169–173.

54. Schupbach P, Guggenheim B, Lutz F. Histopathology of root surface caries. *J Dent Res.* 1990;69:1195–1204.

55. Syed SA, Loesche WJ, Pape HL, et al. Predominant cultivable flora isolated from human root surface caries plaque biofilm. *Infect Immun.* 1975;11:727–731.

56. Katz RV, Hazen SP, Chilton NW, et al. Prevalence and intraoral distribution of root caries in an adult population. *Caries Res.* 1982;16:265–271.

57. Winn DM, Brunelle JA, Selwitz RH, et al. Coronal and root caries in the dentition of adults in the United States, 1988-91. *J Dent Res.* 1996;75(special issue):642–651.

58. Featherstone JDB, Adair SM, Anderson MH, et al. Caries management by risk assessment: consensus statement, April 2002. *CDA J.* 2003;31:257–269.

59. Regezi JA, Sciubba JJ. Salivary gland diseases. In: *Oral Pathology: Clinical-Pathologic Correlations.* 4th ed. Philadelphia, PA: WB Saunders; 2002:183–217.

60. Beck JD, Kohout F, Hunt RJ. Identification of high caries risk adults: attitudes, social factors and diseases. *Int Dent J.* 1988;38:231–238.

61. Jensen ME, Kohout, F. Effect of fluoridated dentifrices on root and coronal caries in an older adult population. *J Am Dent Assoc.* 1998;117:829–832.

62. Wilkins EM. Protocols for prevention and control of dental caries. In: Wilkins EM, ed. *Clinical Practice of the Dental Hygienist.* 11th ed. Baltimore, MD: Lippincott Williams & Wilkins; 2013:377–385.

63. Featherstone JDB. Prevention and reversal of dental caries: role of low level fluoride. *Commun Dent Oral Epidemiol.* 1999;27:31–40.

64. Stamm JW, Banting DW. Comparison of root caries prevalence in adults with life-long residence in fluoridated and non-fluoridated communities [abstract 552]. *J Dent Res.* 1980;59(special issue A):405.

65. Burt BA, Ismail AI, Eklund SA. Root caries in an optimally fluoridated and a high-fluoride community. *J Dent Res.* 1986;65:1154–1158.

66. Leske G, Ripa L, Forte F, et al. Clinical trial of the effectiveness of daily sodium fluoride administration on root caries [abstract 469]. *J Dent Res.* 1988;67(special issue):171.

67. Hunt RJ, Eldredge JB, Beck JD. Effect of residence in a fluoridated community on the incidence of coronal and root caries in an older adult population. *J Public Health Dent.* 1989;49:138–141.

68. Stookey GK, Rodlun CA, Warrick JM, et al. Professional topical fluoride systems vs. root caries in hamsters [abstract 1521]. *J Dent Res.* 1989;68:372.

69. Mattana DJ. Fluorides. In: Wilkins EM, ed. *Clinical Practice of the Dental Hygienist.* 11th ed. Baltimore, MD: Lippincott Williams & Wilkins; 2013:517–541.

70. Jensen ME, Kohout F. The effect of a fluoridated dentifrice on root and coronal caries in an older adult population. *J Am Dent Assoc.* 1988;117:829–832.

71. Wilkins EM. Diet and dietary analysis. In: Wilkins EM, ed. *Clinical Practice of the Dental Hygienist.* 11th ed. Baltimore, MD: Lippincott Williams & Wilkins; 2013:496–516.

72. Graf H, Galasse R. Morbidity, prevalence and intraoral distribution of hypersensitive teeth [abstract 162]. *J Dent Res.* 1977;56(suppl):A89.

73. Klokkevold PR, Takei HH, Carranza FA. General principles of periodontal surgery. In: Newman MG, Takei HH, Klokkevold PR, et al, eds. *Carranza's Clinical Periodontology.* 11th ed. St. Louis, MO: Elsevier Saunders; 2012:525–534.

74. Tilliss TI, Keanting JG. Dentin hypersensitivity. In: Wilkins EM, ed. *Clinical Practice of the Dental Hygienist.* 11th ed. Baltimore, MD: Lippincott Williams & Wilkins; 2013:647–688.

75. Brännstrom M. A hydrodynamic mechanism in the transmission of pain producing stimuli through dentin. In: Andersson DJ, ed. *Sensory Mechanisms in Dentine.* Vol 1. London: Pergamon Press; 1963:73–79.

76. Pillon FL, Romani IG, Schmidt ER. Effect of 3% potassium oxalate topical application on dentinal sensitivity after subgingival scaling and root planing. *J Periodontol.* 2004;75:1461–1464.

77. Fischer C, Wennberg A, Fischer RG, et al. Clinical evaluation of pulp and dentine sensitivity after supragingival and subgingival scaling. *Endodont Dent Traumatol.* 1991;7:259–265.

18

Prognosis and Results After Periodontal Therapy

Dorothy A. Perry and Phyllis L. Beemsterboer

LEARNING OUTCOMES

- Define prognosis.
- Describe the difference between overall prognosis and tooth prognosis.
- Compare the elements of overall prognosis with the elements of tooth prognosis.

- List and describe the factors associated with overall prognosis.
- List and describe the factors associated with individual tooth prognosis.
- Describe the expected outcomes of periodontal therapy.

KEY TERMS

Global prognosis Individual tooth prognosis Overall prognosis Prognosis

The prognosis is the prediction, or forecast, of the extent and duration of disease and its response to treatment. Prognosis is influenced by the pathogenesis of the disease and by individual patient factors, including overall health, risk factors, and compliance. All these factors must be evaluated by the clinician and considered in determining the prognosis for the patient and for specific teeth. Prognosis is a major consideration in treatment planning because all treatment should be based on which intervention is expected to provide the best outcomes.

OVERALL PROGNOSIS

The overall prognosis is the expected outcome for the patient. It is determined on the basis of the specific risk factors that the individual patient presents. For example, a patient with a systemic disease such as type 1 or type 2 diabetes that overlays chronic periodontitis is likely to have a less positive treatment outcome than another patient with the same oral conditions but no systemic disease. Healing and resolution of periodontal disease will be altered for individuals with systemic diseases and conditions because these patients respond differently to bacterial infection. Many factors discussed in Chapters 6, 7, and 9 will alter patient responses and therefore will complicate the overall prognosis. Individuals with systemic diseases and conditions are less likely to follow the course of healing that one would expect—regeneration and repair of periodontal tissues over the days and weeks after treatment.

All information available from the subjective and objective assessment of each patient is applied to formulate the overall prognosis. This prognosis is also sometimes referred to as a global prognosis. Once the overall prognosis is analyzed and determined, an individual tooth prognosis is determined for each tooth.[1] These categories are somewhat arbitrary because some patients may only have a few teeth, so the prognosis for those individual teeth and the global prognosis may be the same.

To determine the overall case prognosis, the following questions need to be addressed[2]:

- Should treatment be undertaken?
- Is treatment likely to succeed (retain the teeth and provide good function)?
- If prosthetic replacements will be made, can the periodontally treated teeth support the burden?

CLINICAL NOTE 18-1 The dental hygienist must consider prognosis as either short-term or long-term. Short-term prognosis usually refers to survival of the teeth for 5 years or less. Prognosis is best considered as a short-term prediction. The accuracy of predictions diminishes with longer time frames because many intervening events, illnesses, and situations can occur.

The factors considered in making an overall prognosis for patients with periodontal disease include age, systemic health, smoking, type of periodontal disease, oral conditions (including inflammation and bone levels), and the attitude and perceptions of the patient. Many clinicians consider the attitude, perceptions, and cooperation of the patient the most critical factors in the lasting success of periodontal treatment.

Prognosis is far from an exact science and research to develop better methods for assigning prognosis based on objective clinical criteria is ongoing.[3]

Age is a significant consideration. Epidemiologic studies (see Chapter 3) show that older patients demonstrate greater periodontal destruction as they age. However, concern arises when younger patients have significant periodontal destruction. In fact, younger individuals are less likely than older individuals with similar amounts of periodontal disease to respond well to treatment because some genetic or unidentified systemic factor is contributing to the advancement of the disease at an early age. Older individuals would have been more resistant and taken years longer to lose the same amount of attachment and support for the teeth. The prognosis for the older person in this case would be better than for the younger person with similar periodontal destruction because of a greater ability to control the disease process in the older person.

Systemic diseases and conditions influence the host's ability to respond to periodontal diseases. These diseases include diabetes, neutrophil defects, and factors associated with immunosuppression such as human immunodeficiency virus (HIV) infection or organ transplantation. Chapter 9 provides an extensive description of systemic diseases that affect periodontal disease and treatment.

Smoking has a direct relationship to the prevalence and incidence of periodontal disease. Smoking affects not only the severity of disease but also the healing potential of the oral tissues. Patients who smoke do not respond as well to periodontal therapy as those who do not.[2,4] Other forms of tobacco, such as cigar smoking and spit tobacco use, probably have the same effect on prognosis, although most research thus far has centered on cigarette smoking.

The type of periodontal disease is extremely important. The prognosis for chronic periodontitis is generally good with treatment, but some patients with clinical signs and symptoms similar to those of chronic periodontal disease have aggressive forms of periodontal disease. In cases of aggressive periodontitis, for reasons likely related to host response and possibly pathogenic bacterial species, healing is not the same as seen in chronic periodontitis. These patients may lose bone and teeth very rapidly over a few months and their prognosis after treatment is poor.

Oral conditions are an obvious consideration. Heavy deposits of plaque biofilm and calculus and severity of inflammation must be factored into the analysis. Clinical attachment loss indicates how much support for the tooth has been lost. This bone loss is significant because the prognosis is adversely affected as the attachment level gets closer to the root apex. Also, teeth weakened by extensive bone and attachment loss may not be serviceable for certain restorative procedures, such as abutment teeth for fixed partial dentures or removable partial dentures. Overall or global prognosis is defined by categories described in Table 18-1.[1,2]

CLINICAL NOTE 18-2 The attitude and perceptions of the patient are critical to the prognosis. The patient must be a partner in treatment, cooperating with appointment regimens and participating actively in improving daily plaque biofilm control to restore health.

TABLE 18-1	**Global Prognosis Categories and Definitions**[1]
PROGNOSIS	**CONDITIONS**
Excellent	No bone loss, excellent gingival condition, no systemic considerations, good patient cooperation
Good	Adequate remaining periodontal support and ease of maintenance, adequate patient cooperation
Fair	Attachment loss and furcation involvement (Class I), patient cooperation likely, systemic factors controlled
Poor	Attachment loss and furcation involvement that can only be maintained with difficulty (Class II or III), tooth mobility, presence of systemic factors
Questionable	Poor crown-to-root ratio, poor root form, root proximity, Class II or III furcations, mobility, presence of systemic factors
Hopeless	Advanced bone loss, inadequate attachment, uncontrolled environmental/systemic factors, tooth should be extracted

INDIVIDUAL TOOTH PROGNOSIS

Overall prognosis for the dentition may differ from that of the individual teeth. It is common to treat a periodontal patient who has one or more teeth with a poor prognosis but an overall prognosis for the dentition that is good. It is also common for successful therapy to include removal of some teeth to preserve the rest and restore the dentition to function and aesthetics.

The prognosis of the individual teeth is evaluated first on the basis of the overall prognosis and then on the status of each tooth according to pocket depths, attachment loss, mobility, amount and location of furcation involvement, tooth morphologic features, bone levels, general condition of the tooth, and ability to modify etiologic factors.

Pocket depths, particularly persistent deep pockets, can harbor pathogenic plaque biofilms and are associated with increased inflammation. The extent that deep pockets exist in the mouth, or remain after Phase I therapy, can adversely affect the prognosis for the tooth. There is also some evidence that persistent deep pockets are an important risk indicator for future periodontal disease destruction not limited to the original site.[1] Deep pockets also generally reflect loss of attachment to the tooth, a further indication that the tooth is weakened and an indicator of a less favorable prognosis. Bleeding is also associated with deep pockets and persistent inflammation. The relationship of persistent bleeding to the progression of periodontal disease is presented in Box 18-1.

Mobility is associated with less favorable periodontal outcomes but is not confirmed as a risk factor. It is caused by inflammation in the periodontal ligament and bone loss. Mobility can result from loss of support for the tooth (bone and clinical attachment loss) or trauma from occlusion. If the mobility can be corrected by altering occlusal forces (see Chapter 11), then it has no detrimental effect on prognosis. However, if the mobility is the direct result of loss of support for the tooth, then the prognosis is less favorable.[1]

BOX 18-1 The Significance of Gingival Bleeding

Gingival bleeding is a risk predictor for patients on periodontal maintenance. Dr. Gary Armitage generated a random effects meta-analysis to analyze the relationship between bleeding on probing and progression of periodontal disease, defined as 2 mm or more of loss of attachment in a 12-month period.[5] The meta-analysis incorporated three studies with a total population of 171 treated and maintained patients diagnosed with chronic periodontal disease. Bleeding on probing data from 14,114 sites were included in the analysis.

All the patients were managed on 3-month recall schedules. Over a 12-month period, it was determined that if sites exhibited bleeding on probing 50% or more of the time, there was a three-fold increased risk for losing an additional 2 mm or more of clinical attachment. The data generated an odds ratio of 2.79 (95% CI 1.03 to 7.57).

The prognosis for patients who continue to have bleeding sites is poor or fair at best. This highlights the importance of excellent nonsurgical periodontal therapy to remove calculus and plaque biofilm, periodontal surgical and adjunct procedures as needed to reduce pockets and control inflammation, maintenance therapy by the dental hygienist, and especially daily plaque biofilm control by the patients.

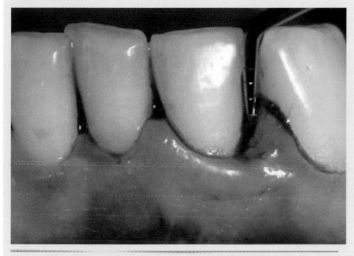

Persistent bleeding on probing in a periodontal case. (Used with permission from Armitage GC. Clinical evaluation of periodontal diseases. *Periodontol 2000.* 1995;7:41.)

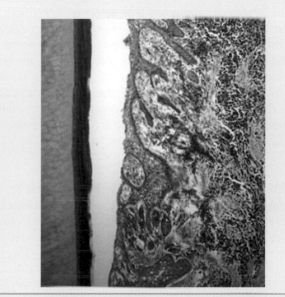

Histologic image of a thinned and ulcerated epithelium lining the pocket wall. Histologic section stained in 0.5% toluidine blue, original magnification ×16.

Furcation involvement has a negative effect on the prognosis for an individual tooth. Access for scaling and root planing and home care is difficult to obtain, so these areas can continue to harbor pathogenic plaque biofilm. The presence of deeper Class II and Class III furcations further diminishes both the dental hygienist's ability to clean the area and the patient's ability to provide adequate plaque biofilm control on a daily basis. Furcations on maxillary first premolars are in the apical third of the root, so when this furcation is exposed, the tooth has lost significant support and its prognosis is generally poor.

Tooth morphologic features can alter the prognosis for specific teeth. Findings such as lingual grooves and cervical projections of enamel lead to isolated pocketing and can permit severe periodontal infections. These are not uncommon findings. Cervical enamel projections are estimated to occur in about 25% of mandibular molars and in 20% of maxillary molars. Some are very small and therefore insignificant; others can extend several millimeters and lead directly into furcation areas (remember there is no soft tissue attachment to enamel surfaces). Lingual grooves are found on about 6% of maxillary lateral incisors and 3% of maxillary central incisors.[2] An example of a long lingual groove and the surgery required to correct the associated periodontal defect is presented in Chapter 14.

Bone level is important for individual teeth because it defines the amount of support remaining for the tooth. Greater bone loss will result in more mobility.[2]

The general condition of the tooth is important to consider individually and for the overall prognosis of the case. Teeth with extensive caries, root caries, endodontic lesions, root resorption, and poor restorations are plaque traps and have less positive prognoses than do intact teeth. Any tooth with extensive caries or other conditions that are likely to need extensive restorative work may not be suitable for the overall treatment plan and may need to be extracted. Sometimes, although the tooth could be saved with periodontal therapy, the restorative treatment plan will require a tooth with more bone support, or less damage to its structure, to serve as an abutment tooth. In these cases, sometimes teeth that could be saved are extracted in light of the overall treatment plan.

CLINICAL NOTE 18-3 Perhaps the most significant consideration for the dental hygienist is the ability to modify etiologic factors presented by the patient. The tooth must be able to be debrided during nonsurgical therapy and maintenance and must be accessible to the patient for plaque biofilm control. If the patient cannot clean the tooth, and it is very difficult and demanding for the dental hygienist to clean, the prognosis is diminished.

PATIENT CONSIDERATIONS

Most often prognosis is determined and the ideal treatment plan is formulated in the best interests of the patient with the intent to preserve all teeth for as long as possible. Occasionally these plans are changed or compromised because the patient views things differently. Sometimes patients choose to follow a treatment plan option where teeth are extracted although they could be saved or to reject treatment altogether. The dental hygienist is dedicated to providing the best possible treatment, and it is sometimes difficult to accept the choice of lesser treatment or loss of teeth, especially because untreated periodontal disease leads to tooth loss.[6] All patients deserve to know the treatment options and how decisions may alter their oral health in the future. Patients may choose not to follow aggressive therapy regimens that include multiple courses of antibiotics and many treatment visits, although they are made aware that these treatment regimens are effective in treating aggressive and refractory periodontal disease.[7] This knowledge must be related through discussion of prognosis and treatment, but in the end the patient is the one who accepts the treatment or chooses to modify it.

PROGNOSES FOR COMMON PERIODONTAL DIAGNOSES

Periodontal diseases are categorized into groups of diseases with generally similar signs, symptoms, and outcomes. Novak and Takei[2] characterized these general disease categories and identified prognoses typical of diseases in the group. This following information is based on their work.

Gingivitis Associated with Dental Plaque Only

Gingivitis associated with dental plaque only is a reversible disease caused by bacterial plaque biofilm. It can occur around teeth with or without attachment loss. The prognosis is good if all contributing factors can be eliminated and the tissue returned to a state of health.[2] A prognosis of excellent should be reserved for gingival disease in which no attachment loss has occurred; thus, healing the gingival inflammation restores the oral condition completely.

Plaque-Induced Gingival Diseases Modified by Systemic Factors

In the case of plaque-induced gingival diseases modified by systemic factors, the host response to the bacterial assault is mediated by other diseases and conditions. Patients tend to have extensive reactions to what seems to be a small amount of plaque. Prognosis depends on both the plaque biofilm control and the control or correction of the systemic situation.[2] An example would be pregnancy gingivitis: the condition is improved with local periodontal therapy and resolves when the systemic condition, the pregnancy, is over. In this example the prognosis would be good to excellent.

Plaque-Induced Gingival Diseases Modified by Medications

The use of drugs such as phenytoin, nifedipine, and oral contraceptives has been shown to be related to gingival conditions.

Some drug-related gingival enlargements are extensive and recur even after surgical correction. Long-term prognoses are related to both plaque biofilm control and long-term use of the medications.[2] It is hard to generalize, but these conditions can be managed with treatment for many years, so the prognosis can be fair to good.

Gingival Diseases Modified by Malnutrition

The prognosis of gingival diseases modified by malnutrition depends on the severity and duration of the deficiency. The condition can be treatable, thus restoring periodontal health, or periodontal support can be so damaged that the teeth are lost.[2] Prognosis can range from hopeless to good.

Chronic Periodontitis

The prognosis for chronic periodontitis is generally good if the inflammation is controlled. Severe attachment loss, furcation involvement, and uncooperative patients will diminish the prognosis to fair or poor.[2]

Aggressive Periodontitis

Aggressive periodontitis occurs as localized or generalized forms and is related to rapid loss of attachment and bone destruction in otherwise healthy patients. It is found as a family trait. The disease is often associated with an infection by *Aggregatibactor actinomycetemcomitans* or *Porphyromonas gingivalis* that results in a much more severe reaction than the amount of plaque biofilm would suggest. The localized form usually appears around the age of puberty and is amenable to periodontal treatment and systemic antibiotic therapy. With proper treatment it has a good to excellent prognosis. Generalized aggressive periodontitis is usually seen in young adults and often has other associated risk factors, such as smoking, and possibly systemic alterations in host defenses. This form of periodontal disease has a fair to poor, or even questionable, prognosis.[2]

Periodontitis as a Manifestation of Systemic Diseases

Typically, patients who display periodontitis as a manifestation of a systemic disease have serious systemic or genetic disorders that limit their ability to respond to the disease. Even with repeated treatment, these patients often have, at best, fair prognoses.[2]

Necrotizing Ulcerative Diseases

Necrotizing ulcerative gingivitis is primarily caused by bacterial plaque biofilm, with secondary factors such as stress or poor nutrition. It is amenable to periodontal treatment, and the prognosis for this disease is good. However, it does result in tissue destruction, and patients commonly have repeated episodes of the disease. Generalized necrotizing ulcerative periodontitis is similar to the gingivitis form except that the tissue damage extends to the deeper supporting structures. These cases are also associated with immunocompromised conditions. The

| BOX 18-2 | Elements for Determining Prognosis in Periodontal Disease |

PROGNOSIS is determined for the overall case and for each individual tooth.

Excellent — Health restored indefinitely with no bone loss or gingival changes

Good — Health restored indefinitely with treatment; some bone and gingival changes persist

Fair — Periodontal condition may worsen in the future

Poor — Treatment efforts might not succeed

Questionable — Teeth are expected to be lost even with treatment

Hopeless — Teeth need to be removed or are expected to be lost

OVERALL PROGNOSIS is affected by many elements, including the following:
- Age
- Systemic health
- Smoking or tobacco use
- Periodontal disease type
- Oral conditions
- Patient attitudes, perceptions, and cooperation

PROGNOSIS FOR EACH TOOTH is affected by many elements, including the following:
- Pocket depths and inflammation
- Mobility
- Extent and location of furcation involvement
- Tooth morphologic features
- Bone level
- General condition of tooth
- Ability to modify etiologic factors

prognosis depends on dealing with both the systemic condition and manifestations of the local periodontal disease, so it is hard to generalize about the prognosis.[2]

A summary of the elements for determining prognosis is presented in Box 18-2.

THE RESULTS OF PERIODONTAL TREATMENT

One straightforward way to assess the results of treatment is to monitor tooth loss in patients with treated periodontal disease. Although there are many factors related to tooth loss, including smoking, deep pockets, systemic disease, and unrestorable teeth, comparing the loss of teeth after periodontal treatment provides the dental hygienist with a sense of long-term preservation of function of the dentition.

A study by Checchi and others[8] evaluated tooth loss compared to individual tooth prognosis for 92 treated periodontal patients over a period of 6.7 years. Throughout the study, patients returned for regular maintenance treatment. Of the 2184 teeth, 44 were lost for periodontal reasons. Relating this finding to the individual tooth prognoses it was found that:

- 0.07% of the teeth with good prognoses (less than 50% bone loss) were lost
- 3.63% of the teeth with questionable prognoses (50% to 75% bone loss) were lost
- 11.34% of the teeth with hopeless prognoses (more than 75% bone loss) were lost

Further, compliant patients who came in for maintenance visits every 3 to 4 months lost fewer teeth and had lower plaque scores than those patients who were less compliant. Not surprisingly, molar teeth were lost more than others, likely due to furcations and anatomy.

Other studies have also shown that after 10 years of maintenance following periodontal therapy certain risk factors are related to tooth loss.[9] Specifically maintenance patients who smoke lost more teeth, as did patients diagnosed at a younger age, and females demonstrated more tooth loss than males over 10 years. Patients who were diagnosed with aggressive or more severe forms of periodontal disease lost more teeth. Similar findings have been reported in a posttreatment population in Norway, with gender and smoking being more significant predictors of tooth loss.[10]

Tooth mortality has been studied by a number of authors and summarized by Merin.[11] Studies involving thousands of teeth were compared, and data revealed that treated periodontal patients lost between 0.72 and 1.6 teeth per person over 10 years, about 1 tooth per year. In contrast, untreated populations lost between 6 to 16 teeth per person.

Although predictions of success of treatment are generally based on tooth loss data, there are many important variables. Patients need to be educated about what they can do to improve their outcomes, for example smoking cessation and good plaque biofilm control. Patient life experience is dynamic and prognosis can change for the better based on compliance, or for the worse, as might be the case with a newly diagnosed systemic illness such as diabetes. In any case, compliance is key to long-term success and maintenance of the teeth. Box 18-3 describes the experience of a single periodontal patient who was treated for over 40 years. This case demonstrates the significance of all aspects of dental hygiene care in managing periodontal disease.

BOX 18-3 30-Year Case Report

The Mayre Heflebower story described by Seibert is a case report documented over a period of 30 years to show the value of maintenance therapy. The success of periodontal treatment and daily oral hygiene in maintaining a comfortable and functional dentition for life is demonstrated in this remarkable patient history.

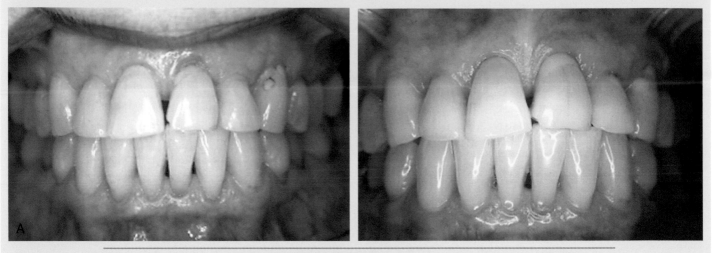

A, Response to periodontal and maintenance therapy. *Left,* Before treatment, note the evidence of gingival inflammation although the tissue is not severely reddened. There is a considerable amount of supragingival plaque biofilm and gingival recession on the facial surface of the mandibular incisors. *Right,* After treatment and 20 years of maintenance therapy, the gingival tissues appear stable and healthy. Note the replacement restorations. (From Seibert JS. *The Mayre Heflebower Story.* Philadelphia, PA: University of Pennsylvania; 1980.)

After the diagnosis of gingivitis with localized areas of periodontitis in 1947, the patient underwent nonsurgical periodontal therapy, including scaling, root planing, and curettage. In addition, she was provided with information and training to control her microbial plaque biofilm and inflammation. This information became the basis of her daily oral hygiene program. Regular professional maintenance visits consisted of a complete oral soft and hard tissue examination, scaling of her teeth as needed, and a dental prophylaxis (polishing).

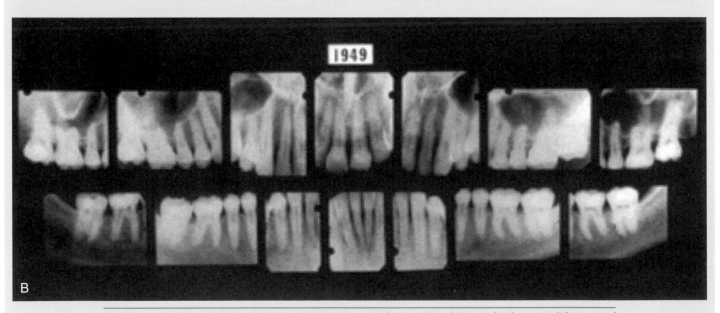

B, Full-mouth radiographs. These were taken in 1949, 2 years after periodontal therapy for the original diagnosis of gingivitis with localized areas of periodontitis in 1947. (From Seibert JS. *The Mayre Heflebower Story.* Philadelphia, PA: University of Pennsylvania; 1980.)

BOX 18-3   30-Year Case Report—cont'd

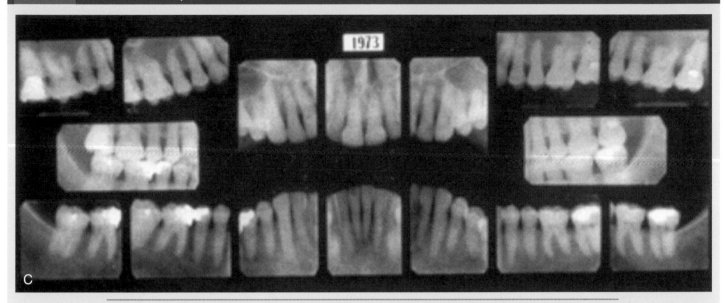

C, Full-mouth radiographs. These were taken in 1973 after 26 years of maintenance therapy that primarily consisted of meticulous daily plaque control and regular maintenance care. Note the preservation of alveolar bone height compared with the radiographs in **B.** (From Seibert JS. *The Mayre Heflebower Story.* Philadelphia, PA: University of Pennsylvania; 1980.)

Success in arresting the progression of disease was apparent 26 years after the initial periodontal therapy, as seen in the clinical health of the periodontal tissues and by comparison of the radiographs taken in 1949 and 1973, illustrated in A, B, and C. No further measurable alveolar bone loss was detected at the time of the patient's death at age 77 years in 1977. The patient's benefit from preventive oral health care is documented in clinical, radiographic, and histologic data. This case provides an opportunity for the dental hygienist to understand the important contribution of prevention and maintenance to lifelong periodontal health.

(From Seibert JS. *The Mayre Heflebower Story.* Philadelphia, PA: University of Pennsylvania; 1980.)

◎ DENTAL HYGIENE CONSIDERATIONS

- Prognosis is the prediction of treatment outcomes.
- Each patient has an overall or global prognosis and prognosis is also determined for each tooth.
- Prognosis is generally defined as excellent, good, fair, poor, questionable, or hopeless.
- Considerations in determining the overall prognosis are age, systemic health, disease type, oral conditions, and patient attitudes and perceptions.
- Considerations for determining the prognosis for each tooth are pocket depths and inflammation, mobility, extent and location of furcation involvement, tooth morphologic features, bone level, and general condition of the tooth.
- Each patient is responsible for treatment choices on the basis of an understanding of the prognosis for treatment alternatives presented, including the prognosis if they choose not to pursue treatment.
- Compliance with regular maintenance care results in lower plaque scores and less tooth loss in patients who have been treated for periodontal diseases.

✷ CASE SCENARIO

Mrs. Smith is 63 years old. She has 5- to 6-mm probing depths throughout her mouth and 5- to 6- mm of clinical attachment loss, and her teeth have shifted position, creating spaces that concern her. Mrs. Smith is seeking dental care because she does not like the spaces that appeared between her front teeth. She is cooperative and has been having her teeth cleaned regularly; her plaque biofilm control is good. The periodontist referred her to you for quadrant scaling and root planing.

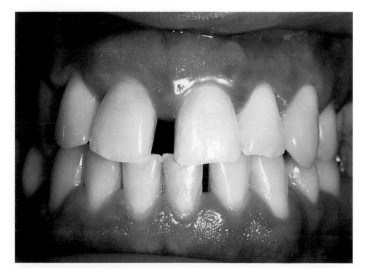

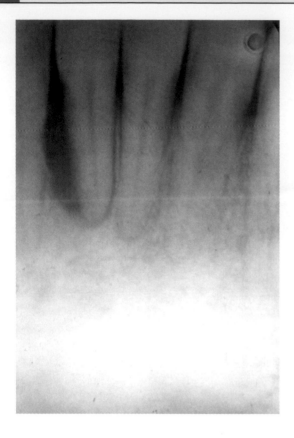

1. The global prognosis for Mrs. Smith is likely to be
   A. excellent.
   B. good.
   C. poor to fair.
   D. questionable.
   E. hopeless.
2. The spaces that appeared between the teeth are likely the result of
   A. bruxism.
   B. systemic factors.
   C. pathologic migration.
   D. primary trauma from occlusion.
   E. secondary trauma from occlusion.
3. Mrs. Smith's prognosis may be more favorable than the deep probing depths suggest because she is older, indicating that the disease has advanced slowly.
   A. Both the statement and reason are correct and related.
   B. Both the statement and reason are correct but NOT related.
   C. The statement is correct, but the reason is NOT correct.
   D. The statement is NOT correct, but the reason is correct.
   E. NEITHER the statement NOR the reason is correct.
4. The radiograph is of Mrs. Smith's mandibular incisor area and #25 is likely to present a combination endodontic and periodontal abscess. The prognosis for this individual tooth is the same as the overall prognosis for the dentition.
   A. Both statements are true.
   B. Both statements are false.
   C. The first statement is true, and the second statement is false.
   D. The first statement is false, and the second statement is true.

MULTIPLE CHOICE

1. The prognosis for aggressive forms of periodontal disease is
   A. unable to be determined.
   B. better than that for chronic periodontitis.
   C. less favorable than that for chronic periodontitis.
   D. exactly the same as that for chronic periodontitis.
2. Global prognosis is the same as the individual tooth prognosis for all patients. The individual tooth prognosis can differ from the overall prognosis.
   A. Both statements are true.
   B. Both statements are false.
   C. The first statement is true, and the second statement is false.
   D. The first statement is false, and the second statement is true.
3. When patients successfully complete periodontal therapy and are compliant with maintenance care, what is the expected rate of tooth loss over 10 years?
   A. One per year
   B. Five to six per year
   C. One per 10 years
   D. Five to six per 10 years
4. In general, the most critical element in determining prognosis is
   A. the attitude of the patient.
   B. dental hygiene care history.
   C. the type of periodontal disease.
   D. the pathogenesis of the disease.
5. Age is a significant factor in determining the overall prognosis because
   A. older people are less likely to cooperate with treatment.
   B. younger people are less likely to cooperate with treatment.
   C. an older individual with significant periodontal destruction is likely to be more susceptible to disease.
   D. a younger individual with significant periodontal destruction is likely to be more susceptible to disease.
6. Mr. Molinas is 38 years old and is HIV-positive. He has necrotizing ulcerative periodontitis characterized by rapid and extensive bone loss. He is very concerned about his overall health and his teeth and he is willing to cooperate with all recommended treatment. The treatment plan is for oral hygiene instruction, quadrant scaling and root planing, and reevaluation for further treatment. The overall prognosis for Mr. Molinas is likely to be
   A. good to excellent.
   B. poor to fair.
   C. questionable.
   D. hopeless.

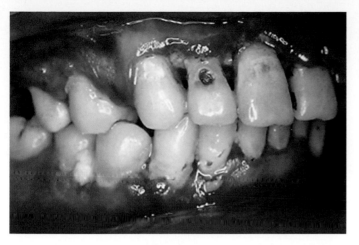

Question 6

7. Ms. Lake is a 43-year-old executive in an advertising agency. She has a very high-stress position and takes little time to have physical examinations or dental check-ups, but she reports that she is in good health. She does not smoke and is a social drinker. She is referred to you by the periodontist for Phase I therapy. Ms. Lake has 8- to 9-mm probing depths throughout her mouth, extreme gingival inflammation, and poor plaque control. What is the likely global prognosis for this patient?
   A. Good to excellent
   B. Poor to fair
   C. Questionable
   D. Hopeless

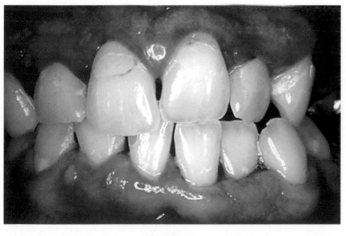

Question 7

8. Mr. Owens is a 13-year-old boy in excellent health. Because he has severe occlusal problems, he has been in orthodontic treatment for the first 6 months of a long treatment plan. He is cooperative with appointments, hates having braces on, and knows that he will be undergoing treatment for several more years. His plaque biofilm control is very poor and he has some supragingival calculus deposits and gingival pockets but no periodontal pocketing. What is the overall prognosis for this patient likely to be?
   A. Good to excellent
   B. Poor to fair
   C. Questionable
   D. Hopeless

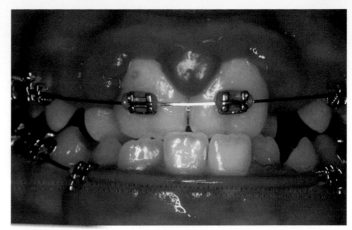

Question 8

SHORT ANSWER

9. Why is the presence of systemic disease so significant for periodontal patients?
10. Why do some teeth that could be treated and saved have to be extracted?

ⓔ Please visit **http://evolve.elsevier.com/Perry/periodontology** for additional practice and study support tools.

REFERENCES

1. Thomas MV, Mealey BL. Formulating a periodontal diagnosis and prognosis. In: Rose LF, Mealey BL, eds. *Periodontics: Medicine, Surgery and Implants.* St. Louis, MO: Elsevier Mosby; 2004:182–199.
2. Novak KF, Takei HH. Determination of prognosis. In: Newman MG, Takei HH, Klokkevold PR, et al, eds. *Carranza's Clinical Periodontology.* 11th ed. Philadelphia, PA: Elsevier Saunders; 2012:373–383.
3. McGuire MK, Nunn ME. Prognosis versus actual outcomes. II. The effectiveness of clinical parameters in developing an accurate prognosis. *J Periodontol.* 1996;67:658–665.
4. Balijoon M, Natto S, Bergstrom J. Long-term effect of smoking on vertical periodontal bone loss. *J Clin Periodontol.* 2005;32:789–795.
5. Armitage GC. Periodontal diseases: diagnosis. *Ann Periodontol.* 1996;1:37–215.
6. Harris RJ. Untreated periodontal disease: a follow-up on 30 cases. *J Periodontol.* 2003;74:672–678.
7. Haffajee AD, Uzel NG, Arguello EI, et al. Clinical and microbiological changes associated with the use of combined antimicrobial therapies to treat "refractory" periodontitis. *J Clin Periodontol.* 2004;31:869–879.
8. Checchi L, Montevecchi M, Gatto MRA, et al. Retrospective study of tooth loss in 92 treated periodontal patients. *J Clin Periodontol.* 2002;29:651–656.
9. Eickholz P, Kaltschmitt J, Berbig J, et al. Tooth loss after active periodontal therapy. 1: patient -related factors for risk, prognosis, and quality of outcome. *J Clin Periodontol.* 2008;35:165–174.
10. Fardal O, Johannessen AC, Linden GJ. Tooth loss during maintenance following periodontal treatment in a periodontal practice in Norway. *J Clin Periodontol.* 2004;31:550–555.
11. Merin RL. Results of periodontal treatment. In: Newman MG, Takei HH, Klokkevold PR, et al, eds. *Carranza's Clinical Periodontology.* 11th ed. Philadelphia, PA: Elsevier Saunders; 2012:756–762.

GLOSSARY

The parenthetical number(s) at the end of each definition refers to the chapter in which the key term is mentioned.

The original source for many definitions was *Mosby's Dental Dictionary*, Mosby, St. Louis; 2004.

Abscess A localized accumulation of pus in a cavity formed by tissue disintegration. (7)

Abutment screw A fastener used to aid in support and retention of a fixed or removable prosthesis. (15)

Access flap procedures Periodontal surgical techniques that provide visualization of the root in conjunction to improve curettage and root planing. Examples include supracrestal, subcrestal full-thickness, and partial-thickness flaps. (14)

Acquired deformities Defects seen in the periodontium related to recession, gingival enlargement, or personal habits that may or may not require therapeutic intervention. (7)

Acquired pellicle A layer of glycoprotein deposited from salivary and crevicular fluids that is strongly bound to the tooth surface. (5)

Acute herpetic gingivostomatitis The manifestations of clinically apparent primary herpes simplex; also called acute herpetic stomatitis. (16)

Acute periodontal abscess An abscess involving the attachment tissues and alveolar bone as a sequela of periodontal disease. The abscess has a short but severe course. (16)

Adherence The act or quality of sticking to something. (4)

Administrator/advocate A person who applies organizational skills, communicates objectives, identifies and manages resources, and evaluates and modifies programs of health, education, or health care. (1)

Aerobe An organism that requires an aerobic or oxygenated environment to survive. (4)

Aggressive periodontitis Periodontal disease that progresses exceedingly rapidly with massive bone loss. (7)

Alveolar bone The specialized bone structure that contains the alveoli or sockets of the teeth and supports the teeth. (2)

Alveolar process The portion of the maxilla or mandible that forms the dental arch and serves as a bony investment for the teeth. (2)

Alveoli Plural form of alveolus; the tooth sockets in the bones in which teeth are attached by means of the periodontal ligament. Each root of a multirooted tooth has its own alveolus. (2)

Amalgam overhang Excess filling material (predominantly mercury) that projects beyond the cavity margins; one of the most common forms of poorly contoured restorations; can cause plaque traps and increased gingival inflammation. (5)

American Dental Hygienists Association (ADHA) A nonprofit professional association of dental hygienists in the United States, created to assist its members in providing the highest professional and ethical care and to serve as an advocate for the advancement of the profession. (1)

Anaerobe A microorganism that can exist and grow only in the partial or complete absence of oxygen. (4)

Anthropology The study of the cultures and characteristics of humanity. (1)

Antibiotic therapy The treatment of disease by the local or systemic administration of antibiotics. (7)

Antibody A specific substance that is produced by an animal as a reaction to the presence of an antigen and that reacts specifically with the antigen in some observable way; also, an immunoglobulin, essential to the immune system, produced by the lymphoid tissue in response to bacteria, viruses, or other antigenic substances. (2)

Anticalculus agents Compounds that inhibit, control, or limit the formation of calculus. (12)

Antigen A substance, usually a protein, that elicits the formation of antibodies when introduced into a foreign body or species. (2)

Apically positioned flap The reflection of gingiva and connective tissue away from the roots of the teeth, and that repositions apically to reduce pocket depths. (14)

Apprenticeship Period during which a person learns by watching and assisting an established dentist. (1)

Assessment The qualified opinion of a health care provider, informed by patient feedback and examination results, with regard to a specific health issue, whether critical, pending, or routine. (10)

Attached gingiva Firm, dense, stippled tissue that extends from the free gingival groove to the mucogingival junction; firmly attached to the bone by collagen fibers. (2)

Attachment apparatus The periodontal ligament, cementum, and alveolar bone. (2)

Attachment loss An increase in the acceptable distance between a structure and its supporting tissues. (14)

Bacterial coaggregation The adherence of certain bacteria to other bacterial species, forming direct attachment between the surface components of the two species and resulting in plaque biofilm accumulation. (4)

Bacterial plaque biofilm A naturally occurring complex microbial ecosystem that adheres to teeth and oral structures and causes inflammation if left undisturbed. (12)

Baltimore College of Dental Surgery The first dental school; officially opened in 1840. (1)

Barber-surgeons Members of a group who were both barbers and also provided bloodletting and tooth extraction services. (1)

Basal lamina A thin flat layer that joins the gingival epithelium and underlying connective tissue. (2)

Bass, Charles C. The person who proposed the importance of plaque removal to oral health, studied the optimum characteristics of toothbrushes, and developed the toothbrushing method most commonly used today. (12)

Bass toothbrushing method A vibratory method of toothbrushing that requires the bristles of a soft multitufted toothbrush to be placed at a 45-degree angle to the long axis of the teeth. A vibratory motion is used to force the bristles into the sulci and between the teeth as effectively as possible. The lingual surfaces of the anterior teeth can be brushed with the heel of the toothbrush for better access and all other areas with the length of the brush head. The occlusal surfaces are brushed with controlled back and forth motions. (12)

Biocompatibility The quality of not threatening or adversely affecting living tissue. (15)

Biologic width The physiologically necessasry area (usually 1 to 2 mm) of connective tissue attachment covered by epithelium between the base of the sulcus or pocket and the alveolar bone; must be considered when estimating the amount of attachment remaining on a periodontally involved tooth. (14)

Biomaterials Biocompatible materials such as gold, stainless steel, cobalt-chromium alloys, bioactive glasses, niobium, hydroxyapatite, tricalcium phosphate, polymers, zirconium, and titanium. (15)

Biteguard An acrylic resin appliance that is fitted over the occlusal and incisal surfaces of the dental arch to stabilize the teeth or provide a flat platform for the unobstructed excursive glides of the mandible. (11)

Bleeding on probing Gingival bleeding that is stimulated by a dental probe. (8)

Blood dyscrasia An abnormal disorder of the blood, such as that found in leukemia and anemia. (9)

Bone loss A decrease in periodontal bone structure or strength, usually as a result of inflammation. (7)

Bruxism The involuntary and often unconscious gnashing, clenching, or grinding of the teeth. (11)

Calculus A concentration composed of calcium phosphate, calcium carbonate, magnesium phosphate, and other elements within an organic matrix composed of desquamated epithelium, mucin, microorganisms, and other debris that adheres to tooth surfaces. (5)

Calculus index (CI-S) The calculus portion of the Simplified Oral Hygiene Index (OHI-S). (3)

Calibrated examiners A team of researchers who are trained to apply the indices to members of a population by use of the same standardized guidelines and definitions. (3)

Cardiovascular disease Disease affecting the cardiovascular system of the body. (9)

Case-control study An investigation using an epidemiologic approach in which previous incidents of a medical condition are used instead of gathering new information from a randomized population. Control is obtained by comparing known cases of the medical condition with a group of persons in whom the condition has not developed. (3)

Cementoenamel junction The junction of the enamel of the crown and the cementum of the root of the tooth. The area above the junction corresponds to the anatomic portion of the tooth; the area apical to the junction constitutes the anatomic root of the tooth. (2)

Cementum A specialized, calcified connective tissue that covers the anatomic root of the tooth and gives attachment to the periodontal ligament. (2)

Charters' toothbrushing method A rotary technique that requires placement of the brush at a 45-degree angle to the tooth surface, with the bristle ends pointing away from the gingiva but toward the interproximal surfaces of the teeth. Essentially, the bristles are repeatedly pressed against the gingival margin and then lifted away to massage the tissue and increase blood flow. The bristles are also pressed into the occlusal surfaces using a slight rotary motion so that they fit into the pits and fissures. (12)

Chemotaxis A signaling process in which inflammatory cells are attracted to areas of the body by stimuli such as trauma or microbial influences. (2)

Chronic periodontal abscess An abscess involving the attachment tissues and alveolar bone as a sequela of periodontal disease. Unlike the acute periodontal abscess, it has a long-lasting course. (16)

Chronic periodontitis The most common form of periodontal disease, with a long slow course. (7)

Clenching Continuous or intermittent closure of the jaws under vertical pressure. (11)

Clinical attachment loss (CAL) A measurement that documents increases in the distance from the cementoenamel junction to the apical depth of the periodontal pocket. The method requires successive measurements over weeks, months, or years. (7)

Clinical examination The visual and tactile scrutiny of the teeth and tissues of the periodontium and the surrounding oral and facial structures; also, the formal testing of the dental hygienist student to determine whether his or her skills meet or exceed established standards. (8)

Clinical jaw function Assessment of jaw function that includes muscle palpation, mandibular movement, joint function, and joint sounds. (11)

Clinician A person who assesses, diagnoses, plans, implements, and evaluates treatment for prevention, intervention, and control of oral diseases while practicing in collaboration with other professionals. (1)

Cohort study A scientific study that focuses on a specific subpopulation, such as children born on a certain date in a specific environment. (3)

Col A slight depression of tissue between the buccal and lingual interdental papillae in posterior teeth. (2)

Combination abscess An abscess of both the periodontal and periapical tissues, which may cause extensive damage, is difficult to diagnose, and requires extensive therapy. (16)

Community Index of Periodontal Treatment Needs (CIPTN) A progressive scale that assigns a numeric score to each tooth. This scale is weighted more toward bone loss than toward gingival inflammation. The score for each tooth is added and averaged by all teeth examined in the individual, providing a score for each person. Population scores are determined by averaging the scores of individuals. (3)

Complement One of eleven complex enzymatic serum proteins. It has many functions, including bacteriolysis (destruction of bacteria) and promotion of the immune response. (2)

Compliance The fulfillment by the patient of the caregiver's prescribed course of treatment; or, the fulfillment of oversight criteria or standards of care necessary for licensure, certification, and accreditation. (17)

Cover screw A device that is placed on top of an implant to protect the internal aspect of the implant from ingrowth of tissue. (15)

Crepitus A crackling sound, such as that produced by the rubbing together of fragments of a fractured bone; in dentistry, it refers to sounds made by the TMJ. (11)

Cross-sectional study The scientific method for the analysis of data gathered from two or more samples at one point in time. (3)

Cytokine A nonantibody protein, such as lymphokine. Cytokines are released by a cell population on contact with a specific antigen. They act as intercellular mediators in the generation of immune response. (2)

Dehiscence A resorbed area of bone over the facial surface of the root that can occur in patients with labially inclined roots. (2)

Dental floss Waxed or plain thread of nylon or silk used to clean the interdental areas. (12)

Dental hygiene care plan See dental hygiene treatment plan. (10)

Dental hygiene process of care An organized systematic group of dental hygiene activities that provides the framework for delivering quality dental hygiene care. (10)

Dental hygiene treatment plan An individualized approach to treatment for a specific patient that details the care to be provided by the dental hygienist. It is a portion of the total treatment plan detailing comprehensive care for the dental patient and is sometimes called the dental hygiene care plan. (10)

Dental plaque biofilm Accumulations of microbes on the surface of the teeth or other solid oral structures, not readily removed by rinsing. (4)

Dental plaque biofilm–induced gingivitis Inflammation of the gingival tissue that is caused by the presence of dental plaque biofilm. (6)

Dentin sensitivity The state of responsiveness of dentin to external influences such as temperature, sugar, and trauma. (13, 17)

Dentinal hypersensitivity A common complaint after periodontal therapy in which the dentin may have been exposed, resulting in tooth pain or sensitivity to heat, cold, and sweet substances. (13, 17)

Dentinal sensitivity A common patient complaint that can often be alleviated. (8)

Dentogingival unit A functional component consisting of an attachment of the junctional epithelium to the root surface that supports the free marginal gingivae and is enhanced by fibers from the connective tissue. (2)

Dermatologic diseases Diseases affecting the skin; often accompanied by pathologic manifestations of various mucosal surfaces such as the oral mucosa, genital mucosa, or conjunctiva. (9)

Developmental anomalies Aberrations or deviations from the normal pattern of development. (7)

Diagnosis The translation of data gathered by clinical and radiographic examination into an organized, classified definition of the conditions present. (10)

Documentation The permanent recording of information properly identified as to time, place, circumstances, and attributes. (8)

Dysfunction A state of morphofunctional disharmony in which the forces developed during function cause pathologic changes in the tissues, which result in abnormal function or pain. The degree of dysfunction can be slight, with no great disturbance to the patient, or significant, making daily activity difficult or impossible. (11)

Early-onset periodontitis (EOP) The term given to periodontal disease affecting children, teens, and young adults. If left untreated, it may cause premature tooth loss; formerly considered prepubertal periodontitis and now considered aggressive periodontitis. (7)

Educator, health promoter A person who uses educational theory and methods to analyze health needs, develop health promotion strategies, and deliver and evaluate the results of attaining or maintaining oral health for individuals or groups. (1)

Effector molecule A molecule that responds to stimulations initiating corrections. The molecule is the smallest particle of an element or chemical compound that is capable of retaining the same chemical identity as the entire substance in mass. (2)

Embrasure Proximal space that is created below the contact areas of the teeth. (2)

Endocrine disturbances and abnormalities Derangements and variations from the normal function of the endocrine system. (9)

Endodontic abscess An abscess involving the dental pulp. (16)

Endoscope An illuminated, flexible optical tube that allows the user to visualize the organs and cavities of the body, and into periodontal pockets. (13)

Endosseous implant An implant that is placed into the alveolar or basal bone and that protrudes through the mucoperiosteum; also called an endosteal implant. (15)

Endotoxin A nondiffusable lipid polysaccharide-polypeptide complex formed within bacteria; when released from the destroyed bacterial cells, it is capable of producing a toxic manifestation in the host. (4)

Enzyme suppression therapy A promising treatment for periodontitis involving antimicrobial doses of doxycycline to produce enzyme inhibition unrelated to antibiotic activity and enhance the results of scaling and root planing in patients with moderate periodontal disease. (7)

Epidemiologic research The inquiry or examination of data, reports, and observations in a search for facts or principles; differs from clinical research in that entire groups are the focus of study, not individuals, and that persons without the disease are included in studies to assess the disease risk among the members of a population. (3)

Epidemiology The study of health and disease in human populations and associated factors. (3)

Episodic periodontal disease Periodontal disease exhibiting occasional bursts of activity followed by periods of remission. During the active phase, bone and other periodontal tissues are lost and the pockets deepen. Active periods are associated with tissue bleeding and provide the opportunity to perform diagnostic tests. During the periods of quiescence (remission), the disease is static and pockets do not deepen. (7)

Evaluation The judgment or appraisal of a condition or situation. In dentistry, it is the clinical judgment of a patient's dental health or an appraisal of staff performance. (8)

Excisional periodontal surgery Periodontal surgical treatment that involves cutting away or taking out periodontal tissue. (14)

Expanded-duty dental hygiene skills The performance by a dental hygienist of skills such as local anesthesia administration, placement and carving of amalgam restorations, placement and finishing of composite restorations, placement and removal of periodontal sutures and periodontal packs, and gingival curettage. (1)

Experimental gingivitis Gingivitis that is induced and studied experimentally in healthy patients by discontinuing all oral hygiene procedures and permitting bacterial plaque to accumulate. (6)

Facultative anaerobe An organism that can use oxygen when oxygen is present but can use anaerobic fermentation when oxygen is absent. It can grow or multiply in both aerobic and anaerobic environments. (4)

Failing implant A device or appliance with associated increasing infection and bone loss. (15)

Fenestration An opening or window in the bone covering the facial surface of a root. (2)

Fiber bundles Connective tissue that is composed of collagen fibrils. (2)

First molar loss syndrome A syndrome that has not been proven to initiate periodontal disease but that is associated with gingival inflammation and pocket formation as the condition progresses. (5)

Fluoride therapy The treatment of disease, injury, or illness with the use of a form of the chemical fluoride. Fluoride is a salt of hydrofluoric acid, commonly sodium or stannous (tin). (17)

Fones, Alfred C. The man who created the role of the dental hygienist and established the first school for dental hygienists in Bridgeport, Connecticut, in 1913. (1)

Food impaction areas Areas of the teeth and oral tissues in which food becomes lodged; generally occur interproximally because of open contact areas, uneven marginal ridge height, or plunger cusps. (5)

Foreign body reaction A reaction caused by an object or substance found in the body in an organ or tissue in which it does not belong. In dentistry, foreign body reactions can cause damage to gingival tissue; for example, impaction from food particles such as popcorn husks or apple skins often results in a lesion. (6)

Free gingiva The unattached coronal portion of the gingiva that encircles the tooth to form the gingival sulcus. (2)

Free gingival groove The shallow line or depression on the surface of the gingiva at the junction of the free and attached gingivae. It most commonly occurs in the mandibular anterior and bicuspid areas. (2)

Fremitus The visible and palpable movement of a tooth during function or parafunction. (11)

Furcation The region of division of the root portion of a tooth. (8)

Generalization The formulation of general principles from sets of information. (3)

Gingiva The fibrous tissue covered by mucous membrane that immediately surrounds the teeth; the visible component of the periodontium inside the mouth. (2)

Gingival abscess A superficial periodontal abscess occurring within the free gingival sulcus surrounding the tooth, frequently caused by food impaction. (16)

Gingival crevicular fluid A serum transudate found in the gingival sulcus. Irritation and inflammation of the gingival tissue increase the flow and alter the constituents of crevicular fluid. (2, 4)

Gingival curettage The process of debridement of the epithelial attachment, the ulcerated and entire (pocket) epithelium, and subjacent inflamed and altered gingival corium; it is a somewhat controversial procedure. (13)

Gingival diseases modified by malnutrition Diseases of the gingiva that are intensified by vitamin deficiencies such as vitamins A, B_1, B_2, B_6, and C. (6)

Gingival diseases modified by medications Diseases of the gingiva that are intensified by use of medications. (6)

Gingival diseases modified by systemic factors Diseases of the gingiva that are intensified by conditions such as endocrine changes or the presence of corticosteroids. (6)

Gingival diseases of fungal origin Diseases of the gingiva that are associated with fungal organisms, most commonly *Candida albicans*. (6)

Gingival diseases of specific bacterial origin Diseases of the gingiva that result from common bacterial infections in the mouth, such as streptococcal infection of the throat and oral tissues (including the gingiva) in young children and sexually transmitted diseases (e.g., meningococcal gonorrhea or syphilis). (6)

Gingival diseases of viral origin Diseases of the gingiva that result from viral infection, such as secondary herpetic infections (e.g., cold sores and fever blisters) and the various types of herpesviruses. (6)

Gingival enlargement A localized deepening of the gingival crevice of 2 mm or more caused by swelling or increase in the volume of the gingiva. (7)

Gingival fluid flow The pattern of movement of gingival fluid. (3)

Gingival index (GI) An assessment tool used to evaluate a case of gingivitis based on visual inspection of the gingivae that takes into consideration the color and firmness of the tissue and the presence of any gingival bleeding during probing. (3)

Gingival lesions of genetic origin Genetically predisposed changes in the gingiva, such as gingival enlargement. (6)

Gingival ligament Fiber bundles that protect and support the junctional epithelium, maintain the tone of the attached gingiva, and protect the periodontal ligament. (2)

Gingival manifestations of systemic conditions Changes in the gingiva that are caused by systemic conditions, such as those related to mucocutaneous disorders, dermatologic diseases, or blood dyscrasias. (6)

Gingival margin The edge of the gingiva next to the teeth. (2)

Gingival recession The apical migration of the gingival crest. (17)

Gingivectomy The surgical excision of unsupported gingival tissue to the level where it is attached, creating a new gingival margin apical in position to the old. (6, 14)

Gingivitis Inflammation of the gingival tissues. (6)

Gingivitis associated with dental plaque biofilm only The most common form of gingivitis; directly related to the presence of bacterial plaque biofilm on the tooth surface; also called plaque-associated gingivitis, or gingivitis. (6)

Gingivoplasty The surgical contouring of the gingival tissues to secure the physiologic architectural form necessary to maintain tissue health and integrity. (14)

Global prognosis The overall prognosis for a patient. (18)

Glucan A polyglucose compound such as cellulose, starch, amylose, glycogen amylose, and callose. (4)

Glycocalyx A structure that contains a network of channels and canals existing within the biofilm, which allows for exchange of nutrients between various microbes and for the removal of their waste products. (4)

Gram-positive and gram-negative cell wall Determined by the use of Gram staining to determine the cell wall structure of a bacterial organism, which often reflects the role of the bacteria in plaque formation and pathogenicity. (4)

Guided tissue regeneration Healing through the repopulation of selected cells. (14)

Hand instrumentation Instruments guided and activated principally by a hand force. (13)

Herpetic whitlow An infection caused by the herpes simplex virus that enters the body through small breaks in the skin; usually appears as cracks in the skin around the fingernails. (16)

Horizontal bone loss A pattern of bone loss in periodontitis in which the marginal crest of the alveolar bone between adjacent teeth is apical to normal bone height and remains level. (14)

Hydrodynamic theory of dentinal sensitivity A theory that attributes tooth sensitivity to the expansion and contraction of fluids within the dentinal tubules, thus causing the nerve endings to trigger pain responses in the tooth pulp. (13)

Hyperfunction An increase in activity of a part or in the stresses applied to a part. (11)

Hyperplasia The abnormal multiplication or increase in the number of normal cells in normal arrangement in a tissue or organ, resulting in a thickening or enlargement of the tissue or organ. (6)

Hypersensitivity reaction Adverse reaction to contact with specific substances in quantities that usually produce no reaction in normal individuals; these adverse reactions can cause cell or tissue damage. (2)

Immediate loading Placement of the restoration at the time of the implant surgery. (15)

Immune system The system of the body responsible for the body's ability to react to assault by bacteria, viruses, tumor growth, injury, and myriad other influences. (2)

Immunoglobulin Serum protein synthesized by plasma cells that act as antibodies and are important in the body's defense mechanisms against infections. The main classes are designated as IgA, IgG, and IgM. (2)

Immunology The study of the immune system and host response. (2)

Implant abutment The portion of an implant that protrudes through the gingival tissues and is designed to support a prosthodontic appliance. (15)

Implant biologic width The dimension of the epithelial and connective tissue attachments. (15)

Implant fixture The root analogue device in the bone. (15)

Incidence The rate of occurrence of new disease in a population over a given period of time. (3)

Incisional periodontal surgery The procedure of choice when excisional periodontal surgery cannot be performed for pocket reduction in which the tissues are pushed away from the underlying tooth roots and alveolar bone, much like the flap of an envelope; also referred to as periodontal flap surgery or flap surgery. (14)

Indexes or indices Systems to quantify periodontal tissues used to define and compare conditions. (3)

Individual tooth prognosis A forecast of the probable outcome of a disease or treatment for a particular tooth. (18)

Infectious disease Pathologic alteration induced in the tissues by the action of microorganisms or their toxins. (9)

Informed consent Permission to proceed with treatment granted by the patient to the health care provider after being told in sufficient detail of the risks of the treatment; can be written or verbal. (9)

Informed refusal Refusal to proceed with treatment given by the patient to the health care provider after being told in sufficient detail of the risks of the treatment; can be written or verbal. (9)

Infrabony pocket A periodontal pocket, the base of which is apical to the crest of the alveolar bone. (14)

Interdental brushes Instruments used to clean between teeth. (12)

Interdental gingiva The soft supporting tissue, consisting of prominent horizontal collagen fibers, that normally fills the space between two contacting teeth. (2)

Intrabony pocket A pocket that extends apically from the crest of the alveolar bone; also called an infrabony pocket. (7, 14)

Irrigation The technique of using a solution to wash or flush debris from the periodontal pocket, a root canal, or a wound. (13)

Joint diseases and disorders Inflammatory, infectious, or functional disorders in a joint. (9)

Jumping distance A gap between the nonengaged implant surface and the inner aspect of the socket wall created during immediate placement of an implant into the extraction socket. (15)

Junctional epithelium A band of epithelial cells that surrounds the tooth and creates a seal at the gingival sulcus to hold it firmly in place. (2)

Keratinization A process that occurs as the keratinocyte migrates from the basal layer to the surface. The cells become increasingly flattened, develop keratohyaline granules in the subsurface, and produce a superficial layer that is similar to skin in which no cell nuclei are present. (2)

Keratinized epithelium An epithelium that has undergone keratinization, which occurs as the keratinocyte migrates from the basal layer to the surface. The cells become increasingly flattened, develop keratohyaline granules in the subsurface, and produce a superficial layer that is similar to skin in which no cell nuclei are present. (2)

Lamina dura A radiographic term denoting the plate of compact bone (alveolar bone) that lies adjacent to the periodontal membrane. It may also be referred to as the cribriform plate on the basis of its histologic appearance of a dense plate of bone with many small holes perforating it. (2)

Lamina propria The connective tissue beneath the gingiva that is made up of two layers: the papillary layer immediately beneath the epithelium, which consists of papillary projections between the rete pegs, and the reticular layer, which extends to the periosteum. (2)

Lingual groove A furrow or channel that forms on the tongue side of selected front teeth. (5)

Lipopolysaccharide A compound or complex of lipid and carbohydrate. (4)

Loading The placement of restorations on the implants. (15)

Localized aggressive periodontitis The periodontal disease associated with young people; in the past it was known as periodontosis or juvenile periodontitis. (3)

Loupe Eyeglass-mounted telescope that magnifies the field of vision up to six times the actual size. (13)

Lysis Cell disintegration caused by a lysin. (2)

Macrophage Any phagocytic cell of the reticuloendothelial system; a cell that takes up antigen and presents it to the lymphocytes. (2)

Magnification The increased visibility of the teeth and tissues during periodontal treatment through a variety of techniques or tools. (13)

Malocclusion A deviation in intramaxillary or intermaxillary relationships of teeth, but not an initiator of pathology. (5)

Masticatory system The coordinated body system that controls the process of chewing food in preparation for digestion. (11)

Materia alba A loosely adherent mass of bacteria and cellular debris around the necks of the teeth; usually associated with poor oral hygiene. (4)

Melanin The dark amorphous pigment of melanotic tumors, skin, hair, choroid coat of the eye, and substantia nigra of the brain. (2)

Microbial succession The changing composition of the biota due to the aging of the plaque. (4)

Microbiota The microscopic organisms living in a particular region. (4)

Microscope An instrument that contains a powerful lens system for enlarging the appearance of and viewing near objects. (13)

Miller Index of Tooth Mobility (MI) The most commonly used technique to quantify tooth mobility, in which two metal instrument handles are placed on either side of the tooth to be tested and the tooth is moved in a facial-lingual direction. Mobility is graded on a scale of 0 to 3 and is often modified with plus or minus signs or identified with Roman numerals. (3)

Mouth breathing The process of inspiration and expiration of air primarily through the oral cavity; leads to localized gingival inflammation that is usually confined to the labial gingiva of the maxillary anterior teeth; also associated with higher levels of plaque and gingivitis. (5)

Mucogingival junction The scalloped linear area denoting the approximation or separation of the gingivae and alveolar mucosa. (2)

Mucogingival surgery A surgical procedure designed to retain a functionally adequate zone of gingiva after surgical pocket elimination, create a functionally adequate zone of attached gingiva, alter the position of or eliminate a frenum, or deepen the vestibule. (14)

Myalgia Pain in the muscles. (11)

Necrotizing ulcerative gingivitis (NUG) An inflammation of the gingivae characterized by necrosis of the interdental papillae, ulceration of the gingival margins, appearance of a pseudomembrane, pain, and a fetid odor. (16)

Necrotizing ulcerative periodontitis (NUP) The most appropriate term for the massive tissue-destroying process that is an extension of acute necrotizing ulcerative gingivitis. By definition, when bone loss and loss of connective tissue attachment to the root surface are present, the disease is periodontitis, not gingivitis. Therefore, most cases of necrotizing ulcerative disease should be considered NUP rather than gingivitis. (7, 16)

Neurologic disorder Condition affecting the neurologic system of the body. (9)

Nightguard An acrylic resin appliance that is worn at night to stabilize the teeth; see also bite guard. (11)

Nonplaque biofilm–induced gingival lesion Lesion that originate from a source other than plaque biofilm on the gingivae. (6)

Nonspecific plaque hypotheses Early theories about the etiologic role of dental plaque in periodontal disease, suggesting that the severity of inflammation was directly related to the quantity of plaque in the mouth, based on the belief that plaque was a homogeneous bacterial mass and that all plaques in all mouths have equal potential to cause disease. (4)

Nonsubmerged protocol See also submerged protocol. Similar to the two-stage submerged procedure except that after implant placement, the tissues are closed either around the specially designed transmucosal portion of the implant or around the healing abutment, which eliminates the need for a second surgery to uncover the implant and thus may reduce both treatment time and patient discomfort. (15)

Nonsurgical periodontal therapy Procedures performed to treat gingival and periodontal diseases including scaling, root planing, oral hygiene instruction, and possible use of antimicrobial agents. (13)

Obligate anaerobe An organism that cannot survive in an aerobic environment. (4)

Occlusal function Activities such as talking, chewing, and swallowing. (11)

One-month evaluation Sometimes called reevaluation or tissue check; the observation and evaluation of tissue healing and the patient's progress toward effective plaque control about 4 weeks after the debridement sequence is completed. (10)

Operculum A flap of tissue over a partially erupted tooth, particularly a third molar that can result in pericoronitis. (16)

Oral cancer Malignancies indicative of unchecked cell growth that may be found in and around the oropharynx, gingiva, alveolar and buccal mucosae, lower mouth, lips, and tongue. (9)

Oral epithelium The epithelial covering of the oral mucous membranes. (2)

Oral hygiene assessment The qualified opinion of a health care provider regarding a patient's state of oral health, based on examination and patient feedback. (8)

Oral mucosa The lining of the oral cavity, composed of stratified squamous epithelium and the underlying lamina propria. (2)

Oral prophylaxis The cleaning of the teeth to prevent oral disease. (1)

Orange complex bacteria Bacteria that have been characterized as late colonizers and tend to reside in the biofilm closest to the soft tissue lining of the pocket. (4)

Orthodontic appliance Device used for influencing tooth position; long associated with increased plaque accumulation, gingivitis, and caries susceptibility in children and adolescents. (5)

Orthofunction A state of morphofunctional harmony in which the forces developed during function are within an adaptive physiologic range and there are no pathologic changes in the oral tissues. (11)

Osseointegration The growth action of bone tissue as it assimilates surgically implanted devices or prostheses to be used as either replacement parts or anchors. (15)

Osseous defects A concavity in the bone surrounding one or more teeth, resulting from periodontal disease. (14)

Osseous surgery The therapeutic surgical measures used and designed to eliminate osseous deformities or create a favorable environment. (14)

Ostectomy The excision of a bone or portion of a bone. (14)

Osteoplasty A surgical procedure to modify or change the configuration of a bone. (14)

Overall prognosis See global prognosis. (18)

Overcontoured crowns Crowns in which the natural anatomy has been altered by the use of too much restoration material; associated with gingival inflammation and periodontal disease. (5)

Overcontoured restoration Restoration containing so much excess restorative material that the normal anatomic structure is altered; linked to periodontal inflammation. (5)

Papillae Gingiva that fill the embrasure spaces between teeth. (2)

Parafunctional activity Movements that are considered outside or beyond function and that result in wear facets, such as teeth grinding or clenching. (11)

Parakeratinized epithelium Epithelium that shows signs of partial keratinization. (2)

Pathogenesis The course of an illness or condition, from its origin to manifestation and outbreak. (7)

Pathogenicity The ability to cause disease. (4, 7)

Patient motivation The patient's stimulus or incentive to act or react in a certain way. (12)

Pellicle A film or membrane. (4)

Periapical abscess An acute or chronic inflammation of the periapical tissues characterized by a localized accumulation of pus at the apex of a tooth. (16)

Pericoronitis Inflammation of the operculum or tissue flap over a partially erupted tooth, particularly a third molar. (16)

Peri-implant disease Disease that occurs in the area around an implant and its investing tissues. (15)

Peri-implant mucositis Inflammation of the mucous membrane around the area of a dental implant that is reversible. (15)

Peri-implantitis Inflammation in and around the mucosa and bone of a dental implant that may also affect abutment areas. (8, 15)

Periodontal abscess An acute, localized, purulent infection of the periodontium. (7, 15)

Periodontal assessment The examination of the periodontal and gingival tissues. (8)

Periodontal bone loss The loss of crestal alveolar bone through the inflammatory process. (7)

Periodontal debridement The removal of foreign material and damaged tissue from areas surrounding the tooth. (13)

Periodontal disease Any of a group of inflammatory and infectious diseases affecting the gums and supporting tissues of the teeth. (7)

Periodontal Disease Index (PDI) An assessment of gingival condition based on probe depths and attachment loss in six teeth as representative of the entire dentition: #3, the maxillary right first molar; #9, the maxillary left central incisor; #12, the maxillary left first premolar; #19, the mandibular left first molar; #25, the mandibular right central incisor; and #28, the mandibular right first premolar.

Periodontal dressing A protective obtundent dressing covering of the gum and periodontal tissues used after periodontal surgery. (14)

Periodontal flap surgery The surgical reflection of a portion of periodontal tissue to provide access for debridement of the teeth. (14)

Periodontal ligament The mode of attachment of the tooth to the alveolus; the investing and supporting mechanism for the tooth. (2)

Periodontal maintenance Keeping the periodontium in a functional state or in the correct location. (10, 17)

Periodontal plastic surgery The surgical alteration, replacement, restoration, or reconstruction of the periodontium for structural or cosmetic purposes. (14)

Periodontal pocket A pathologically deepened gingival sulcus. (7)

Periodontal Screening and Recording (PSR) A screening system developed by the American Academy of Periodontology and the American Dental Association that enables the clinician to identify which patients need a full examination and which patients require only a screening examination in the private practice setting. (3)

Periodontal surgery Surgical work performed on the periodontium. (14)

Periodontics The study of the examination, diagnosis, and treatment of diseases affecting the periodontium. (1)

Periodontitis Alterations in the periodontium resulting from inflammation or any chronic progressive disease of the periodontium. (1, 7)

Periodontoclasia An old term for destructive or degenerative disease of the periodontium. (1)

Periodontology The science of periodontics. (1)

Permeability The degree to which one substance allows another to pass through it. (12)

Phagocytize The act of ingesting or engulfing microorganisms, cells, or other substances by another cell. (2)

Phase I treatment The etiologic treatment of a condition. (10)

Phase II treatment The surgical treatment of a condition. (10)

Phase III treatment The restorative treatment of a condition. (10)

Phase IV treatment The maintenance treatment of a condition. (10)

Physiologic mesial migration The gradual, mesial tooth movement that occurs throughout life. (2)

Physiologic mobility The normal slight movement of the teeth. (11)

Physiologic occlusion An occlusion that operates in harmony and presents no pathologic manifestation; an acceptable occlusion. (11)

Plaque control The regular removal of plaque. (12)

Plaque Index of Silness and Löe (PI) An index that places the most significance on the amount of plaque at the gingival margin because of the importance of the proximity and relationship of plaque in that location to gingival inflammation, which is measured clinically by bleeding. (3)

Pocket elimination surgery The use of surgery to obtain a healthy gingival attachment and an intact, functioning attachment apparatus with reduced probing pocket depths. (14)

Pocket reduction surgery The use of surgery to reduce the depth of an existing pocket. (14)

Polishing The use of abrasive agents to remove stains and supragingival plaque biofilm from the teeth. (13)

Postoperative instructions The detailed information given to a patient after surgery or other invasive treatment. (14)

Postoperative procedures Treatment that is performed after surgery or other invasive procedures. (14)

Powered instrumentation The use of instruments applied with a nonhand force. (13)

Powered toothbrushing The use of a powered or mechanical toothbrush, such as one operated by batteries. (12)

Preceptor A clinician-teacher. (1)

Pregnancy tumor A specific type of gingival lesion that is actually not a tumor but a localized area of pyogenic granulation tissue, aggravated by hormonal changes during pregnancy; usually resolves after the baby is born but may require surgical removal of a residual enlargement. (6)

Preliminary phase Immediate treatment whose purpose is to bring all emergency and other critical situations under control. (10)

Prepubertal periodontitis A very rare condition among children that may be localized or generalized and may affect both the primary and secondary dentitions; usually involves severe gingival inflammation, rapid bone loss, and early tooth loss. (7)

Prevalence The number of cases of a disease present in a given population at one time. (3)

Primary traumatic occlusion Injury to tissues and bones caused by heavy occlusal forces exceeding the adaptive range in a normal periodontium. (11)

Probing measurements Measurements of sulcus or pocket depths taken while using a periodontal probe. (8)

Profession A calling, vocation, or means of livelihood or gain. (1)

Prognosis The foretelling of the probable course of a disease or regimen of treatment. (10, 18)

Progress notes Also called chart notes; the documentation of treatment at each visit. (10)

Prophylaxis The prevention of disease; in dentistry, refers to the routine cleaning and polishing procedures. (13)

Pseudopockets A pocket formed by gingival hyperplasia and edema without apical migration of the epithelial tissue. (7)

Purulence Pus, also referred to as exudate or purulent exudate. (16)

Pyorrhea alveolaris Another name for periodontoclasia, suggested by F. H. Rehwinkel in 1877. This name was never totally accepted because it was descriptive of only one aspect of pathology, bone loss. However, pyorrhea became a commonly used term that is still heard today. (1)

Pyrophosphate A compound found in parotid saliva that helps delay calcification of bacterial plaque; also, the active ingredient of commercially available tartar-control oral hygiene products. (5)

Radiographic examination The study and interpretation of radiographs of the mouth and associated structures. (8)

Rapidly progressing periodontitis Periodontitis that occurs in young adults, usually between 20 and 30 years old, and causes rapid and severe gingival inflammation. (7)

Recall The procedure of reminding or advising a patient to have the oral health reviewed and examined; an important part of preventive dentistry. (17)

Recession In the gingiva, refers to location of the margin of the tissue, not its condition. Recession can occur in periodontal disease or can be associated with clinically healthy tissue. (6)

Recurrent periodontitis Periodontal disease that returns after a completed treatment sequence, or episodic periodontal disease. (17)

Red complex bacteria Bacteria that have been characterized as late colonizers and virulent, and that tend to reside in the biofilm closest to the soft tissue lining of the pocket. (4)

Reevaluation A follow-up appraisal or clinical opinion. (10)

Refractory periodontitis Periodontal disease that does not respond to appropriate treatment. (7)

Regeneration surgery The surgical renewal or repair of lost or damaged tissue. (14)

Researcher A person who applies the scientific method to select appropriate therapies, educational methods, or content, interprets and applies findings, and solves problems. (1)

Rete pegs Ridges of epithelium that serve as a connection between the free and attached gingiva and the underlying connective tissue. (2)

Risk factors Exposures, behaviors, and characteristics associated with a disease. (3, 5, 7)

Risk indicator A behavior that causes a person to have a greater likelihood of a disease. (5)

Roll toothbrushing method The technique in which the teeth are brushed the way they grow: down on the upper teeth and up on the lower teeth. Bristles are placed next to the gingiva and the handle of the toothbrush is turned to stroke the bristles along the sides of the teeth. This action is repeated several times in each location, moving around the arches, until all of the teeth are brushed. The technique requires a fair amount of concentration to apply the brush to each area and sufficient dexterity to "roll" the brush on the buccal and lingual surfaces. In addition, the rolling strokes must be performed slowly so that the gingival third of the teeth will be adequately cleaned. (12)

Root caries Tooth decay occurring on a portion of the root. (17)

Root planing A procedure that smoothes the surface of a root by removing abnormal toxic cementum or dentin that is rough, contaminated, or permeated with calculus. (13)

Rubber tip stimulators Convenient inexpensive devices that are used in interdental plaque biofilm removal, consisting of a conical piece of firm rubber or plastic several millimeters long that is placed proximally, resting the side of the cone of rubber on the gingiva, and worked in a small circular motion. (11)

Russell Periodontal Index (PI) A progressive scale that assigns a numeric score to each tooth. This scale is weighted more toward bone loss than toward gingival inflammation. The score for each tooth is added and averaged by all teeth examined in the individual, providing a score for each person. Population scores are determined by averaging the scores of individuals. (3)

Salivary calculus Another name for supragingival calculus (reflecting the source of the mineral content). (5)

Salivary glycoproteins The adsorption (attachment) of glycoproteins from saliva, probably the result of an ionic interaction between the calcium and phosphate ions of the hydroxyapatite and the oppositely charged groups of the salivary glycoproteins. (4)

Sample A selected part of a population that is taken to be representative of the whole population. (3)

Scaling The removal of calcareous deposits from the teeth by use of suitable instruments. (13)

Scrub toothbrushing method The simplest brushing technique, consisting of merely placing the bristles next to the teeth and moving them back and forth, or scrubbing. It does not focus cleaning at the gingival margin and may miss many areas of plaque biofilm. Extremely vigorous scrubbing, especially with a stiff-bristled brush, can also lead to gingival trauma and recession. (12)

Secondary traumatic occlusion Occlusion that occurs when normal occlusal forces exceed the capability of a periodontium that is already affected by periodontal disease. (11)

Serumal calculus Another name for subgingival calculus (because of the source of the mineral content). (5)

Severity The level of disease. (3)

Sharpey's fibers Collagenous fibers that become incorporated into the cementum. (2)

Simplified Oral Hygiene Index (OHI-S) Has both a debris index (DI-S) for plaque and a calculus index (CI-S). The scores can be used singly to provide a plaque index or a calculus index, or they may be combined to provide an oral hygiene index. (3)

Site-specific Localized to a particular area. (7)

Sonic instrumentation See ultrasonic instrumentation. (13)

Specific plaque hypothesis The idea that as many as a dozen microbial species may be responsible for most cases of periodontitis, compared with the nonspecific plaque hypothesis. (4, 13)

Splint A device used to protect the teeth and provide a stable position for them. (11)

Stage I gingivitis The initial stage of gingivitis; occurs in the first few days of contact between microbial plaque biofilm and the gingival tissues. This stage is an acute inflammatory response that is characterized by dilation of the blood vessels and increased blood flow. (6)

Stage II gingivitis Also referred to as early gingivitis. These lesions begin to form 4 to 7 days after plaque has accumulated in the gingival sulcus. (6)

Stage III gingivitis Characterized by the gingival inflammation reaching an established stage (after 15 to 21 days). (6)

Stage IV gingivitis The advanced stage of gingivitis in which the inflammatory processes have extended beyond the gingiva and into the other periodontal tissues. (6)

Stillman toothbrushing method A massaging technique reputed to fill the gingival blood vessels with oxygenated blood, requiring placement of the bristles pointing apically but not at right angles to the gingiva to minimize puncture. Pressure is placed on the bristles, causing them to flex and the tissue to blanch, and then the pressure is released. The procedure is repeated for all teeth in all areas of the mouth while the brush is rinsed several times with a salt water and sodium bicarbonate solution. This technique most likely results in improved gingival health because of plaque removal. (12)

Stippled gingiva Gingiva having an orange peel appearance; believed to result from the bundles of collagen fibers that enter the connective tissue. (2)

Subgingival calculus Calculus deposited on the tooth structure and found apical to the gingival margin within the confines of the gingival cervix, gingival pocket, or periodontal pocket. (5)

Subgingival irrigation The flushing of liquid with a handheld device to remove bacterial plaque biofilm from dental surfaces beneath the gum line. (12)

Subgingival plaque biofilm Plaque biofilm that is located in the gingival sulcus or periodontal pocket. (4)

Submarginal calculus Another term for subgingival calculus (because of its location). (5)

Submerged protocol An implant technique that requires two surgical procedures before fabrication of the restorations that will be placed on the implants. The first surgery places the implant fixture within bone, followed by a second surgery 3 to 6 months later to uncover the implant so that it can be accessed through the mucosa. (15)

Subperiosteal implant An appliance consisting of an open-mesh frame designed to fit over the surface of the bone beneath the periosteum. (15)

Substantivity Pertaining to the capability of an oral antimicrobial agent to continue its therapeutic activity for a prolonged period of time. (12)

Sulcular epithelium The stratified squamous epithelium forming the covering of the soft tissue wall of the gingival sulcus, or crevice. (2)

Sulcus Bleeding Index (SBI) A measure of bleeding on probing, in which measurements are taken at four points around each tooth: the mesial, distal, buccal, and lingual surfaces. A probe is gently inserted in the sulcus areas across a quadrant and withdrawn and the gingival units are scored 30 seconds after probing to allow time for bleeding to become visible, which is important in evaluating less inflamed tissue. (3)

Suppuration The formation and discharge of pus. (7, 16)

Suprabony pockets Periodontal pockets that occur above the crest of the alveolar bone. (7, 14)

Supracontact An area on a tooth that may prevent well-distributed, stable contact between the maxillary and mandibular teeth, such as an occlusal interference. (11)

Supragingival calculus Calculus deposited on the teeth occlusal or incisal to the gingival crest. (5)

Supragingival irrigation The flushing of liquid with a handheld device to remove bacterial plaque from dental surfaces above or even with the gum line. (12)

Supragingival plaque biofilm Plaque biofilm that is deposited on the clinical crowns of the teeth. (4)

Supramarginal calculus Another name for supragingival calculus. (5)

Superstructure A term for a restoration most commonly referred to when describing restoration of an implant or implants. (15)

Tartar The common name for dental calculus, often used by patients when referring to calculus. (5)

Temporomandibular disorder (TMD) Disorder associated with one or both of the temporomandibular joints. (11)

Temporomandibular disorder screening examination Assessment of a patient's risk for TMD. (11)

Titanium A highly reactive yet biocompatible metal that is the material of choice in osseointegration. (15)

Tobacco use The practice of purposefully using tobacco for its perceived physical and psychological benefits, such as mental alertness, relaxation, or weight control. (9)

Tooth mobility The loosening of a tooth or teeth; an important diagnostic sign. (8)

Tooth root proximity A close distance between roots. (2)

Tooth wear A loss of substance or a diminishing of the teeth through use, friction, or other destructive factors. (8)

Toothpick A wood sliver used to cleanse the interdental space. (12)

Toxicity The ability of a drug or poison to cause harm, especially to cause permanent injury or death. (12)

Transosteal implant An implant that traverses the mandible in an apicocoronal direction and protrudes through the gingival tissues into the mouth for prosthesis anchorage. Its use is limited to the mandible, where it is commonly referred to as a staple implant. (15)

Traumatic lesion Lesion pertaining to or caused by an injury. (6)

Traumatic occlusion An occlusion that has caused injury to the teeth, muscles, or temporomandibular joint. (11)

Treatment sequence The order of occurrence of procedures and appointments required to restore the oral health of a patient. (10)

Trismus Spasms of the muscles of mastication resulting in the inability to open the mouth; often symptomatic of pericoronitis. (11)

Ultrasonic instrumentation Devices that use high-energy and high-frequency vibrations for calculus, plaque, and stain removal. (13)

Vertical bone loss An abnormal decrease in the alveolar crestal bone height indicated by a visible loss of bone on one tooth's proximal surface compared with the tooth on the adjacent side. (14)

Virulence The power of a microorganism to produce disease. (4)

Volpe Manhold Index (VI) An index that measures supragingival calculus; was originally designed to measure the mandibular incisors but also has been applied to other teeth and studies of tartar control toothpastes. (3)

Xerostomia Dryness of the mouth resulting from functional or organic disturbances of the salivary glands and lack of the normal secretion, often caused by prescribed medications. (17)

INDEX

Page numbers followed by "f" indicate figures, "t" indicate tables, and "b" indicate boxes.